Burn Care and Rehabilitation: Principles and Practice

Contemporary Perspectives in Rehabilitation

Steven L. Wolf, PhD, FAPTA
Editor-in-Chief

PUBLISHED VOLUMES

The Biomechanics of the Foot and Ankle
Robert Donatelli, MA, PT, OCS

Pharmacology in Rehabilitation
Charles D. Ciccone, PhD, PT

Wound Healing: Alternatives in Management
Luther C. Kloth, MS, PT, Joseph M. McCulloch, PhD, PT, and Jeffrey A. Feedar, PT

Thermal Agents in Rehabilitation, 2nd Edition
Susan L. Michlovitz, MS, PT

Electrotherapy in Rehabilitation
Meryl R. Gersh, MMSc, PT

Dynamics of Human Biologic Tissues
Dean P. Currier, PhD, PT, and Roger M. Nelson, PhD, PT

Concepts in Hand Rehabilitation
Barbara G. Stanley, PT, CHT, and Susan M. Tribuzi, OTR, CHT

Cardiopulmonary Rehabilitation: Basic Theory and Application, 2nd Edition
Frances J. Brannon, PhD, Margaret W. Foley, MN, Julie Ann Starr, MS, PT, and Mary Geyer Black, MS, PT

Rehabilitation of the Knee: A Problem-Solving Approach
Bruce H. Greenfield, MMSc, PT

Burn Care and Rehabilitation: Principles and Practice

Reginald L. Richard, MS, PT
Burn Clinical Specialist
Miami Valley Hospital
Adult Regional Burn Center
Dayton, Ohio

Marlys J. Staley, MS, PT
Supervisor, Occupational and Physical Therapy
Shriners Burns Institute
Cincinnati, Ohio

F. A. DAVIS COMPANY • Philadelphia

F. A. Davis Company
1915 Arch Street
Philadelphia, PA 19103

Printed in the United States of America

Last digit indicates print number: 10 9 8 7 6 5 4 3 2 1

Senior Allied Health Editor: Jean-François Vilain
Senior Allied Health Developmental Editor: Ralph Zickgraf
Production Editor: Gail Shapiro
Cover Design By: Steven Ross Morrone

As new scientific information becomes available through basic and clinical research, recommended treatments and drug therapies undergo changes. The author(s) and publisher have done everything possible to make this book accurate, up to date, and in accord with accepted standards at the time of publication. The authors, editors, and publisher are not responsible for errors or omissions or for consequences from application of the book, and make no warranty, expressed or implied, in regard to the contents of the book. Any practice described in this book should be applied by the reader in accordance with professional standards of care used in regard to the unique circumstances that may apply in each situation. The reader is advised always to check product information (package inserts) for changes and new information regarding dose and contraindications before administering any drug. Caution is especially urged when using new or infrequently ordered drugs.

Library of Congress Cataloging-in-Publication Data

Richard, Reginald L, 1951–
Burn care and rehabilitation : principles and practice /
Reginald L. Richard, Marlys J. Staley.
p. cm.
Includes bibliographical references and index.
ISBN 0-8036-7361-2 :
1. Burns and scalds—Patients—Rehabilitation. 2. Burns and scalds. I. Staley, Marlys, 1958– . II. Title.
[DNLM: 1. Burns—Therapy. 2. Burns—Rehabilitation. WO 704 R5136 1993]
RD96.4.R53 1993
617.1′106—dc20
DNLM/DLC
for Library of Congress 93-8304
CIP

Dedication

To: Reg, my life partner, for his unending love and patience, not only during this collaboration, but always; my parents, for caring; Dr. Robert Gillespie and the burn unit staff at St. Elizabeth's Community Health Center, for initiating me to burn care and helping me grow; the staff at Santa Clara Valley Medical Center, for sharing their knowledge and friendship; and the administration at Shriners Burns Institute, Cincinnati Unit, especially Dr. Glenn Warden and Mary Beth Daugherty, for their guidance and support.

MJS

To: My co, Marlys, for her diligence and committment to this book and our life together; my boys, Brett and Adam, and my parents and family for their understanding love; Drs. Sidney F. Miller and Robert K. Finley, Jr., for their continuous support and encouragement for more than 17 years; and the administrators of Miami Valley Hospital, in particular Joe Tod, for all the opportunities they have afforded along the way.

RR

Foreword

To describe a book as "comprehensive" connotes inclusive and complete coverage of the content area. When the content is so defined and presented at a level appreciated by the reader, then a work of immeasurable aid and purpose is born. Such is the case with this mammoth effort of Reginald L. Richard and Marlys J. Staley. To understand the unique pathophysiological consequences and rehabilitation needs of the burn patient is incumbent upon all students in the health care professions. To commit to the treatment and restitution of function among this special class of patient evokes a calling for exceptionally gifted and dedicated clinicians. But whether one is a student or a clinician, the comprehensive nature of this book yields an insight never before captured in print.

Burn Care and Rehabilitation: Principles and Practice fulfills all the criteria of preceding texts in the *Contemporary Perspectives in Rehabilitation* series. The content is written by highly qualified and knowledgeable people, many of whom are clinicians sensitive to the instructional needs of students and clinicians alike. The entire text is well-referenced and incorporates challenging case studies for the reader in a problem-solving format. But perhaps the most significant feature of this book is the fact that it was written with a sensitivity for the special needs of burn patients. This sensitivity transcends educational bounds and, in unequivocal fashion, allows the reader to (re)learn the extraordinary, but often overlooked, considerations demanded in the care, rehabilitation, and management of multiplexed problems in this patient group. For students or clinicians, from assistants to therapists, this text will serve as a well-orchestrated and complete companion.

As Marlys and Reg note in their Preface, the text is divided into four portions. The first addresses "The Fundamentals" including the anatomy and physiology and pathological, biophysical, and healing properties of skin after burns. Section II, "The Care" explores such issues as triage and resuscitation, wound care, and surgical management. In this section the first in a series of case histories is presented, within Chapter 8, "Burn Wound Care." Perhaps Section III, "The Rehabilitation," is most exciting, because each author provides clear insights into thinking processes leading toward treatment progression and decision determinants. The broad range of coverage, which includes evaluation, positioning, splinting, exercise and ambulation, scar management, applications of physical agents, and follow-up plans, is thought provoking and clearly presented.

Last, the unique and exceptional Section IV, "The Concerns," covers such singular management issues as pain symptomatology, children, the hand, chemical and electrical burns, and other, frequently overlooked issues, such as neuromuscular/

musculoskeletal complications and unusual skin disruptions. A particular strength of this book is the extensive list of appendices providing information that would otherwise require multiple resources to retrieve. Thus readers have at their disposal a compendium of information on burn care products, moisturizers, positioning devices, splints, and bandaging materials.

While we believe that this book will be welcomed by all professionals concerned with or treating burn patients, no text is ever totally complete, despite the best intentions and conscientious efforts of its authors. We see this book as belonging to you! We invite you to enjoy its content and to learn from it and to offer us input should your special needs not be addressed in this first edition.

Steven L. Wolf, PhD, FAPTA
Series Editor,
Contemporary Perspectives in Rehabilitation

Preface

The development of a nationwide system of designated burn centers means that today most individuals who suffer a major burn injury receive quick, highly effective treatment in one of these specialized centers. As a result, survival rates for patients with major burn injuries have improved significantly over the past 20 years, to the point that a person with burns over as much as 70 percent of the total body surface area now has a 50 percent chance to survive such an injury. Once healed, however, many patients return to their local communities for continued rehabilitation and follow-up care. The phase of patient recovery after hospitalization for a burn is a critical period, because most burn scar contractures and hypertrophic scars occur during this time. Given these circumstances, there is an increased likelihood that physical and occupational therapists in the patients' local communities will be challenged to provide continued rehabilitation services to these major burn survivors.

In April, 1990, after speaking at the Ohio APTA State Conference, we were given the opportunity to co-edit a book on burn care for therapists. At that point, we had only an inkling of the enormously time-consuming and gratifying task we were about to undertake. This book is the culmination of approximately 3 years of intensive work, not only by us, but by each of the contributors.

Our goal, in order to set the book apart from other quality texts on burn care and rehabilitation, was to provide a text that was comprehensive in both breadth and depth of information. We sought to provide information from which students as well as therapists and therapist assistants with all levels of burn care experience could benefit.

In order to be as comprehensive as possible, we asked 25 of the most knowledgeable and experienced clinicians in the field of burn care to contribute. This group of individuals, including ourselves, represents over 300 years of combined burn experience. The reader will notice that with one exception every chapter has been authored or co-authored by at least one therapist. We felt that if information was to be useful to therapists it should be presented from a therapist's viewpoint. In addition, the majority of our reviewers were therapists, either clinicians or academicians, which helped keep the text pertinent to and understandable by therapists.

The book is divided into four sections: The Fundamentals; The Care; The Rehabilitation; and The Concerns. The Fundamentals includes a history of burn rehabilitation and covers the basic sciences as they relate to burn care. This section supplies the knowledge of skin anatomy, burn pathophysiology, and skin and scar biomechanics essential for the intelligent application of rehabilitation techniques. The Care focuses on resuscitation of the patient and care of the burn wound itself. The Rehabilitation takes a comprehensive look at a multitude of therapeutic interventions, from patient evaluation through discharge and follow-up care. The Concerns address areas of burn care which either require special management principles or are less commonly encountered by therapists. These chapters provide therapists with a source of information they can use as a reference for topics typically not found in other burn texts. In addition, there is an abundance of tables, figures and references, as well as an extensive glossary and many appendices, to help make this a useful reference book.

Some chapters build on the information presented in related chapters, while others stand alone. The reader may notice some repetition of material. For the most part, such duplication was intentional, either for clarification or emphasis. Recognizing that repetition is a means to learn and that different authors have assorted methods of explaining information, we elected to leave some potentially duplicate material to enhance the book.

Reginald L. Richard
Marlys J. Staley

Acknowledgments

The Editors wish to express their sincere appreciation to: Jeffrey E. Falkel, PhD, PT, for presenting us with the opportunity to undertake such an endeavor; all chapter authors, for their knowledgeable contributions; the F. A. Davis staff, in particular Jean-François Vilain, Ralph Zickgraf, and Ona Kosmos, for their invaluable assistance; Steven Wolf, CPR Series Editor, for his guidance and direction; the Visual Arts Department at the Shriners Burns Institute, Cincinnati Unit, especially Kati Ackley and Carol Meyer; the Miami Valley Hospital library staff, especially Sally Sexton and Shirley Sebald, for their perpetual assistance in all our projects; Dr. Dave Greenhalgh, for his "spur-of-the-moment" technical explanations; and John Ford and Cindy Ratermann of the Medical Photography Department at Miami Valley Hospital.

Finally, we wish to thank the following educators and clinicians, whose careful reading of and thoughtful comments on the manuscript helped us immeasurably in shaping the text: Nancy A. Bookstein, MS, PT; Rhea Cohn, MS, PT; Christopher E. Duncan, MS, PT; Steven Fisher, MD; Carole L. Johnson, PhD, PT; Clyde Killian, PhD, PT; Maude Malick, OTR, ASHT; Joseph McCulloch, PhD, PT; Susan Michlovitz, MS, PT; Frank Pierson, PT, Professor Emeritus; and Brian V. Reed, PhD, PT.

Contributors

Lois M. Apfel, OTR
Principal Occupational Therapist
Regional Burn Center
UCSD Medical Center
San Diego, California

Judith A. Carr-Collins, OTR
Burn Clinician
Westchester Burn Center
Valhalla, New York

Mary Beth Daugherty, OTR
Rehabilitation Services Department Manager
Shriners Burns Institute
Cincinnati, Ohio

Kristi Dutcher, PT
Physical Therapy Supervisor
University of Washington Burn Center
Seattle, Washington

John J. Everett, PhD
Department of Psychiatry
Harvard Medical School
Cambridge, Massachusetts

Jeffrey E. Falkel, PhD, PT
Director of Clinical Research
Therex Physical Therapy
Englewood, Colorado

Robert K. Finley, Jr., MD, FACS
Co-Director
Miami Valley Hospital Regional Adult Burn Center
Professor of Surgery
Wright State University School of Medicine
Dayton, Ohio

David G. Greenhalgh, MD, FACS
Assistant Chief of Staff
Shriners Burns Institute
Cincinnati Unit
Assistant Professor of Surgery
University of Cincinnati
Cincinnati, Ohio

Julianne Wright Howell, MS, PT, CHT
Owner/Director
Hand Management Specialists
Richmond, Virginia

Cathy Neville Humphrey, PT
University of Alabama at Birmingham
Birmingham, Alabama

Christy P. Irwin, OTR
Occupational Therapy Department
University of California
San Diego Medical Center
San Diego, California

Carole Johnson, PhD, PT
Fall City, Washington

Cheryl J. Leman, MA, OTR/L, FAOTA
Burn Rehabilitation Specialist Consultant
The Burn Center at the Washington Hospital Center
Washington, DC

Kevin McDonald, RPT
Director of Physical Therapy
Rehabilitation Hospital of Colorado Springs
Colorado Springs, Colorado

Sidney F. Miller, MD, FACS
Director
Miami Valley Hospital Regional Adult Burn Center
Professor of Surgery
Wright State University School of Medicine
Dayton, Ohio

Barry F. Moss, PhD
Department of Rehabilitation Medicine
University of Washington School of Medicine
Seattle, Washington

David R. Patterson, PhD
Associate Professor
Department of Rehabilitation Medicine
University of Washington School of Medicine
Seattle, Washington

Sandra Utley Reeves, OTR/L
Senior Occupational Therapist
Shands Hospital at the University of Florida
Gainesville, Florida

Reginald L. Richard, MS, PT
Burn Clinical Specialist
Miami Valley Hospital Regional Adult Burn Center
Dayton, Ohio

Nanci Ricks, PT
Private Physical Therapist
Littleton, Colorado

Jeffrey R. Saffle, MD, FACS
Associate Professor of Surgery
University of Utah Medical Center
Director
Intermountain Burn Center
Salt Lake City, Utah

Margaret Schmitt, PT
Baltimore Regional Burn Center
Francis Scott Key Medical Center
Baltimore, Maryland

W. Andrew Schnebly, PT
Doxey-Hatch Medical Center
Salt Lake City, Utah

Marlys J. Staley, MS, PT
Supervisor
Occupational and Physical Therapy
Shriners Burns Institute
Cincinnati, Ohio

R. Scott Ward, PT
Assistant Professor
Division of Physical Therapy
University of Utah Health Sciences Center
Salt Lake City, Utah

Glenn D. Warden, MD, FACS
Chief of Staff
Shriners Burns Institute
Cincinnati Unit
Professor of Surgery
University of Cincinnati
Cincinnati, Ohio

Margaret I. Wittman, PT
Supervisor, Burn Trauma Team
North Carolina Jaycee Burn Center
UNC Hospitals
Chapel Hill, North Carolina

Contents

SECTION I

The Fundamentals

Learning is finding out what you already know.
Doing is demonstrating that you know it.
Teaching is reminding others that they know just as well as you.
We are all learners, doers, teachers.

Richard Bach

CHAPTER 1

The Evolution of Burn Rehabilitation Management

Reginald L. Richard, MS, PT
Marlys J. Staley, MS, PT
Robert K. Finley, Jr., MD, FACS

Humans have used fire since the dawn of history. Along with fire's use came treatment of the body's devastation associated with its misuse. As fire is a physical entity, it is natural that physical measures have been used to counteract fire's deleterious effects on humans. The purpose of this chapter is to expose the therapist to the major changes that have occurred from premedieval times up to the present in the care and rehabilitation of burn patients.

FROM PREHISTORY THROUGH THE MIDDLE AGES

There is anthropologic evidence that fire was used by ancient Peking man in China as far back as 250,000 B.C.[1] As the world's population grew, the incidence of burn injuries presumably did so as well. Burn injuries became so widespread that Neanderthal man of 60,000 B.C. sought a remedy for this malady and used herbs as a treatment method. In approximately 1600 B.C., the first written record of the treatment of burn injuries appeared in the Ebers Papyrus.[2]

By the first century A.D., the problem of scar contracture following a burn had become so common that Aurelius Cornelius Celsus, a medical encyclopedist, described this condition in his book *DeMedicina*. According to Haynes,[2] Celsus recorded one of the earliest references of surgical excision for the correction of burn scar contracture. Later, during the Byzantine Empire of 625 A.D., Paulus of Aegina, a Greek physician and author, described the use of water immersion therapy for the treatment of burn wounds.[3]

FROM THE FIFTEENTH TO THE NINETEENTH CENTURY

The recommendation of elevating the hand, presumably to aid healing and control edema, was first written down by Lanfranco Da Milan in his 1498 *Chirurgia parva*. Robotti[4] reported that Ambroise Pare, the famous barber-surgeon, first mentioned the use of a splint to keep the digits in forced flexion after excision of a scar in 1545. Pare also warned against the development of flexion contractures of the hand, axilla, arm, and knee stating that "these parts should not stick together." In 1591, William Clowes wrote the first book dedicated to the treatment of burns entitled *A Profitable and Necessary Book of Observations for All Those That Are Burned*.[4,5] In his book he describes the mismanagement of a patient leading to scar formation by writing, "Nevertheless there was left behinde an ill-formed circatrise [scar] by reason of the ill handling at the first, which after by no means possible could be prevented or amended."[5]

In 1607, Fabricious Hildanus wrote in his text *DeCombustionibus* how he was successful in apparently correcting an extreme case of a dorsal hand and finger contracture. He accomplished this correction "by dividing the scar with transverse incisions followed by splinting to avoid recurrence."[2] Interestingly, leather straps were incorporated into Hildanus's early form of hand splint rendering the splint adjustable! Fabry of Hilden also is credited with prescribing the use of massage with an ointment "as a tanner stretches hides" for lessening contractures.[2] Richard Wiseman (1622 to 1676) advanced Fabry's use of splints by incorporating them earlier in the course of patient treatment "to avoid contractures of joints."[5]

Approximately 150 years later, J. W. Turner (1790 to 1836), professor of surgery at the Royal College of Surgeons of Edinburgh, espoused the benefits of range-of-motion exercises ". . . so as not to cause pain. If some movement appears bound to be lost, or a position inevitably maintained, one must use all one's art to maintain the most favorable position and the most useful motion." Hence, he had conceptualized the "position of function."[5] During this same period, the use of pressure on wounds and scars first emerged. In his "Essay on Burns" in 1797, Edward Kentish, a surgeon, described a type of pressure dressing that relieved pain.[5]

THE NINETEENTH CENTURY

Rayer, in 1835, also recognized the positive effect that pressure had on scars;[6] however, it was not until 1881 that Unna began applying his well-known pressure dressing to burn scars.[6] In addition, James Syme (1799–1870), who opened the first hospital dedicated to burn care in 1848, advocated the use of "pressure" on wounds.[5]

Later that century, G. D. Pollock, an English surgeon who believed that skin grafting would correct scar contractures, "advocated early grafting to . . . prevent contracture and deformity."[3] In the February 15, 1879, issue of *Medical Record*, J. M. Taylor,[7] a surgical resident at The Children's Hospital in Philadelphia, described the treatment of a ten-year-old boy who had an elbow flexion contracture with a type of serial bandage or splint using an oakum (hemp fiber) pad insert.

In 1884, Frank C. Wilson,[8] reporting in *Medical News*, wrote of an extremely interesting case involving a young female patient with a 64-month-old unhealed burn. The patient is described as having a 150 degree elbow flexion contracture, possibly from heterotopic ossification; a severely deformed hand and fingers, as well as presumably suffering from what we term today as reflex sympathetic dystrophy. During the course of her successful recovery, the patient received massage, daily manipulation of her joints by "a skillful manipulator," splinting, and electrical stimulation![8]

THE EARLY TWENTIETH CENTURY

According to an article by two physicians, Seeger and Schaefer,[9] the use of "ambrine," or paraffin wax, as a method to treat burn wounds was introduced by Barthe de Sandfort in 1914. This article, published in 1934, also holds the distinction of being the first publication on the topic of burns to appear in an exclusively "therapy" journal, *The Physiotherapy Review* (forerunner to *Physical Therapy*).

In 1915, two years prior to the formation of the American Occupational Therapy Association and six years before the American Physical Therapy Association was founded, physician Charles A. Parker[10] from Chicago described the basics of proper positioning for the burn patient. Also, he used casting material for splints and fabricated what is more popularly known today as the "airplane" splint for axillary burns.

Although Sterling Bunnel[4,11] is credited with describing the principles of dynamic splinting, V. P. Blair,[12] in 1923, was incorporating the use of rubber bands into hand splints for patients undergoing reconstructive surgery. However, Bunnell and Koch[4] had to stress the importance of hand splinting before dynamic splinting became "universally accepted."

In the 1930s, immobilization of the extremities, in conjunction with proper positioning, was emphasized to prevent scar contracture deformity.[13-15] There was a growing realization that contracture prevention was better than a cure. Also, at that time, the controversy over whether to apply pressure to a wound arose and continues even today.[16] Advocates stated that pressure assisted with skin graft adherence while opponents believed that such pressure would cause shearing and tissue necrosis.[13] During this same time, Seeger and Schaefer[9] began using ultraviolet light to stimulate epithelial growth.

In 1943, Hamilton and Barnett[17] reportedly prescribed the use of corrective splints, active motion, and early intervention of both occupational and physical therapy. This "early" time frame for therapy to begin spanned 22 days to 8 weeks after the burn injury occurred as evidenced by the case presentation included in their article. Furthermore, A. B. Wallace, credited by Cockshot[5] as founding the exposure method of wound treatment, emphasized "all that is necessary are exposure and immobilization when treating burns." This delay in therapy intervention appears to have persisted throughout the decade.[17] However, an exception is noted in an article written by H. C. Wilson in 1945.[18] Wilson, a physical therapist with the Australian military and the first therapist found to author an article regarding burns, guardedly wrote of beginning active hand movements after the initial period of burn patient shock.

FROM MIDCENTURY TO THE PRESENT

By the end of the 1950s, burn patients were allowed minimal active movement before skin grafting. However, patients essentially were kept immobile and nonambulatory until all wounds had healed.[19-22] For example, the *Physical Therapy Review*[23] in 1958 published a case report in which therapy was initiated on the 45th day after the burn when the skin grafts "were sufficiently healed so that they would not be disturbed by physical therapy procedures."

Ironically, in that same year, John Moncrief,[24,25] eventual third president of the American Burn Association, wrote two articles that probably influenced the delivery of rehabilitation treatment more than any other publication to that time. In the *Annals of Surgery*, Dr. Moncrief wrote, "In patients having joint involvement, active motion and physiotherapy should be instituted initially and continued for as long as improvement occurs"; furthermore, ". . . it is important that active physiotherapy be instituted as soon as possible in order to prevent the loss of increased range gained by the operative procedure."[24] This postoperative time frame was defined and re-emphasized in the same year in his *American Journal of Surgery* article as "A patient begins physiotherapy eight to ten days after grafting. It is imperative for this therapy to be carried out at such an early date in order to increase the range of motion as rapidly as possible."[25]

By 1961, Irving Feller[26] at the University of Michigan was reporting the application of splints "in the operating room at the time of grafting," and in 1964, Gronley was performing range-of-motion exercises to the hands on the sixth to eighth day following skin grafting.[27] E. B. Evans,[28] in 1966, wrote, "Ideally, physical therapy should begin on the day of the burn," and two years later he suggested the use of isometric exercises to areas supporting recent skin grafts.[29]

In 1967, the American Burn Association was formed and led by Curtis P. Artz as the first president.[30] The development of this association over the years has epitomized the concept of the "burn team," as put forth by Feller,[31] to embrace the contributions of therapists and other health care members to the specialized field of burn treatment. One of the most influential leaders, on behalf of all burn therapists, has been Carole L. Johnson. Johnson was the first therapist to serve in the capacity of at-large member to the board of trustees of the association after the establishment of such a position in 1974. She was instrumental in establishing the PT/OT Forum specialty section of the *Journal of Burn Care and Rehabilitation* at the time of her appointment as Associate Editor to the journal in 1984. And, in recognition of her continued efforts and many contributions to burn care and the association, she was honored in 1989 as a recipient of the Curtis P. Artz Distinguished Service Award, the highest recognition of a nonphysician extended by the American Burn Association.

Since the 1970s, advances in burn rehabilitation have escalated as patient survival rates continued to improve. In 1970, George Koepke[32] from the University of Michigan, one of the earliest physiatrists actively involved in burn care, was the first to advocate range-of-motion exercises while the patient was under anesthesia to lessen the risk of contractures. In that same year, Larson[33] was encouraging limited joint motion "on the fifth postgraft day," and one year later was applying splints to patients "within one hour of admission."[34] Also, as a result of other work by Larson on hypertrophic scarring, the first customized pressure garment became commercially available in 1972.

One of the most in-depth articles investigating the effects of rehabilitation on burn patients was written by Dobbs and Curreri in 1972.[35] This classic article was one of the earliest attempts to investigate critically the outcomes of burn patients on a comprehensive scale, and much of the information still is applicable today. In this extensive patient review, the unequal contribution of partial- and full-thickness burns, the effect of immobilization, and the proximity of the burn to the joint in the formation of scar contractures were reported. Also, the incidence of contractures at specific joints were presented in this comprehensive work.

The use of thermoplastic materials for splinting burn patients was popularized by Willis in 1970.[36–38] By 1977, Newmeyer and Kilgore[39] had reduced the immobilization period of patients following skin grafting to 3 to 5 days. In 1979, the transparent face mask for the control of hypertrophic scars was first reported.[40]

A resurgence in the interest of modalities other than hydrotherapy to treat burn patients also appeared during this time. Paraffin, functional electrical stimulation, continuous passive motion machines and transcutaneous electric nerve stimulation all were used effectively.[41–49]

In the 1980s, a further reduction in the amount of time patients were immobilized following skin grafting occurred as Richard et al.[50,51] reported on satisfactory patient outcomes with range-of-motion exercises performed on the first day after skin grafting. Concurrently, Nicosia and Petro[53] and Hammond and Ward[52] were recommending that the rehabilitation therapist be considered part of the operating room team. In 1991, Schmitt, French, and Kalil[54] wrote on decreasing the bed rest time for ambulating patients with lower-extremity skin grafts from 10 to 6 days, which was reduced further to 1 day as reported by Burnsworth, Krob, and Langer-Schnepp.[55]

SUMMARY

Burn injuries have occurred ever since the discovery of fire. Early intervention was directed at treating the burn wound. However, as the deleterious effects of burn scar contractures became manifest, a concerted effort began to manage this problem. Burn scar contractures were first treated by excision, which was then combined with splints. Massaging and stretching of burn scars soon followed but were used for correction instead of prevention.

Splinting and proper positioning of patients were started earlier in the course of patient treatment, after which the benefits of applying pressure to burn wounds and scar were recognized. A variety of treatments ensued, including serial splinting and modalities. However, patient immobilization until all wounds were healed became the protocol for treatment before therapy was allowed to begin.

In the mid-1940s, patients were performing active range-of-motion exercises earlier in their course of treatment, but it took the influence of John Moncrief[24] in the late 1950s to emphasize the need for early therapy intervention. From that point forward, an emphasis on burn patient rehabilitation began. From admission, splints, positioning, and exercise all became part of the patient's daily routine.

Pressure garments to control hypertrophic scarring became available in the early 1970s, and as the therapist became more involved in the physical management of the burn patient, rehabilitation was further advanced.

In spite of the deformities from burn scars that continue to plague burn patients and frustrate their caregivers, many beneficial changes have taken place in the rehabilitation of burn patients up to the present time. However, only by knowing what has transpired in the past can therapists advance the rehabilitation of burn patients in the future.

REFERENCES

1. Braidwood, RJ: Prehistoric Men. Scott, Foresman, Glenview, 1967, pp 45–46.
2. Haynes, BW Jr: The history of burn care. In Boswick, JA Jr, (ed): The Art And Science of Burn Care. Aspen, Rockville, 1987, pp 3–9.
3. Freshwater, MF and Krizek, TJ: Skin grafting of burns: A centennial. J Trauma 11:862–865, 1971.
4. Robotti, EB: The treatment of burns: An historical perspective with emphasis on the hand. Hand Clinics 6:163–190, 1990.
5. Cockshot, WP: The history of the treatment of burns. Surg Gynecol Obstet 85:116–124, 1956.
6. Huang, TT, Blackwell, SJ, and Lewis, SR: Ten years experience in managing patients with burn contractures of axilla, elbow, wrist, and knee joints. Plast Reconstr Surg 61:70–76, 1978.
7. Taylor, JM: Serious burn followed by contraction of tissue cured by nitrate of silver and pressure carefully applied by means of rollers. Med Rec 16:154, 1879.
8. Wilson, FC: A case of extensive burn, unhealed after six years, permanently cured by massage and skin grafting. Med News 44:237–239, 1884.
9. Seeger, SJ and Schaefer, AA: The treatment of burns. Physiother Rev 14:174–176, 1934.
10. Parker, CA: Treatment of burns of the extremities with special reference to the prevention of deformities and preservation of function. JAMA 65:16–20, 1915.
11. Colditz, JC: Low profile dynamic splinting of the injured hand. Am J Occup Ther 37:182–188, 1983.
12. Blair, VP: Restoration of the burnt child. S Med J 16:522-527, 1923.
13. Coughlin, WT: Contractures due to burns. Surg Gynecol Obstet 68:352–361, 1939.
14. Mixter, CG: Contractions of the neck following burns. N Engl J Med 208:190–196, 1933.
15. Kazanjian, VH: The repair of contractures resulting from burns. N Engl J Med 215:1104–1120, 1936.
16. Engrav, LH, MacDonald, LB, and Covey MH: Do splinting and pressure devices damage new grafts? J Burn Care Rehabil 4:107–108, 1983.
17. Hamilton, JE and Barnett, LA: The treatment of war burns. Surg Clin North Am 23:1575–1588, 1943.
18. Wilson, HC: Physical therapy in a plastic surgery unit. Physiother Rev 25:3, 1945.
19. Miller, H and Posch, JL: Acute burns of the hands. Am J Surg Nov 80:784–789, 1950.
20. Prior, MM and Jaeger, L: Physical therapy in the treatment of burns. Phys Ther Rev 32:510–513, 1952.
21. Holland, EF: Role of physical therapy in the rehabilitation of burned patients. Phys Ther Rev 32:244–246, 1952.
22. Rhoads, JE: The management of burns with special reference to rehabilitation. Phys Ther Rev 33:5–9, 1953.
23. Adams, RH and MacTaggart, L: Physical therapy in the treatment of burns. Phys Ther Rev 38:481–482, 1958.
24. Moncrief, JA: Complications of burns. Ann Surg 147:443–475, 1958.
25. Moncrief, JA: Third degree burns of the dorsum of the hand. Am J Surg 96:535–544, 1958.
26. Feller, I, Koepke, G, and Drew D: The management of extensive full-thickness thermal wounds. Surg Clin North Am 41:1177–1189, 1961.
27. Gronley, JK: Early intensive physical therapy for the burned hand. Phys Ther 44:875–880, 1964.
28. Evans, EB: Orthopaedic measures in the treatment of severe burns. J Bone Joint Surg 48-A:643–669, 1966.
29. Evans, EB, Larson, DL, and Yates S: Preservation and restoration of joint function in patients with severe burns. JAMA 204:843–848, 1968.
30. Heinrich, JJ: Personal communication, June, 1991.
31. Feller, I, et al: The team approach to total rehabilitation of the severely burned patient. Heart Lung 2:701–706, 1973.
32. Koepke, GH: The role of physical medicine in the treatment of burns. Surg Clin North Am 50:1385–1399, 1970.
33. Larson, DL, et al: Repair of the boutonniere deformity of the burned hand. J Trauma 10:481–487, 1970.
34. Larson, DL, et al: Techniques for decreasing scar formation and contracture in the burned patient. J Trauma 11:807–823, 1971.
35. Dobbs, ER and Curreri, PW. Burns: Analysis of results of physical therapy in 681 patients. J Trauma 12:242–248, 1972.
36. Koepke, GH, Feallock, B, and Feller, I: Splinting the severely burned hand. Am J Occup Ther 24:147–150, 1963.
37. Willis, B: The use of Orthoplast isoprene splints in the treatment of the acutely burned child: Preliminary report. Am J Occup Ther 23:57–61, 1969.
38. Staley, MJ, et al: A comprehensive evaluation of available splinting materials. Proc American Burn Association, Baltimore, Maryland, 1991, 23:178.
39. Newmeyer, WL and Kilgore, ES: Management of the burned hand. Phys Ther 57:16–23, 1977.
40. Rivers, EA, Strate, RG, and Soeem, LD: The transparent face mask. Am J Occup Ther 33:108–113, 1979.

41. Head, MD and Helm, PA: Paraffin and sustained stretching in the treatment of burn contractures. Burns 4:136–139, 1978.
42. Apfel, LM, et al: Functional electrical stimulation in intrinsic/extrinsic imbalanced burned hands. J Burn Care Rehabil 8:97–102, 1987.
43. Chu, Chi-Sing, et al: Weak direct current accelerates split-thickness graft healing on tangentially excised second-degree burns. J Burn Care Rehabil 12:285–293, 1991.
44. Covey, MH, et al: Efficacy of continuous passive motion (CPM) devices with hand burns. J Burn Care Rehabil 9:397–400, 1988.
45. McAllister, LP and Salazar, CA: Case report on the use of CPM on an electrical burn. J Burn Care Rehabil 9:401, 1988.
46. Daugherty, MB: Adolescent burn patient benefits from shoulder CPM. In-Motion 1:3, 1988.
47. Richard, RL, Miller, SF, and Staley, MJ. The physiologic response of a patient with critical burns to continuous passive motion. J Burn Care Rehabil 11:554–556, 1990.
48. Kimball, KL, et al: Use of TENS for pain reduction in burn patients receiving Travase. J Burn Care Rehabil 8:28–31, 1987.
49. Lewis, SM, et al: Effects of auricular acupuncture-like transcutaneous electric nerve stimulation on pain levels following wound care in patients with burns: A pilot study. J Burn Care Rehabil 11:322–329, 1990.
50. Richard, RL, Miller, SF, and Finley, RK Jr: Restoration of normal function involving herniated quadriceps muscles following electric burn. J Burn Care Rehabil 6:347–349, 1985.
51. Richard, RL, et al: Early range of motion following skin grafting. Proc American Burn Association, New Orleans, 1989, 21:136.
52. Nicosia, JE and Petro, JA: Manual of Burn Care. Raven Press, New York, 1983, p 89.
53. Hammond, J and Ward, CG: Surgical fixation of skin grafts. J Burn Care Rehabil 9:516–517, 1988.
54. Schmitt, MA, French, L, and Kalil, ET: How soon is safe? Ambulation of the burn patient following lower extremity skin grafting. J Burn Care Rehabil 12:33–37, 1991.
55. Burnsworth, B, Krob, MJ, and Langer-Schnepp, M: Immediate ambulation of patients with lower-extremity grafts. J Burn Care Rehabil 13:89–92, 1992.

CHAPTER 2

Anatomy and Physiology of the Skin

Jeffrey E. Falkel, PhD, PT

The skin is the largest organ of the human body, averaging over 2 m^2 in surface area, and yet in most places is less than 2 mm in thickness.[1] Burn injury primarily involves a destruction and disruption of the normal anatomy and physiologic function of the skin. Although the burn therapist is intimately familiar with the abnormal anatomy and physiology of the skin after a burn injury, the therapist should be aware of normal skin structure and function. Therefore, the purpose of this chapter is to review the basics of normal anatomy and physiology of the skin to promote understanding of how this large, complex organ system functions prior to a burn injury. This chapter will present an integrated approach to the anatomy and structure of the various skin layers, the function of each component within these layers, and the physiologic interactions of the skin with the environment.

THE EPIDERMIS

The epidermis consists of four distinct layers: the stratum corneum, or horny layer; the stratum granulosum, or granular layer; the stratum spinosum, or spinous layer; and the stratum basale, or basal cell layer.[2] A fifth layer, the stratum lucidum, is found in the skin on the soles of the feet and the palms of the hands as a thin eosinophilic band that is located at the base of the stratum corneum.[2] Figure 2–1 presents a schematic diagram of the structures present in the skin and Figure 2–2 is a photomicrograph of the structures of the epidermis. The stratum corneum is the outermost covering, and consists of 15 to 20 layers.[3] The second layer of the epidermis is the stratum granulosum. This layer consists of flattened nucleated cells containing distinctive cytoplasmic inclusions called *keratohyalin granules.*[1] This stratum also serves as a transition layer between the stratum corneum and the lower layers of the epidermis that produce keratinocytes.[1,2,4] The stratum spinosum is comprised of

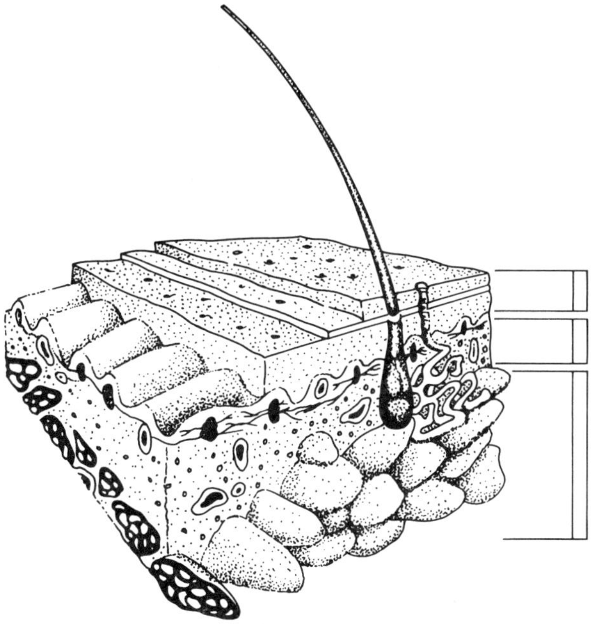

FIGURE 2–1. Cross section of the skin. (From O'Sullivan, SB and Schmitz, TJ (eds): Physical Rehabilitation: Assessment and Treatment. FA Davis, Philadelphia, 1988, p 516, with permission.)

several layers of a polyhedral type cell that lie above the germinal layer of cells.[1] The stratum basale or basal cell layer of keratinocytes is the germinative layer of the epidermis.[1] The basal keratinocytes are structurally cuboidal or low columnar in shape, with a basal surface that conforms to the supporting dermal tissue.[1,2] These keratinocytes contain various cytoplasmic structures and organelles, such as mitochondria, endoplasmic reticulum, rosettes of ribosomes, Golgi complexes, and prominent nucleoli.[1]

The keratinocytes are attached to each other by desmosomes, which are highly developed cellular attachments located at the periphery of each keratinocyte.[1,2] There are subtle, structural differences of the desmosomes as the basal keratinocytes differentiate through the various layers of the epidermis,[1,5,6] The attachment of the desmosomes to the keratinocytes can be broken and re-formed, which allows maturing keratinocytes to migrate toward the stratum corneum.[2] The desmosomes of the stratum corneum are degraded prior to desquamation,[1] which is the process of shedding the outer layers of the epidermis as the lower layers move toward the surface. The desmosome system appears to minimize the effects of mechanical stress on the epidermis and prevents a shearing of the epidermal cells.[2] Glycocalyx is a substance located between the keratinocytes and it is probably the substance to which various circulating antibodies attach.[2]

The epidermis is normally in a constant balance between the production of keratinocytes and the desquamation of the outer layers of the stratum corneum. The keratinocyte cells will differentiate in the direction toward the surface of the epidermis to produce the cornified surface layer.[7] The average "transit time"[8] from the basal layer outward to the stratum corneum is approximately 26 to 42 days.[1,2,7,8] The outermost cells of the stratum corneum undergo desquamation while the lower layers are

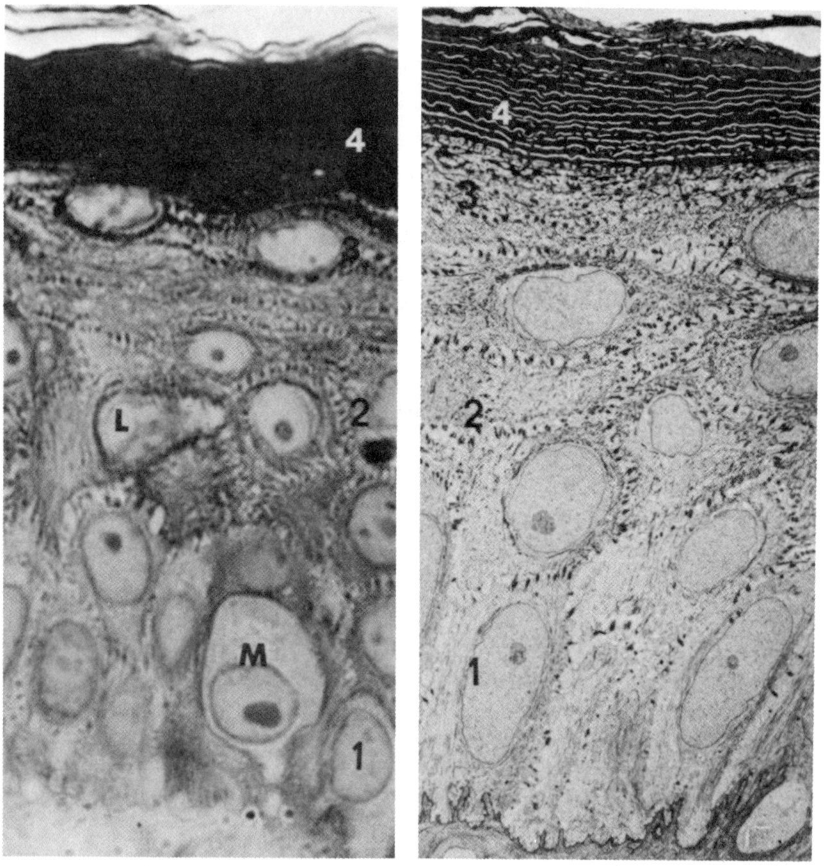

FIGURE 2–2. (*Right*) Photomicrograph of human epidermis showing conventional layers of keratinocytes: (1) basal cell layer, (2) stratum spinosum, (3) stratum granulosum, (4) stratum corneum. (*Left*) Two types of immigrant cells: melanocyte (M) in the basal layer and Langerhans cell (L) in the suprabasal region. (From Goldsmith,[1] p 6, with permission.)

replaced from below. The transit time from the lowest layer of the stratum corneum to its desquamation is approximately 14 days.[1] Thus, normal epidermis completely replaces itself in 45 to 75 days.[1,8,9]

Epidermal Structures

There are a variety of cellular structures other than keratinocytes located in the epidermis. These structures function within the epidermis, and with the cutaneous epidermal structures (to be discussed later), make the epidermis a metabolically active and essential component of the skin.

MELANOCYTES

Melanocytes are dendritic cells that produce pigment granules known as melanosomes, which contain the pigment melanin.[2,7] Melanocytes are located at the dermoepidermal junction, although there are some melanocytes located in the dermis. The distribution of melanocytes varies throughout the body and changes with age. There is about 1 melanocyte for every 5 epidermal cells on the face, but only 1 melanocyte for every 20 cells on the buttocks. The normal ratio of melanocytes to keratinocytes varies between 1:4 to 1:10, depending on the region of the body.[7] The ratio decreases with increasing age. Melanosomes are thought to be transferred through melanocytic dendrites into the adjacent keratinocytes secondary to phagocytic activity of the melanin pigment.[2] Patterson and Blaylock[2] suggested that each melanocyte serves approximately 36 keratinocytes, resulting in a functional system called the *epidermal-melanin unit.*

The relative number of melanocytes is approximately equal for both men and women and for all races.[7] The variation in the coloration between and within races is not due to differences in the number of melanocytes, but rather to the activity, rate, and production of melanin.[2,7] For example, dark-skinned individuals tend to have fully melanized and very large melanosomes that are singly dispersed within the keratinocytes. However, fair-skinned people have much smaller and less melanized melanosomes that tend to be grouped into melanosome complexes.[2] The above findings must be considered when choosing a donor site after a full-thickness burn injury. A difference in coloration will occur when skin from areas of low melanosome content is grafted to burned areas that had a higher number of melanocytes.

Melanin functions to protect the epidermis from the harmful effects of ultraviolet light by forming a protective cap around the keratinocyte nuclei to prevent ultraviolet damage to the DNA in the nucleus.[2] Melanogenesis occurs within the melanosome and involves the conversion of the colorless amino acid tyrosine into a brown-black polymer of melanin.[7] The amount of melanin and the process of melanogenesis also acts to protect the skin from a superficial burn (that is, sunburn) when exposure to sunlight is gradually increased.

LANGERHANS CELLS

The Langerhans cells are another type of dendritic cell found in the epidermis. They are similar to melanocytes, except they lack pigment.[2,10] The true function of the Langerhans cells was unknown until recently. Original research suggested that the Langerhans cells were involved in the organization and function of the squamous epidermis.[10–12] Whether the Langerhans cells are responsible for the control of the proliferation of keratinocytes and the pattern of epidermal cell columns is open to debate.[10,13,14] Langerhans cells might be concerned with the breakdown or loosening of the intercellular connections by the desmosomes.[10,15] More recent research findings have determined that the Langerhans cells are active as phagocytes[2,10] and their major functions are to provide a "reticuloepithelial trap" for various contact antigens and to present them to T cells for destruction.[2,10] Langerhans cells assist in one of the primary functions of the skin, to protect the internal structures from potential infectious agents in the external environment. Several investigators have determined that Langerhans cells are reduced in number and may be damaged by excessive exposures to ultraviolet light.[10,16,17]

Cutaneous Appendages of the Epidermis

Several other structures that significantly affect the function and physiology of the human skin are epidermal in origin. These structures, seen in Figure 2–3, are the hair follicles, the sebaceous and apocrine glands, and the eccrine sweat glands.

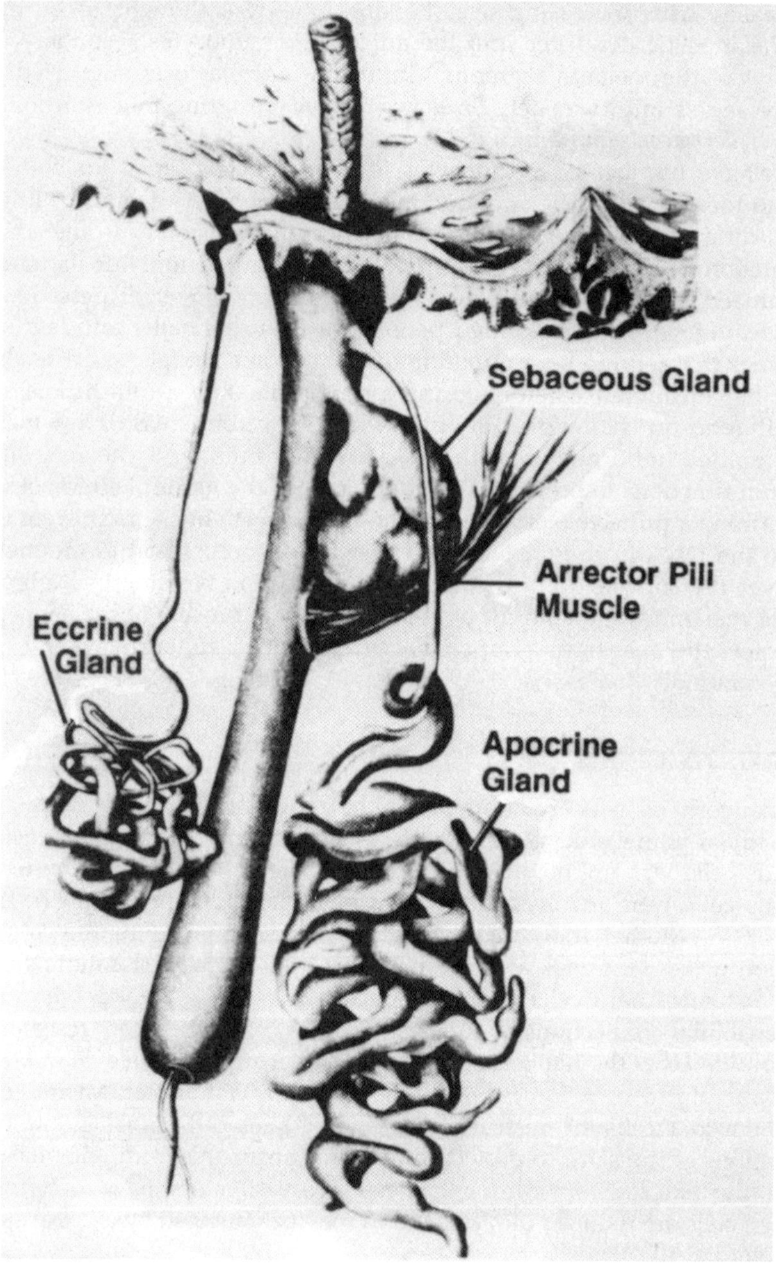

FIGURE 2–3. Drawing of the relationship of a hair follicle and eccrine, apocrine, and sebaceous glands. (From Goldsmith,[1] p 40, with permission.)

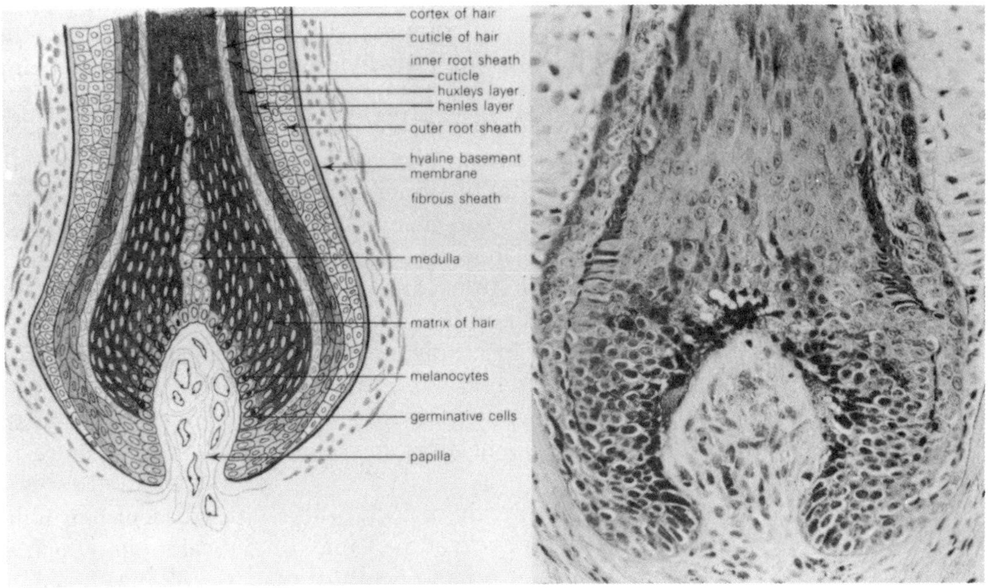

FIGURE 2–4. (*A*) As shown in this diagram, the cells of the hair matrix differentiate along six separate lines. From the outside inward, they are: the Henle's layer, the first to cornify and only one cell thick; Huxley's layer, characterized by brightly eosinophilic-staining trichohyaline granules and two cells thick; cuticle of the inner root sheath; cuticle of the hair; hair cortex; and hair medulla. Surrounding the central core of the matrix products is the pale, staining, relatively broad, outer root sheath. Through a narrow outlet at the distal end of the bulb, the papilla emerges to become continuous with the connective tissue sheath that envelops the entire follicle. (*B*) A photomicrograph of the hair matrix. (From Moschella, Pillsbury, Hurley,[7] p 40, with permission.)

HAIR FOLLICLES

The hair follicles consist of "pockets of epithelium" which are continuous with the superficial epidermis.[10] The hair follicle can be divided into three portions: the infundibulum, which is the most superficial and primarily epidermal; the isthmus, which comprises the tissue between the entry into the follicle of the sebaceous gland and the insertion of the arrector pili muscle; and the inferior portion, which gives rise to the hair bulb including the hair papilla and matrix.[2] Since the hair follicle is composed of primarily epidermal tissue it has a significant function in the re-epithelialization of the burn wound. Unless the burn depth is very deep partial or full thickness, epidermal tissue will be available in the wound site from which epidermal skin buds will generate new epithelium.

Figure 2–4 is a photomicrograph of the cross section of the distal end of the hair. Hairs produced in the hair follicle are keratinous fibers growing out from the epithelial follicles that are distributed universally over the skin surface, with the exception of the soles of the feet and the palms of the hand.[1,2,4,7] The terminal hair follicle has a regular, three-cycle growth phase. The active phase is called the *anagen*; the *catagen* is the involuting phase, and the *telogen* is the resting phase.[2] The proportion of follicles in a particular phase is partly dependent on their location. Over 85 percent of scalp hairs are in the anagen phase at any time, whereas a significant percentage of eyelash hairs are in the telogen phase.[2] At the lowest portion of the follicle, an area is dilated into a bulb of epithelium that is enclosed by a connective tissue papilla.[1] The cells in this bulb are undifferentiated and are rapidly dividing. In fact, the mitotic rate of the matrix of the hair follicle is among the most rapidly dividing tissue in the body, being replaced completely every 12 to 24 hours.[1,2,7] The products of the matrix, which are the inner root sheath and hair, move outward toward the surface of the skin by passing over the stationary outer root sheath. The cuticle of the inner root sheath connects with the cuticle of the hair so that the inner root and the hair ascend toward the surface at the same rate of speed.[7] The hair shaft consists of dead cornified structures that extend from the follicle above the skin surface.[7] The shaft contains three compartments: an inner medulla, a cortex, and an outer cuticle. The color of the hair depends on the distribution and amount of melanin within the cortex.[7] Blond hair produces fewer melanosomes, or incompletely melanized melanosomes. Red hair has melanin that is chemically different from that of black hair, with the melanosomes possibly having some iron-containing pigment that causes the reddish coloration. Gray hair has an absence of melanosomes due to a relative absence of melanocytes.[7]

Hair follicles produce hair independently of each other, with adjacent hair follicles being in different phases of the hair cycle at the same time.[7] Scalp hair, which is primarily composed of protein, grows at a rate of approximately 0.35 mm per day, with a total, daily manufacture of almost 100 feet of scalp hair![7] The growth of hair is dependent on numerous factors, such as hormones, temperature, nutrition, and light exposure.[1,2,7]

Human hair has several distinct physiologic functions. Nerve endings are connected to hair follicles that participate in the sensory system of the skin. The hair traps air and serves as a source of insulation, although this is primarily effective on the scalp. Hair also serves to combat infection by trapping infectious organisms and keeping them at a distance from the skin surface.[1]

SEBACEOUS GLANDS

These glands arise from an epithelial bud from the outer hair root sheath at the junction of the infundibulum and isthmus of the hair follicle.[7] Sebaceous glands are distributed over the entire body, with the exception of the plantar and dorsal surface of the foot and the palms of the hands.[7] The secretion from the sebaceous glands is classified as holocrine, because the entire cell is "cast off," in a manner similar to the desquamation of the cornified cells of the epidermis.[2,7] The sebum or secretory product is emptied into the hair follicle.[2] The sebaceous glands change size throughout the lifespan. They are relatively large in the new born, diminish in size during childhood, and enlarge again during adolescence.[2] The role of the sebaceous glands is much greater in animals than in humans. The sebum coats the animals fur to protect the skin and assist in insulation. Human sebaceous glands act primarily to secrete sebum to assist in keeping the skin moist and supple. If the sebaceous glands are damaged or destroyed as the result of a burn injury, the new skin cover may not have the ability to secrete enough sebum to keep the skin moist, and may require frequent applications of moisturizing creams. Other hypothesized functions of sebum include: (1) barrier protection against germs, (2) regulation of percutaneous absorption, (3) antimicrobial activity, and (4) a vitamin D precursor. However, speculation about the exact function of sebum in humans still exists.[7,18]

APOCRINE SWEAT GLANDS

The apocrine sweat glands are found primarily in the axillae and pubic region. The mammary gland is considered to be histochemically an apocrine gland.[2,7] An apocrine gland consists of a coiled secretory gland located in the lower portion of the dermis and a straight excretory duct that empties onto the infundibular component of the hair follicle, which is normally adjacent to the sebaceous gland.[7] The lining of the apocrine duct and secretory coil consists of columnar or cuboidal epidermal cells.[7] The production of apocrine sweat consists of secretion, which is a continuous process, and excretion, which occurs when a reservoir of apocrine secretion is propelled upward.[7] The quantity of apocrine sweat produced daily is generally small. The apocrine secretion is sterile and odorless within the duct. However, once the apocrine secretion combines with bacteria on the surface of the skin, the bacteria degrade the apocrine sweat, resulting in body odor.[2,7] Most of the underarm deodorants contain some type of antibacterial agent that eliminates the offending organisms.[7] The apocrine glands have no known function in the human.[2,7]

ECCRINE SWEAT GLANDS

The eccrine sweat gland is composed of epidermal skin layers.[1,2,7,8] The eccrine sweat glands are located throughout the body, with the highest concentrations located on the forehead, axillae, and palms and soles of the feet, and the lowest concentrations located on the arms and legs.[2,7] There are approximately 3 million eccrine sweat glands present at birth, and no additional eccrine glands are formed throughout the rest of the lifespan.[7]

The eccrine sweat gland unit consists of a coiled gland and three sections of an eccrine duct. The coiled dermal duct lies with the coiled gland in the dermis and gives rise to a straight duct. This straight duct connects with the spiral duct, located in the epidermis, and the spiral duct exits to the skin surface.[2,7] The gland is innervated extensively by unmyelinated nerve fibers, with the initiation of sweating being mediated by acetylcholine and inhibited by atropine.[7] The eccrine gland also responds to sympathetic and parasympathetic stimulation.

Eccrine sweat is a colorless, odorless hypotonic solution that is approximately 99 percent water by weight, with the remaining 1 percent containing various solutes of electrolytes, lipids, minerals, and amino acids.[7] The primary stimulus for the production of eccrine sweat is heat. The thermoregulatory center in the hypothalamus is responsible for triggering sweat production. The hypothalamus acts as a "neural thermostat" by integrating the impulses of rising skin temperature and blood temperature with the production of sweat. A rise of as little as 0.5°C will activate the hypothalamus to initiate the action of the sweat glands.[7] All eccrine sweat glands do not function at one time, and the total amount of sweat produced by each gland is relatively small. However, the total sweat production in the adult can reach levels in excess of 2 to 3 liters per hour, and the evaporation of each liter removes 540 calories of heat from the body.[7,19]

Sweating is the most effective way for the body to dissipate heat. As the body temperature rises, either due to external or internal factors, the hypothalamus initiates the sweating mechanism. As the body temperature rises, such as during exercise, the increase in blood temperature perfusing the hypothalamus continues to activate the sweating response.[7,19] With prolonged exposure to a hot environment, the body will begin the process of acclimation. The sweating mechanism will adjust so that smaller increases in body temperature will result in the production of a given amount of sweat production. The levels of the solutes, primarily electrolytes, in the sweat also will be reduced after a period of acclimation.[7,19] For the sweating mechanism to be effective in cooling the body, the sweat must evaporate. Evaporation of sweat will cool the skin surface and create a thermal gradient to dissipate the heat from the core, working muscles, and tissues out to the skin. This process is most effective in hot, dry conditions. Environmental conditions that are hot and humid cause reduced evaporation of the produced sweat, because the air around the skin is also saturated with moisture. Thus, the sweat seems to "drip" off the body rather than evaporate. The loss of the thermal gradient from the core to the skin creates an increase in the rise of core temperature, which could reach dangerous levels with even minimal exertion in unacclimated individuals.[19]

The loss of eccrine sweat glands with deep partial-thickness and full-thickness burns can have serious consequences for the rehabilitation of the patient with a burn injury. If a significant percentage of eccrine sweat glands are lost, the patient must rely on the remaining sweat glands for thermoregulation. Studies have shown that persons who have sustained a full-thickness burn to a significant percent of their body have a total sweat production similar to subjects without burn injury.[20] However, because the number of eccrine glands is reduced with a full-thickness burn injury, the sweating rate is inefficient, with a concomitant rise in core temperature. Secondly, the loss of sweat glands reduces the effective sweating area and decreases the thermal gradient between the core of the body and the skin. A third concern for the patient with a full-thickness burn injury is the problem with exercise in a hot, humid environment. As mentioned above, hot and humid environmental conditions do not allow the effective evaporation of sweat for thermoregulation. Consequently, the patient with reduced sweat glands is further compromised by the lack of evaporative sweating, which results in an even greater rise in core temperature. The ability to sweat and the amount of skin that has the capacity for sweating are important considerations in the recreational, vocational, and exercise prescription for patients with deep partial- and full-thickness burn injuries.

BASEMENT MEMBRANE

There are a variety of connective tissue fibers located in an subjacent to the epidermis known as the *basement membrane*.[1] The basal lamina consists of grooves on the epidermis, or epidermal ridges, which fit intimately with projections from the dermis, termed *dermal papillae*. Microfilaments of 10 to 12 nm in diameter insert into the basal lamina and are aggregated in the subjacent papillary dermis. The resultant structure that is formed, referred to as rete pegs, acts as a series of "hills and valleys" to increase the surface area and to resist shearing forces between the epidermal and dermal layers. Blisters may occur if there is a defect in this interface. Following a burn injury, regenerated epidermis lacks these interconnections for a prolonged time and the skin is prone to abrasion with only minor trauma.

THE DERMIS

The dermis is composed primarily of extracellular proteins and a dense fibroelastic connective tissue that is made of collagen, elastic fibers, and an interfibrillar gel substance.[1,2,7] The thickness of the epidermis is approximately equal to the thickness of this piece of paper, but it can vary from 0.04 mm on the eyelids to 1.6 mm on the palms of the hands.[7] The thickness of the dermis is approximately 15 to 40 times greater than that of the epidermis, depending on its location.[7] The most dominant structural elements of the dermis are produced and monitored by the fibroblast.[1] Weinstein and Boucek[21] identified collagen as the component that accounts for approximately 77 percent of the fat-free dry weight of the dermis. Collagen is the element responsible for the tensile strength of the dermis. Type I collagen accounts for the majority of collagen in the dermis, and type III collagen represents approximately 15 percent.[1,21] Elastic fibers are interwoven into the network of collagen to restore the normal array of fibrous tissue following its deformation by external mechanical stresses and forces.[1] Fibroblasts are considered the "master cells" of the dermis.[1,2,21] They produce reticular collagen, elastic fibers, and the ground substance that comprise the dermis. The dermis contains the vast vascular network and nervous innervation of the skin, as well as the epidermal appendages.[1]

The dermis is divided into two distinct strata: the papillary dermis, which is the thinner and more superficial portion, and the reticular dermis, which is the thicker portion interfacing with the subcutaneous tissue. Figure 2–5 is a photomicrograph of a cross section of the two strata of the dermis.

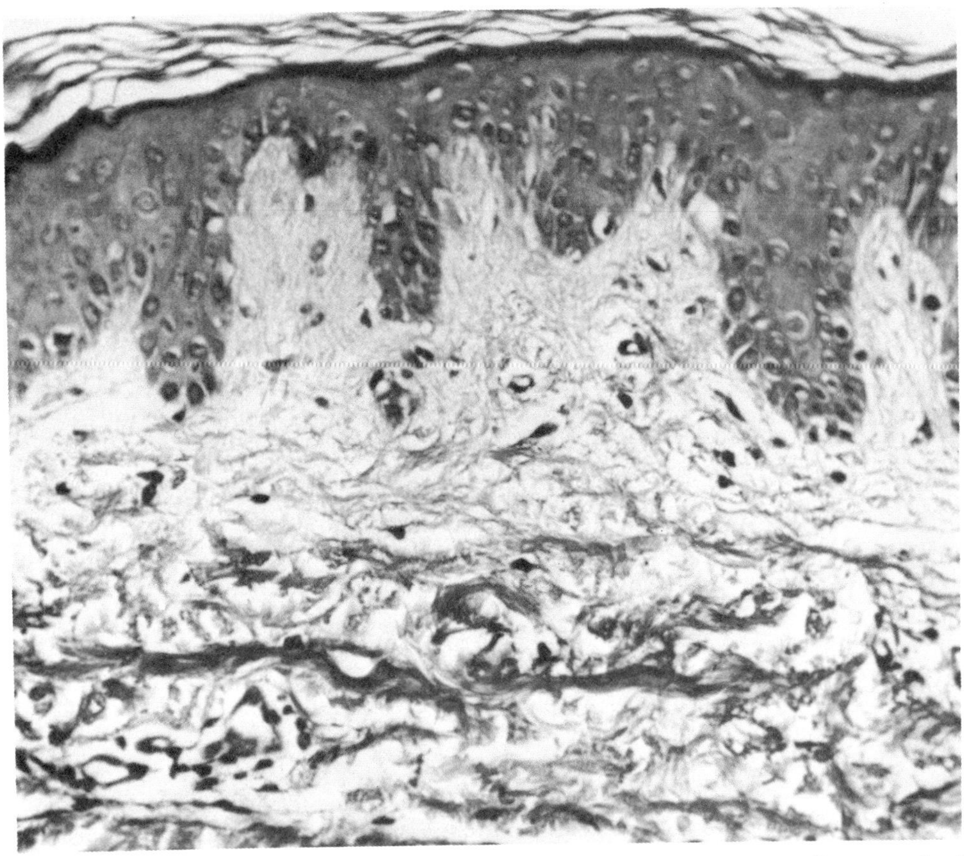

FIGURE 2–5. The superficial (papillary) dermis is composed of thin, haphazardly arranged collagen fibers in contrast to the deeper (reticular) dermis which is formed by thick collagen bundles (×374). (From Moschella, Pillsbury, Hurley,[7] p 11, with permission.)

Papillary Dermis

The papillary dermis is molded against the overlying epidermis and conforms to the basal layer ridges, grooves, and appendages of the epidermis.[1] The papillary dermis comprises primarily smaller, loosely distributed elastic and collagen fibrils. It also contains a substantially greater proportion of interfibrillar gel and connective tissue that supports and encloses the superficial aspects of the microcirculation and lymphatic network just below the papillary projections of the dermis.[1] Brown[22] has determined that the thickness of the collagen fibers in the papillary dermis ranges from 0.3 to 3 μm in diameter.

Reticular Dermis

The deeper and thicker component of the dermis is the reticular dermis. The reticular dermis is somewhat more acellular and avascular as compared to the papillary dermis and contains elastic fibers and dense collagen bundles of approximately 10 to 40 μm in diameter.[1,7] The total thickness of the reticular dermis may be up to 4 or 5 mm. These collagen bundles are arranged primarily parallel to the skin surface,[7] although some of the collagen also is arranged in a perpendicular orientation that forms a "lattice work."[1,7,23] The function of this arrangement of parallel and tangential collagen fibers in the reticular dermis is to provide the skin with preferential direction of extensibility.[1] When the reticular dermis is injured, punctured, or displaced, the collagen fibers will return to their original state and become aligned parallel to the direction of the least amount of extensibility.[1,24] This functional orientation of the reticular collagen will play a significant role in the healing and possible hypertrophic scarring that occurs after a burn injury. The reticular dermis interfaces with the subcutaneous tissue is composed of varying amounts of subcutaneous fat, striated muscle, and fascial structures.

Dermal Structures

Similar to the epidermis, there are several different types of structures contained within the dermis that manifest their function throughout the skin organ system. These structures include the smooth muscle of the arrector pilorum; blood, lymphatic vessels, and microvasculature; and a network of nervous structures and organs.

SMOOTH MUSCLE

The arrector pilorum muscles arise in the dermis and insert upon the hair follicles below the sebaceous duct.[2] The muscle is able to cause the hair follicle to elevate when contracted, causing "goose flesh" of the skin. This muscle contraction results in an increase in the metabolic rate of the skin and is an attempt by the skin to assist in maintaining the necessary thermoneutral environment of the body during exposure to cold.[19]

BLOOD VESSELS AND MICROCIRCULATION

The blood supply to the skin is derived from the cutaneous branches of the subcutaneous musculocutaneous arteries.[1] Figure 2–6 depicts the microcirculation of the skin. The branches from the cutaneous arteries become a distinctive small-vessel plexus which lies in the deep layer of the reticular dermis. Small arteries and arterioles then ascend toward the surface as small perforating arteries into the papillary dermis, where they branch again into terminal arterioles.[1] At this level, the microcirculation network of arterioles, capillaries, and venules provides a vast quantity of blood to the dermal layers. Compared to the microcirculation in other regions of the body, the arterioles, capillaries, and venules of the skin are distinguished by a relatively thicker vessel wall.[1] This thicker vessel wall has been attributed to a thicker basement membrane. The additional elastic fibers and collagen located in these vessel walls serve to "protect the skin vasculature from damage due to their relatively superficial location."[1] In addition, extensive arteriovenous anastomoses are present in the skin, particularly in the digits.[7] These anastomoses serve as preferential channels to move blood past the capillary bed more rapidly for purposes of thermoregulation, increased metabolic demand, and alterations in the distribution of cardiac output.[25] The venules then descend toward the lower level of the reticular dermis, draining the small venules into muscular veins and they finally connect with the subcutaneous venous system.[1]

Thermoregulation is the "cardinal function" of the cutaneous vasculature.[7] Another vital function of the cutaneous vasculature is to provide nutrition to the skin.[7] The vast number of capillaries in the dermis provide more than an adequate blood

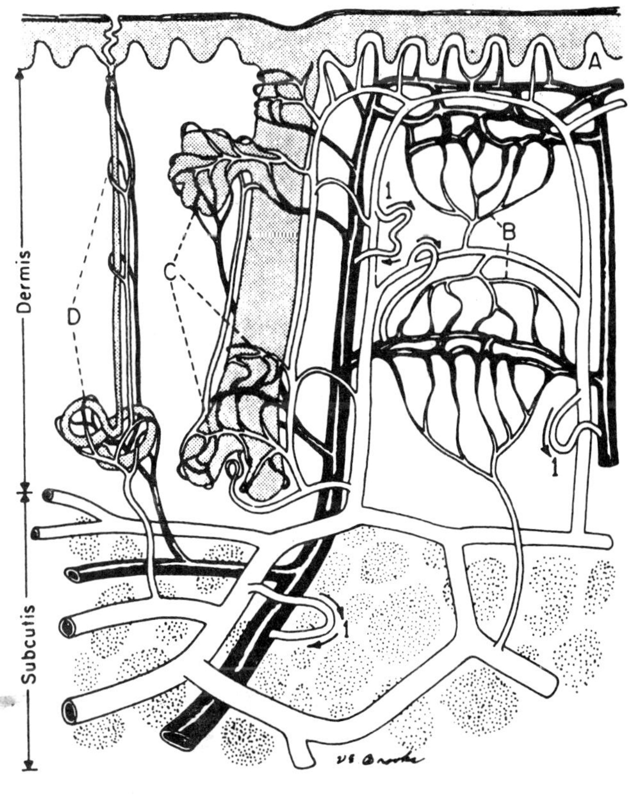

FIGURE 2–6. Schematic depiction of the microcirculation units of the skin. The arterial vessels are shown in white and the veins are in black. (*A*) the papillary dermis; (*B*) the reticular dermis; (*C*) the pilosebaceous apparatus; and (*D*) an eccrine sweat gland and duct. 1 identifies some arteriovenous communications at different levels in the skin and subcutaneous tissue. (From Goldsmith,[1] p 26, with permission.)

supply for the epithelial appendages, whose metabolic demand is greater than that of the connective tissue of the skin.[7] The vasculature of the skin also plays a major role in the inflammatory process. The erythema seen in the skin as part of the inflammatory process, either due to histamine, bradykinins, or other inflammatory by-products, is a function of the quantity of blood in the microcirculation of the skin. One of the limiting factors in the healing of the burn wound is the amount of damage that occurs to the microcirculation and vascular network of the skin due to the burn trauma. Partial-thickness burns that do not involve the deeper structures of the dermis and the majority of the vascular bed of the skin have the potential to heal rapidly because the integrity of the microvascular circulation remains intact. As the burn wound heals, care must be taken in dressing changes, debridement, splinting, and exercise activities to "protect" the microcirculation from damage as it supplies the re-epithelialization process.

LYMPHATIC VESSELS

The structure of the lymphatic vessels consists of a single endothelial layer, containing a system of valves, and a discontinuous layer of basal laminar material.[1,7] The function of the lymphatic vessels within the skin is to transport particulate and liquid matter from the extravascular compartments of the skin.[7,26] The collecting and transportation vessels descend to the lower level of the reticular dermis and accompany the venous blood vessels away from the skin.[7]

NERVE SUPPLY TO THE SKIN

The skin serves as one of the major sensory organs of the body and provides constant feedback to the nervous system about the nature and stress of the human environment. The skin may be innervated with more than one million afferent nerve fibers.[10,16] The skin contains sensory organs for all of the principle sensations of touch, pain, warmth, cold, itch, tickle, and pressure.[1,7,8] Weddell et al.[27] and Sinclair[28] have identified an extensive branching of myelinated sensory nerve endings in two main plexuses in the dermis. The lowermost plexus is deep in the reticular layer, which is orientated in a parallel fashion with the surface of the skin. This plexus sends fibers upward to form a more superficial plexus that is made up of both myelinated and unmyelinated nerves.[1] Most of the nervous structures and fibers end in the dermis, and some penetrate into the basement membrane. However, very few fibers travel very deep into the epidermis.[7] The motor innervation of the skin is accomplished by the autonomic nervous system, specifically the sympathetic fibers.[1] These motor nerves are responsible for vasomotor control of the microvasculature, pilomotor function of the arrector pili muscles attached to the hair follicles, and the secretion of the eccrine sweat glands.[1,7,8]

SENSORY RECEPTORS

Figure 2–7 presents a diagram of the orientation and variety of sensory organs found in the skin. Because of the importance of the sensations that the skin transmits to the nervous system and the impact that the environment has on these sensory organs, each structure will be briefly reviewed in this section (Table 2–1).

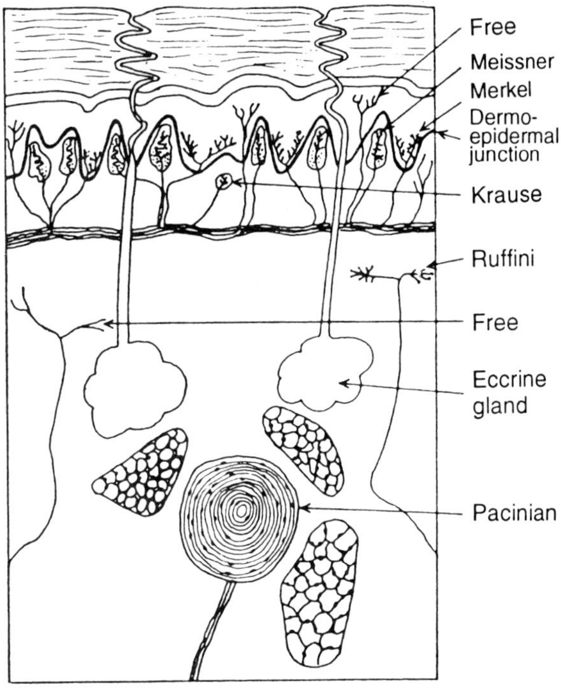

FIGURE 2–7. Diagrammatic section showing various nerve endings in the skin of the finger tip. (From Rook, A, et al,[10] p 24, with permission.)

TABLE 2–1. Sensory Receptors in the Epidermis and Dermis of Human Skin

Structure	Location	Function
Free terminals	Epidermis, dermis	Sensations of itch and pain; fine discrimination for sensory stimuli in the digits
Merkel cell endings	Epidermal ridge	Mechanoreceptor for the sensation of touch
Meissner touch corpuscles	Papillary dermis of palm of hand and sole of foot	Sensation of touch and relative amounts of pressure associated with sensation of touch
Pacinian corpuscles	Deep layers of palmar dermis, palmar subcutaneous tissue, and near periosteum of proximal phalanges	Sense of vibration, signals local changes in blood flow
Pilo-Ruffini corpuscles	Encircling the hair follicles	Slow-reacting mechanoreceptor that responds to changes in pressure sensed by hair follicles; Ruffini end organs also responsible for sensation of warmth
Krause end bulb	Superficial layers of the dermis	Sensation of cold

Free Terminals

The majority of the sensory receptors found in the epidermis and dermis are classified as "free" nerve endings or terminals, which do not have any specific morphologic function.[29] Receptors presumably are related to the sensations of itch and pain.[1] These types of receptors are classified as "free" in that one or more axons are enclosed in an extension of the Schwann cell, which is then covered with a basal lamina.[1,29] In the skin of the digits, the terminal Schwann cell may sheathe one or more axonal branches of a single nerve, which may either terminate within the dermal papilla or send a terminal axon into the epidermis.[1] This arrangement accounts for the fine discrimination of sensory stimuli in the digits as compared to other areas of the skin that have few free nerve endings.

Merkel Cell Endings

A Merkel cell is a specialized cell, larger than the keratinocyte, which lies at the base of the epidermal ridge.[1,7] Merkel cells have attachments next to the keratinocytes. The dermal surface of the Merkel cell is enclosed in Schwann cell membranes whose basal lamina are continuous with the epidermal basal lamina.[1] Merkel cells are believed to function as a form of mechanoreceptor for the sensation of touch.[1,7,8]

Meissner's Touch Corpuscles

These oval or elongated structures, approximately 20 to 40 $\times$ 150 μm in size, are found predominately in the digits and volar pads.[7,8] They are most dense in the papillary dermis of the palm of the hand and sole of the foot. Their anatomic structure consists of a "coil or tangle" of terminal axons covered by basal laminar cells that are interspersed with flattened laminar cells.[7] The Meissner's touch corpuscles are responsible for the sensation of touch and the relative amounts of pressure associated with the sensation of touch.[8]

Pacinian Corpuscles

These structures are rather large, 0.5 to 4 mm in length, and 0.3 to 0.7 mm in diameter, and are found in the deep layers of the palmar dermis, palmar subcutaneous tissue, and near the periosteum of the proximal phalanges.[1] Morphologically, the pacinian corpuscle is a multilaminar capsule with an unmyelinated axon at its core. The pacinian corpuscle has long been associated with the sensation of vibration;[1,30] however, it has been theorized that it is also a mechanism to signal local changes in blood flow.[1,30] Cauna and Mannan[30] have suggested that when the arteriovenous anastomosis is open, the increased venous pressure is sensed by the pacinian corpuscles and this activates local changes in blood flow through the skin.

Pilo-Ruffini Corpuscles

These sensory receptors are cylindrical encapsulated nerve endings that encircle the hair follicles.[1,7] These receptors are thought to be slow-reacting mechanoreceptors that respond to changes in pressure on the skin, specifically sensed by movement of the hair follicles.[1,8] The Ruffini corpuscle is somewhat unique in regards to the other sensory receptors in the skin, because its terminal nerve branch is enclosed in a specialized connective tissue compartment of collagen fibrils, elastic fibers, and connective tissue cells called septal cells.[1] This specialized compartment may respond to the mechanical stresses on the skin for longer periods of time, and thus allows the receptor more time to provide information to the nervous system about the force, direction, and magnitude of the pressure on the skin.[31] The Ruffini end organs also are responsible for the sensation of warmth.[10]

Krause End Bulb

The Krause end bulb is an encapsulated swelling on myelinated fibers that are located in the superficial layers of the dermis.[10] This receptor is the end organ for cold sensation and is widely distributed in the connective tissue of the dermis.

In summary, the skin possesses an intricate network of a variety of nerve receptors that allow this organ system to function and provide feedback based on the environmental stimuli that are presented to it. Patients with moderate to severe burn injuries may lose some or all of these receptors. As a result, the return of sensation and the ability to discriminate various intensities and durations of sensation needs to be assessed in the rehabilitative phase of recovery.

FUNCTIONS OF THE SKIN

The primary functions of the skin are to: (1) serve as a barrier to prevent the penetration of foreign objects, material, and radiation; (2) function as part of the immune system to prevent various organisms from gaining exposure to internal organs; (3) serve as a water barrier; (4) regulate heat exchange and assist in body temperature homeostasis; (5) transmit sensory feedback from the environment; (6) resist mechanical stresses; (7) provide a cosmetic covering for personal identity; and (8) allow for the absorption of selected substances.[1,2,7,8,10] The skin also functions as a site for endocrine function and interaction.[1,7,8]

The function and ability of the skin to allow selective permeability is an important factor to consider. The skin, as suggested by Hurley,[32] should be viewed as a structure that will limit water loss and as a membrane that will protect the body from the penetration of water and other chemicals. However, the skin is one of the primary sources for the introduction of a variety of medications into the body. Thus, the skin must possess the ability for selective permeability. There is a morphologic paradox to the amount of permeability that is permitted by the skin. The stratum corneum serves a dual role: first, as one of the most important structures serving as a barrier to absorption;[7] and second, as one of the three possible pathways, with the hair follicles and the eccrine glands, for percutaneous absorption.[7,10] As with most substances, a concentration gradient is necessary to allow and drive the percutaneous absorption of substances across the stratum corneum. Thus, Hurley[32] suggested that the relative hydration of the stratum corneum will have a dramatic impact on the ability of the stratum corneum to act effectively during percutaneous absorption.

Other factors that impact on the skin's ability to repel or absorb a particular substance include the temperature of the skin, the changes in pH of the skin and the substance, and the chemical nature of the substance. Lipids and lipid-soluble compounds will pass through the skin relatively easily, whereas hydrophilic organic compounds have a much more difficult time crossing the skin barrier.[7] Various gaseous compounds, like carbon monoxide, will pass through the skin when present in high enough concentrations.

REGIONAL VARIATION IN THE SKIN

Figure 2–8 depicts the differences in the regional thicknesses of the epidermis and dermis in selected regions of the body. Klingman[33] has described in great detail the regional differences in a variety of structures that occupy the skin. These findings, along with current histochemical, histopathologic, biochemical, and bacteriologic studies, suggest there is tremendous variation in the different regions of the body so that generalizations about one region may not be applicable to another.[10,33] There is a direct application and need for the burn therapist to appreciate that these regional variations in the structure and composition of the skin do exist. A split-thickness skin graft may not retain many of the original region's structural and functional variations. When this occurs, the burn therapist needs to be aware of the potential alterations in function, sensation, or characteristics that the newly grafted skin will demonstrate. Therefore, a brief overview of some of these regional variations follows.

The thickness of the epidermis varies greatly from the extensive, compact, thick stratum corneum of the soles, palms, and other areas of high friction to the very thin epidermis of the eyelids. The thickness of the stratum corneum will have a direct influence on the ability of the skin to resist physical and chemical trauma and will alter the permeability of the region.[10]

The distribution of the various appendages, such as hair follicles, sebaceous glands, apocrine glands, and eccrine glands varies greatly throughout the body. The number of hair follicles remains relatively unchanged until midlife, but the alteration of the microclimate surrounding each region of the body will result in dynamic changes in the relative distribution and activity of the hair follicles.[10] The activity of the eccrine glands is dependent on environmental stress.[10,25] For example, individuals who have been raised in northern climates will have a reduced number and size of the effective eccrine sweat glands when compared to those people who have grown up in the much hotter southern climates. These warmer climates necessitate a more efficient utilization of the eccrine sweat glands for effective thermoregulation.

The distribution, function, and productivity of the melanocytes is altered based on the region and age of the individual. The environmental stresses of ultraviolet light, heat, and humidity also will impact the amount of melanocyte activity.

There is a marked variation in the structure of the epidermal-dermal junction.[10,34] The number and type of epidermal appendages, and the sculpturing of the under-

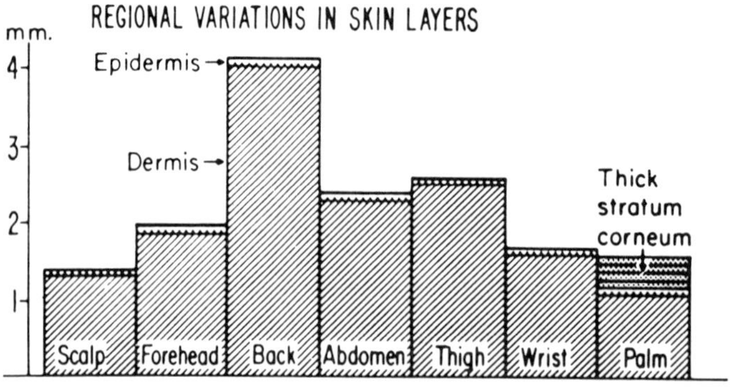

FIGURE 2–8. Diagram showing the regional variation in the thickness of the skin. (From Goldsmith,[1] p 5, with permission.)

surface of the epidermis is directly related to the ability of the region to withstand mechanical stresses.[10]

The dermis, as shown in Figure 2–8, varies greatly in depth throughout the body. This depth variation is based in part on the functional requirements of the regions of the skin. The size and arrangement of the elastic and collagen fibers also will vary and impact significantly on the amount and time frame of scarring after a burn injury or harvesting of a skin graft.[10]

There are marked variations in the blood supply to the different regions of the skin. These variations are based not only on the functional structure of the tissue in the region but also on the components of the skin in that area. For example, the highly distensible skin over the eyelids has a dramatically different amount of microvasculature and subsequent blood flow as compared to the more rigid regions over the finger tips.[10]

There are differences in the relative amounts of histamine, prostaglandin, bradykinins, and other locally reactive chemical substances that are found in a particular region of the skin. These three substances are very active in the skin's role of thermoregulation by their vasodilation effects on the vascular smooth muscles contained in the arterial and capillary beds of the skin. In addition, histamine and prostaglandins play a role in the pain and inflammatory responses after injury to the skin. Rook et al.[10] described the areas of the eyelids and upper lip as regions of very high histamine content, with the chest and abdomen having substantially lower amounts of this chemical.

The percutaneous absorption ability of the skin in a particular region is an area being investigated.[10] There are many potential anatomic barriers that may influence the skin's capacity for absorption. The thickness of the stratum corneum, the size and distribution of hair follicles, the relative amount of microvasculature, and the structure and composition of the dermis all have a dramatic influence on how well a particular area is able to absorb a given type of substance.

There is considerable regional variation in a number of components of the skin. The burn therapist needs to be cognizant of these potential differences in regional variation as they work with patients who have suffered various types and depths of burn injuries.

SUMMARY

The skin is an active organ of the body that directly impacts the ability of other organ systems to function normally. There are significant regional variations in the amount, structure, and function of the epidermal and dermal layers. These differences permit the physiologic and functional capacities of the skin to exist. The skin is one of the most dynamic organ systems of the body in its ability to adapt to the environment. When the skin is subjected to a trauma, such as a burn injury, it has the ability to adapt to this stress as well. However, the nature, extent, depth, and condition of the burn greatly affect the healing of the skin. This chapter has provided information by which the burn therapist can compare the alterations and modifications of the healing burned tissue to the normal structure and function of the skin.

REFERENCES

1. Goldsmith, LA (ed): Biochemistry and Physiology of the Skin. Oxford University Press, New York, 1983, pp 3–63.
2. Patterson, JW and Blaylock, WK: Dermatology. Medical Examination Publishing, New York, 1987, pp 1–15.
3. Holbrook, KA and Odland, GF: Regional differences in the thickness (cell layers) of the human strateum corneum: An ultrastructural analysis. J Invest Dermatol 62:415–422, 1974.
4. Elias, PM: Epidermal lipid, membranes and keratinization. J Dermatol 20:1–19, 1981.
5. Raknerud, N: The ultrastructure of the interfollicular epidermis of the hairless (hr/hr) mouse. III. Desmosomal transformation during keratinization. J Ultrastruc Res 52:32–51, 1975.
6. Odland, GF and Reed, TH: Epidermis. In Zelickson AS (ed): Ultrastructure of Normal and Abnormal Skin. Lea & Febiger, Philadelphia, 1967, pp 54–75.
7. Moschella, SL, Pillsbury, DM, and Hurley, HJ (eds): Dermatology, Vol. 1. WB Saunders, Philadelphia, 1975, pp 1–77.
8. Halprin, KM: Epidermal "turnover time"—a re-examination. Br J Dermatol 86:14–19, 1972.
9. Bergstresser, PR and Taylor, JR: Epidermal "turnover time"—a new examination. Br J Dermatol 96:503–509, 1977.
10. Rook, A, et al (eds): Textbook of Dermatology. Blackwell Scientific Publications, Oxford, 1986, pp 5–38.
11. Riley, PA: The epidermis. In Jarrett, A (ed): The Physiology and Pathophysiology of the Skin, Vol. 3. Academic Press, London, 1974, pp 1101–1106.
12. Wolff, K and Schreiner, E: Uptake, intracellular transport and degradation of exogenous protein by Langerhans cell. An electron microscopic-cytochemical study using peroxidase as tracer substance. J Invest Dermatol 54:37–47, 1970.
13. Schweizer, J and Marks, F: A developmental study of the distribution and frequency of Langerhans cells in relation to formation of patterning in mouse tail epidermis. J Invest Dermatol 69:198–204, 1977.
14. Mackenzie, IC: The role of the keratinocyte and the Langerhans cells. Am J Anat 144:127–131, 1975.
15. Prunieras, M: Interaction between keratinocytes and dendritic cells. J Invest Dermatol 52:1–17, 1969.
16. Aberer, W, et al: Ultraviolet light depletes surface markers of Langerhans cells. J Invest Dermatol 76:202–210, 1981.
17. Okamoto, H and Horio, T: The effect of 8-methoxypsoralen and long-wave ultraviolet light on Langerhans cells. J Invest Dermatol 77:345–346, 1981.
18. Klingman, AM and Shelley, WB: An investigation of the biology of the human sebaceous gland. J Invest Dermatol 30:99–105, 1958.
19. Pandolf, KB, Sawka, MN, and Gonzalez, RR (eds): Human Performance Physiology and Environmental Medicine at Terrestrial Extremes. William C Brown, Dubuque, 1988.
20. Shapiro, Y, et al: Thermoregulation responses of patients with extensive healed burns. J Appl Physiol 53:1019–1022, 1982.
21. Weinstein, GD and Boucek, RJ: Collagen and elastin of human dermis. J Invest Dermatol 35:227–229, 1960.
22. Brown, IA: Scanning electron microscopy of human dermal fibrous tissue. J Anat 113:159–168, 1972.
23. Langer, K: On the anatomy and physiology of the skin. I. The cleavability of the cutis. Br J Plast Surg 31:3–8, 1978.
24. Gibson, T and Kenedi, RM: The structural components of the dermis and their mechanical characteristics. In Montagna W et al (eds): Advances in Anatomy, Embryology and Cell Biology. Appleton-Century-Crofts, New York, 1970, pp 19–38.
25. deVries, HA: Physiology of Exercise, ed 4. William C Brown, Dubuque, 1986, pp 135–136.
26. Horstmann, E: The lymph vessels of skin. Die Ernahrungsindustrie 68:379–383, 1966.
27. Weddell, G, et al: The morphology of peripheral nerve terminations in the skin. Q J Microscop Sci 95:483-501, 1954.
28. Sinclair D: Nerves and the skin: Normal anatomy of sensory nerves and receptors. In Jarrett, A (ed): The Physiology and Pathophysiology of the Skin, Vol. 2. Academic Press, New York, 1973, pp 348–402.
29. Cauna, N: Fine morphological characteristics and microtopography of the free nerve endings of human digital skin. Anat Rec 198:643–656, 1980.
30. Cauna, N and Mannan, G: The structure of human digital Pacinian corpuscles (corpuscula lamellosa) and its functional significance. J Anat 92:1–20, 1958.
31. Biemesderfer, D, et al: The pilo-Ruffini complex: A non-sinus hair and associated slowly-adapting mechanoreceptor in primate facial skin. Brain Res 142:197–222, 1978.
32. Hurley, HJ: The permeability of the skin. In Moschella, SL, Pillsbury, DM, and Hurley, HJ (eds): Dermatology, Vol. 1. WB Saunders, Philadelphia, 1975, pp 64–67.
33. Kligman, AM: Regional skin variations. In Mailbach, HI and Hidlick-Smith, H: Skin Bacteria and Their Role in Infection. McGraw-Hill, New York, 1965, pp 13–30.
34. Montagna, W and Parakkal, PF: The Structure and Function of the Skin, ed 3. Academic Press, New York, 1974, p 23.

CHAPTER 3

Pathologic Manifestations of Burn Injury

Carole Johnson, PT, PhD

Each year approximately 7500 people die and 310,000 are seriously injured in fires.[1] Burns are also the leading cause of accidental deaths in the home for children between the ages of 1 and 14. This statistic assumes greater significance when years of continuing rehabilitation are necessary for the survivors. Although the most obvious insult to the body from a burn injury is to the skin, a cascade of multiorgan responses also occurs.

The therapist providing optimal care should understand the systemic as well as local effects of burn injury. Cardiovascular, gastrointestinal, respiratory, and renal systems as well as responses of the immune system are altered and influence the patient's capability for rehabilitation. The purposes of this chapter are to provide detailed information about the acute burn wound, offer pertinent information about systems affected by the injury, and conclude with aspects of the healed burn wound.

THE INTEGUMENTARY SYSTEM

Mechanism of Injury

Although normal skin anatomy and physiology have been reviewed, a few salient features need to be emphasized for the pathophysiology to be understood clearly. The skin varies considerably over different parts of the body in overall thickness of both the epidermis and dermis, water and oil content, vascularity, and subcutaneous fat. Therefore, similar temperatures produce different depths of injury to different body parts. For example, the same temperature applied to the skin on the medial aspect of the forearm will create a deeper burn than to the considerably thicker skin of the back of the same person. In addition, the pediatric and the geriatric populations have fewer protective layers of epithelium, so the same intensity of heat applied to these patients will create deeper burns.

The skin, as an organ, dissipates heat maximally in areas with greatest vasculature. However, if absorption of heat exceeds the rate of dissipation, cellular temperature will rise and destruction will occur. This increase in temperature causes a series of reactions in the underlying vasculature of the skin. Clinically these reactions are observed by changes in the appearance of the burned skin, for example, in the common sunburn. Regardless of the location on the body, an extreme temperature rise produces immediate cellular death on the surface.

In addition to location and temperature, duration of the applied heat source is critical. The longer a hot or even warm material contacts the skin, the more severe the tissue destruction. A good example is the patient who arrives in the outpatient physical therapy department with a mottled and sensitive back due to a burn caused from lying on a heating pad. Individuals are surprised that such a low heat could create a burn, but they are unaware of the effects of duration of heat.

Diller[2] analyzed burns caused by long-term exposure to a heating pad. He stated that care should be taken when heat therapy is applied, even when a conventional heating pad is used. This warning is particularly germane when areas of the body in which the skin is thin are treated with heat or when heat is used with patients who have impaired cutaneous circulation.

Although heat transfer to the skin is complex, three components are critical: the location of the area injured; the temperature at the location; and the duration of exposure. These components result in varying depths of injury, from which classifications of injury have been devised.

Classification of Burns

The traditional classification of burn depth has been first, second, and third degree. This classification system generally has been replaced by the terms superficial, partial thickness, and full thickness (Table 3–1). The latter classification better describes clinical findings and implies potential healing time and subsequent scarring. However, a major difficulty with these classifications is that burn wound depth is seldom uniform. Although a contact wound may have the most heterogeneous-appearing surface, most burns typically look like an archery target (Fig. 3–1). The most severe burns are located centrally and less severe burns located peripherally. A classification of burns based on zones evolved from this concept.[3]

The zone of coagulation represents the bull's eye of the target and is the area of greatest destruction. Irreversible cellular death has occurred from thermal coagulation. The area appears white and leathery because all viable tissue has been destroyed.

The zone of coagulation merges with the zone of stasis, which is perhaps the most critical zone. The stasis zone is damaged and temporarily lacks a normal blood supply, but the zone is not avascular. With appropriate protection and treatment, vascular restoration can occur and damage minimized. If the wound is subject to drying, further trauma, or infection, normal circulation may not be re-established and the zone of coagulation may be extended. Thus, a potentially viable area is converted to an irreversibly necrotic area.

TABLE 3–1. Burn Wound Classification

Severity	Cause	Surface Appearance	Color	Sensation	Histologic Depth	Healing
			Superficial			
All are minor except if person is under 18 months or over 65 years or with severe loss of fluids.	Sunburn Ultraviolet exposure Short flash	Dry, no blisters Edema—amount variable	Erythematous	Painful	Epidermal layers only	3–7 days with peeling. No scarring. May have discoloration.
			Partial-Thickness			
Minor Adults < 15% Children < 10%	Superficial Scald Short exposure	Blistered Weeping Moist blebs	Superficial Red	Very painful Sensitive to temperature	Superficial Epidermis, some papillary dermis	Superficial 7–21 days, no grafting No/minimal scarring Pigment changes
Moderate Adults 15–30% Children 10–30% Minor chemical or electrical < 15% but involves face, hands, feet or perineum.	Deep Immersion scald Flame	Blisters are large, thick-walled, will usually increase in size.	Deep Mottled white (pale), pink to cherry red		Deep Epidermis, papillary and reticular layers of dermis, may include fat domes of subcutaneous layer	Deep 21–35 days if no infection, if infected, may convert to full-thickness
Severe > 30%		Normal to firm texture	Red, will blanch with pressure and refill.			May develop severe hypertrophic scarring
			Full-Thickness			
Minor < 2%	Chemical Electrical Flame Scald	Dry, leathery or nonpliable until debridement	Mixed white, waxy, pearly	Little or no pain Hair pulls out easily Anesthetic to temperature	Down to and includes subcutaneous tissue May include fascia, muscle, tendon, and bone	Large areas require grafting, or requires many months to heal. Small areas may heal from edges after weeks.
Moderate 2–10% any involvement of face, hands, feet, or perineum.	**Time** — **Temperature** 1 sec — 158F 2 sec — 150F 10 sec — 140F 30 sec — 130F 1 min — 127F 10 min — 120F	Charred, blood vessels visible under eschar. If red, will not blanch with pressure.	Dark khaki, mahogany			
Severe > 10%	Major chemical or electrical	Usually no blisters, but if present, thin-walled and will not increase in size.	Charred			

From Johnson, C: Update on burn wounds. Wounds: A Compendium of Clinical Research and Practice, 4:142, 1992, with permission.

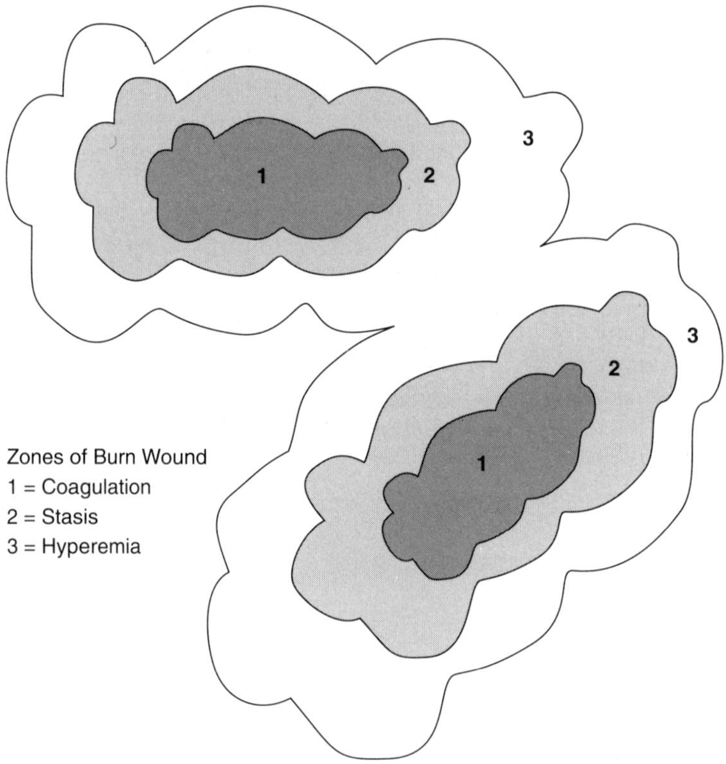

FIGURE 3–1. Most burns represent a mosaic of injured tissue. The deepest injury or burn is at the center in the zone of coagulation, while the more superficial burns are at the periphery in the zone of hyperemia. The intermediate zone of stasis may convert to a deeper burn with inappropriate treatment.

The zone of stasis initially is moist, red, blistered, and blanches on pressure, the typical description of a partial-thickness burn. Usually within minutes following the injury, "stasis" occurs as the flow of blood ceases to move through the capillaries as a result of multiple vascular changes (see Chapter 5). An abnormal aggregation of platelets and leukocytes develops in the underlying capillaries causing thrombosis. Vasoconstriction and platelet aggregation further decrease blood flow to this zone. Almost immediately post burn, cellular destruction begins in direct response to the heat and indirectly as a response to vascular occlusion.

This zone of stasis may be further divided into two areas, a superficial zone of early stasis and a deeper zone of delayed stasis. Injury is most severe in the superficial zone and the area becomes ischemic in 2 hours or less but not immediately. Injury is less severe in the more deeply situated zone of delayed stasis and becomes ischemic between 4 and 16 to 24 hours post burn. In contrast to the zone of early stasis, some hair follicle epithelial cells may remain viable in the deeper zone. If drying or other injury is avoided, these epithelial cells appear able to migrate and repopulate hair follicles in all levels.[3]

Burns have a third or outer zone, the zone of hyperemia. Since this area is furthest from injury, vascular integrity is maintained and blanches on pressure. No cell death occurs and the area appears pink. In other words, it is equivalent to a superficial burn.

Various clinical criteria are used in the assessment of burn depth. These include cause of the burn, wound appearance, sensation (pinprick test), blanching under pressure, and hair follicle integrity. Clinical observation continues as the standard for diagnosis. Very shallow burns that heal in less than 2 weeks and very deep full-thickness burns are relatively easy for even the inexperienced observer to determine. Unfortunately, many burns represent injury whose depth is intermediate between these obvious ones. Evaluation by an experienced surgeon as to whether an apparent deep dermal burn will heal in 3 weeks has an accuracy of about 50 percent.[5] As discussed in other chapters, burns that take longer than 3 weeks to heal often scar and lead to functional impairment.

Aggressive surgical intervention, including early excision and skin grafting of burns of intermediate depth has demonstrated shortened hospital stay and duration of illness and improved function and appearance, especially with burns of the face, hands, and feet. Because of this intervention, accurate and reliable methods for assessing the depth of burn injury have been pursued.

Four categories of methods include the detection of: (1) changes in blood flow (fluorescein, laser doppler, thermography); (2) dead cells or denatured collagen (biopsy, ultrasound, vital dyes); (3) color changes of the wound (light reflectance); (4) physical changes such as edema (nuclear magnetic resonance imaging).[5] In theory, all of these diagnostic techniques have merit.

For example, thermography studies[6,7] found that superficial burns were warmer than the adjacent unburned skin and deep dermal and full-thickness burns were colder than adjacent unburned skin. Laser doppler studies[8] found that superficial burns sometimes had a minimum blood flow in the first 24 to 48 hours post burn, then the blood-flow levels were elevated. Deeper wounds exhibited severely depressed cutaneous flow, although the pattern was not always clear.

Burn depth at the time of injury is difficult to determine and the initial static picture may change. Desiccation, mechanical injury, and infection can cause a deeper injury. If the appearance of the burn wound changes to a deeper classification, then a longer healing time is expected and greater scarring and functional impairment are anticipated. Frequent observations of the wound under the dressing are valuable for effective patient care. Thinking in terms of burn wound dynamics, rather than a classification system, assists therapists to understand the actual damage the burn injury has caused.

Infection

A function of the integumentary system is to protect the body against bacterial invasion. Because of the removal of this protection, infection remains the most common cause of morbidity and mortality.[9] Instead of an intact skin barrier, a covering of eschar lies on the surface of the burn wound. Eschar is a nonviable biologic material. The denatured protein is a rich pabulum for microbial growth and proliferation.[9] In addition, eschar is avascular because of thermal thrombosis. This avascular eschar denies delivery of cellular components from the host defense system. The microcirculation to the underlying wound also has been altered, limiting bloodborne antibiotics to the area.

Alexander[9] reported that burn wounds are never sterile, despite claims made to the contrary. Methods developed to detect wound colonization include quantitative swab and smear cultures,[10] quantitative biopsy,[11] and biopsy for histopathology.[12] According to Taddonio et al.[13] in a survey of wound monitoring, 92 percent of the responding burn facilities monitor burn wounds for microbes, and this monitoring typically was done at least twice weekly by either surface swab or quantitative biopsy.

Although initially the burn wound has only a few organisms, this usually progresses to heavy colonization during the first few days following injury. Colonization may progress to infection. Quantitative cultures of the wound surface or of a wound biopsy appear to be helpful in confirming the absence of wound infection, but are of little help in confirming the presence of infection.[14] Quantitative cultures of wound biopsy specimens that show bacterial counts less than 10^6 organisms per gram of tissue correlate well with absence of infection on histologic examination. Conversely, less than 50 percent of quantitative cultures, showing growth of 10^6 or more bacteria per gram of tissue, are associated with histologic evidence of infection.

Infection still is clinically detected by local signs at the burn wound. Focal dark discoloration of the burn, conversion of an area of partial-thickness injury to full-thickness necrosis, green discoloration of subcutaneous fat, the appearance of vesicular lesions in healing or recently healed partial-thickness burn, and unexpectedly rapid separation or sloughing of the eschar suggest infection. If the increase in microorganisms is limited primarily to the burn eschar, the infection is described as noninvasive. If the microorganisms invade the underlying viable tissue, the infection is described as invasive.

Pruitt and McManus[14] described criteria for staging the microbial status of burn wounds (Table 3–2). The stages represent the progression of bacterial spread. As the numerical stage increases, so does the mortality of the burn patient.

Bacteremia is the presence of viable bacteria in the circulating blood and septicemia is a systemic disease caused by the presence of microorganisms or their toxins in the circulating blood. Any sudden decline in the patient's general state must be suspected as being caused by septicemia. If a patient is responsive in the morning and appears disoriented and agitated in the afternoon, the therapist should suspect that a septic episode is occurring and should notify the appropriate medical staff.

Topical chemotherapy, prompt excision of eschar, and timely closure of the burn wound have significantly reduced the occurrence of invasive burn wound infection and its related mortality. However, the type of organisms present in the eschar strongly influence the incidence of infection. For example, enzymes and other meta-

TABLE 3–2. Criteria for Staging the Microbial Status of Burn Wounds

Stage I: Colonization	
A. Superficial	Sparse microbial population on burn wound surface
B. Penetration	Microorganisms present in variable thickness of eschar
C. Proliferation	Dense population of microorganisms at nonviable-viable tissue interface
Stage II: Invasion	
A. Microinvasion	Microscopic foci of microorganisms in viable tissue immediately subjacent to subeschar space
B. Generalized	Widespread penetration of microorganisms deep into viable subcutaneous tissues
C. Microvascular	Involvement of lymphatics and microvasculature

From Pruitt, B and McManus, A,[14] with permission.

bolic products produced by *Pseudomonas* species, as well as their flagellum-imparted motility, enhance the invasive potential of those organisms and the rapid spread of infection. Conversely, wound infections caused by staphylococci tend to remain superficial and localized. The invasive potential and characteristics of nonbacterial wound infections also are organism specific.

Age also affects the incidence of infection. In patients over 60 years of age the incidence increases dramatically. The overall medical and nutritional status of the patient influences the host response to injury. Hospital infection control programs have been effective in minimizing endemic organisms that possess broad antimicrobial resistance, thereby preventing the establishment of newly introduced resistant organisms.

The most common mode of spreading infection within burn units is through contact from hospital personnel. Hand washing remains the most effective means of minimizing cross-contamination. Because therapists move from patient to patient, they must practice optimum infection control by performing repeated hand washing. While treating a burn patient, the therapist may contact urinary and intravenous catheters, tracheostomies, and other invasive devices. These are potential entries and outlets for microorganisms and must be handled with care to promote proper infection control.

Therapists are aware of this important aspect of burn care and have addressed such issues as autocontamination in hydrotherapy[15] to cleaning methods for splints.[16] Some facilities limit the amount of equipment therapists can take into a patient's room or where patients can be treated until the burn wound is closed, because of the concern for infection. The burn wound should be totally re-epithelialized before concerns for infection can be reduced.

THE CARDIOVASCULAR SYSTEM

Pre-existing Cardiac Conditions

Cardiac disease can significantly alter the management, morbidity, and mortality of patients with burns.[17] Because heart disease is a major health problem and more than half of all reported deaths in the United States are due to cardiovascular disease, its occurrence in a burn unit population should be anticipated.

Goff et al.[17] reviewed 2477 consecutive acute burn admissions to determine the types and incidence of cardiac complications. One hundred-fifteen patients had a history of cardiac disorders. Forty-six percent of these patients with cardiac history manifested some form of cardiac dysfunction, most frequently arrhythmias during hospitalization. The mortality rate in the group with cardiac history was 30 percent, but death was not directly related to a cardiac event in all cases.

Only 6 percent of patients without prior history manifested cardiac dysfunction. The in-hospital mortality rate after myocardial infarction for both groups was 3½ to 4 times greater than for patients without burns. If prior cardiovascular disease is documented, the history is particularly significant to the therapist. The subsequent burn treatment will continue to stress an already impaired system and modification of treatment may be required.

Acute Burn Injury Effects

Hypermetabolism is one initial insult to the cardiovascular system. The hypermetabolic state is directly proportional to the size of the burn and may reach 2 to 2½ times the basal metabolic rate in patients with burns greater than 50 percent total body surface area.[17] Hypermetabolism is evidenced by increased oxygen consumption, cardiac output, minute ventilation, and core temperature.

This response coincides with and may be mediated by increased catecholamine production and release. Catecholamines are substances with chemical structures similar to epinephrine and norepinephrine and are monitored as a guide to adrenal activity or to a stress syndrome. The myocardium is one of the end organs affected by catecholamines and the increased catecholamine stimulation causes increased myocardial oxygen consumption. This increased consumption is a major factor in the pathogenesis of myocardial dysfunction.

The most immediate life-threatening response to burn injury is shock. The primary cause of shock in the burn patient is usually hypovolemia, or loss of circulating fluid. Shock is detected by a drop in blood pressure accompanied by an increased pulse rate and decreased urine output.[18] The extent and depth of the burn, age, and general physical condition influence the severity of shock. For example, a 70-year-old overweight individual with high blood pressure may exhibit shock with a burn covering 10 percent of body surface area, while a 20-year-old individual in good physical and mental health may not exhibit shock with 25 percent of body area burned.

Burn shock reflects an acute peripheral circulatory failure. The most significant component is the loss of large volumes of plasma and extracellular fluid. Following minor burns, the immediate vascular response is confined to the burn area, but with involvement of more than 30 percent of the body surface, increased capillary permeability becomes a systemic problem.

Hypovolemia results from shifts and losses of fluid from the circulation. These changes may result in sometimes dramatic edema and one of the therapist's first responsibilities may be positioning the patient to help reduce or resolve this edema.

Fluid Balance

NORMAL

Approximately 70 percent of the body's weight is water. Fifty percent of this water is distributed within the cells as intracellular fluid (Fig. 3–2). Fifteen percent of the fluid bathes the cells as interstitial fluid. Plasma or intravascular fluid accounts for 5 percent. Normally fluid passes between the capillaries, the interstitial spaces, and the cells through a process of diffusion and filtration. The net exchange of fluids between intracellular and extracellular compartments is usually small.

What mechanisms maintain this normal fluid balance? Figure 3–3 focuses on some of the forces involved in these mechanisms. Hydrostatic pressure is the pressure exerted by a fluid. For example, water in a garden hose exerts a certain amount of pressure against the walls of the hose. Conversely, osmosis is the tendency for water to move from a region of low particulate concentration to a region of high concentration. The hydrostatic difference between the capillary blood pressure and interstitial fluid pressure favors the filtration of protein-free plasma out of the capillary. The

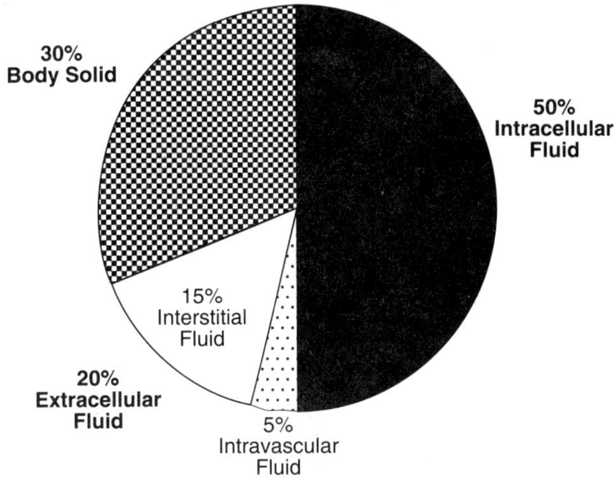

FIGURE 3–2. Fluid compartments of the body. Approximately 70 percent of body weight is water. The cells contain 50 percent of the water distributed in the body. The fluid around the cells represents another 15 percent. The fluid in the vasculature amounts to 5 percent.

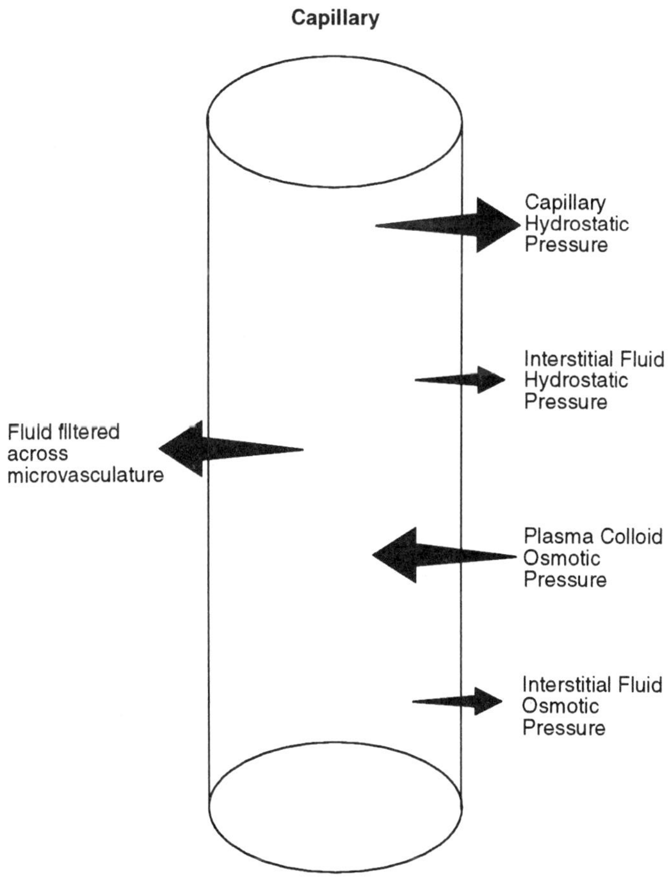

FIGURE 3–3. Forces are exerted on the capillary wall that determine the filtration of fluids from the microvasculature. Edema occurs when an imbalance of these forces favors movement of fluid to the extravascular space.

protein concentration difference between the plasma and interstitial fluid favors the osmotic movement of interstitial fluid into the capillary.[19] These two opposing forces act to move fluid across the capillary wall. For these forces to work normally, the structure of the microvessel wall must be intact.

ABNORMAL

Direct thermal injury results in an immediate decrease in blood flow to the involved tissues to slow blood loss in the affected areas. Initial vasoconstriction is mediated by norepinephrine and usually lasts from a few seconds to a few minutes. The constriction is prolonged by the release of serotonin. Serotonin is contained in the granules of mast cells in connective tissue and in platelets released into the interstitial fluid when injury and bleeding occur (Fig. 3–4).

The vasoconstriction is followed by pronounced arteriolar vasodilation in the microcirculation that remains patent. Histamine is released into the area from mast cells, basophils, and platelets. These substances act to increase capillary permeability and permit whole plasma to be released into the burn wound. Electron micrographs have demonstrated the formation of gaps between normal endothelial cells as well as destruction of endothelial cells. Consequently, the vessels become "leaky" and an immediate imbalance occurs in the forces maintaining capillary flow.

The intravascular fluid is the first to be depleted in burns. The next fluid lost is interstitial, and the most stable fluid is intracellular.[18] The intravascular loss or plasma volume reduction is accompanied by an increased hematocrit, blood cell agglutina-

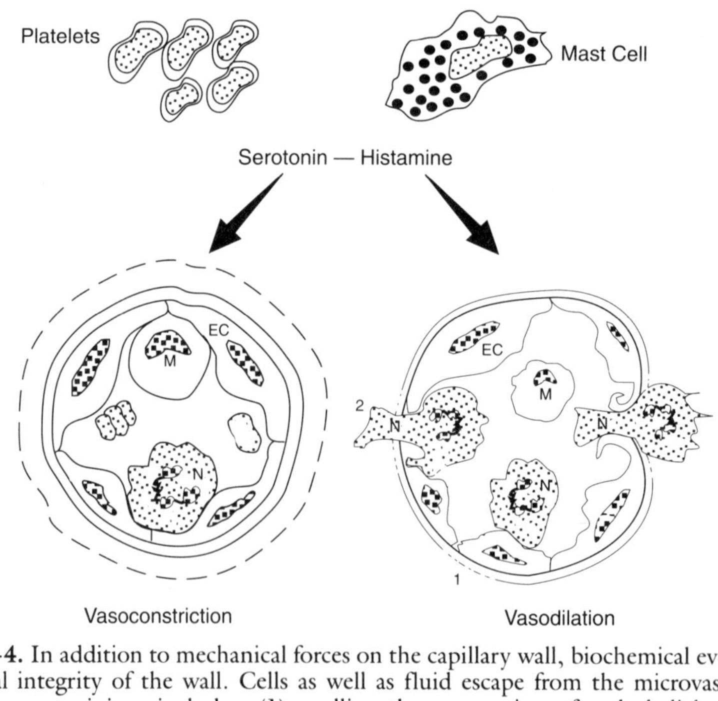

FIGURE 3–4. In addition to mechanical forces on the capillary wall, biochemical events influence the structural integrity of the wall. Cells as well as fluid escape from the microvasculature. The vascular response to injury includes: (1) swelling then separation of endothelial cells (EC), (2) blood cells (RBC) leave blood vessel by "diapedesis," and (3) migration of leukocytes (M = monocyte; N = neutrophil) to the wounded area.

tion, and sludging or stasis of the microcirculation. Hematocrit is the volume percentage of red blood cells to whole blood and normal ranges are 40 to 45 percent in men and 35 to 45 percent in women. The hematocrit rises immediately after a severe burn and then decreases to preburn levels with adequate fluid replacement. Without fluid substitution, burn injuries can result in hypovolemic shock.

The protein composition of edema fluid in a full-thickness burn is exactly the same as plasma.[4] Edema fluid is initially a clear, serous fluid. With increased migration of leukocytes and lower-molecular-weight plasma proteins like albumin, the interstitial fluid becomes a cellular aggregate. Edema develops when the rate that fluid is filtered from the microvessels exceeds the rate lymphatic vessels drain the same tissue mass.[20] Fluid resuscitation may markedly aggravate edema formation.

The formation of edema is one of the first burn sequelae the therapist treats. Appropriate positioning and/or splinting of the involved area can facilitate the resolution of edema. Elevation of hands and feet may minimize edema fluid, but the patient must be monitored carefully and consistently for decreased blood flow. External pressure from positioning devices and internal pressure from excessive interstitial fluid may develop and cause occlusion of small vessels.

Acute edema in the first few days after burn injury creates a stiffness in the joints, while chronic edema can lead to further limitation of joint range of motion.[21] The presence of edema also compromises circulation. If thick inelastic eschar is circumferential, an escharotomy is performed to allow for expansion of the compressed tissues.

Guidelines for activities for edematous areas are basically empirical. Most therapists try to promote active exercise two to three times each day to maintain joint mobility. Other therapists think gentle passive motion is beneficial. Escharotomies usually are not a deterrent to exercise.

Cardiovascular Rehabilitation

Significant cardiovascular complications may result from prolonged bed rest and deconditioning.[22] Saltin et al.[23] observed five normal subjects confined to bed for 20 consecutive days and calculated approximately a 1 percent decrease in physiologic function each day. The maximum oxygen consumption decreased a total of 25 percent accompanied by similar decrements in maximal stroke volume and cardiac output.

The most commonly accepted method of assessing functional capacity of the cardiovascular system is the use of MET values for any level or intensity of activity. MET is a metabolic equivalent system that was derived from the resting oxygen consumption for a 70-kg, 40-year-old man. One MET is equivalent to 3.5 ml of oxygen consumption per kilogram of body weight per minute of activity. Physical activity is assessed as a multiple of the MET value. A MET is also an estimate of basal metabolic rate. The American College of Sports Medicine has published MET equivalents for a variety of recreational and occupational activities.[24]

If burn patients have a cardiovascular functional capacity that is greater than 8 METs, formal cardiovascular rehabilitation may not be necessary unless the demands of their job or leisure activities require a higher MET capacity. However, patients who are unable to achieve 8 METs should be placed in a formal rehabilitation program to improve their functional capacity. This type of rehabilitation program involves the progressive stressing of the cardiovascular system using aerobic conditioning principles to create a "training effect" of the central cardiac function and peripheral delivery and utilization of oxygen.

A variety of other physiologic changes have been described as the result of inactivity. Loss of vasomotor reflexes and increased blood viscosity as a result of decreased plasma volume and venous return to the heart cause patients to experience orthostatic hypotension and excessive tachycardia with minimal exertion.

Prolonged inactivity also may cause altered psychologic responses that can limit the patient's recovery.[25] Anxiety, depression, and denial are associated with dependency and loss of control of the environment. These responses can lead to prolonged anguish and psychologic disability, in addition to physical cardiovascular disability.

Therapists must have an understanding of the potential effects a burn injury can have on the cardiovascular system. In addition to the immediate effects of burn shock and edema, knowledge about pre-existing cardiac conditions should be obtained. The patient's rehabilitation and return to previous life-style will be strongly influenced by the cardiovascular resources that have been preserved following burn trauma.

THE RESPIRATORY SYSTEM

The respiratory system can be affected by an inhalation injury or infection. The lungs in patients with both an inhalation injury and a burn are in double jeopardy,[26] and this combined injury may accelerate multiple organ failure.

Smoke inhalation is defined as airway or pulmonary parenchymal injury resulting from the inhalation of toxic combustion products. The incidence of smoke inhalation in all hospitalized burn patients varies from 5 to 35 percent. Without thermal injury, the mortality rate is less than 10 percent. With a thermal injury, the mortality rate is reported from 25 to 65 percent.[26]

Smoke inhalation may present as three separate injuries: carbon monoxide intoxication, upper airway obstruction, or a chemical pneumonitis.[27] Carbon monoxide has a half-life of 4 hours on room air and is diagnosed by measuring carboxyhemoglobin. In carbon monoxide intoxication, carbon monoxide combines with myoglobin in the muscles and the cytochrome oxidase system in the brain.

A variety of conditions may indicate upper airway obstruction: fire in a closed space, burns of the face and neck, singed nasal hair, blisters and redness of the posterior pharynx, and such physical signs as increased rate of breathing, shallow respiration, increasing hoarseness, and increased amounts of sputum. Patients who have a large quantity of carbonaceous sputum on the second or third day may lack adequate oxygenation and show late development of adult respiratory distress syndrome (ARDS). A chemical injury to the lung is difficult to diagnose, but the patient also may present with ARDS.

Pneumonia is now the predominant type of infection in burn patients.[14] The organisms that cause infections at any given burn center change with time. In 1982, *Pseudomonas aeruginosa* was the organism most often present in cultures of airway secretion. In contrast, in 1989, *Staphylococcus aureus* was the cause of 48 percent and *P. aeruginosa* the cause of only 16 percent of the pneumonias.

Good pulmonary toilet is essential in all patients with respiratory problems. Adequate oxygenation will be impaired with accumulation of mucus and debris in the lung. For the nonintubated patient, oxygenation can be improved with coughing, deep breathing, and incentive spirometry. For the intubated patient, oxygenation may be improved with adequate suctioning. For both groups of patients, oxygenation will improve with frequent changes in position and out-of-bed activity.

In a review of the literature, there is a glaring absence of studies on burn patients in terms of their cardiorespiratory response to exercise. However, one of the most recent was a case study of a patient during the use of continuous passive motion (CPM).[28] Heart and respiratory rates and blood pressure were recorded from post-burn day 0 to 6 before the initiation of CPM on day 7. For a 54-year-old woman with a 39 percent total body surface burn (23.5 percent full-thickness) before CPM, the average heart rate was 118.4 beats per minute, average respiratory rate was 22.1 respirations per minute, systolic blood pressure was 119.5 mm Hg and diastolic blood pressure was 62.1 mm Hg. No statistical difference was observed in any of the study parameters after the initiation of CPM.

THE GASTROINTESTINAL SYSTEM

A major advance in the care of burn patients occurred with the recognition that stresses on the gastrointestinal tract, hypermetabolism, and subsequent weight loss needed to be treated. Burn patients often complain of having insufficient energy for activities or exercise and this may reflect their elevated metabolic state. The therapist with limited knowledge in this area may make overwhelming demands of the compromised patient.

Hypermetabolism

Over 50 years ago Cuthbertson[29] described the metabolic responses of patients following injury. Increased urinary losses of nitrogen, potassium, phosphorus, and other intracellular constituents indicate an accelerated catabolism or breakdown of compounds in the body. The breakdown of muscle components, particularly protein used to generate energy, leads to muscle atrophy and a consequent loss of body weight. The nitrogen metabolized from amino acids is excreted as urea, and the body is described as being in a negative nitrogen balance. Normal nitrogen loss through the urine in the adult male usually is minimal. In a severely burned or infected patient, nitrogen loss may increase to 30–40 g/day.[30] Approximately 90 percent of the nitrogen loss occurs through the urine and about 10 percent is lost in wound exudate.[18]

Other metabolic changes include an increased rate of glucose production and utilization and a decreased rate of lipid metabolism. These alterations can effect other physiologic parameters, including the immune system. Large quantities of calories and protein are necessary to achieve positive nitrogen balance. The larger the total body surface affected by the burn, the greater the body's caloric and protein requirements. These requirements may exceed a normal adult's by two to three times in patients with burns involving 50 percent of the total body surface area. If the burn size exceeds approximately 50 to 60 percent, there appears to be minimal further increases.[31]

In addition to the size of the burn, the estimate of energy and protein requirements will vary according to the patient's preinjury nutritional status, age, sex, weight, and height. Also, the patient's response to the injury varies with the previous state of nutrition. For example, a recent study showed that a group of obese patients required significantly more days on mechanical ventilatory support systems and their incidence of clinical sepsis was greater.[32] Therefore, nutritional support plays a vital role in the survival and well-being of burn patients from multiple aspects.

Nutritional Support

Methods of delivering nutritional support in order of normal preference are: (1) hospital diet, (2) oral supplements, (3) tube feeding formulas, (4) peripheral intravenous supplements, and (5) total parenteral nutrition (TPN) through a central venous catheter.[33]

Many nutritional formulas have been derived from studies of burn patient populations surviving their injury. These formulas serve as guidelines for the amount of calories the patient needs each day. However, patients with burn injuries between 20 and 30 percent of total body surface area may be able to meet nutritional goals through oral nourishment.[33]

As in other forms of trauma, gastric dilation and paralytic ileus occur in response to burn shock, pain, or fear. In the past, patients were given nothing by mouth for the first 72 hours, or until bowel sounds were heard by stethoscope. When the bowel became active, clinicians thought that the patient could safely be given liquids and progress to a full diet as tolerated. More recent studies have indicated that the ileus is confined to the stomach and colon and that the small intestine continues to function normally.[31] As such, immediate postburn enteral nutrition is possible through the use of a feeding tube inserted through the nose, past the stomach, and into the small bowel. Diarrhea has been a common complication with enteral tube feedings. However, this incidence is decreased in patients who receive tube feedings within 48 hours of burn injury and when the tube feedings are continuous rather than intermittent.

The use of TPN has been shown to result in atrophy of the intestinal mucosa and elevation of serum insulin, hence decreasing fat mobilization. Elevation of insulin also causes the body to utilize more protein for energy and thereby increases protein catabolism. Because of the complications with the use of TPN, initiating enteral feedings as early as possible in the postburn period are becoming more the rule than the exception.

Vigorous physical therapy promotes preservation of muscle bulk and function. Supervised activity must be provided daily to all patients subjected to prolonged immobilization or inactivity. The use of skeletal traction and air-fluidized beds encourages immobility and loss of lean body mass. Active isometric exercises should be performed by these patients.

THE RENAL SYSTEM

The measurement and evaluation of components of urinary output from the burn patient is important to assess the adequacy of fluid therapy. An understanding of some common terms is helpful (Table 3–3). Renal output can be affected by: (1) initially rapid changes in blood volume from the shift of plasmalike exudate into the

TABLE 3–3. Terms Used in Assessing Renal Function

Abnormal contents of urine	
Hematuria	Presence of blood in the urine may be caused from blood in kidneys
Hemoglobinuria	Presence of free hemoglobin in the urine usually the result of damage outside the renal system
Myoglobinuria	Presence of myoglobin in the urine occurs with extensive muscle damage
Amount (average amount excreted by a healthy adult in 24 hours varies from 1000–1500 ml, although much greater variations can occur for short periods of time)	
Anuria	No urine output
Oliguria	Decreased amount of urine output in relation to fluid intake
Polyuria	Increased amount of urine output in relation to fluid intake

burned area, (2) massive fluid therapy to correct hypovolemia, (3) hemoglobinuria from red blood cell destruction, (4) cardiovascular changes, and (5) hormonal changes. Damage to the renal tubules can occur due to free hemoglobin from extensive red blood cell damage, which could ultimately lead to necrosis.

RESPONSES OF THE IMMUNE SYSTEM

A major focus of research is directed toward understanding how the body protects itself from infection. The subject is complicated and seems to revolve around a myriad of cascades. However, the immunologic competence of the burn patient is severely depressed for many reasons and understanding some basic concepts can give the therapist an appreciation of the efforts required to bolster a patient's immune capabilities.

Leukocytes are white blood cells that use blood vessels as a means of being transported to the extravascular space in response to tissue injury and inflammation. The two classes of leukocytes are polymorphonuclear leukocytes (granulocytes) and mononuclear cells. Granulocytes include neutrophils, eosinophils, and basophils. A general abbreviation for polymorphonuclear cells is PMNs. Mononuclear cells include monocytes and lymphocytes.

In the initial inflammatory phase, the neutrophil is one of the most predominant cells present in the interstitial fluid. Their function is phagocytosis of debris. Phagocytosis is a process of engulfing or ingesting microorganisms, cells, or foreign particles. When neutrophils are lysed, or broken down, proteolytic and collagenolytic enzymes are released that begin an early autolytic debridement process of solubilizing necrotic protein and collagen.

Monocytes leave or emigrate from the capillary into the tissue spaces and are then called macrophages. This cell is considered the most important regulatory cell in the inflammatory reaction for tissue healing. Macrophages also are phagocytic, but they tolerate severe hypoxia very well. This may explain why they are present in chronic inflammation. In addition, macrophages release factors or chemicals that attract fibroblasts to the area, and they influence collagen deposition substantially.

Lymphocytes have subsets of cells called T-lymphocytes and B-lymphocytes. Both T-cells and B-cells are derived from a common bone marrow stem cell. Cells that mature under the influence of the thymus differentiate into mature T-lymphocytes while B-lymphocytes avoid thymus influence. Lymphocytes are the only cells capable of recognizing an antigen as foreign and of initiating specific mechanisms to dispose of the invader.

An antigen is any of a variety of material (microorganisms, toxoids, foreign proteins) that, as a result of contact with appropriate tissues of the body, stimulate an immune response. After a latent period, this response can be manifested by the appearance of circulating antibodies that react with the antigen; some degree of immunity to infectious disease if the antigen was a microorganism or its products; or an increased reaction, as in hypersensitivity.

The altered immune response following thermal injury is a complex interaction involving the components of the immune system as well as interaction of the metabolic alterations and the burn wound environment.[34] Immunosuppression following burn injury probably contributes to invasion of microorganisms into the burn wound and the spread of infection to distal sites.

Depending on the background and interest of the therapist, understanding the mechanisms of immune responses may seem irrelevant. However, an appreciation for the complexity of the problem is important. A significant focus of research is to determine how these immune responses affect the burn patient and how the medical profession can amplify the responses to better protect the patient from infection.

THE HEALED BURN WOUND

Several aspects of the healed burn wound need to be addressed as a pathologic result of the injury. Although patients may be relieved to have the burn wound ultimately healed, the tissue coverage will not duplicate their original skin and they should be educated about the changes.

Sensory Changes

Clinicians know that burn patients suffer decreased sensation after their injuries. Ward et al.[35] studied the loss of cutaneous sensation after skin grafting in 60 burn patients who had applied for impairment assessment. Ninety-seven percent demonstrated markedly diminished or absent responses to sharp/dull, hot/cold, and light touch stimuli over skin grafted areas. All but one patient had intact perception over donor sites and healed (ungrafted) partial-thickness burns. Deep touch sensation was intact over both grafted and ungrafted areas in all patients. Depth of burn injury appears to be the best predictor of altered sensation.

The decrease in sensation that was observed rarely contributed significantly to the long-term impairment rating of the patients. For this study group, mean impairment was 14 percent (range 0 to 78 percent). Objective and subjective evaluation of abnormal sensibility contributed, at most, 5 percent impairment.

One of the most frequent complaints of patients with sensory abnormalities was increased sensitivity to ambient temperatures. This was also the most frequent problem when patients with outside jobs returned to work. Fifty percent of the patients had this complaint, and of these, 66.6 percent reported more sensitivity to cold, as opposed to a warm environment.

Other patient complaints included chronic itching, pain, feeling of tightness in the skin, numbness, tingling, and a burning sensation (not pain). These complaints were related to injuries to nociceptors. A nociceptor is a peripheral nerve receptor that is stimulated by injury, itching (pruritus), or pain.

These changes are important for the therapist to anticipate, because scar management programs could be delayed if the patient's skin is hypersensitive. Traditional desensitization programs should be instituted early, so that when the appropriate time for wearing a pressure garment occurs, the patient is prepared both physically and psychologically. For some patients, the application of pressure promotes desensitization, although the mechanism is not well understood.

Skin Changes

Skin changes can be categorized in terms of integrity, pigmentation, and lubrication. Healed burned skin may be very fragile and tolerate only a minimum amount of friction or irritation. In some cases, the motion at a joint can create enough skin friction to cause blisters. Normally the rete pegs are anchoring devices to maintain the cohesiveness of the epidermis and dermis, but the interface between the two tissues frequently appears very flat in newly healed skin. Unfortunately, no predictive marker exists to determine which patients will blister. Minimizing skin irritation, including avoidance of improperly fitted clothes or prolonged soaking of the healed area in water, is an important measure for maintaining the integrity of newly healed skin.

Some patients heal with either hyperpigmentation or hypopigmentation. Discoloration of the healed area may be emotionally traumatic depending on the location. Not only does the intensity of the color change from day to day, but the overall color of skin changes gradually over several months. The lasting changes relate to the amount of melanin in the surviving skin, which is directly related to the depth of injury.

Since pigmentation is a significant safety factor in protection from the sun, the patient needs to be advised about exposure to the sun. The use of sunscreens can be helpful, but they need to be carefully tested on small areas of skin to avoid an allergic reaction. The newly healed skin is highly susceptible to additional injury from prolonged exposure to the sun.

Vascularity also influences skin coloring. Placing an extremity in a dependent position increases the redness in the scars. Wearing pressure garments may minimize these changes for dependent extremities as well as other body areas.

Skin lubrication usually needs to be augmented, since destruction of sebaceous glands severely impairs the normal mechanism of lubrication. Without adequate moisturizing, cracking and further skin breakdown can frustrate the patient, especially if the patient has recurrent blisters. Gentle massaging when applying a cream may help promote a more pliable tissue surface. However, massaging too long or too hard may create macerated areas. The patient should be reminded that on fragile tissue "more is not necessarily better" regarding the application of cream or massage.

Scar Contracture

From the context of burn wound pathophysiology, two aspects of scarring are significant. One is scarring's effect on range of motion (ROM), and the other is its effect on appearance.

For the burn patient, the phase of wound healing may be a time of intense pain that strongly inhibits movement. The patient tends to assume a comfortable position. This position may predispose the new collagen fibers in the wound to fuse together in a shortened length becoming a solid mass of collagen. The combination of immobilization and fusing collagen across joint creases may limit range of motion and result in contracture formation.

As described previously, the pattern of a burn is usually a mosaic, so not all joints may be equally restricted. An individual joint may have full ROM. Adjacent joints also may exhibit full isolated ROM. However, when the patient attempts to move both joints simultaneously, the tight scar tissue may restrict full range. For example, full elbow extension may be obtained as long as the patient is not asked to abduct the shoulder or flex the wrist.

If the burn wound is treated appropriately, the wound ultimately will achieve a covering. However, the tissue covering the wound may not necessarily be normal, even if scarring appears minimal. The therapist needs to remember that the patient may feel a tightness with a newly healed burn. For professionals to think of their own "skinned knee" or "scab across the knuckle," might provide some empathy for the patient's concern or frustration in achieving or maintaining full ROM.

Scar contractures can continue to form throughout the scar remodeling phase, regardless of the patient's activity level. Patient persistence with stretching and exercise is necessary to combat this relentless process until maturation is achieved.

In most western cultures, emphasis is placed on a person's beauty, including a smooth-textured skin with a blemish-free appearance. For persons who have been burned, the remnants of the injury continues in the form of a scarred appearance.

Burn scars can present as hypertrophic or keloid, flat but with an altered texture, or with an irregular contour if the burn was covered with a mesh skin graft. In addition to altered surface texture, the hue of the skin can be marred by hyperpigmentation or hypopigmentation. With either surface appearance or skin tone changes, these alterations remain with the patient. Even with exceptional results from plastic surgery, burn scars never disappear completely.

SUMMARY

The purpose of this chapter is to provide therapists with the information to increase their knowledge and understanding regarding the pathophysiology of the burn injury. The integumentary system sustains the most obvious insult. Information is provided regarding the mechanism of injury, how the burn injury is classified, and the role infection plays in the healing process.

Burn shock, edema, and additional stress on pre-existing cardiac conditions strongly influence the cardiovascular system. The respiratory system can be affected by inhalation injuries or by infection. Hypermetabolism in response to injury and the necessary nutritional support taxes the gastrointestinal system while assessment of the functioning of the renal system indicates the success of resuscitation. The role of the immune system continues to be defined, but seems to extend to most aspects of burn care.

Beginning with the insult to the skin and ending with the maturation process of the healed burn wound, the rehabilitation process challenges the therapist to maximize cosmetic and functional outcome of these very complex patients.

REFERENCES

1. Silverstein, P and Lack, B: Epidemiology and prevention. In Boswick, J (ed): The Art and Science of Burn Care. Aspen, Rockville, 1987, p 12.
2. Diller, K: Analysis of burns caused by long-term exposure to a heating pad. J Burn Care Rehabil 12:214–217, 1991.
3. Zawacki, B: The local effects of burn injury. In Boswick, J (ed): The Art and Science of Burn Care. Aspen, Rockville, 1987, pp 25–32.
4. Dimick, A: Pathophysiology. In Fisher, S and Helm, P (eds): Comprehensive Rehabilitation of Burns. Williams & Wilkins, Baltimore, 1984, p 16.
5. Heimbach, D et al: Burn depth: A review. World J Surg 16:10–15, 1992.
6. Cole, R, Jones, S, and Shakespeare, G: Thermographic assessment of hand burns. Burns 16:60–63, 1990.
7. Cole, R, et al: Thermographic assessment of burns using a nonpermeable membrane as wound covering. Burns 17:117–122, 1991.
8. Green, M, Holloway, G, and Heimbach, D: Laser doppler monitoring of microcirculatory changes in acute burn wounds. J Burn Care Rehabil 9:57–62, 1988.
9. Alexander, J: The role of infection in the burn patient. In Boswick, J (ed): The Art and Science of Burn Care. Aspen, Rockville, 1987, p 104.
10. Levine, M, Lindberg, R, and Mason, A: The quantitative swab culture and smear: A quick simple method for determining the number of viable aerobic bacteria on open wounds. J Trauma 16:89–94, 1976.
11. Baxter, C, Curreri, P, and Marvin, J: The control of burn wound sepsis by the use of quantitative bacteriologic studies and subeschar clysis with antibiotics. Surg Clin North Am 53:1509, 1973.
12. Kim, S, et al: Frozen section technique to evaluate early burn wound biopsy: A comparison with the rapid section technique. J Trauma 25:1134–1137, 1985.
13. Taddonio, T, et al: A survey of wound monitoring and topical antimicrobial therapy practices in the treatment of burn injury. J Burn Care Rehabil 11:423–427, 1990.
14. Pruitt, B and McManus, A: The changing epidemiology of infection in burn patients. World J Surg 16:57–67, 1992.
15. Richard, R, et al: Autocontamination of the burn patient by hydrotherapy. Bull Clin Rev Burn Inj 1:40, 1984.
16. Wright, M, et al: The microbiology and cleaning of thermoplastic splints in burn care. J Burn Care Rehabil 10:79–83, 1989.
17. Goff, D, et al: Cardiac disease and the patient with burns. J Burn Care Rehabil 11:305–307, 1990.
18. Feller, I and Jones, C: Nursing the burned patient. Braun-Brumfield, Ann Arbor, 1974, pp 50–54.
19. Vander, A, Sherman, J, and Luciano, D: Human Physiology, The Mechanisms of Body Function. McGraw-Hill, New York, pp 293–295.
20. Lund, T, Onarheim, H, and Reed, R: Pathogenesis of edema formation in burn injuries. World J Surg 16:2–9, 1992.
21. Pullium, G: Splinting and positioning. In Fisher, S and Helm, P (eds): Comprehensive Rehabilitation of Burns. Williams & Wilkins, Baltimore, 1984, p 65.
22. Adams, R, et al: Cardiovascular rehabilitation of patients with burns. J Burn Care Rehabil 11:246–255, 1990.
23. Saltin, B, et al: Response to exercise after bedrest and after training: A longitudinal study of adaptive changes in oxygen transport and body composition. Circulation (Suppl) 7:1–78, 1968.
24. American College of Sports Medicine: Guidelines for Exercise, Testing and Prescription. Lea & Febiger, Philadelphia, 1991.
25. Razin, A: Psychosocial intervention in coronary artery disease: A review. Psychosom Med 44:363–387, 1982.
26. Clark, W: Smoke inhalation: Diagnosis and treatment. World J Surg 16:24–29, 1992.
27. Moore, S and Marvin, J: Monitoring the burn patient. In Boswick, J (ed): The Art and Science of Burn Care. Aspen, Rockville, 1987, pp 221–230.
28. Richard, R, Miller, S, and Staley, M: The physiological response of a patient with critical burns to continuous passive motion. J Burn Care Rehabil 11:554–556, 1990.
29. Cuthertson, D: The disturbance of metabolism produced by bone and non-bony injury, with notes on certain abnormal conditions of bone. Biochem J 24:1244–1263, 1930.
30. Baxter, C: Metabolism and nutrition in burn patients. Compr Ther 13:36–42, 1987.
31. Waymack, J and Herndon, D: Nutritional support of the burned patient. World J Surg 16:80–86, 1992.

32. Baumer, T, et al: Significance of obesity of nutritional, immunological, hormonal and clinical outcome parameters in burns. Proc American Burn Association 1991, 23:189.
33. Wachtel, T: Nutritional support of the burn patient. In Boswick, J (ed): The Art and Science of Burn Care. Aspen, Rockville, 1987, pp 203–220.
34. Warden, G: Immunologic response to burn injury. In Boswick, J (ed): The Art and Science of Burn Care. Aspen, Rockville, 1987, p 113.
35. Ward, R, et al: Sensory loss over grafted areas in patients with burns. J Burn Care Rehabil 10:536–538, 1989.

CHAPTER 4

Biophysical Aspects of Normal Skin and Burn Scar

Reginald L. Richard, MS, PT
Marlys J. Staley, MS, PT

The integument, or skin covering the human body, is an organ system that frequently is taken for granted. One of the many vital functions of skin is to allow unrestricted movement of the body. The ability to perform functional and meaningful tasks with the limbs and trunk is attributed in part to the pliable quality of the skin. When the normally pliable skin is replaced by scar tissue following a burn injury, functional impairments can occur in the form of scar tissue contractures.

The therapist should have a basic understanding of how normal skin functions from a biophysical perspective to assist the burn patient in averting the formation of scar contractures. These same principles then can be applied to the pathologic burn scar when planning and implementing a burn patient treatment program. For the burn therapist, knowledge of tissue biomechanics should serve as the basis for evaluation, the development of treatment techniques, and for monitoring treatment programs.[1]

This chapter will focus on the complex biomechanic interaction that occurs within the skin and subsequent burn scar tissue. However, the intent of this chapter is to be a primer for therapists interested in this topic or seeking to understand the basic workings of skin and scar rather than to answer the many questions surrounding this highly technical and variable subject.

EARLY INVESTIGATIONS OF SOFT TISSUE BIOMECHANICS

The application of mechanical engineering principles to medicine and surgery is not new.[2] The mechanical properties of tissue have attracted the attention of researchers for more than a century.[2,3] However, only in the 1960s did major improvements in mechanical testing of tissue begin.[4] This fact makes biomechanics, the application of mechanical engineering principles to living tissue, a relatively new topic of study.[5]

Over the time in which engineering principles have been applied to biologic tissue, scientists accumulated much information and insight into the mechanics of various tissues. However, in 1981, Kennedi and Gibson[6] stated that "retrospective evaluation highlights the shortcomings of present-day efforts in analyses" of biologic materials by mechanical means. They further stated, "it now seems clear that present attempts to describe the biomechanical behavior of such living entities in terms of mathematical concepts and techniques used for nonbiological materials have failed."

The reason why early experiments performed on skin and other soft tissues "failed" is because studies fell short of accounting for the many variables that since have been recognized as necessitating attention. Factors such as subjects' age and gender, the physical environment in which the investigation was performed (e.g., the effect that humidity has on tissue specimens), and other factors were recognized only later as having an impact on testing results. Also, much tissue experimentation was performed on animals, which is of questionable applicability to humans.

What this observation means for therapists is that many treatment questions still need answers. Despite the depth of present-day knowledge, a greater understanding of tissue biomechanics is needed before definitive applications of this information can be made. Nonetheless, in defense of the earlier investigators' attempts to understand the biomechanical nature of tissues, they chose to undertake experimentation on one of the body's most highly complex tissues, namely the skin.

Evans, as cited by Kennedi,[7] has classified body tissues into a hierarchy of categories according to the complexity of their structure and behavior: tissues with a relatively simple structure and one dominant component such as tendon; tissues with a relatively complex microarchitecture whose mechanical response is dominated by only one component, as in the case of fascia; and tissues with both a complex structure and an interactive component behavior such as skin.

SKIN AND SCAR MORPHOLOGY

Skin is a difficult tissue to evaluate and understand due to its complex structure. Categorically, the skin consists of two main layers: the thin, partially keratinized cellular epithelial top layer, and the thicker, deeper layer of the dermis[8] (see Chapter 2). The dermis is a multicomponent structure, the basic elements of which are five intertwined networks consisting of collagen fibers, elastic fibers, nerve fibers, small blood vessels, and lymphatics.[1] Additionally, hair shafts and the ducts of sweat and sebaceous glands also reside in the dermis. Surrounding all of these constituents is a gel-like amorphous matrix called the ground substance.[1,8]

The role of the epidermis as related to the mechanical behavior of the skin usually is disregarded by investigators. Also, tissue cells, by themselves, provide little or no contribution to the mechanical properties of skin.[4] Likewise, many investigators ignore the influence that blood vessels, lymphatics, glands, and nerves have on the mechanical properties of skin.[8] However, therapists should remember that blood vessels, nerves, and lymphatics are intimately enmeshed within the fibrous networks and contribute to ischemia, pain, and swelling, respectively.[1] The special mechanical contributions of structures, such as hair shafts that act to transfix the skin at various intervals, have been assessed elsewhere[1,4,6] and an in-depth presentation about their contribution is beyond the scope of this chapter. Therefore, only the fibrous networks of collagen, elastin, and the ground substance will be given serious consideration.

The primary mechanical behavior of the skin takes place in the dermis, particularly in the deeper reticular layer, between the mobile collagen and elastic fibers and the lubricative ground substance.[8,9] Thus, skin is described as being a viscoelastic structure.[4,9,10] For clarification, this viscoelastic characterization of tissue is so labeled because of the viscous property of the semi-liquid ground substance and the combined elastic or stretchable property of both collagen and elastin rather than just the latter as the name may imply.

Biomechanically, intact skin is composed of collagen and elastin fibers surrounded by ground substance. However, scar tissue is composed primarily of collagen fibers and ground substance and lacks elastic fibers. Following a burn injury, elastin is not readily replaced and plays practically no role in wound repair.[11] Collagen, elastin, and ground substance will be described separately before their combined physical interaction is discussed.

Collagen

Collagen is the basic structural fibrous protein found in soft and hard tissues, is present in most of the body's supportive tissues,[3,5] and is the most abundant fibrous component of skin and scar tissue.[4] The structural formation of dermal collagen is distinctively different at three levels: the network of fibers, the fibers themselves, and the fibrils that constitute the fibers as depicted in Figure 4–1.[12] As described in Chapter 6, the collagen fibers of the dermis are aggregates of a large but variable number of collagen fibrils, which in turn are supercoils of filaments constructed from a basic trihelical spiral of amino acid chains.[1,5,12] Collagen fibrils appear to be cross-striated and form a light and dark pattern (Fig. 4–2) that, when seen in a tendon, is interpreted as representing the sinusoidal pattern of the collagen fiber (Fig. 4–3).[5] Collagen fibers found in the reticular layer of the dermis are highly undulated fibers and lie in a planar array without orientation (Fig. 4–4).[2,12,13] These convoluted fibers are separated from each other by an amorphous ground substance in the relaxed state (Fig. 4–5).[2,9,12–14] Collagen bundles in normal dermis are wavy and contain ample interstitial space.[15] Collagen in burn scar is arranged in a whorl-like pattern and is tightly woven (Fig. 4–6).[16]

Collagen fibers of the dermis are unbranched and extremely long structures when compared to their diameter.[2,9,12,15] In connective tissue, collagen fibers probably vary considerably in length.[5] With no evidence of any firm attachments between adjacent fiber bundles, collagen fibers seem free to move relative to each other.[2]

Collagen is the main load-carrying element in skin, tendons, and scar. Collagen provides strength to the tissue, thus the tissue with the highest percentage of collagen has the greatest strength.[5,17] Its role in all connective tissues appears to be that of the major element to resist stress.[4] While collagen fibers provide the tensile strength of tissue, the elastic fibers are responsible for the skin's deforming qualities.

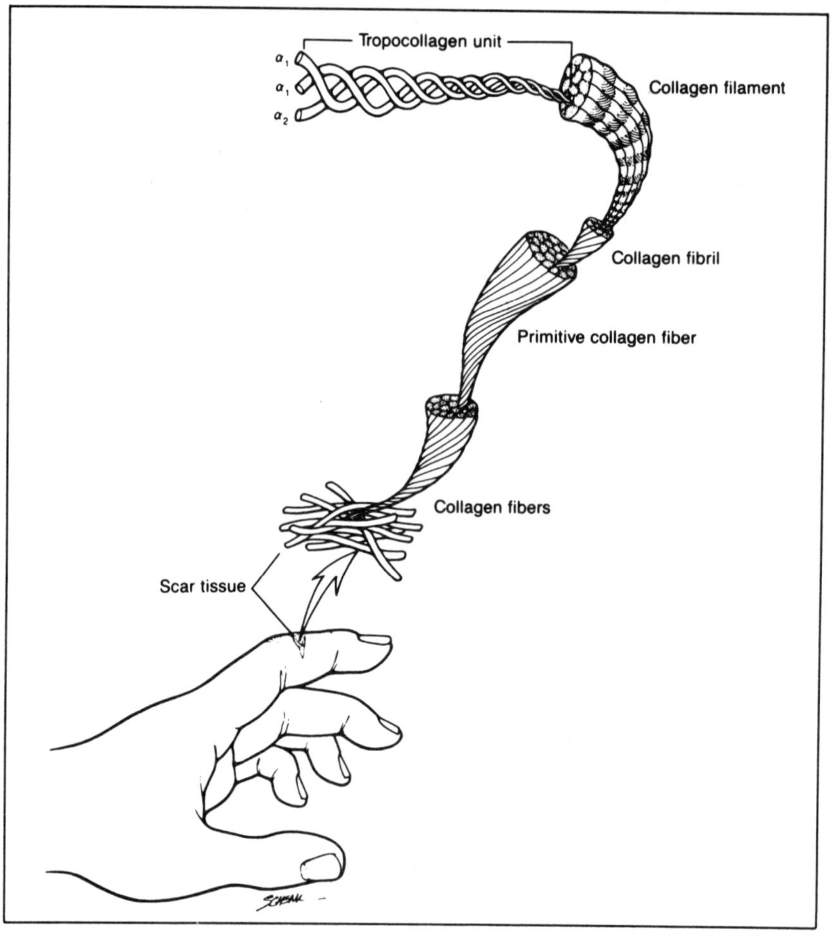

FIGURE 4–1. Structural composition of collagen displaying the various levels of tissue organization. (From Hardy, MA: The biology of scar formation. Phys Ther 69:1014–1024, 1989, p 1019, with permission.)

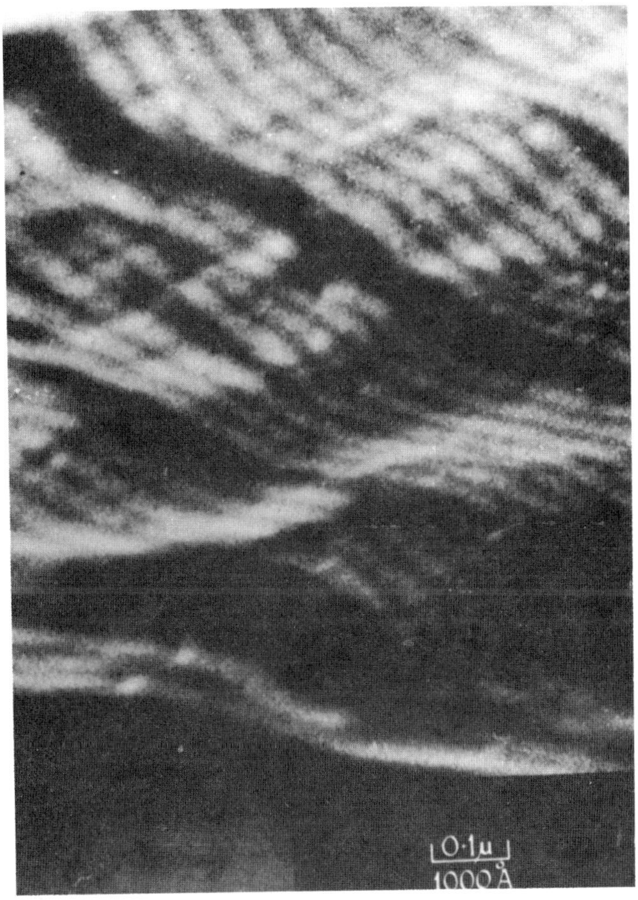

FIGURE 4–2. Cross striations of collagen fibrils interpreted as ordered alignment of collagen subunits. (From Gibson,[9] p 24, with permission.)

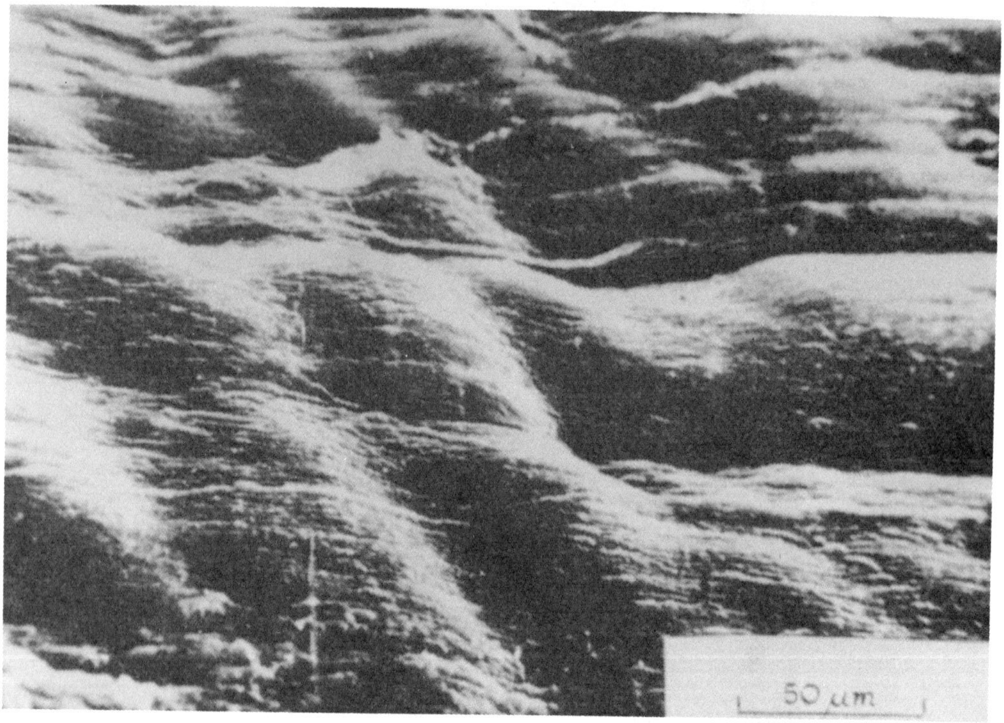

FIGURE 4–3. Wavy appearance of tendon surface. (From Barbenel,[24] p 166, with permission.)

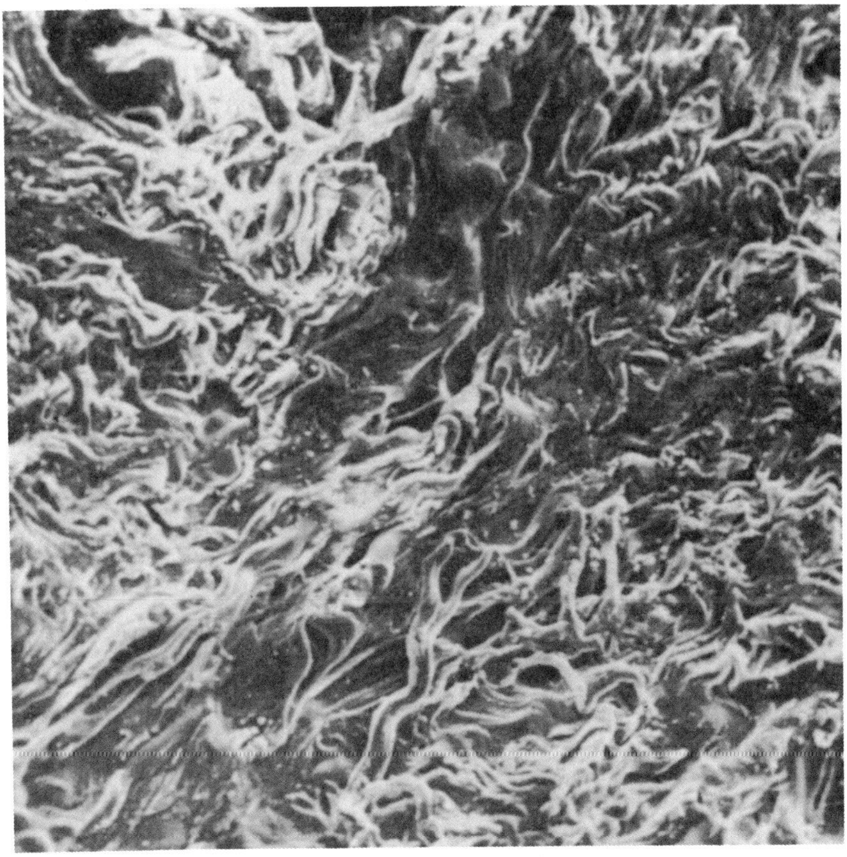

FIGURE 4–4. Collagen fibers of dermis lying in random orientation. (From Gibson, T and Kennedi, RM: Factors affecting the mechanical characteristics of human skin. In Dunphy, JE and VanWinkle, W (eds): Repair and Regeneration. McGraw-Hill, New York, 1963, p 92, with permission.)

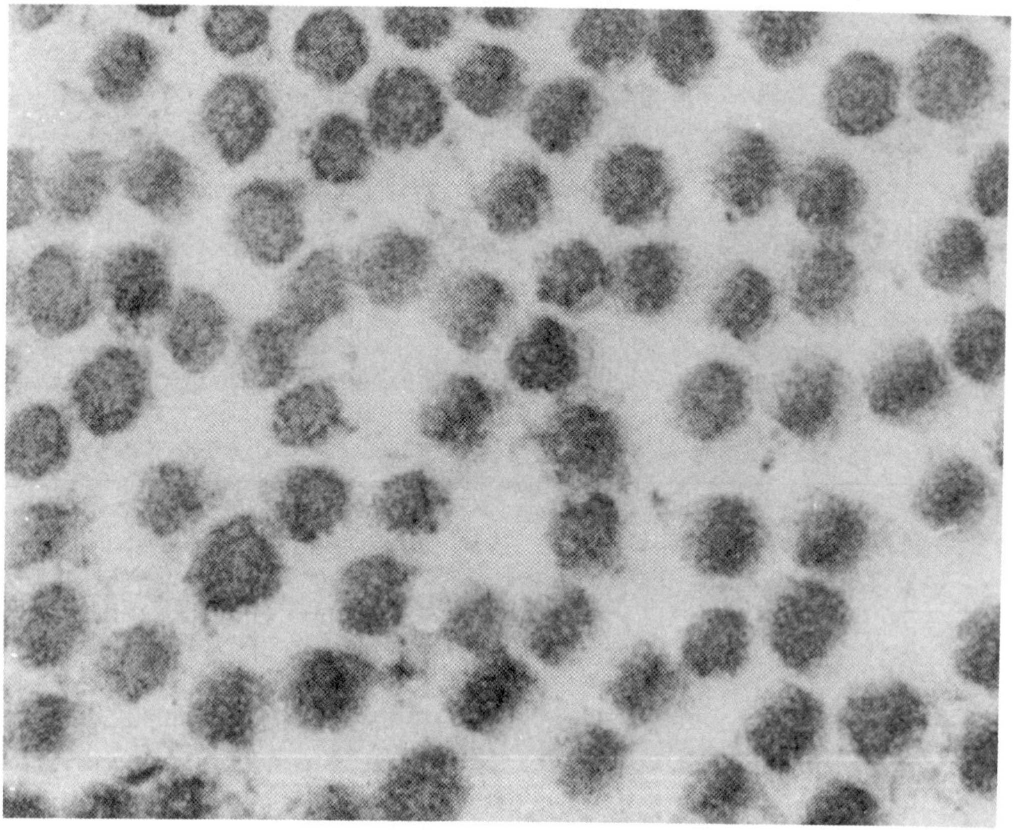

FIGURE 4–5. Cross section of collagen fiber showing ground substance (white) surrounding the dark-stained collagen fibrils. (From Gibson, T and Kennedi, RM: Factors affecting the mechanical characteristics of human skin. In Dunphy, JE and VanWinkle, W (eds): Repair and Regeneration. McGraw-Hill, New York, 1969, p 94, with permission.)

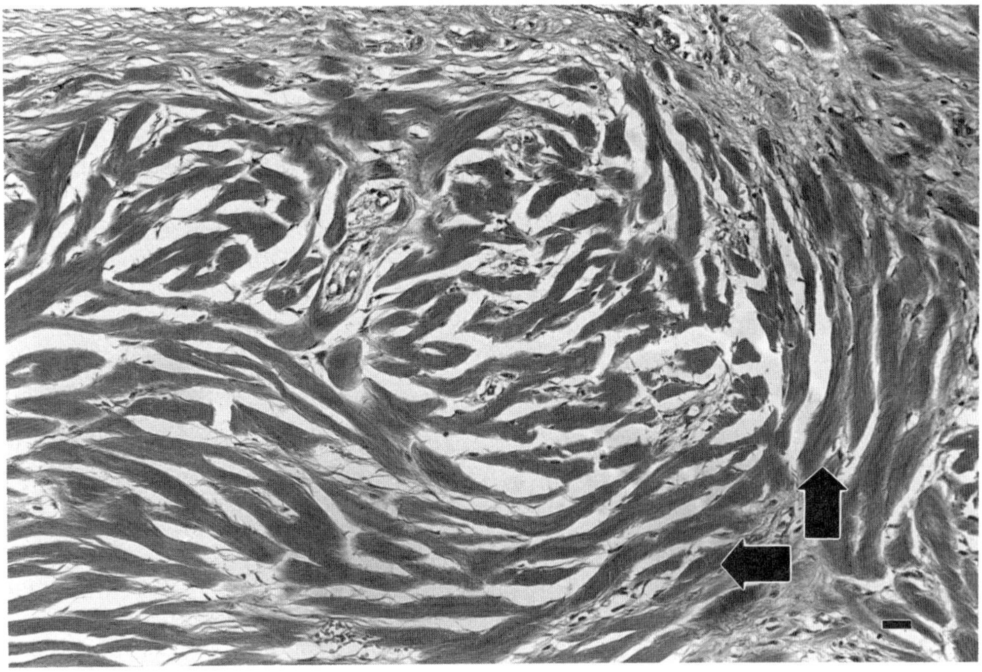

FIGURE 4–6. Whorl-like configuration of burn scar collagen. Direction of arrows demonstrates the mixed orientation of the collagen bundles. Scale bar = 0.1 mm. (Courtesy of Steve Boyce, 1991).

Elastin

Skin possesses a degree of elasticity due to the presence of elastic fibers.[18] In addition, the elastic fibers maintain the skin in a state of constant tension (Fig. 4–7).[18] Elastic fibers in connective tissues do not show a distinctive pattern of orientation. They appear to exist as either long, branched, and randomly coiled chains or as straight fibers.[5,11,13,15,19] In skin, the branching, netlike characteristic of elastic fibers is

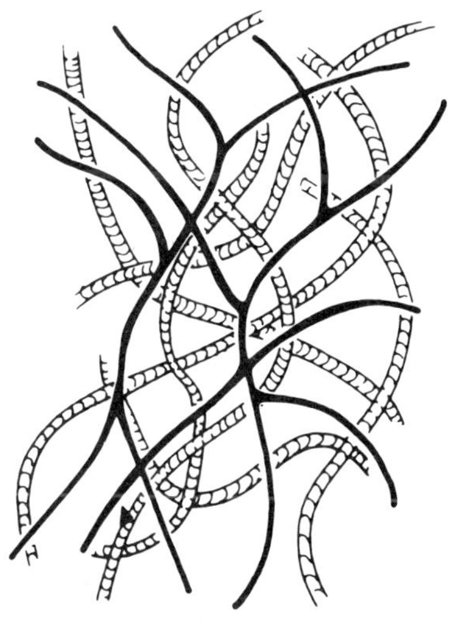

FIGURE 4–7. Schematic drawing of collagen and elastin weave in normal skin. Note that the collagen strands are individual while the elastin is branched. Dark lines—elastic fibers. Striated lines—collagen fibers. (From Brody, GS, Peng, STJ, and Landel, RF: The etiology of hypertrophic scar contracture: Another view. Plast Reconst Surg 67: 673–684, 1981, p 682, with permission.)

particularly apparent.[11] The elastic fibers have end-to-side junctions that attach to one another, whereas collagen fibers are independent from each other.[2,9,12,15] The fixed points of attachment that exist in the elastic fiber network act to deform adjacent fibers when elongated.[2,12] Cross-linking of elastin is very similar in its mechanical properties to what occurs in collagen. However, cross-linking in elastin is perhaps more widespread.[11]

Elastic fibers are closely associated with collagen fibers,[11] but are scattered,[19] sparse,[20] and much finer than collagen fibers.[9,12] They form a delicate network between the collagen fibers with many of the elastic fibers looped spirally around the collagen in relaxed skin.* Elastic fibers add little to the tensile strength of skin.[9,12,19] Rather, they are regarded as springlike energy-storing devices responsible for the recoiling mechanism of returning stretched aligned collagen to its resting state.†

Ground Substance

As stated previously, the ground substance is an amorphous, gel-like component found in between, surrounding, and throughout the fibrous network of collagen and elastin[8,9] (see Fig. 4–5). Dense connective tissue contains a very small amount of ground substance; loose connective tissue contains much more.[5] The composition of the ground substance varies with the tissue but contains interstitial fluid and a group of high-molecular-weight substances, the mucopolysaccharides (MPS),[4,5,9] which more recently have been referred to as glycosaminoglycans (GAGs).[8,22,23]

The GAGs are very large macromolecules composed primarily of carbohydrates associated with varying amounts of protein.[4,23] One function of the GAGs probably is related to the provision of normal suppleness and turgor of the skin.[4] There are approximately seven such substances in connective tissue.[23] In human dermis, there are three major GAGs: hyaluronic acid, dermatan sulfate, and chondroitin sulfate[4] (Table 4–1). The proportions of hyaluronic acid and dermatan sulfate are highest during adolescence[4,24] and change by only a few percentage points throughout life. Conversely, chondroitin sulfate is 8 percent of the total in early childhood and decreases thereafter.[4] Burn scar contains approximately six times the amount of chondroitin 4-sulfate found in normal skin. Interestingly, of the GAGs mentioned, chondroitin 4-sulfate is the only one found in bone. This finding may be partly responsible for the firmness of burn scar.

TABLE 4–1. Percent of Glycosaminoglycans in Normal Skin and Hypertrophic Scar

	Hyaluronic Acid	Dermatan Sulfate	Chondroitin 4 Sulfate
Normal skin	41.5	54.0	4.5
Hypertrophic scar	18.5	55.1	26.4

Adapted from Kischer, Shetlar, and Shetlar,[15] p. 64, Copyright 1975, American Medical Association.

*References 2, 9, 11, 12, 15, 18, 21.
†References 2, 3, 9, 11, 12, 15, 16, 19.

The viscosity of the ground substance is related to the content of the GAGs.[25] The GAGs are very hydrophilic and bind most of the tissue fluid.[8] Hyaluronic acid has a large molecular weight and is associated with very small amounts of protein.[23]

GAGs are highly charged molecules and can be measured biochemically.[4,23] In skin, the variable quantities of dermatan sulfate and chondroitin sulfate provide the negative charges for ionic bonding to positive ions.[4] The general pattern that seems to emerge is that the less highly charged GAGs, such as hyaluronic acid, tend to decrease during the early stages of wound healing, while the more highly charged GAGs, like the chondroitin sulfates, tend to increase.[23] The time at which these changes occur varies according to the time of healing and may play a role in the inelasticity of burn contractures.[23]

BIOMECHANICS

The combination and interaction of the three viscoelastic components of collagen, elastin, and ground substance characterizes the soft tissues of the body from a mechanical perspective. Normal skin lies in a state of constant tension schematically represented by the well-known Langer's lines (Fig. 4-8). Collagen fibers lie in a convoluted state in both the normal state of skin as part of the dermis and in the pathologic state as part of burn scar. The elastic fibers in normal skin partly are responsible for these coils and cause the tension in skin. However, relaxed tendon tissue also lies in a wavy state naturally without elastic fibers. Very little elastin is regenerated in scars during the wound-healing process, so it is unclear as to what causes the whorls in burn scars.

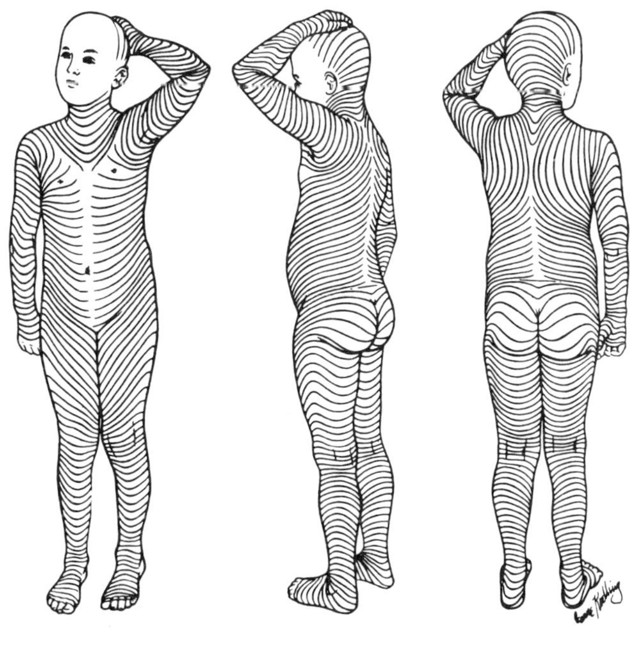

FIGURE 4–8. Langer's lines of the body which represent lines of maximal tension. (From Manteuffel, SV and Berkich, EJ: The burn patient. Management and operating room support. Ethicon, Inc., Somerville, NJ, p 30, with permission.)

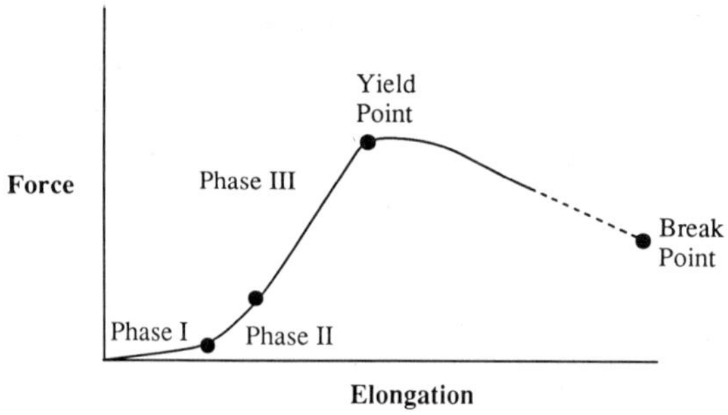

FIGURE 4–9. Typical stress-strain curve for tissues of the body showing various phases and critical points. See text for explanation of terms.

Stress-Strain Curve

One of the primary patient interventions used in burn rehabilitation is "stretching" of burn scar to regain range of motion and function. A stress-strain curve (Fig. 4–9) will be used to diagrammatically represent the biomechanics of skin and scar and to illustrate what occurs within these tissues when a stretching or elongating force is applied.

Technically, stress is defined as the ratio of force (F) or load to a given cross-sectional area (A) of tissue where load is the measured total force applied to the specimen, stress is recorded as the force per unit area when measured at right angles to the line of action.[4]

$$\text{Stress} = \frac{F}{A} \tag{1}$$

Strain, on the other hand, refers to the ratio of the relative change or increase in tissue length to the original length of the tissue.[25]

$$\text{Strain} = \frac{\text{Change in length}}{\text{Original length}} \times 100 \tag{2}$$

Descriptively, stress is defined as the force or load applied to a tissue, while strain is stated in terms of extension or elongation of a tissue expressed as a percent of increased tissue length.[4] Reviewing the literature on this topic can be confusing, as stress carries many values or units of measure such as newtons per square meter (N/m^2), dynes per centimeter squared (d/cm^2), or pounds per square inch (psi). For the purpose of this chapter, the terms of force or load for stress and percent (%) elongation for strain are used.

To describe the action of tissues, the stress-strain or force-elongation curve can be conveniently divided into three phases as follows (see Fig. 4–9).[2,15]

PHASE I

As a given magnitude of force is applied to a tissue, the tissue begins to elongate. With skin, the initial portion of the stress-strain curve is relatively flat and considerable tissue extension occurs from the application of minimal force.[9,12,26,27] During phase I, the combined elastic-collagen fiber weave is lengthened by the applied stretching force. The elastic fibers simply elongate due to their elastic nature and the collagen

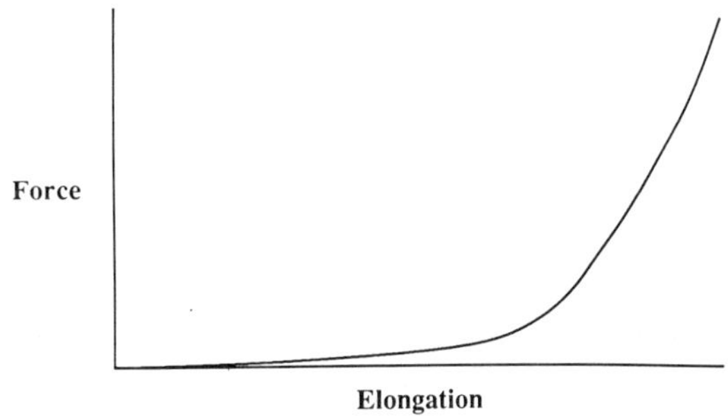

FIGURE 4–10. Stress-strain curve for ligamentum flavum. Note the amount of elongation requiring a minimal force.

fibers begin to uncoil and straighten. During this time of fibrous elongation, the elastic fibers are noted to be "slipping through" the ground substance, while the unfurling of the collagen fibers begins to displace the ground substance. In both cases, the fibers become parallel and elongate in the direction of stretch. Due to the random orientation of the collagen fibers, some fibers lie in the direction of stretch, while others need to change direction to become aligned. This phase represents "taking up the slack" of the tissue.[27]

In contrast to skin, the ligamentum flavum is highly elasticized and exhibits an extremely long phase I as seen in Figure 4–10. Conversely, tendon and burn scar are composed primarily of collagen bundles, so the first part of the curve is abbreviated due to the lack of elastic fibers and decreased pliability of these two tissues. The relative compliance of phase I, during which elongation of the tissue is produced by applying a low load, is followed by a progressive stiffening of the tissue with increased elongation.[28]

PHASE II

Phase II is referred to as the transitional phase and represents tissue stiffening as elongation progresses.[4] This portion of the curve is the range in which tissues usually function under normal physiologic conditions.[5] If skin or scar is to elongate further, an increasing amount of load or force becomes necessary as more and more collagen fibers begin to align themselves in the direction of stretch. There is a need to impart an increased force in phase II due to the increased cross-sectional area of the tissue as additional fibers become aligned in the direction of stress. During this "elbow" portion of the curve, the load increases exponentially with increasing elongation.[5,15,29] An additional factor contributing to the need for increased force is the further extrusion of the ground substance from between the fibers as they become more parallel to one another.

PHASE III

Phase III is a continuation of phase II, where significant increases in loading produce little further tissue elongation. Restated, this concept means that only a minimal amount of tissue length is achieved by considerably increasing the load.[9,12,15,26] As tension applied to a tissue is increased, more and more fibers become aligned and take up the load until all fibers are oriented in a parallel manner. In the case of skin, the relative inextensibility of collagen is demonstrated by a small increase in tissue length when increasingly greater loads are applied.[12]

During phase III, the load-elongation relationship is virtually linear.[15,27] This linear portion of the curve is a function of the fully oriented collagen fibers and the further thickened cross-sectional area of the combined fibers.[5,9] The more closely the slope of the line approaches vertical, the greater is the tissue stiffness.[26] This "high-stiffness" phase III is commonly referred to as terminal stiffness.[4,15,26] During this period, the fully oriented and close-packed formation of the collagen displaces the remaining ground substance from between its fibers. The terminal portion of the curve for skin is similar to the stress-strain curve configuration obtained with pure collagen only. This linear resemblance indicates that the collagen fibers are primarily responsible for the high resistance and tensile strength of skin.[12,15]

YIELD POINT

The tissue has reached the peak of functional elongation at its yield point (see Fig. 4–9). Actual changes in the physical constitution of the tissue begin to occur beyond this point. Because of being unable to absorb any additional force, tissue begins to break down. The tissue suddenly starts to elongate further with little or no additional application of force. As the tissue continues to degrade and less and less force is required for additional elongation until the tissue physically comes apart at its breaking point. The start of the stress-strain curve up to the yield point is known as the physiologic or elastic portion of the curve, whereas beyond the yield point is referred to as the nonphysiologic or plastic portion.

HYSTERESIS

Upon release of a stretched tissue in the physiologic range of elongation, the tissue will tend to return to its original length. However, this "unloading" curve is different from the loading curve and the curves are described as being noncoincident, as seen in Figure 4–11.[4,9]

When the load causing the elongation of the tissue is released, there is an immediate decrease in the tissue tension but a delay in the retraction of the tissue to a shorter length. This hysteresis, or lagging behind, of the tissue may be due to several factors. There may be only a partial release of the energy absorbed by the tissue during extension.[9] Also, hysteresis is strongly influenced by the maximum amplitude of stretch and the extent to which the tissue specimen is actually elongated.[30]

Hysteresis of a tissue appears to be a reversal of the tissue fiber–ground substance interaction. As described previously, in the linear portion of phase III, all the tissue fibers are aligned tightly in the direction of stretch and the ground substance is

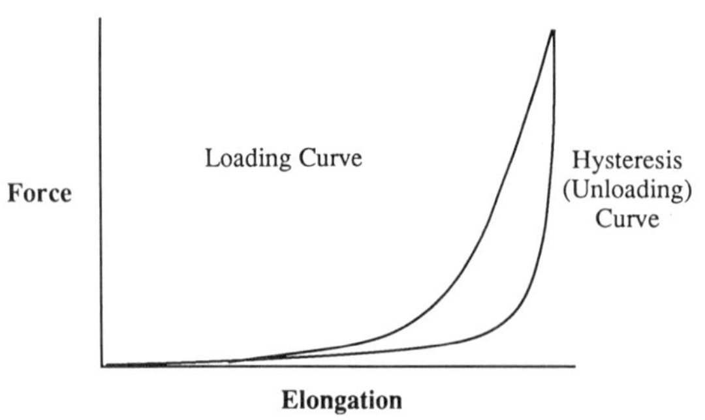

FIGURE 4–11. Stress-strain or tissue loading curve displaying hysteresis upon unloading of an elongated tissue.

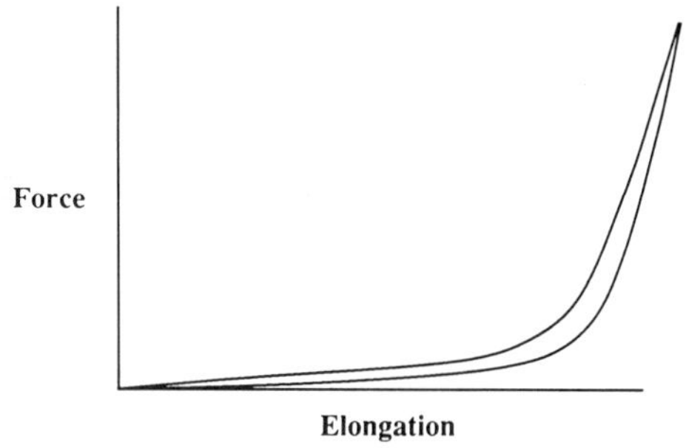

FIGURE 4–12. Hysteresis curve for the ligamentum flavum. Notice how closely the hysteresis curve follows the loading curve.

displaced from between the fibers. When the tissue relaxes, the ground substance reinfiltrates between the fibers as they resume their coiled state. Hence, there is a delay in the tissue retraction process while the fibers again displace the ground substance and the ground substance refills the area between the fibers.

The hysteresis curve is different for various tissues. For example, with tendon there is significant hysteresis while the stress-strain curve obtained from the ligamentum flavum shows no appreciable hysteresis when load-cycled (Fig. 4–12). This latter example confirms the assumption that hysteresis of skin is a function of the collagen fibers in its network rather than the elastic fibers.[9]

Additionally, many tissues are anisotropic, that is, having unequal properties in different directions. The principle mechanical difference associated with anisotropic tissue appears to be an increased deformation at low loads.[24] Skin is anisotropic and viscoelastic. Thus skin's nonlinear properties are directional as well as load- and strain-rate dependent.[26,31]

MECHANICAL PRINCIPLES APPLIED TO BURN REHABILITATION

Successive Length Induction

In addition to tissues displaying hysteresis, repeated stress-strain curves of the same tissue sample also change with successive stretching (Fig. 4–13). Each time a force is applied in succession to a tissue, the elongation of the tissue in phase I will be increased before entering into phase II.[4] Likewise, at a specific peak force, the tissue length is greater at the end of phase III. Only after several cycles, reportedly 6 to 10, does the specimen become stable and the curve reproducible.[3,4,5,9,32]

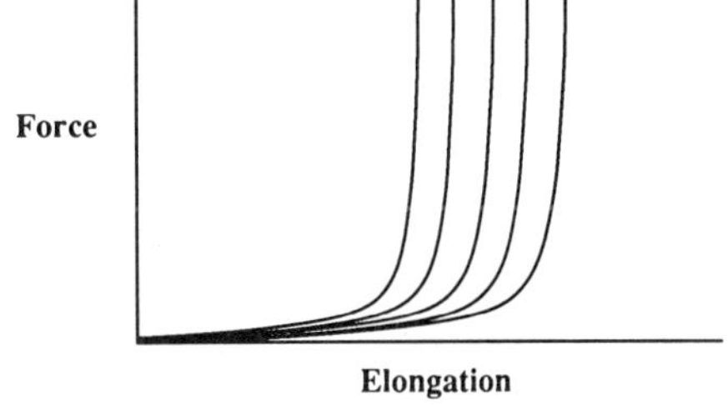

FIGURE 4–13. Successive elongation graph displaying an increase in tissue length with repeated stretching to the same amount of terminal force.

An initial period of length adjustment seems common to all tissues.[5] In mechanical terms, the process is called *preconditioning*,[4,5,32] and in engineering terms, *load cycling*.[9] The precise reason why there is an increase in tissue length with successive stretching is not known.[9] One explanation is the internal structure of the tissue may change with the cycling.[5] This "stress softening" also could result from a temporary fatigue or damage of the tissue components or from blood being expressed from the tissue as it is continuously stretched.[30]

By repeated cycling, eventually a steady state is reached at which no further elongation will occur unless the cycling routine is changed.[5] This steady state depends upon the amount of force and the extent to which the tissue is allowed to relax or recover between stretches. Changing the upper and lower limits of the cycling, by either increasing the force or lengthening the time between repetitions, alters the internal structure and the specimen will need to be preconditioned again.[5]

The property of successive length induction in tissue is an important concept for use in a burn patient's treatment program. Before a force of any magnitude is applied to tight scar tissue, the optimal tissue length should be gained through repeated cycles of stretching. Clinically, a newly fabricated splint may appear to need readjusting if, when the splint was originally made, the patient's scar tissue was at an optimal length following preliminary stretching but the splint was not worn for several hours afterward. In this case, the patient's scar should be repeatedly stretched again until the tissue resumes its original optimal length for reapplication of the splint.

Creep

This term, extrapolated from polymer physics, describes the progressive elongation of a material when it is stretched with the force kept constant.[9,33] Therapists knowingly or unknowingly use this principle everyday. When a biologic tissue is loaded to a predetermined level and the load maintained as a constant, the amount of tissue elongation will increase with time, and the tissue is said to undergo "creep" (Fig. 4–14).[2,4,9,24] The progressive elongation of tissue length, measured as a function of time, reflects the viscoelastic behavior of the tissue.[4,34]

In burn rehabilitation, the interventions of dynamic splinting and isotonic stretching best exemplify this principle.[35,36,37] With dynamic splinting (see Chapter 11), a constant force is applied to the shortened tissue. As the tissue elongates from the applied load, the applied force continues via the dynamic component of the splint, that is, the rubber bands, wires, or force springs. With isotonic stretching, the therapist applies a constant load to the tight tissue either manually or through the

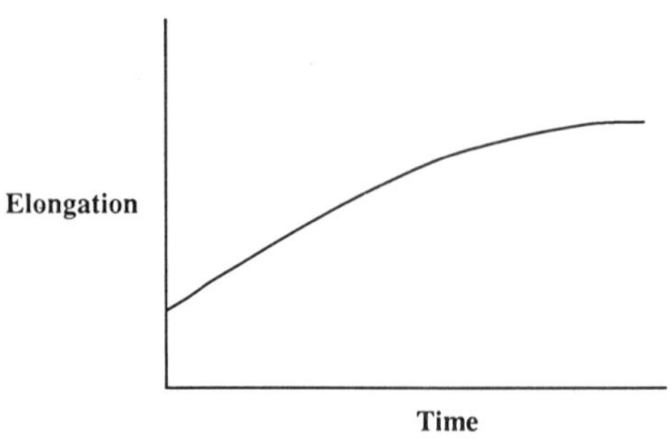

FIGURE 4–14. Creep is the progressive elongation of tissue over time with the application of a constant force.

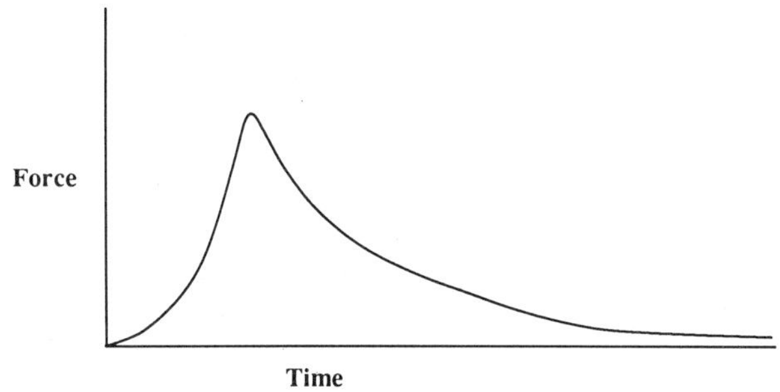

FIGURE 4–15. Stress relaxation curve from peak application of stress demonstrating a decrease in force over time required to maintain a tissue at a given length.

use of weights with gravity assisting. When manually applying a constant tension, the therapist continually increases the range of motion of the limb as the tissue elongates. Using a weight, the force is kept constant as the scar tissue elongates. For example, a cuff weight attached to the wrist can be used to stretch an elbow flexion contracture.

Stress Relaxation

Another characteristic of viscoelastic materials is the principle of stress relaxation.[5,9,33] Stress relaxation is the progressive reduction in force required to keep a specimen extended at a given length[9] (Fig. 4–15). In stress relaxation tests, the specimen is stretched to a given length and the load on the tissue is measured over time.[4,12,24] The greater the force, the greater the amount of stress relaxation that occurs.[12,17] This reaction is understandable, because with lower loads there is a slight shift in ground substance and, as the load increases, the shift of ground substance increases.[12]

For tendon, there is a larger reduction in stress (force) level than relaxation, suggesting that some other factor is present besides a reduction in effective viscosity (i.e., ground substance fluid shift). Theoretically, there may be a reduction in the amount of cross-linking between the collagen fibrils caused by the ground substance GAGs, or possibly the behavior of collagen may be time dependent.[17]

Tissue relaxation, in response to a constant stress, is another factor that is directly applicable to the clinical situation. Burn therapists capitalize on this response with many of the commonly used techniques described elsewhere in this book. Positioning, static splinting, and serial casting are all examples. With each of these patient interventions, a stretching force is applied to the scar tissue of a patient within a moderately tolerable range. Shortly thereafter, the level of patient discomfort decreases as the tissue accommodates to the load.

Strain Rate

Another important factor to consider when applying therapeutic techniques that utilize either creep or stress relaxation is how fast or quickly the load used to elongate the tissue is applied. By definition, strain rate is the amount of tissue elongation per unit time.[17] Concisely stated, the more quickly a strain is applied, the greater

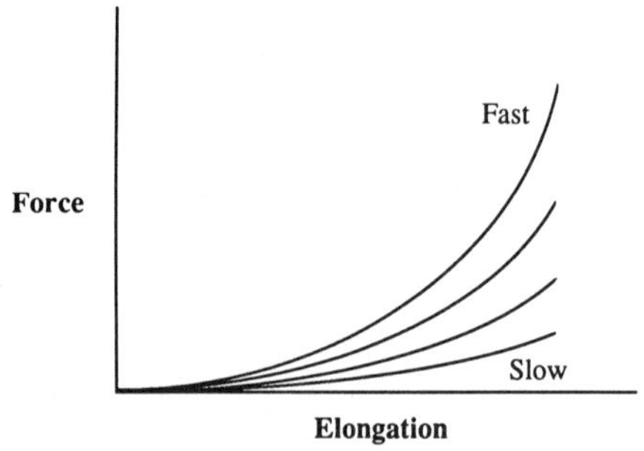

FIGURE 4–16. Reaction of tissue at different strain rates. Notice the same endpoint of tissue elongation for fast or slowly applied force but the greater amount of force required when a faster strain rate is applied.

the tissue deformation.[9] However, although more tissue deformation occurs with a greater strain rate, a faster application of strain has less appreciable effect on tissue elongation than one might expect (Fig. 4–16).

Fung[5] reported that various tissues demonstrate a strain rate insensitivity; that is, there is a disproportionately small amount of tissue length gained when attempting to elongate tissue at increasing rates. In tests on cartilage, four specimens were subjected to cyclic tests at different strain rates varying from 0.04 percent per second to 4 percent per second. Within this range of strain rates, the hysteresis loop and the peak stresses increased only slightly with increased strain rates. Likewise, McEllnany, as cited by Fung,[5] showed only a 2.5-fold increase in stress of muscle at any given strain when the strain rate was increased from 0.001 to 1000 per second, an increase of 10^6.

Besides the mechanical results of strain rate, there are biologic effects on tissue to consider as well. The application of a load too suddenly may cause tissue rupture; however, if the same load is applied slowly, rupture may be avoided.[9] Likewise, using too high a strain rate when applying a force to burn scar contracture can cause the tissue to separate. Clinically, a desired amount of tissue elongation is achievable using a reduced strain rate and a lower force if an adequate amount of time is budgeted for patient treatment.

This reduced stress level is an important consideration from a clinical and humanitarian perspective. Because of the amount of pain usually involved in burn rehabilitation treatments, patients can tolerate a slower strain rate better than one applied too quickly. In addition, the risk of tissue damage is lowered if a more gentle approach is used.

Time Dependence

All viscoelastic tissues of the body are time dependent.[10,14] This means that when the principles of creep and stress relaxation are used, the duration of time that a force is applied to a tissue is of utmost importance.

To achieve a 20 percent reduction in force during a stress relaxation test of skin under a normalized load, Barbenel, Evans, and Finley[24] reported that 1000 seconds (>16 minutes) was required.[24] In tests of stress relaxation on articular cartilage, Woo[5] reported that 15 minutes were needed to reach a relaxed state with only a 5 percent tissue elongation. In addition, for cartilaginous tissue elongated between 16 and 29 percent, stress relaxation did not plateau even after 100 minutes. Creep tests on

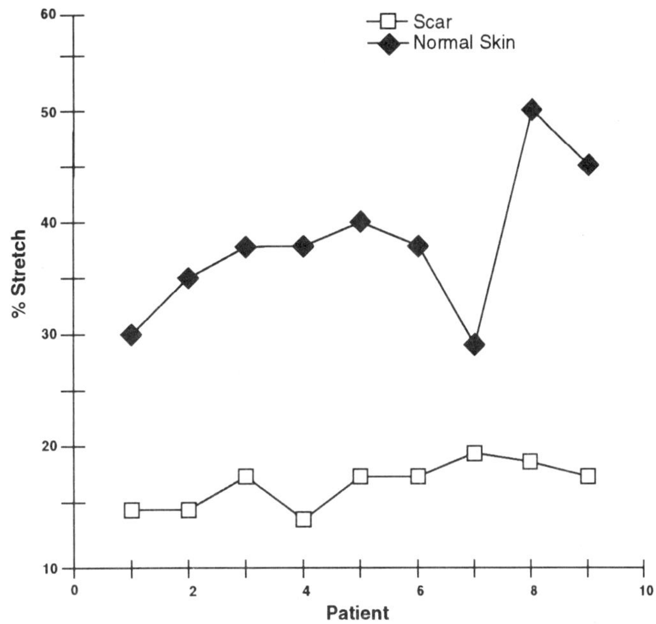

FIGURE 4–17. Comparison of tissue elasticity of normal skin and burn scar. (From Bartel et al,[38] p 659, with permission.)

costal cartilage required 1000 minutes (>16 hours) to gain an approximate 85 percent elongation.[9]

Both skin and cartilage are much more extensible than burn scar. The upper limit for burn scar elongation is approximately 16 percent (Fig. 4–17).[38] Therefore, scar tissue requires an excessive amount of time to elongate.

In both stress relaxation and creep, the fundamentally critical factor is allowing a sufficient amount of time to elapse for the results to occur. Often therapists are said to need an "aggressive" approach in rehabilitating burn patients. However, this treatment approach should be tempered with adequate consideration given to the time factor required for tissue adaptation. Therefore, in light of the biophysical considerations presented in this chapter, patience and persistence appear to be necessary ingredients in the burn rehabilitation program for optimal patient outcomes.

SUMMARY

This chapter integrates the disciplines of biologic science and mechanical engineering to describe the intimate relationship that exists between the physical properties and characteristics of living tissue and the physical principles governing their action in burn rehabilitation. Collagen, elastin, and ground substance are the main constituents of skin and burn scar. Their structure and interaction with each other are described. The biomechanics of living tissue are represented with the use of a stress-strain curve. This curve illustrates what occurs with tissues when an elongating force is applied. Successive length induction, creep, stress-relaxation, and time rate are mechanical principles that are described and then applied to burn rehabilitation techniques.

Utilization of the information presented will assist the therapist in gaining an understanding of the principles that should be applied in the treatment of the burn patient.

REFERENCES

1. Kennedi, RM, et al: Tissue mechanics. Phys Med Biol 20:699–717, 1975.
2. Gibson, T and Kennedi, RM: Biomechanical properties of skin. Surg Clin North Am 47:279–294, 1967.
3. Viidik, A: On the rheology and morphology of soft collagenous tissue. J Anat 105:184, 1969.
4. Millington, PF and Wilkinson, R: Skin. Cambridge University Press, Cambridge, 1983.
5. Fung, YC: Biomechanics: Mechanical Properties of Living Tissues. Springer-Verlag, New York, 1981.
6. Kennedi, RM and Gibson, T: Experiments and analysis: A retrospect. In Marks, R and Payne, PA (eds): Bioengineering and the Skin. MTP Press, Boston, 1981, pp 3–7.
7. Kennedi, RM: The load-deformation characteristics of connective tissues. J Biomed Mater Res Symp, 5:427–434, 1974.
8. Oomens, CWJ, vanCampen, DH, and Grootenboer, HJ: A mixture approach to the mechanics of skin. J Biomechanics 20:877–885, 1987.
9. Gibson, T and Kennedi, RM: The structural components of the dermis and their mechanical characteristics. In Montagna, W, Bentley, JP, and Dobson, RL (eds): The Dermis. Advances in Biology of Skin. Appleton-Century-Crofts, New York, 1970, pp 19–34.
10. Forrester, JC, et al: Mechanical, biochemical and architectural features of repair. In Dunphy, JE and VanWinkle, W (eds): Repair and Regeneration. McGraw-Hill, New York, 1969, pp 71–85.
11. Peacock, CC: Wound Repair. WB Saunders, Philadelphia, 1984.
12. Gibson, T and Kennedi, RM: Factors affecting the mechanical characteristics of human skin. In Dunphy, JE and VanWinkle, W (eds): Repair and Regeneration. McGraw-Hill, New York, 1969, pp 87–98.
13. Lanir, Y: The fibrous structure of the skin and its relation to mechanical behavior. In Marks, R, and Payne, PA (eds): Bioengineering and the Skin. MTP Press, Boston, 1981, pp 93–96.
14. Gibson, T, Kennedi, RM, and Craik, JE: The mobile microarchitecture of dermal collagen. Br J Surg 52:764–770, 1965.
15. Kischer, CW, Shetlar, MR, and Shetlar, CL: Alteration of hypertrophic scars induced by mechanical pressure. Arch Dermatol 111:60–64, 1975.
16. Larson, DL, et al: The Prevention and Correction of Burn Scar Contracture and Hypertrophy. Shriners' Burns Institute, Galveston, 1973, pp 1–23.
17. Minns, RJ, Soden, PD, and Jackson, DS: The role of the fibrous components and ground substance in the mechanical properties of biological tissues: A preliminary investigation. J Biomechanics 6:153–165, 1973.
18. Converse, JM: General principles. In Converse, JM (ed): Reconstructive Plastic Surgery. WB Saunders, Philadelphia, 1977, pp 3–68.
19. Oxlund, H, Manschot, J, and Viidik, A. The role of elastin in the mechanical properties of skin. J Biomechanics 21:213–218, 1988.
20. Ryhanan, L and Uitto, J: Elastic fibers of the connective tissue. In Goldsmith, LA (ed): Biochemistry and Physiology of the Skin. Oxford University Press, Oxford, 1983, pp 433–447.
21. Oxlund, H: Changes in connective tissue during corticotropin and corticosteroid treatment. Dan Med Bull 31:187–206, 1984.
22. Jeanloz, RW: The nomenclature of mucopolysaccharides. Arthritis Rheum 3:233–237, 1960.
23. Bentley, JP: Mucopolysaccharide synthesis in healing wounds. In Dunphy, JE and VanWinkle, W (eds): Repair and Regeneration. McGraw-Hill, New York, 1969, pp 151–160.
24. Barbenel, JC, Evans, JH, and Finley, JB: Stress-strain-time relations for soft connective tissues. In Kennedi, RM (ed): Perspectives in Biomedical Engineering. University Park Press, London, 1973, pp 165–172.
25. Sears, FW, Zemansky, MW, and Young, HD: College Physics. Addison-Wesley, Reading, Mass., 1974, pp 167–170.
26. Stark, HL: Directional variations in the extensibility of human skin. Br J Plast Surg 30:105–114, 1977.
27. Grahamme, R: A method for measuring human skin elasticity "in vivo" with observations on the effects of age, sex, and pregnancy. Clin Sci 39:223–238, 1970.
28. Ferguson, J and Barbenel, JC: Skin surface patterns and the directional mechanical properties of the dermis. In Marks, R and Payne, PA (eds): Bioengineering and the Skin. MTP Press, Boston, 1981, pp 83–92.
29. Oxlund, H and Andreassen, TT: The roles of hyaluronic acid, collagen and elastin in the mechanical properties of connective tissues. J Anat 131:611–620, 1980.

30. Chu, BM and Brody, G: Nondestructive measurements of the properties of healing burn scars. Med Instrum 9:139–142, 1975.
31. Clark, JA, et al: Mechanical characterization of human postburn hypertrophic skin during pressure therapy. J Biomechanics 20:397–406, 1987.
32. Barbenel, JC and Evans, JH: The time-dependent mechanical properties of skin. J Invest Dermatol 69:318–320, 1977.
33. Elden, HR: Biophysical properties of aging skin. In Montagna, W, Bentley, JP, and Dobson, RL (eds): The Dermis. Advances in Biology of Skin. Appleton-Century-Crofts, New York, 1970, pp 240–252.
34. Escoffier, C, et al: Age-related mechanical properties of human skin: An in vivo study. J Invest Dermatol 93:353–357, 1989.
35. Richard, RL: Use of the Dynasplint to correct elbow flexion burn contracture: A case report. J Burn Care Rehabil 7:151–152, 1986.
36. Richard, RL, et al: Treatment of exposed bilateral achilles tendons with use of the Dynasplint. Phys Ther 68:989–991, 1988.
37. Richard, R and Staley, MJ: Dynamic splinting: Basic science and modern technology. Phys Ther Forum 11:32–33, 1992.
38. Bartell, TH, Monafo, WW, and Mustoe, TA: A new instrument for serial measurements of elasticity in hypertrophic scar. J Burn Care Rehabil 9:657–660, 1988.

CHAPTER 5

Burn Wound Healing

David G. Greenhalgh, MD
Marlys J. Staley, MS, PT

Wound healing is the normal reparative response to injury. Simpler animal species, such as salamanders, have the ability to regenerate tissues to their normal state. Their small size and relative simplicity allow for re-creation of normal tissues, such as limbs, within a reasonable amount of time. Larger and more complex species have lost this regenerative capacity, probably because of the pressures of the environment. Re-creation of a limb in a large mammal would most likely require months to years. In that time, the larger species would either starve to death or die from infection. For these reasons, organisms have evolved a relatively rapid and efficient process to cover an open wound. Unfortunately, to accomplish the goal of repairing injured tissue efficiently, more complex animals are forced to replace normal tissue with scar. Instead of regenerating an arm, the body rapidly closes the residual limb to prevent blood loss and infection. Scar tissue is never quite like the tissue it replaces, but in most cases it is an adequate substitute. Sometimes the healing process leads to excessive scarring that can cause more problems than the original injury. Pathologic scarring in the burn patient can lead to such problems as hypertrophic scars, keloids, scar contractures, pulmonary fibrosis, and other complications.

Therapists frequently deal with problems in healing. The ultimate goal of wound management is to allow a wound to close as rapidly as possible, resemble the original tissue as much as possible, and produce the least amount of scarring. The best way to optimize wound repair is to understand the actual mechanisms of healing. Much progress has been made in the understanding of wound repair. Investigators are starting to understand the controls of wound repair down to the molecular level. Although this review will not examine healing to this level of complexity, many of the cellular and molecular controls will be discussed. The goal is to enable the therapist to use this knowledge to better understand why specific treatments and dressings are used, why some patients scar more than others, why specific treatments for scarring are performed, and why healing fails. The therapist will learn that there are still many aspects of wound repair that are not yet understood.

TYPES OF WOUND REPAIR

Wound repair can be categorized into three distinct processes: scar formation, epithelialization or re-creation of a cellular barrier, and contraction. All injured tissue undergoes some combination of all three of these repair processes. Each type of repair process may influence the extent of the other to affect the ultimate outcome. For instance, if an open wound re-epithelializes quickly, the scarring may be less than if the wound takes a long time to close. The different processes will be described separately, but a close interrelationship exists. For the most part, the descriptions will relate to wound healing in skin, but the same principles apply to all types of tissue.

Scar Formation

Scar formation essentially is the repair of damaged connective tissue, or for skin the re-creation of the dermis. Connective tissue is the substance that gives strength to all tissues, and its main components are the extracellular matrix proteins such as collagens and glycosaminoglycans (GAGs). The most important protein for the strength of tissue repair is collagen, and for the most part scar formation concentrates on new collagen development. Connective tissue is alive and is dependent on many types of cells for its development and maintenance.

Early wound healing investigations concentrated on the changes in the strength of incisions over time. Based on incisional strengths, three phases were consistently found and have been used to describe scar formation in all tissues (Fig. 5–1).[1] For the first few days after wounding, little incisional strength is gained, so this phase is called the *lag, substrate,* or *inflammatory phase.* After 4 to 5 days, incisional strength improves in a linear fashion and this improvement is proportional to the increasing production of collagen. This phase is called the *proliferative, fibroblastic,* or *collagen*

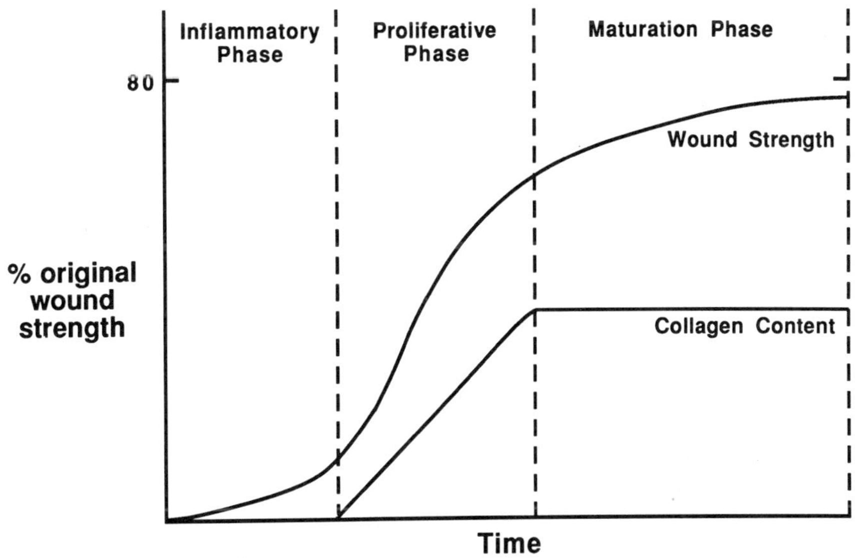

FIGURE 5–1. The three phases of wound healing; both wound strength and collagen content increase over time.

phase. After a few weeks, the amount of collagen in the wound plateaus, but the incisional strength continues to improve at a more gradual rate. The *maturation phase* begins when no increase in collagen occurs and lasts for months until the scar becomes flat, white, and inactive. Interestingly, the scar replacing normal dermis never completely regains the same strength as dermis, but instead reaches about 80 percent of the original skin strength.[2]

INFLAMMATORY PHASE

Vascular Response

After injury, the signals initiating wound repair start immediately. The inflammatory phase (also called lag phase) is essentially a preparatory phase that helps prepare the wound for repair. The major function is to rid the wound of foreign tissue and start the inflammatory reaction to help fight infection. The first part of the lag phase is the vascular response, where the main task is to stop hemorrhage. Release of local mediators, such as catecholamines (epinephrine and norepinephrine), produces vasoconstriction for the first 5 to 10 minutes to shut down blood flow. At the same time, collagen and other molecules exposed after tissue damage activate platelets and initiate the clotting cascade to prevent further bleeding (Fig. 5–2). Damage to cell membranes activates enzymes that stimulate synthesis of prostaglandins and leukotrienes, which participate in the immediate response to injury. After approximately 10 minutes, local tissue cells, the cells lining blood vessels (endothelial cells), and serum release mediators that increase permeability in postcapillary venules. Endothelial cells contract in response to these mediators, especially histamine, to create gaps between these cells and allow for leakage of macromolecules into the local tissue (Table 5–1).[3–6] The increased permeability and edema formation appear to occur in two phases. Initial edema formation is completed within minutes and is probably due to histamine and other local mediators.[7,8] A second increase in permeability that continues for hours is caused by other mediators (see Table 5–1).[9–13]

Cellular Response

All the local vascular changes set the stage for the next phase of the inflammatory phase of wound healing, the *cellular response.* The cellular response is essentially a controlled form of inflammation. Vasodilation and increased permeability allow easier access for inflammatory cells to enter the injured tissue. Current research is concentrating on how the information that an area of the body has been injured is communicated to these cells. Cellular communication is performed by various proteins, called *cytokines,* that act as chemical messengers. Cytokines are released from damaged or activated cells, and the surrounding tissues, and then diffuse out to other cells. When cytokines bind to receptors on the responding cells, messages are sent to the intracellular structures, especially the nucleus, to change the actions of that cell. The messages sent to responding cells vary according to the type of cytokine and the type of cell receiving the message. One type of message directs the cell to go toward the highest concentration of the cytokine, which in this case is the injured tissue. This type of directed movement is called *chemotaxis* and is the main way that inflammatory cells are attracted to the wound. After inflammatory cells arrive at the site of injury, they adhere to the cellular lining of the local capillaries and migrate through the vessel wall into the wound by a process called *diapedesis.* The injury induces endothelial cells to produce proteins that act as "adhesion molecules" to bind

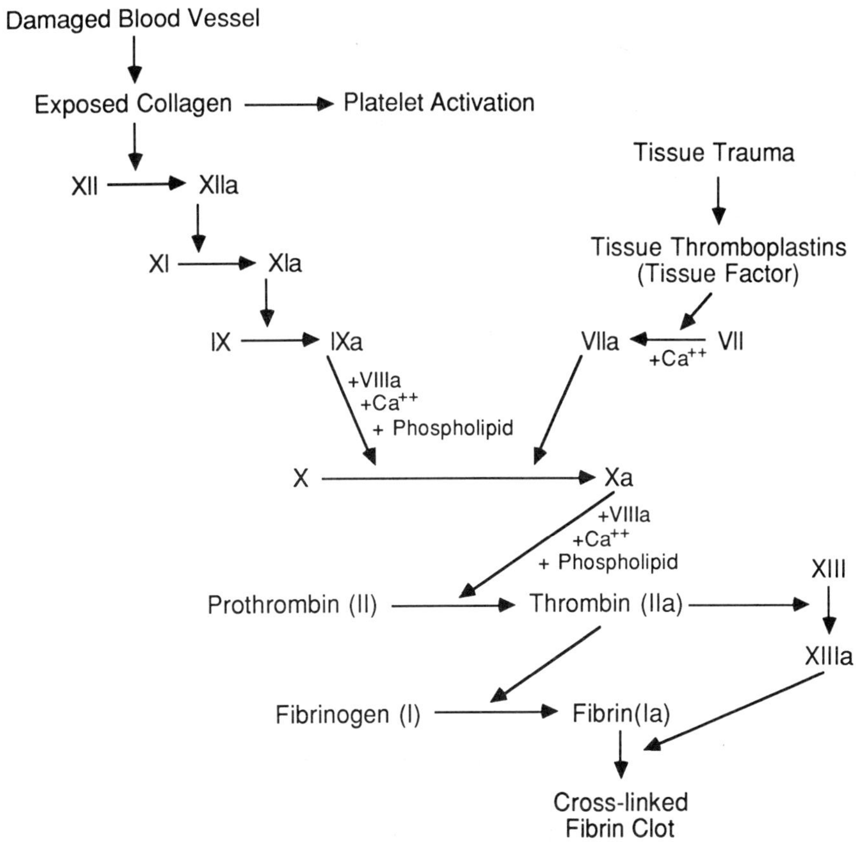

FIGURE 5–2. The clotting cascade is intimately involved with the initiation of wound healing. Several different products attract the cells involved in the healing process. The end product, fibrin, weakly holds the wound together and acts as a scaffold for cell migration. The Roman numerals correspond to the different factors (proteins) involved in the cascade.

TABLE 5–1. Mediators of the Vascular Response to Injury

Local Response	Mediator
Vasoconstriction	Epinephrine, norepinephrine, prostaglandins, serotonin, leukotrienes
Vasodilation	Histamine, prostaglandins, kinins, nitric oxide, and others
Early increase in permeability (early edema)	Histamine, serotonin, kinins, prostaglandins
Late increase in permeability (late edema)	Leukotrienes, platelet activating factor, complement fragments, and others
Platelet activation	Exposed collagen, ADP, prostaglandins, thrombin, immune aggregates
Initiation of clotting cascade	Exposed collagen, tissue thromboplastin, endotoxin, interleukin-1, Hageman factor

with other specific adhesion molecules on the surface of white blood cells to make them adhere so that diapedesis can occur.

An important subclass of cytokines, called *growth factors,* stimulate cells to divide and proliferate. Many types of growth factors have been found to play a major role in wound healing by attracting cells into the wound and stimulating their proliferation. The proteins also stimulate other cells to increase extracellular matrix protein synthesis (Table 5-2). The release of growth factors and other cytokines occurs within seconds of injury. Platelets carry many proteins in vesicles called *alpha granules,* which assist in hemostasis when they are released on contact with damaged tissues. The alpha granules have been found to contain many different types of growth factors.

Platelets are not the only part of the clotting cascade that help in the initiation of wound healing. Thrombin also has been shown to have growth factor activities and may potentiate the effects of other growth factors. Fibrin and its by-products not only attract neutrophils and macrophages, but fibrin and another protein called fibronectin act as the "glue" to hold the wound together until the appearance of collagen. Because these proteins have relatively weak binding capabilities, incisions have almost no strength, hence the origin of the name "lag phase." Migrating cells use the fibrin and fibronectin as scaffolding to migrate into the wound. If too much fibrin is depos-

TABLE 5-2. Growth Factor Actions Related to Wound Healing

Growth Factor	Action Related to Wound Healing
Platelet-derived growth factor (PDGF)	Chemotaxis: fibroblasts, smooth muscle cells, monocytes?, neutrophils? Mitogen: fibroblasts, smooth muscle cells, chondrocytes Increased collagen, collagenase, and GAG synthesis
Basic fibroblast growth factor (bFGF)	Chemotaxis: endothelial cells, fibroblasts Mitogen: endothelial cells, fibroblasts Angiogenesis is major function Increased collagenase and proteinase production
Epidermal growth factor (EGF)	Enhanced motility of epithelial cells Mitogen: all epithelial cells (keratinocytes), endothelial cells Angiogenesis Increased hyaluronic acid production Increased proteinase inhibitor production
Transforming growth factor-alpha (TGF-α)	Enhanced epithelial migration Mitogen: epithelial cells (keratinocytes) Angiogenesis
Transforming growth factor-beta (TGF-β)	Chemotaxis: monocytes, fibroblasts Mitogen: fibroblasts Inhibits proliferation: keratinocytes, endothelial cells, and many other cell types Enhances differentiation of keratinocytes Increased collagen, fibronectin, GAG production Inhibits breakdown of extracellular matrix
Insulin like growth factor I, II (IGF-I, IGF-II)	Mitogen: fibroblasts and other cells, mostly through synergistic actions with other growth factors

ited, cells have difficulty entering the wound. The white, "cheesy" layer that is commonly seen on the surface of burns is actually a combination of fibrin and the topical antimicrobial agent (silver sulfadiazine). The fibrinous layer of chronic wounds or burns is debrided to assist in cellular migration and improve wound healing.

Tissue injury activates several serum mediators that also attract inflammatory cells into the wound. Leukocytes and bacterial breakdown products are both strong stimuli for neutrophil migration into a wound.[14-16] If infection develops, the continued release of these mediators leads to an excessive number of neutrophils that if allowed to accumulate become pus.

Early studies of wound histology revealed a consistent sequence of cell migration into the wound. Neutrophils came first, followed by macrophages and lymphocytes, and after a few days fibroblasts appeared. After the emergence of fibroblasts, the wound appeared to develop collagen and tensile strength. At the same time as the arrival of fibroblasts, new capillaries invaded the wound. Eventually, the cells seemed to leave the wound in the same order that they arrived.

In the mid-1970s researchers concentrated on determining which cell types played important roles in wound healing. Simpson and Ross[17] eliminated neutrophils from a wound and demonstrated that unless a wound became infected, healing proceeded without problems. The main function of neutrophils is to fight infection, and they do not appear to be an important regulator of wound repair. By eliminating macrophages and monocytes, Leibovich and Ross[18] were able to markedly impair wound healing. Several other investigators have confirmed that macrophages are key regulators of wound repair.[19-23] Macrophages appear to be the ideal cell for regulating wound repair since they appear in the wound soon after injury and remain until the wound nears maturity. Macrophages are one of the few cells that are able to survive in the harsh environment of a wound. They can live with very low oxygen and high lactate levels. They also produce many growth factors and cytokines that act to stimulate and also inhibit wound healing. Macrophages also produce collagenases to help break down collagen and probably participate in the regulation of collagen deposition.

The role of lymphocytes in wound repair is less clear. An early study demonstrated that eliminating lymphocytes did not alter wound repair.[24] More recent studies suggest that lymphocytes probably do influence wound repair by producing many substances that have the potential to influence the actions of macrophages and fibroblasts.[25-28] Lymphocytes also produce factors that may play a role in inhibiting cellular proliferation and collagen production. The *interferons,* especially gamma interferon, are one of the classes of messengers sent from lymphocytes that may act as negative-feedback mechanisms to limit the amount of collagen produced in the wound.[29-32] The most likely scenario is that all of the cell types have complex interactions that regulate the healing process. These interactions not only stimulate the healing process but also turn off the inflammatory and healing processes when they are no longer needed. When these cellular communications go awry, such complications as fibrosis, hypertrophic scars, or keloids may develop. Essentially, the cells do not get the message to stop the scarring process, and without negative feedback the production of collagen continues beyond its need. An understanding of these complex interactions is in development. The eventual goal of scar management will be to understand the mechanisms that control wound healing well enough to have some control over it.

Classical Components of Inflammation

All the classical components of inflammation (redness, heat, swelling, and pain) can be observed in this early phase of wound healing. The erythema (redness) and local warmth (heat) are caused by the local vasodilation, and edema (swelling) results from the increased permeability caused by the response to local injury. Pain is also caused by the release of local mediators that activate local pain nerve fibers. The inflammatory response prepares the injured tissue for the reparative processes of the next phase.

PROLIFERATIVE PHASE

In addition to cleaning the wound of debris and fighting infection, a major role of the inflammatory phase is to attract fibroblasts into the wound. Once the fibroblasts arrive and produce collagen, the proliferative phase begins. The various interactions between the inflammatory cells persist after the arrival of fibroblasts, but the focus of this phase is to create new collagen for improving the strength of the wound. During this phase, the breaking strength of an incision increases in proportion to the amount of collagen formed in the wound (see Fig. 5–1). Much of the discussion in this section will concentrate on how collagen and other components of the extracellular matrix are produced. The other important aspect of this phase is called *angiogenesis,* or re-creation of a blood supply. Revascularization is needed to supply the oxygen and nutrients to allow for the synthetic activities of the fibroblasts.

Extracellular Matrix

The main components of extracellular matrix (ECM) include collagen, elastin, and GAGs.[33,34] Collagen is an extremely strong fibrous material that creates the strength of tissue. Elastin is another fibrous but elastic protein that gives the elastic characteristics to tissue. GAGs are a class of molecules that consist of a protein core with polysaccharides attached to them. They are the "ground substance" that "fill in" the spaces between collagen, elastin, and cells. These substances are all produced by fibroblasts during the proliferative phase. The combination of new and loosely organized collagen, other proteins, GAGs, the cells of tissue repair, and new capillaries is called *granulation tissue.* Granulation tissue is the red and moist tissue that is seen in the bottom of wounds that have been open for a period of time. Granulation tissue acts as the precursor to the formation of scar tissue.

Collagen Biosynthesis

The predominant protein found in scar is collagen. Peacock[33] states that greater than 50 percent of the protein in repair tissue may be collagen. Collagen biosynthesis is a complex process that starts with the creation of peptide chains of repeating amino acid triplets inside the fibroblast (Fig. 5–3). Three peptide chains then intertwine to form a helix. The small glycines allow for tight α-helix formation and the prolines in the X positions stabilize the helix. The hydroxyl groups on the hydroxyprolines, occupying the Y positions, create intramolecular bonds between three α-helices to form a "superhelix" of procollagen. After the procollagen molecules are secreted from the cell, the propeptide ends are cleaved to form insoluble tropocollagen molecules. The tropocollagen molecules line up and intermolecular bonds form to further stabilize the microfibrils. Microfibrils combine to form fibrils that in turn weave to create collagen fibers. Detailed reviews that give excellent descriptions of collagen biosyn-

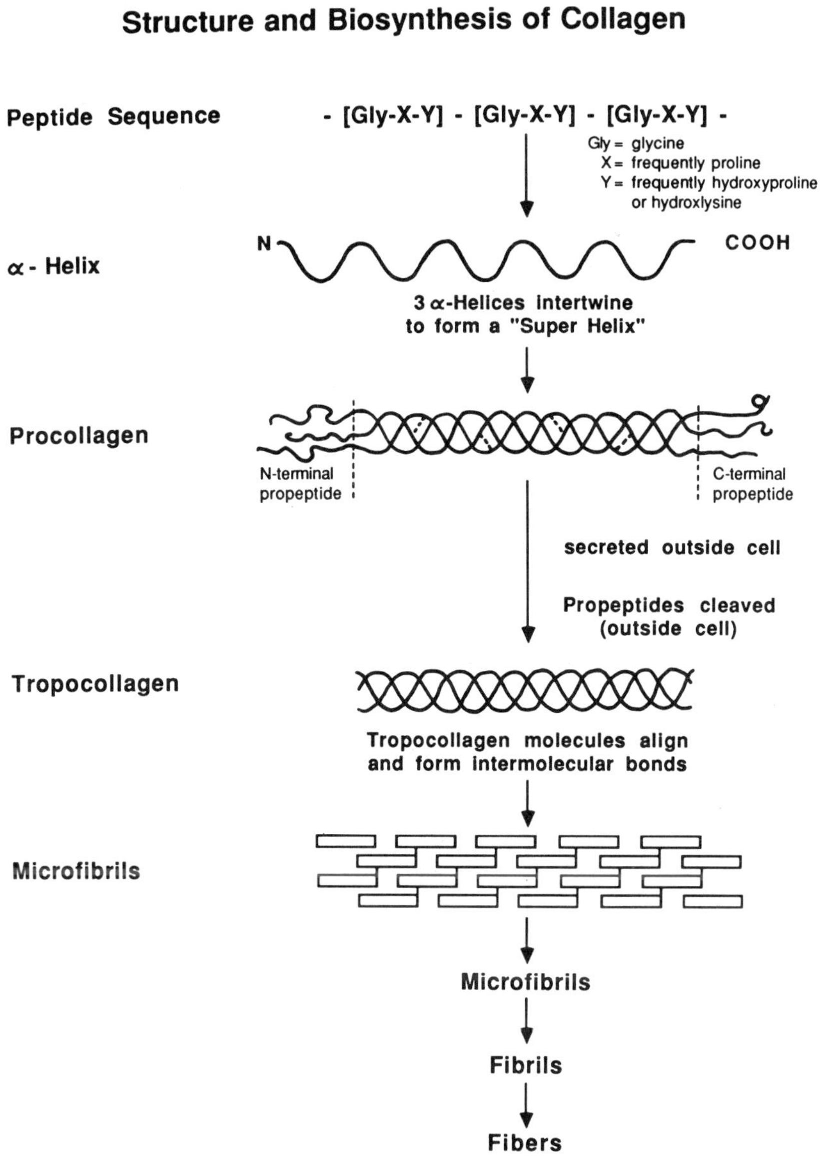

FIGURE 5–3. Illustration of collagen biosynthesis.

thesis are available.[34-40] All forms of collagen (there are at least 10 types) have characteristics that are unique to the collagen family (Table 5–3). The most striking characteristic is the presence of high amounts of hydroxyproline and hydroxylysine, which are the amino acids proline and lysine with the addition of a hydroxyl group (—OH). The "hydroxylated" amino acids are rarely found outside of collagen molecules and are important for creating cross-linkages that increase the strength of the molecule. The addition of the hydroxyl group is one of the most important steps in the biosynthesis of collagen. The enzyme controlling the reaction, protocollagen hydroxylase or prolyl/lysyl hydroxylase, requires oxygen, ascorbic acid (vitamin C), ferrous iron (Fe^{2+}) and α-ketoglutarate to function (Fig. 5–4). Fibroblasts that lack oxygen, iron, or

TABLE 5–3. Types of Collagen

Type	Localization in Tissue
I	Dermis, tendon, bone, scar, other tissues
II	Cartilage
III	Dermis, cardiovascular, and gastrointestinal systems
IV	Basement membranes of all tissues
V	Lamina reticularis of muscle, skin; basal lamina of kidney, lung, and other organs
VI	Lamina reticularis of dermis and other tissues
VII	Anchoring fibrils of skin
VIII	Endothelial cells, ligamentum nuchae fibroblasts
IX	Cartilage
X	Cartilage

vitamin C produce abnormal collagen that leads to impaired healing, such as scurvy for vitamin C deficiency. Other nutrients are important for different biosynthetic steps, and healing abnormalities related to these nutrient deficiencies will be discussed later.

Angiogenesis

The other important component of the proliferative phase of wound healing is the creation of a new blood supply called *angiogenesis*. Angiogenesis may begin as early as 1 to 2 days after wounding, but primarily occurs during the proliferative phase. Initially, the wound has a relatively hypoxic environment. The lack of oxygen stimulates inflammatory cells to utilize the glycolytic pathway for energy, and the end product is lactic acid. Both hypoxia and lactic acid stimulate macrophages to release "angiogenic factors" that help initiate the ingrowth of new capillaries.[41] Angiogenic factors stimulate endothelial cells to release substances, probably collagenases, that break down the postvenule basement membrane. Endothelial cells then detach and migrate toward the angiogenic stimulus. As the cells migrate, they form a line of endothelial cells called a capillary "sprout." These cells proliferate in the venule and the sprout to form a column of cells that eventually develops a lumen. When two sprouts anastomose to each other, they form a capillary loop that is capable of transporting blood. The endothelial cells synthesize a new basement membrane and, finally, supporting cells or pericytes grow around the new blood vessel.[42]

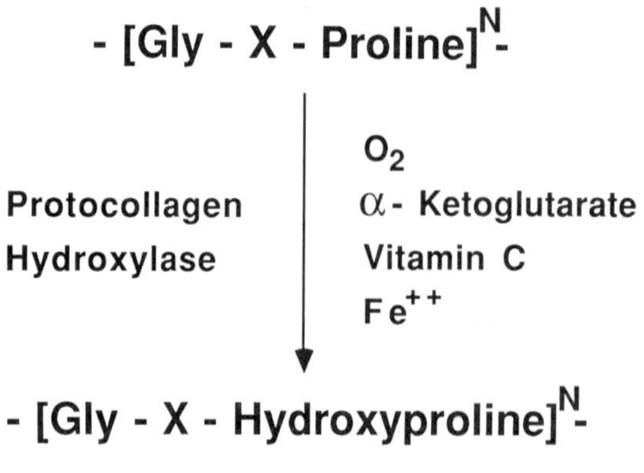

FIGURE 5–4. Hydroxylation of proline is a key regulatory step in the biosynthesis of collagen.

MATURATION PHASE

Scar Maturation

In the final phase of scar formation, the strength of the wound continues to improve but the actual collagen content does not change (see Fig. 5–1). Measured collagen content does not change because a dynamic balance is developed where collagen synthesis equals collagen degradation. The scar eventually becomes less erythematous, flattens, and appears to "mature," thus the name maturation phase. This phase begins after a few weeks and may last for years. The final phase ends when the wound becomes pale and stops changing in form. The number of cells in the wound markedly decreases, but a few cells always remain. Fibroblasts continue to produce collagen, but other cells, including macrophages, fibroblasts, endothelial cells, and others secrete collagenases, elastases, and other proteolytic enzymes that break down extracellular matrix proteins. Wound tensile strength continues to increase because collagen fibers are aligned along lines of stress. Most fibers that are not stressed are degraded while new fibers are synthesized in areas of increased tension. During the maturation phase more cross-linkages between collagen molecules are formed to increase the strength without increasing the quantity of collagen. By microscopic evaluation, collagen fibers are much smaller in the fresh wound when compared to more mature wounds.[43] Initially, more type III collagen is present in the scar, but with maturation, more of the collagen is replaced by type I. The other extracellular matrix proteins also are modified in the maturation phase.

Resolution of Inflammation

Another main component of the maturation phase of scar formation involves the resolution of inflammation and angiogenesis. Much more is known about what initiates the healing process than what turns it off. First, the stimulus for inflammation has to be eliminated to stop production of any cytokines. When the wound becomes vascularized, the elevated levels of oxygen and normalized lactic acid levels remove the stimulus for release of angiogenic factors by macrophages.[44] When the wound is covered with epithelial cells, the stimulus for creating granulation tissue seems to dissipate. Keratinocytes, the cells that make up the majority of epidermis, have been found to release a factor that inhibits fibroblast growth.[45] Macrophages and lymphocytes similarly release cytokines that have inhibitory actions on inflammatory cells and fibroblasts.[25,26,28] Although many interactions are probably involved, cytokines (transforming growth factor-β and the interferons) are likely candidates for the downregulation of the healing process.[29,46,47] Edema fluid is resorbed and excess debris gradually is consumed by phagocytic cells. Eventually, the number of cells and the vascularity of the wound decrease to the point where a mature wound is dominated by collagen fibers and little else.

Pathologic Scar Formation

During scar formation, altered regulation of the reparative processes can lead to abnormal healing. A wound that for any reason fails to become covered with epithelium will continue to have an inflammatory reaction. With chronic inflammation wounds develop thick, exuberant granulation tissue that essentially consists of disorganized collagen, neutrophils, macrophages, and capillaries. Clinically, the granulation tissue, commonly called "proud flesh," is red, friable, and raised. Wounds that remain unhealed longer are susceptible to developing thicker and more erythematous scars. Partial-thickness burn wounds that take longer to heal will lead to thicker and redder scars than those that heal faster. The prolonged exposure to the environment leads to a greater inflammatory reaction, which tends to potentiate the stimulus for collagen synthesis and angiogenesis. The thickening of "hypertrophic" scars appears to result from an imbalance of collagen synthesis and degradation.[48-50] When hypertrophic scars become even larger and seem to grow beyond the boundary of the original wound they are called *keloids*. Extensive efforts have been devoted to differentiating between hypertrophic scars and keloids. For practical purposes, they can be considered differences along the continuum of collagen production/degradation imbalance. For the most part, the cause of hypertrophic scarring is unknown. Certainly, different people with the same wound and time for healing will have completely different degrees of scarring. Differences in split-thickness donor site scarring exemplify this point. Some patients heal with nearly invisible donor sites, while others develop unsightly keloids. The differences appear to be somewhat related to ethnic heritage, age, and the site of the wound. As stated previously, anything that prolongs the healing process seems to predispose the wound to an increased tendency for hypertrophic scarring. Anything that causes a persistence in the inflammatory process probably also contributes to excessive scarring. Chronic scratching of a wound frequently will cause small breaks in the epithelial barrier, lead to persistent inflammation and more scarring. Excessive tension on the wound is another factor that seems to potentiate scarring, probably by causing minute amounts of damage and persistent inflammatory activation. All of the hypotheses, however, do not explain all of the quirks of hypertrophic scarring.

Epithelialization

FUNCTION AND ANATOMY OF EPIDERMIS

The second important function of wound repair is to re-create the epithelial barrier. An epithelium is any aggregate of cells that group together to form a protective barrier over a large surface.[51] For the purpose of this review, the epidermis will be used as the representative epithelial tissue, but re-epithelialization of all tissues is similar. Epidermis functions to protect the underlying tissues from invasion of microorganisms and prevents the loss of bodily fluids. Covering open wounds, such as burns, with new epithelium is one of the major goals in wound repair. The epithelium alone, however, lacks durability and thus needs to be associated with the resiliency of dermis or scar. If only the epidermis and superficial dermis are damaged, as in partial-thickness burns or split-thickness donor sites, then only epidermal regeneration is vital. When both epidermis and dermis are destroyed, as in full-thickness burns, then the regeneration of a dermal-like base (scar tissue) and re-epithelialization are both important. Placing only cultured keratinocytes on full-thickness wounds results in a barrier that lacks durability and blisters easily.

Epidermis is composed of many different layers of cells (Fig. 5–5). The bottommost layer, called the basal layer, contains the most undifferentiated cell type. The basal cells are the cells that proliferate to replace epidermal cells that die. As the cells move farther away from the basal layer, they become more differentiated and eventually die to produce a keratinized layer called the stratum corneum. The stratum corneum thickens in response to stress to produce calluses.

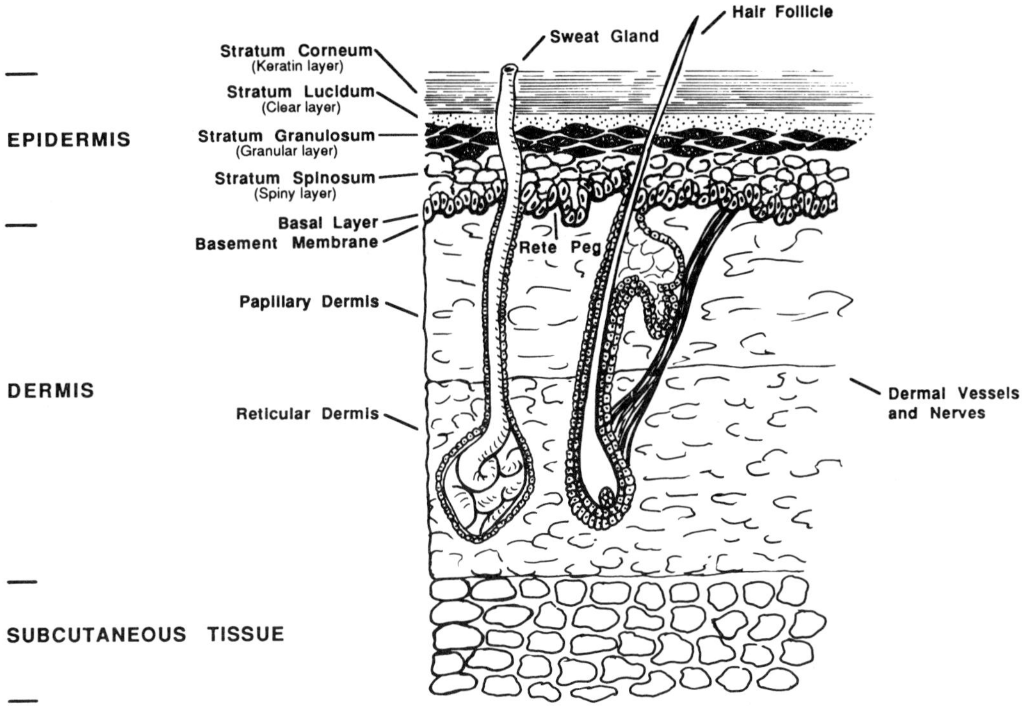

FIGURE 5–5. Anatomy of the skin. Normal skin has an epidermis that is composed of five layers. The basement membrane separates the dermis from the epidermis. The cells of the epidermal basal layer continue into the dermis as they line the hair follicles and other skin appendages.

BASEMENT MEMBRANE

To act as a barrier, epidermal cells have to bind tightly to each other and to the tissue beneath them. Junctions, called *desmosomes,* form between the keratinocytes, and hemidesmosomes help bind the cells to the dermis. The actual binding of the basal layer to the dermis is quite complex, but a knowledge of this binding is helpful in understanding several aspects of epidermal healing. Basal cells attach to a complex of extracellular matrix proteins called the basement membrane. By electron microscopic analysis, the basement membrane is composed of a *lamina lucida,* a lucent layer adjacent to the basal layer. The next layer is electron dense and therefore is called the *lamina densa.* A *sub-lamina densa zone* or *lamina fibroreticularis* lies just above the dermis. The biochemical makeup of each of these layers is beginning to become elucidated and is depicted in Figure 5–6.[52–54] Toxic epidermal necrolysis (TEN) and *Staphylococcus aureus*-scalded skin syndrome are two examples where a toxin causes disruption of the bonds between the dermis and epidermis. These patients suffer from sloughing of their epidermis. Normally the epidermis and dermis do not bind together in flat sheets. They coapt through a series of hills and valleys called "rete pegs" that help prevent shear injuries between the two layers. After a partial-thickness burn injury, the new epithelium grows across the dermis in a flat sheet that lacks resistance to shear. Therefore, healed partial-thickness burns or donor sites are prone to blistering until the rete pegs redevelop.

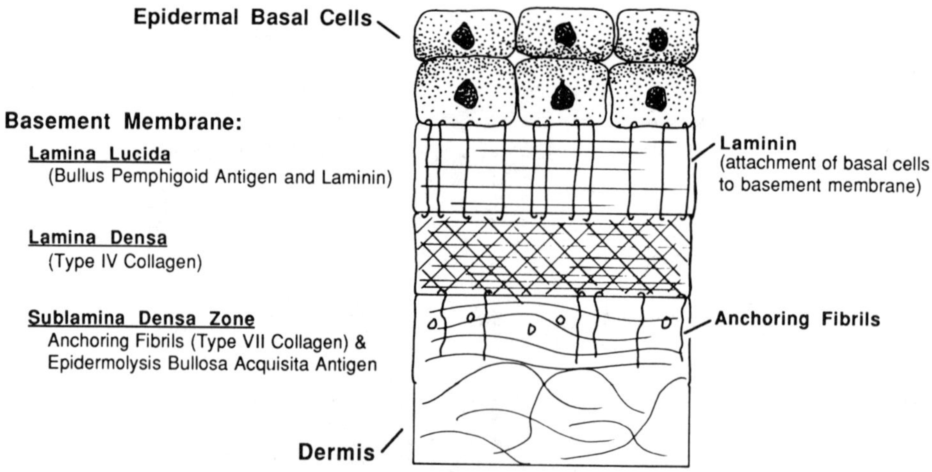

FIGURE 5–6. Structure of the basement membrane at the epidermal-dermal junction. The basement membrane is composed of a lamina lucida that attaches the basal cells to the next layer called the lamina densa. Anchoring fibrils in the sub-lamina densa bind the type IV collagen of the basement membrane to type I collagen in the dermis.

EPIDERMAL REGENERATION

If the epithelium is injured but the basement membrane is spared, the basal cells increase their rate of proliferation and migrate away from the basement membrane to replace those lost. If the basement membrane is damaged, the basal cells on the edge lose cell-cell contact and become exposed to the proteins (fibrin; fibronectin; types I, III, and IV collagen) of the wound. In vitro studies reveal that loss of cell-cell contact inhibition and the proteins commonly found in wounds are all stimuli for keratinocyte migration.[52,54,55] At the same time, macrophages and other cells in the wound release several growth factors, such as epidermal growth factor, transforming growth factor α, and transforming growth factor β that also stimulate keratinocyte migration and proliferation.[56–58] Cells on the wound edge migrate, but do not proliferate, while the cells inside the wound edge divide to replace the cells that travel. The cells at or just above the basal layer on the wound margin flatten in the direction of the wound and change form to allow motility. The desmosomes, hemidesmosomes, and basement membrane attachments dissolve and the cells start migrating across the wound bed. When the cells migrate, they maintain connections with the cells behind them so that they close the wound as a sheet. One hypothesis is that the cells leading the migration attach to the exposed collagen, fibronectin, and fibrin to pull themselves over the wound bed in what is called the *sliding model*.[52,55,59] The other hypothesis is called the *leapfrog* or *rolling model* of epithelial travel.[52,55,59] Because the epidermal cells travel as a multilayered unit, the leading cells may attach and the cells just behind them roll over these leading cells to attach to the wound surface. Although the actual mechanism of cellular motion is not known, both models probably apply in different situations.

Epithelial cells secrete enzymes, such as collagenases and other proteases, during their migration. Woodley et al.[52,55] suggest that the leading edge of the migrating cells attaches to the exposed damaged tissue. As the cell pulls itself over the wound surface, collagenases are needed to allow detachment so that the cells can continue to migrate. Collagenases and other proteases are also important since the cells need to migrate on live, moist tissue. When the wound is exposed to air a scab is formed. Epithelial cells have to digest the bonds between the scab and the viable tissue using these enzymes in order to re-epithelialize the wound. The scab will fall off after the epithelial cells have covered the wound and broken all the bonds holding the scab in place. Several studies have demonstrated that epithelial closure is faster if the wound remains moist and no scab forms,[60–62] which is a rational for keeping a wound moist instead of allowing it to dry. Donor sites, for example, heal faster if they are kept moist with saline-soaked gauze or bathed in their own fluids as under a biologic dressing than if allowed to dry after being covered with fine-mesh gauze.

Once the epithelial cells from all sides of the wound meet in the middle, migration stops by a process called *cell-cell contact inhibition*. The actual messages that tell a keratinocyte to stop migrating are not known. Possibly growth factors or other cytokines are released upon contact to "tell" the leading cells to stop migrating and start proliferating. The keratinocytes proliferate and differentiate to reproduce a stratified and keratinized epithelium. Once the epithelium covers a wound, the inflammatory process seems to decrease rapidly. Eisinger et al.[45] have shown that extracts from epidermal cells, called *epidermal cell–derived factors* (EDF), inhibit fibroblast function. In vitro studies[45] demonstrated that EDF inhibited fibroblast-induced contraction in collagen sponges. Clinically, a burn wound that is covered faster with new epithelium appears to scar less than those that remain open for longer periods. Eventually, the new epithelium resembles the original epidermis except that all of the epithelial appendages, such as hair follicles and sweat glands, are never regenerated in a full-thickness injury. The epithelial cells lining the appendages extend far below the dermal-epidermal junction. In a partial-thickness injury, the appendages not only survive but provide many sources for new epithelial buds. As the epithelial cells migrate out of the appendages, they can be seen as the white dots on the surface of a healing partial-thickness injury (Fig. 5–7). The epithelial cells lining the appendages explain why a person can heal a large partial-thickness burn.

Wound Contraction

MECHANISMS OF WOUND CONTRACTION

During wound contraction, the edges migrate toward the center to "shrink" the wound. The extent of contraction is dependent on the looseness of the surrounding skin. Rodents have very mobile and redundant skin and therefore close 90 percent of their wounds with contraction. The same is true in humans but to a lesser degree. Areas of loose skin, such as in the buttock region, will contract nicely, but less mobile areas, such as over the ankle, cannot contract as much. Contraction is independent of epithelial migration and relies on the presence of wound granulation tissue. Results from several studies have shown that removal of granulation tissue in the middle of a wound will temporarily halt contraction until more granulation tissue develops.[63-65] Collagen production is not necessary since wounds in guinea pigs that are deficient in vitamin C still contract.[66] Many aspects of contraction parallel scar formation. A contracting wound has a "lag phase" that is followed by a relatively rapid decrease in wound size, which in turn is followed by a period of slower contraction until closure (Fig. 5–8). The lag phase correlates with the entry of fibroblasts into the fresh wound

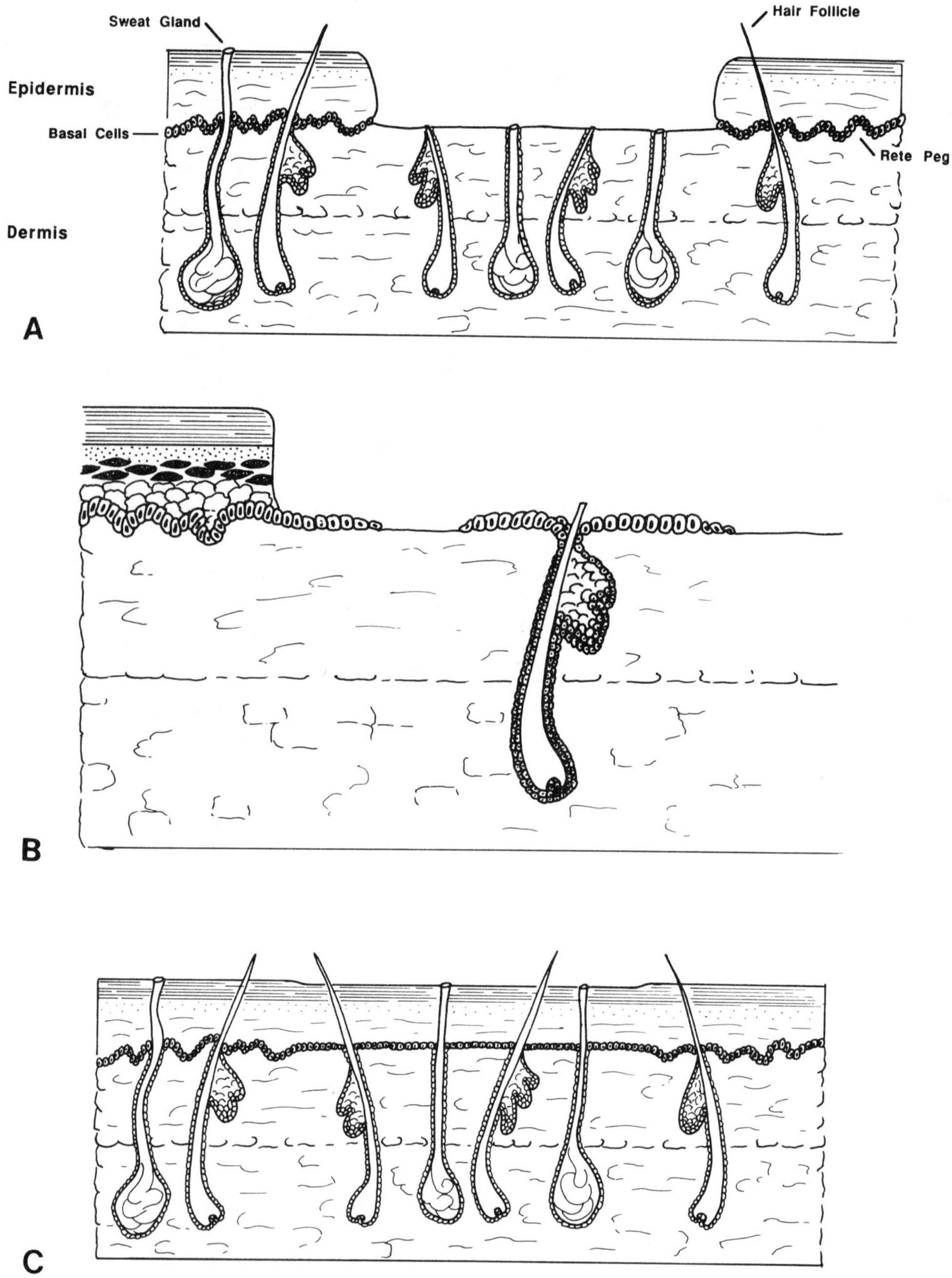

FIGURE 5–7. (*A*) After a partial-thickness injury, some of the dermis and its skin appendages remain. (*B*) The basal cells adjacent to the wound and in the appendages lose cell-cell contact inhibition and migrate across the viable wound surface. Migrating cells are replaced by proliferating basal cells at the wound edge and in the appendages. (*C*) After migrating epidermal cells meet, cell-cell contact inhibition stops migration. Basal cells differentiate to re-create the different layers of the epidermis. The healed skin blisters easily because rete pegs do not redevelop for several months.

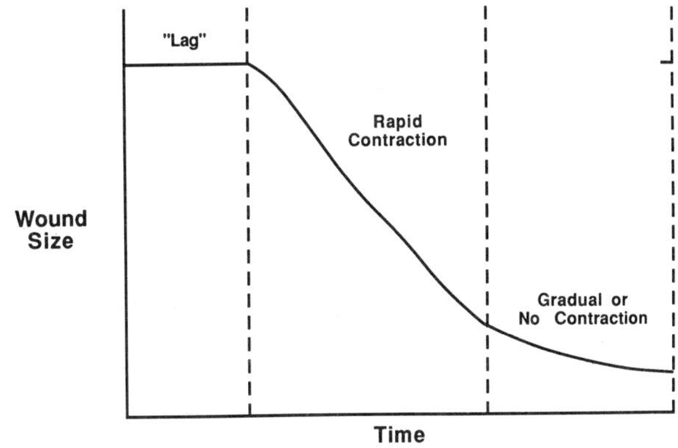

FIGURE 5–8. The rate of wound contraction varies in a manner similar to the phases of scar formation. A lag phase lasts a few days as the fibroblasts enter the wound. Rapid contraction takes place for the next few weeks as the contractile cells shrink the wound. Finally, a phase of gradual or no change in wound size completes contraction.

and fibroblasts appear to be the cells responsible for wound contraction. Electron microscopic evaluation of granulation tissue reveals a population of cells that have musclelike components (myosin and actin). These cells have been called *myofibroblasts* because they resemble both muscle cells and fibroblasts.[67] All fibroblasts have the capability to develop contractile elements; therefore, myofibroblasts are probably just a variant of fibroblasts.[68] Contraction occurs rapidly and usually is completed in 2 to 3 weeks. Collagen synthesis frequently continues long after contraction has been completed.

Several theories have been developed to explain the mechanisms of wound contraction. The two most accepted hypotheses are called the *picture frame* theory and the *pull* theory.[69,70] In the picture frame hypothesis, the cells in the wound margin migrate toward the middle of the wound and pull the wound edge with it. To support this hypothesis, Watts, Grillo, and Gross[71] removed granulation tissue up to 0.5 to 1.0 mm from the wound edge and did not notice any decrease in the rate in wound closure. Excising the wound edge for only 0.5 mm stopped contraction. The other theory, the pull hypothesis, suggests that the granulation tissue inside the wound exerts tension on the wound edge and pulls it toward the middle. Support for this theory came from experiments where contracting wounds were splinted open. When the splint was removed, the wound would contract rapidly unless the central portion of the granulation tissue was excised.[72] Measurements of wound tension were also determined and declined to zero if the central granulation tissue was excised.[73] These two hypotheses are unimportant because all of the fibroblasts extending from the central aspect of the wound to the wound margin probably participate.

WOUND CONTRACTURE

A distinction must be made between wound contraction and wound contracture. *Wound contraction* involves the active movement of wound edges over the wound surface and is a process that is completed in a few weeks. *Wound contracture* is the shrinkage of a scar through the process of collagen remodeling. Contractures develop over the entire maturation phase of scar formation and therefore can intensify over months. Both processes probably involve the contractile properties of fibroblasts but are unrelated at least in timing after wounding.

TYPES OF WOUND CLOSURE

Primary Closure

In any discussion of wound healing different types of wound repair should be defined. A wound that is reapproximated by suture or tape is called a *primary closure.* Any wound that is closed primarily has to be relatively free of contamination and debris or else it will become infected. The longer a wound is left open, the greater the chance of infection. The risk of infection also is dependent on the blood supply to the area. A vascular area is more resistant to infection than an avascular region, which is why closure of most wounds is inadvisable after 6 to 8 hours following injury, except in regions around the face where the increased vascularity affords more protection. The vascularity of the rectal region also explains why wounds (i.e., hemorrhoids) can be closed primarily in the presence of significant bacterial contamination. Clearly there are cosmetic advantages to a primary closure, which will result in a narrow linear scar.

Closure by Secondary Intent

If a wound is contaminated, primary closure increases the risk for wound infection. To prevent infection, or if closure of a wound is not desirable for other reasons, allowing the wound to granulate and re-epithelialize is called *healing by secondary intent.* By keeping the wound open and frequently covering the wound with any moist dressing, the bacterial numbers are kept in check. To maximize healing, saline is used to allow for the best environment for epithelial closure. Any fibrinous exudate or necrotic tissue that collects will interfere with epithelial travel and needs to be debrided. If granulation tissue grows excessively, producing a heap of raised and dark red tissue, the tissue should be trimmed back either sharply or with silver nitrate cauterization to the level of epithelial travel. Epithelial cells have difficulty "climbing over" these raised areas of "proud flesh." Healing by secondary intent takes more time and usually produces a more unsightly scar than primary closure, but the wound generally does not become infected. For example, when a patient suffers a small full-thickness electrical burn on a finger tip, grafting and primary closure are not possible. These wounds are allowed to heal by secondary intent and usually do fine. They may, however, require weeks to heal.

Delayed Primary Closure

A compromise between the above methods is called a *delayed primary closure.* A wound felt to be contaminated, such as after performing an escharotomy, can be treated initially by secondary intent to eliminate the excess bacteria. After a few days of treating the open wound, the wound then can be closed primarily. Interestingly, waiting a few days does not impair the strength of the wound but instead may even enhance wound strength.[74] Apparently, the time the wound is left open corresponds to the lag phase, so the wound becomes "primed" while being left open.

Skin Grafting

For large, open surface defects such as after full-thickness burns, normal healing processes are incapable of closing the wound expeditiously. Tissue has to be transferred from another source to cover the wound. The simplest form of transfer is skin grafting. The healing of skin grafts can be divided into three phases[75,76] (Fig. 5–9). The first, the phase of serum imbibition, begins immediately after placing the graft on the wound bed.[77] Because there are no vascular connections, nutrients are supplied by diffusion of serum from the bed. The graft is held in place only by weak fibrin and fibronectin bonds. Penetration of new capillaries into the graft marks the phase of revascularization. After 24 to 48 hours, endothelial cells start migrating into the graft and form new capillaries in a process similar to angiogenesis in other wounds. Investigators also have found evidence that some of the newly formed capillaries can connect directly to capillaries remaining in the graft in a process called *inosculation*.[78] Most likely, however, the major portion of revascularization involves ingrowth of new capillaries and not inosculation. Complete clinical revascularization takes 4 to 6 days. Maintaining the delicate vascular connections until the graft becomes more firmly attached is important because any shearing between the two will lead to bleeding, hematoma formation, and frequently graft loss. Therefore, most grafted areas are immobilized initially with stents or splints. The phase of organization starts at about 4 days when fibroblasts migrate into the graft. The fibroblasts then lay down collagen along the fibrin scaffolding to increase the resistance of the graft to shearing. Unless supported by immobile dressings, the graft is too delicate to allow movement of the wound bed until after 5 days when enough collagen bridges have formed to increase resistance to shear. The graft then matures in a manner that parallels wound scar maturation as described earlier. Collagen within the graft and the collagen binding the graft to the bed align along lines of stress, and unneeded collagen is degraded. The process of maturation is quite vascular, leading to the appearance of redness in recent grafts. Eventually, the extra vascularity and fibroblast number decline to produce a graft that resembles normal skin. Just like scar maturation, graft maturation requires months for completion.

Flaps

Other forms of tissue transfer are used to cover large surface defects. Flaps involve transferring tissue that contains its own blood supply. Because they do contain a blood supply, flaps are effective in covering areas that are relatively avascular (over bone and tendon), where skin grafts are ineffective.[79] Flaps also are thicker than skin grafts because skin, subcutaneous tissue and sometimes muscle are transferred. The edges of the flap heal by primary intent to the edges of the new wound bed. Since the entire thickness of tissue will not survive from diffusion of nutrients from the wound bed, the flap requires a blood supply from the portion that remains attached. This blood supply must be adequate enough to maintain viability in the distal flap until primary closure is complete. At this time, dermal vessels will invade the distal flap to maintain viability.

A local flap involves moving tissue to a neighboring wound by rotating, advancing, or transposing the tissue. Part of the skin has to remain attached to maintain its

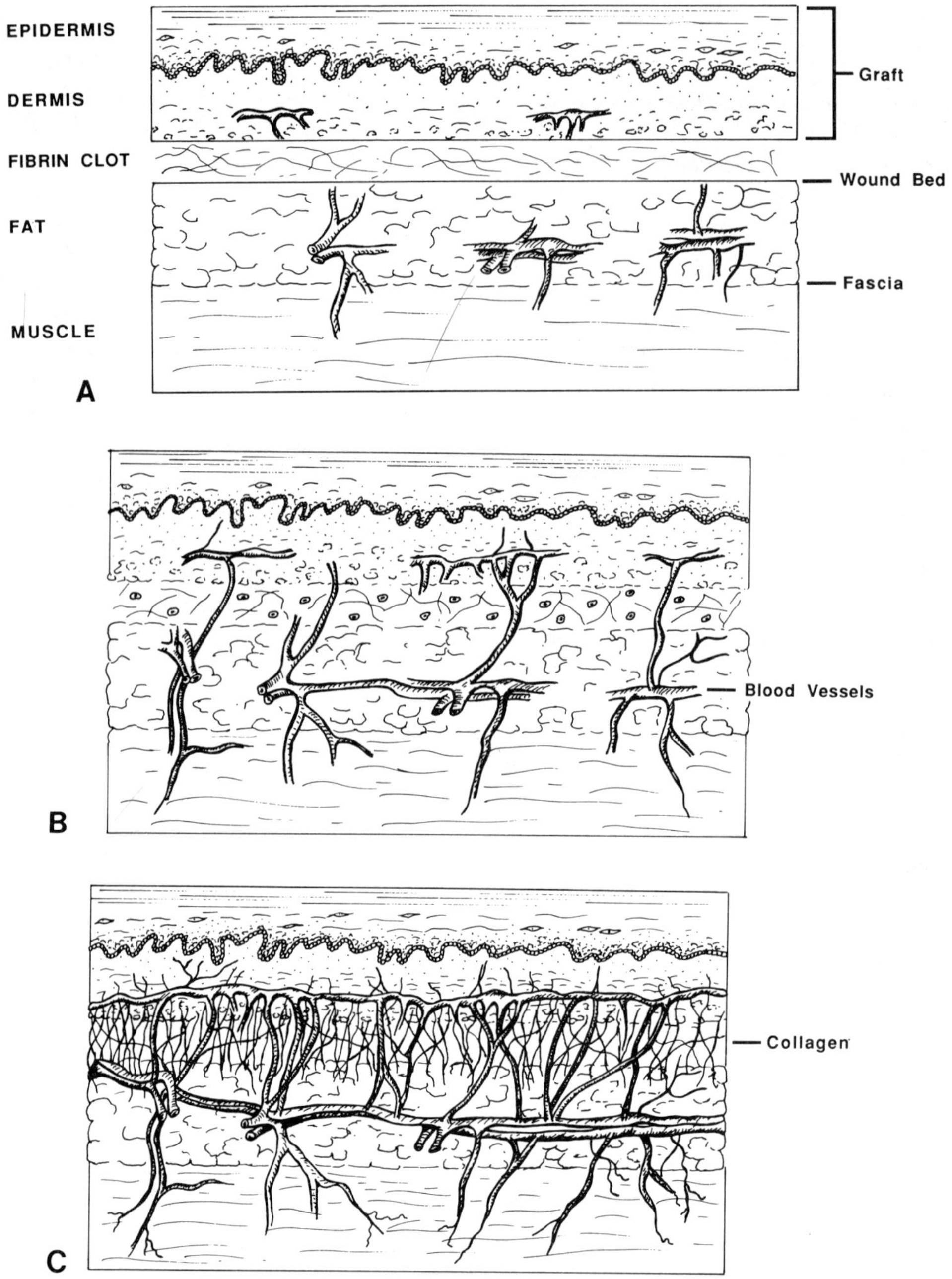

FIGURE 5–9. The healing of skin grafts involves three phases: (*A*) In the phase of serum imbibition the graft sticks on the wound bed by weak fibrin bonds. The cells survive by diffusion of nutrients from the wound bed. (*B*) At 24–48 hours, new capillaries start invading the skin graft, marking the phase of revascularization. (*C*) The phase of organization starts at 4–5 days when collagen linkages are made between the wound bed and the graft to create firm attachments.

blood supply. Many local flaps are supplied only by the dermal plexus in what is called a "random" blood supply. The base of the flap, that part remaining attached, has to be relatively wide compared to the length of the flap or the tip will die. A local flap, such as a groin flap, also can have its blood supplied by a single, larger vessel, which permits a longer flap in relation to the base. The blood supply is based on an "axial" pattern. Other flaps are based on the knowledge that the muscle underlying a region of skin is supplied by a limited number of blood vessels. Myocutaneous flaps are based on this blood supply and allow transfer of muscle, fat, and skin as a unit. Current microsurgical techniques allow for these myocutaneous units to be disconnected from their vasculature and reconnected to arteries and veins at distant sites. These free flaps allow for coverage of large defects in areas where local transfers are not possible, especially in the distal extremities and head. The more difficult techniques require extensive skill in microvascular and plastic surgery.

Meshed Skin Grafts

Very large surface areas of open wounds, such as in major burns, make rapid coverage difficult. Skin grafts that are placed as a sheet are superior as far as cosmesis is concerned but require an equally large area of donor skin. For covering larger areas, donor skin can be "meshed" to allow for varying amounts of expansion. Usually skin is meshed 1.5:1 or 3:1 to cover relatively large areas. Two types of healing occur with meshed grafts. The donor skin attaches and adheres just like any graft. The interstices heal by re-epithelializing over granulation tissue. The larger the mesh, the more the graft heals by secondary intent and the greater the extent of scarring. Because meshed grafts heal by these two processes, the meshed pattern persists as a permanent scar. If possible, placing a graft as a sheet results in the least scarring and the closest resemblance to noninjured skin.

FACTORS AFFECTING WOUND HEALING

This section will briefly describe several factors that either beneficially or adversely affect wound repair. These factors should be kept in mind when evaluating any patient with a healing impairment. Clinically, most healing failures involve some form of host impairment such as infection; malnutrition; diabetes; or treatment with steroids, chemotherapy, or radiation. Any attempt to prevent healing complications or to improve healing should concentrate on the causes of the impairment.

Age

Age affects many aspects of wound repair. Overall, the rate of healing appears to slow with increasing age. Several investigators have documented that fibroblasts proliferate at a slower rate in older animals and individuals.[80-82] Older cells also have decreased synthetic capability. The characteristics of collagen also change in elderly skin. Soluble collagen decreases while insoluble collagen increases.[80] The amount of elastin increases but the number of elastic fibers decreases to make skin less elastic.[80]

With decreasing GAGs older skin loses its ability to retain water and tends to be thin and wrinkle.[80] Wound contraction also proceeds at a slower rate in the elderly.[83-84]

The depth of a burn is dependent on four factors: (1) the temperature of the contacting agent, (2) the duration of contact, (3) the thickness of the skin, and (4) the blood supply of the skin. Elderly patients tend to have deeper burns because they have thinner skin and a poorer blood supply that lends to a decreased ability to dissipate heat. The elderly also tend to have altered sensation and may not sense pain as well, or lack the quickness to stop the burning process leading to prolonged exposure to the heat.[85-86] Burns in the elderly take longer to heal but they tend to scar less than younger patients. The looser and thinner skin allows for less resistance to contraction. The thinness of the skin may account for a full-thickness donor site being created accidentally when the intention was to harvest a partial-thickness donor site.

There is recent interest in healing in the very young and even in fetal healing. Young animals appear to form granulation tissue faster than adults and have more rapid gain in incisional strength than adults.[87] Their wounds also have more rapid fibroblast proliferation and greater collagen synthesis.[88] Although some feel that younger animals scar less than adults,[82] the amount of scarring in children relative to human adults is less clear and needs to be studied. Infants and children suffering from burns do develop significant scarring that is not obviously different from that seen in adults. Clearly, scars do not enlarge as the rest of the body grows. Even if a scar is not a functional problem when a child is young, the scar fails to lengthen as the rest of the body grows and may result in a contracture. An infant usually requires several contracture releases until growth has been completed. Interestingly, wound repair in fetuses has been examined and appears to result in minimal scarring.[89] Possibly, in the earlier stages of life, wound healing more closely resembles tissue regeneration seen in simpler animals.

Infection

Although infection classically has been associated with wound healing problems, not all bacterial contaminations are harmful. The effects of infection on tissue repair can be divided into its local or systemic effects. As early as 1916, Carrel and Hartmann[90] found that infection in the wound impaired wound contraction. Since then, many other investigators have demonstrated that wound infections impair healing.[91-94] Bucknall[95] examined the effects of several different species of bacteria and found that *Pseudomonas* followed closely by *Staphylococcus aureus* produced the greatest reduction in wound bursting strength.[95] Clinically, these two organisms are the most common contaminants of burn wounds and clinical experience suggests that the combination of *Pseudomonas* and *Staph. aureus* is the most common cause of skin graft loss. In contrast, just as many investigators have found that localized infections improve wound repair. Tenorio et al.[96] improved incisional tensile strengths with 10^8 to 10^9 *Escherichia coli, Pseudomonas, Proteus mirablis,* and *Streptococcus fecalis* singularly or in combination. Other investigators found similar improvements with *E. coli*[97] and different strains of *Staph. aureus.*[98-101]

Why does there seem to be such a discrepancy? The most likely explanation is that bacterial contamination leads to an increased inflammatory response with release of more cytokines to attract more of the cells needed for wound repair. If, however, the wound becomes overwhelmed with virulent microorganisms, then bacterial proteases and the products of inflammatory cells lead to local tissue damage. Since bacteria are never eliminated from a wound, especially a burn wound, the goal of wound management is to use topical antimicrobials to keep the bacterial numbers at a low enough level to prevent impaired healing and systemic invasion.

Studies show that the host's response to infection may be as important as the infection itself in influencing healing.[102-107] An infection near or distant from the wound alters systemic metabolic activity and nutritional intake and can alter healing. The hypermetabolic activity seen in burn patients is at least partially caused by the inflammatory response in the wound. Long-term responses also are influenced. Burn wounds that become infected but eventually do heal frequently scar more than those wounds that heal rapidly. The increased scarring probably results from the increased inflammatory response caused by the infection.

Nutrition

PROTEIN AND CALORIE DEPLETION

As previously alluded to, nutrition is of extreme importance in wound healing. Malnutrition can be divided into total protein and calorie deficiency (marasmus) or just protein insufficiency (kwashiorkor). Total starvation producing protein-calorie malnutrition is relatively obvious, demonstrated by weight loss and muscle wasting. Protein insufficiency alone is less obvious. People who eat foods high in fat and carbohydrates but deficient in proteins are frequently obese but nonetheless malnourished and at risk for healing complications. As early as 1942, protein depletion was found to impair healing[108] and several studies support this finding.[109-111] Total protein-calorie malnutrition also impairs many aspects of healing.[112] Even partial starvation beginning after the wound has been created can significantly weaken an incision and may be at least a partial explanation of healing impairments related to burns and infection.[107]

Patients with large burns develop a hypermetabolic state that can approach twice that of an unburned person. Despite aggressive attempts at nutritional supplementation, burn patients frequently lose weight and have signs of malnutrition. The increased metabolic needs along with the associated immunosuppression increase the risk for wound healing complications in burn patients. One of the major breakthroughs in burn patient survival has been made possible through aggressive nutritional support. Starting nutritional support as soon as possible after injury helps to prevent wound healing problems.[113-115] Bozetti, Terno, and Longoni demonstrated that hydroxyproline levels were lower in wounds of patients given low-protein and low-calorie fluids when compared to those patients given intravenous nutritional supplementation.[116] Current standards of therapy dictate that patients with any significant signs of malnutrition be given nutritional supplementation prior to any surgical procedure if at all feasible. A weight loss of approximately 20 percent should alert the clinician to increased risk of wound repair complications.

VITAMINS

Some vitamins are clearly important for normal tissue repair (Table 5–4). Vitamin C has already been discussed as being vital to normal collagen synthesis. The dy-

TABLE 5–4. The Effects of Vitamins on Wound Healing

Vitamin	Action Related to Wound Healing
C	Required for protocollagen hydroxylase function. This intracellular enzyme creates intramolecular bonds between collagen α-helices. Deficiency (scurvy) results in abnormal collagen synthesis, markedly weakened wounds, and scar breakdown.
A	Induces fibroblast differentiation and increased collagen synthesis. It counteracts the ill effects of steroids and local radiation on wound healing.
E	The role of this superoxide scavenger in wound healing is uncertain. Some studies suggest that vitamin E may inhibit healing.
B_1 (thiamine)	Required for normal cell energy metabolism. Thiamine deficiency may inhibit wound healing.
B_5 (pantothenic acid)	Required for metabolism of carbohydrates, proteins, and fats. Pantothenic acid deficiency may inhibit wound healing.

namic balance of collagen breakdown and synthesis persists after maturation of the wound and can explain why old scars break down in diseases such as scurvy. With severe vitamin C deficiency, collagen synthesis stops but collagenases continue to degrade the collagen until scars weaken to the point of disruption.[117] The other important vitamin that has significant effects on healing is vitamin A. Several investigators have reported that feeding animals extra vitamin A may reverse healing impairments caused by various factors.[118-121] Vitamin A induces fibroblasts to differentiate and increase collagen synthesis.[122] Topical application of vitamin A also may improve healing.[123] The role of other vitamins in tissue repair is less clear. Vitamin E is frequently applied topically on healing burn wounds, but actual studies do not support its role in improving healing and some suggest that vitamin E impairs healing.[124-126] Thiamine and pantothenic acid are other vitamins that may result in impaired healing when deficient.[127,128]

TRACE ELEMENTS

Deficiencies in trace elements also may cause clinical healing problems (Table 5-5). These trace elements are actually metals that are needed for enzyme functions. Iron already has been discussed as being required for the hydroxylation of proline and lysine in collagen synthesis, but levels do not become low enough to alter collagen synthesis until anemia becomes life threatening. Anemia, at levels consistent with life, has not been found to impair wound repair. Zinc is an element that is required for about 120 enzyme reactions.[129] Many of the reactions necessary for DNA and RNA synthesis require zinc, so that any deficiency leads to decreased proliferative capabilities and impaired protein synthesis. More specifically, zinc in low or excessively high levels decreases the activity of lysyl oxidase, an enzyme required for the cross-linking between collagen molecules.[130] Interestingly, zinc also is involved in the activity of collagenase. Several investigations have demonstrated that zinc deficiency leads to impaired wound healing.[131-136] Copper is another trace metal that is essential to reparative processes. Lysyl oxidase contains and requires copper for its actions in cross-linking collagen molecules.[137,138] Manganese is needed for the addi-

TABLE 5–5. The Effects of Trace Elements on Wound Healing

Trace Element	Action Related to Wound Healing
Iron	Required for protocollagen hydroxylase function. This intracellular enzyme creates intramolecular bonds between collagen α-helices. Anemia has to become severe before wound healing is affected.
Zinc	Required for numerous enzyme reactions, including DNA and RNA synthesis. Zinc is required for proliferation of the reparative cells. It also is necessary for lysyl oxidase function, the enzyme responsible for intermolecular collagen bond formation (between tropocollagen molecules) and is important in scar maturation.
Copper	Required for lysyl oxidase activity to form intermolecular collagen cross-linkages. As with zinc, copper is important for collagen maturation.
Manganese	Required for galactosyl and glucosyl transferase, which add carbohydrate side chains to collagen α-helices. These carbohydrates stabilize collagen molecules.
Calcium*	Required for the endopeptidases that cleave the nonhelical ends (propeptides) from procollagen to form tropocollagen. Calcium has numerous other physiologically important functions.
Magnesium*	Required for enzymes that participate in protein synthesis. Magnesium has many other activities that are related to those of calcium.

*Calcium and magnesium are electrolytes that exist in relatively high concentrations in the body and are not really "trace elements."

tion of carbohydrates to proteins and may affect collagen synthesis and cartilage growth.[139,140] Although shortages in trace elements may contribute to impaired healing, these are unusual cases. For most healthy patients that consume a relatively normal diet, shortages in these metals are unusual.

Oxygen

Physicians have known for centuries that an adequate blood supply is essential for healing wounds. Patients with wounds in areas suffering from poor vascularity frequently fail to heal and are much more apt to require amputation. Re-establishing an adequate blood supply often is needed for healing of these problem wounds. Poor vascularity essentially translates into hypoxia. Oxygen is required to supply the energy for the high metabolic needs of a healing wound. LaVan and Hunt[141] suggest that oxygen may be the rate-limiting substrate in many wounds. As stated earlier, oxygen is required for the hydroxylation of proline and lysine in collagen synthesis (see Fig. 5–4). At the low levels of oxygen observed in wounds (PO_2 between 0 and 50 mm Hg) the hydroxylation reaction is proportional to the oxygen delivery.[142] Fibroblasts that are cultured in a hypoxic environment tend to have the same abnormalities in collagen synthesis as those seen in vitamin C deficiency.[143] The tensile strength of wounds has been found to be proportional to the oxygen delivery to a wound.[144,145]

The delivery of enough oxygen to a wound depends not only on blood oxygen levels but also on the perfusion to the wound. When blood volume decreases, the body compensates for the insufficiency by limiting blood flow to less necessary tissues. The selective vasoconstriction that funnels blood preferentially to vital organs, such as the brain and heart, is essential to survival during any form of shock. One of the first tissues to be sacrificed is the skin. Unfortunately, the skin is the most common site of wounds and burns. Inadequate perfusion frequently causes healing abnormalities and may increase the extent of injury.[146] Burns may become deeper if patients are inadequately resuscitated during burn shock. Inadequate resuscitation leads to poor perfusion and ultimately to insufficient oxygen delivery to the burned tissues.

Oxygen is so essential to healing that some researchers have felt that high levels of oxygen may be even more beneficial. The treatment of wounds with hyperbaric oxygen is based on this hypothesis. Several noncontrolled studies suggest that hyperbaric oxygen improves healing,[147–152] but just as many have found no improvement[144,153–155] (see Chapter 15). Although oxygen is needed for healing, the efficacy of delivering high levels is not clear. High levels of oxygen may lead to the formation of oxygen free radicals that have the potential to damage tissues.[156] High oxygen levels have been associated with pathologic scarring.[157] The question of whether a high level of oxygen in the wound improves healing needs to be resolved.

Diseases Causing Impaired Wound Healing

Diabetes mellitus is well known as being associated with altered healing.[158–166] The causes of healing problems in diabetics are multifactorial and complex.[167,168] Diabetes is associated with increased vascular insufficiency involving vessels ranging from large arteries to the capillaries. Even when palpable pulses are present, microvascular disease may contribute to altered oxygen and nutrient delivery to a wound. Secondly, diabetic neuropathy allows for small injuries to go unnoticed and become chronic. Finally, diabetic wounds are less likely to resist infections, and as a result diabetics are more likely to require amputations than nondiabetics. Adequate glucose control has been shown to improve healing[159,169] and several animal models suggest that growth factors have the potential to improve diabetic healing.[166,170–173]

Other chronic diseases are associated with wound healing problems. Chronic renal failure and liver failure predispose patients to impaired healing.[165] Malignancy also contributes to healing abnormalities, probably by indirectly competing for nutrients.[174,175] Any disease that is associated with malnutrition will predispose the patient to abnormal healing.

Other Causes of Impaired Healing

STEROIDS

Several common drugs impair tissue repair. The most notorious drugs associated with altered healing are steroids. Steroids are powerful inhibitors of the inflammatory response and therefore are potent inhibitors of healing.* Collagen synthesis and fibrosis also are inhibited with steroid use.[176,179] The effects of steroids on healing have been shown to be at least partially reversed with vitamin A[118] or growth factors.[179–181]

*References 118, 123, 176–178.

CHEMOTHERAPY AGENTS

Chemotherapy agents act by killing rapidly growing cells with the hope of eliminating proliferating cancer cells. Unfortunately, the healing wound also requires cellular proliferation. Several investigators have reported that most forms of chemotherapy agents given locally or systemically impair healing.[182–187] As with other toxic substances, nutritional alterations may contribute to the impairment.[188] Topical application of recombinant growth factors has been found to reverse some healing abnormalities.[189,190]

RADIATION

The healing impairment found after acute radiation exposure also is due to inhibition of proliferating cells.[185,191,192] As for other healing impairments, vitamin A or growth factors may ameliorate the altered healing.[120,193] Delayed healing or even chronic wounds may result from previous radiation therapy. Radiation may cause a chronic vasculitis that impairs local blood supply and predisposes the patient to impaired healing.[191,192] Chronic wounds in areas of previous radiation are extremely difficult to manage.

DRUGS THAT ALTER THE IMMUNE SYSTEM

Drugs that alter the immune system also may affect healing through the interactions of macrophages, lymphocytes, and fibroblasts. Drugs used for immunosuppression are essential for organ or tissue transplantation but may alter healing. Cyclosporine has been found to impair healing in higher doses,[194] but in lower doses had no effect.[195] This finding is important since some institutions are treating patients with large burns with allografts and cyclosporine to prevent graft rejection.[196]

FUTURE GOALS

A great deal is now known about the cellular controls of wound repair, and every day more is discovered about the actual molecular aspects of healing. This knowledge is being used to determine ways to improve healing through the use of recombinant cytokines such as growth factors. Animal models clearly indicate that healing impairments can be reversed and that to some extent healing can be stimulated.* Clinical studies using growth factors are being performed and preliminary findings are encouraging.[207–209] In the burn field, studies have demonstrated improvements in healing relatively small donor sites, but the benefit has not been great[210] and already has been disputed.[211] The stimulated healing of small donor sites is not of clinical value since they heal so fast. Of greater importance would be to accelerate the healing of donor sites in patients with large burns so that the donor site could be reharvested faster. Growth factors do have the potential to help in this situation and also may be of value for improving skin graft adherence.

Another area of current interest in burns is the development of skin substitutes. Much progress already has been made, but skin substitutes still lack the durability

*References 166, 170–173, 179–181, 189–190, 193, 197–206.

and resistance to infection that autografts possess. In the future, skin substitutes may not only have a closer resemblance to skin but may even contain pigment and skin appendages.

Burn care has advanced to the point of greatly improving the survival of burn patients. The next goal is to improve the cosmetic and functional results of the survivors. A great deal is known about how to improve healing, but little is known about inhibiting excessive healing. Extensive investigation is needed to understand the cellular and molecular controls of what turns off healing. Hopefully the control of scarring then will be possible.

SUMMARY

The mechanisms of wound healing have been described down to the cellular and molecular level. The three types of wound repair: scar formation, epithelialization, and wound contraction have been reviewed separately but, in actuality, they proceed simultaneously. Scar formation involves three phases that start with an inflammatory phase that is characterized by cellular migration and proliferation. The proliferative phase is dominated by collagen deposition and angiogenesis, and finally, the maturation phase involves resolution of inflammation and scar maturation. The regeneration of the epidermis involves migration of keratinocytes across the wound bed and re-creation of the basement membrane. The theories of how fibroblasts or myofibroblasts cause wound contraction has been reviewed. The difference between wound contraction and contracture was emphasized.

The strategies for closing wounds ranging in size from a small incision to the entire surface of the body were described. Many factors can adversely affect wound healing. Age and infection are important factors to remember when trying to heal a wound. Nutritional factors including protein and calorie intake as well as vitamins and trace elements are extremely important. Many obstacles to adequate healing include impaired oxygenation; diabetes; chronic diseases; or treatment with steroids, chemotherapy agents, radiation, or drugs that affect the immune system. Dealing with these problem wounds is a major goal for health care providers. Many of these healing difficulties are being overcome by new and exciting techniques.

REFERENCES

1. Mast, BA: The skin. In Cohen, IK, Diegelmann, RF, and Lindblad, WJ (eds): Wound Healing. Biochemical and Clinical Aspects. WB Saunders, Philadelphia, 1992, pp 344–355.
2. Peacock, EE, Jr: Wound Repair, ed 3. WB Saunders, Philadelphia, 1984, p 108.
3. Peacock, EE, Jr: Wound Repair, ed 3. WB Saunders, Philadelphia, 1984, pp 2–7.
4. Williams, TJ: Factors that affect vessel reactivity and leukocyte emigration. In Clark, RAF and Henson, PM (eds): The Molecular and Cellular Biology of Wound Repair. Plenum Press, New York, 1988, pp 115–147.
5. Bergstrom, S, et al: Observations on the effects of infusion of prostaglandin E in man. Acta Physiol Scand 45:145–151, 1959.
6. Majno, G, Shea, SM, and Leventhal, M: Endothelial contraction induced by histamine type mediators: An electron microscopic study. J Cell Biol 42:647–672, 1969.
7. Williams, TJ and Morley, J: Prostaglandins as potentiators of increased vascular permeability in inflammation. Nature (Lond) 246:215–217, 1973.
8. Moncada, S, Ferreira, SH, and Vane, JR: Prostaglandins, aspirin-like oedema of inflammation. Nature (Lond) 246:217–219, 1973.
9. Voelkel, NF, et al: Nonimmunological production of leukotrienes induced by platelet activating factor. Science (USA) 218:286–288, 1982.

10. Lin, AH, Morton, DR, and Gorman, RR: Acetyl glyceryl ether phosphorylcholine stimulates leukotriene B_4 synthesis in human polymorphonuclear leukocytes. J Clin Invest 70:1058–1065, 1982.
11. Hahn, F and Oberdorf, A: Antihistaminica and anaphylaktoide. Z Immunitaetsforsch 107:528–538, 1950.
12. Foreman, JC, et al: Structure-activity relationships for some substance-P related peptides that cause wheal and flare reactions in human skin. J Physiol (Lond) 335:449–465, 1983.
13. Williams, TJ: Vasoactive intestinal polypeptide is more potent than prostaglandin E2 as a vasodilator and oedema potentiator in rabbit skin. Br J Pharmacol 77:505–509, 1982.
14. Snyderman, R, Phillips, J, and Mergenhagen, SE: Polymorphonuclear leukocyte chemotactic activity in rabbit serum and guinea pig serum treated with immune complexes: Evidence for C5a as the major chemotactic factor. Infect Immun 1:521–525, 1970.
15. Ford-Hutchinson, EW, et al: Leukotriene B, a potent chemokinetic and aggregating substance released from polymorphonuclear leukocytes. Nature (Lond) 286:264–265, 1980.
16. Showell, HJ, et al: The structure-activity relations of synthetic peptides as chemotactic factors and inducers of lysosomal enzyme secretion for neutrophils. J Exp Med 143:1154–1169, 1976.
17. Simpson, DM and Ross, R: The neutrophilic leukocyte in wound repair: A study with antineutrophil serum. J Clin Invest 51:2009–2023, 1972.
18. Leibovich, SJ and Ross, R: The role of the macrophage in wound repair. A study with hydrocortisone and antimacrophage serum. Am J Pathol 78:71–100, 1975.
19. Leibovich, SJ and Ross, R: A macrophage-dependent factor that stimulates the proliferation of fibroblasts *in vitro.* Am J Pathol 84:501–513, 1976.
20. Clark, RA, et al: Role of macrophages in wound healing. Surg Forum 27:16–18, 1976.
21. Korn, JH, Halushka, PV, and LeRoy, EC: Mononuclear cell modulation of connective tissue function. J Clin Invest 65:543–554, 1980.
22. Diegelmann, RF, Cohen, IK, and Kaplan, AM: The role of macrophages in wound repair: A review. Plast Reconstr Surg 68:107–113, 1981.
23. Riches, DWH: The multiple roles of macrophages in wound healing. In Clark, RAF and Henson, PM (eds): The Molecular and Cellular Biology of Wound Repair. Plenum Press, New York, 1988, pp 213–239.
24. Morris, PJ and Burke, JF: Antilymphocyte serum and Staphylococcal infection. Nature (Lond) 214:1138–1139, 1967.
25. Wahl, SM, Wahl, LM and McCarthy, JB: Lymphocyte-mediated activation of fibroblast proliferation and collagen production. J Immunol 121:942–946, 1978.
26. Wahl, LM and Wahl, SM: Lymphokine modulation of connective tissue metabolism. Ann NY Acad Sci 332:411–422, 1979.
27. Fishel, RS, et al: Lymphocyte participation in wound healing: Morphologic assessment using monoclonal antibodies. Ann Surg 206:25–29, 1987.
28. Barbul, A: Role of T cell-dependent immune system in wound healing. Prog Clin Biol Res 266:161–175, 1988.
29. Jimenez, SA, Freundlich, B, and Rosenbloom, J: Selective inhibition of human diploid fibroblast collagen synthesis by interferons. J Clin Invest 74:1112–1116, 1984.
30. Rosenbloom, J, et al: Inhibition of excessive scleroderma fibroblast collagen production by recombinant gamma-interferon. Arthritis Rheum 29:851–856, 1986.
31. Granstein, RD, et al: The systemic administration of gamma interferon inhibits collagen synthesis and acute inflammation in a murine skin wounding model. J Invest Dermatol 93:18–27, 1989.
32. Granstein, RD, et al: A controlled trial of intralesional recombinant interferon-gamma in the treatment of keloidal scarring. Clinical and histologic findings. Arch Dermatol 126:1295–1302, 1990.
33. Peacock, EE, Jr: Wound Repair, ed 3. WB Saunders, Philadelphia, 1984, pp 56–101.
34. Grant, ME and Prockop, DJ: The biosynthesis of collagen. Part I. N Engl J Med 286:194–199, 1972.
35. Grant, ME and Prockop, DJ: The biosynthesis of collagen. Part II. N Engl J Med 286:242–249, 1972.
36. Grant, ME and Prockop, DJ: The biosynthesis of collagen. Part III. N Engl J Med 286:291–300, 1972.
37. Uitto, J and Lichtenstein, JR: Defects in the biochemistry of collagen in diseases of connective tissue. J Invest Dermatol 66:59–79, 1976.
38. Prockop, DJ, et al: The biosynthesis of collagen and its disorders. Part I. N Engl J Med 301:13–23, 1979.
39. Prockop, DJ, et al: The biosynthesis of collagen and its disorders. Part II. N Engl J Med 301:77–85, 1979.
40. Prockop, DJ and Kivirikko, KI: Heritable diseases of collagen. N Engl J Med 311:376–386, 1984.
41. Folkman, J and Klagsbrun, M: Angiogenic factors. Science (USA) 235:442–447, 1987.
42. Folkman, J: Toward an understanding of angiogenesis: Search and discovery. Perspect Biol Med 29:10–36, 1985.
43. Peacock, EE, Jr: Wound Repair, ed 3. WB Saunders, Philadelphia, 1984, pp 118–120.
44. Knighton, DR, et al: Oxygen tension regulates the expression of angiogenesis factor by macrophages. Science (USA) 221:1283–1285, 1983.

45. Eisinger, M, et al: Growth regulation of skin cells by epidermal cell-derived factors: Implications for wound healing. Proc Natl Acad Sci USA 85:1937–1941, 1988.
46. Massague, J: The TGF-β family of growth and differentiation factors. Cell 49:437–438, 1987.
47. Sporn, MB and Roberts, AB: Transforming growth factor-β. Multiple actions and potential clinical applications. JAMA 262:938–941, 1989.
48. Ketchum, LD, Cohen, IK, and Masters, FW: Hypertrophic scars and keloids. Plast Reconstr Surg 53:140–154, 1974.
49. Ketchum, LD: Hypertrophic scars and keloids. Clin Plast Surg 4:301–310, 1977.
50. Rockwell, WB, Cohen, IK, and Ehrlich, JP: Keloids and hypertrophic scars: A comprehensive review. Plast Reconstr Surg 84:827–837, 1989.
51. Bloom, W and Fawcett, DW: A Textbook of Histology. WB Saunders, Philadelphia, 1975, p 83.
52. Woodley, DT, O'Keefe, EJ, and Prunieras M: Cutaneous wound healing: A model for cell-matrix interactions. J Am Acad Dermatol 12:420–433, 1985.
53. Woodley, DT and Briggaman, RA: Re-formation of the epidermal-dermal junction during wound healing. In Clark, RAF and Henson, PM (eds): The Molecular and Cellular Biology of Wound Repair. Plenum Press, New York, 1988, pp 559–586.
54. Furthmayr, H: Basement membranes. In Clark, RAF and Henson, PM (eds): The Molecular and Cellular Biology of Wound Repair. Plenum Press, New York, 1988, pp 525–558.
55. Woodley, DT, Bachman, PM, and O'Keefe, EJ: The role of matrix components in human keratinocyte re-epithelialization. Prog Clin Biol Res 365:129–140, 1991.
56. Barrandon, Y and Green H: Cell migration is essential for sustained growth of keratinocyte colonies: The roles of transforming growth factor-α and epidermal growth factor. Cell 50:1131–1137, 1987.
57. Hebda, PA: Stimulatory effects of transforming growth factor-beta and epidermal growth factor on epidermal cell outgrowth from porcine skin explant cultures. J Invest Dermatol 91:440–445, 1988.
58. Gherhardi, E, et al: Purification of scatter factor, a fibroblast-derived basic protein that modulates epithelial interactions and movement. Proc Natl Acad Sci (USA) 86:5844–5848, 1989.
59. Stenn, KS and DePalma, L: Re-epithelialization. In Clark, RAF and Henson, PM (eds): The Molecular and Cellular Biology of Wound Repair. Plenum Press, New York, 1988, pp 321–335.
60. Eaglstein, WH: Experiences with biosynthetic dressings. J Am Acad Dermatol 12:434–440, 1985.
61. Dyson, M, et al: Comparison of the effects of moist and dry conditions on dermal repair. J Invest Dermatol 91:434–439, 1988.
62. Bolton, L, et al: Dressings' effects on wound healing. Wounds 2:126–134, 1990.
63. Lindquist, G: The healing of skin defects. An experimental study in the white rat. Acta Chir Scand 94(suppl):163, 1946.
64. Abercrombie, M, Flint, MH, and James, DW: Collagen formation and wound contraction during repair of small excised wounds in the skin of rats. J Embryol Exp Morph 2:264–274, 1954.
65. Montandon, D, D'Andiran, G, and Gabbiani, G: The mechanism of wound contraction and epithelialization. Clin Plast Surg 4:325–346, 1977.
66. Abercrombie, M, Flint, MH, and James, DW: Wound contraction in relation to collagen formation in scorbutic guinea pigs. J Embryol Exp Morphol 4:167–173, 1956.
67. Gabbiani, G, et al: Granulation tissue as a contractile organ. J Exp Med 135:719–734, 1972.
68. Eddy, RJ, Petro, JA, and Tomasek, JJ: Evidence for the nonmuscular nature of the "myofibroblast" of granulation tissue and hypertrophic scar. An immunofluorescence study. Am J Pathol 130:252–260, 1988.
69. Van Winkle, W, Jr: Wound contraction. Surg Gynecol Obstet 116:131–142, 1967.
70. Peacock, EE, Jr: Wound Repair, ed 3. WB Saunders, Philadelphia, 1984, pp 38–55.
71. Watts, GR, Grillo, HL, and Gross, J: Studies in wound healing—II, the role of granulation tissue in contraction. Ann Surg 148:153–160, 1958.
72. Abercrombie, M, James, DW and Newcombe, JF: Wound contraction in rabbit skin. J Anat (Lond) 94:170–182, 1960.
73. Higton, DIR and James, DW: The force of contraction of full-thickness wounds of rabbit skin. Br J Surg 51:462–466, 1964.
74. Johnson, BW, et al: Primary and secondary healing in infected wounds. An experimental study. Arch Surg 117:1189–1193, 1982.
75. Converse, JM and Rapaport, FT: The vascularization of skin autografts and homografts. An experimental study in man. Ann Surg 143:306–315, 1956.
76. Barratt, GE and Koopmann, CF: Skin grafts: Physiology and clinical considerations. Otolaryngol Clin N Am 17:335–351, 1984.
77. Converse, JM, Uhlschmid, GJ, and Ballantyne, DL, Jr: "Plasmatic circulation" in skin grafts. The phase of serum imbibition. Plast Reconstr Surg 43:495–499, 1969.
78. Converse, JM, Smahel, J, and Ballantyne, DL, Jr: Inosculation of vessels of skin graft and host bed. A fortuitous encounter. Br J Plast Surg 28:274–282, 1975.
79. Hidalgo, DA: Plastic surgical reconstruction. In Wilmore, DW, Brennan, MF, Harken, AH, Holcroft, JW, and Meakins, JL (eds): American College of Surgeons: Care of the Surgical Patient. Scientific American, New York, Sec. XI, part 3.

80. Carrel, A and Ebeling, AH: Age and multiplication of fibroblasts. J Exp Med 34:599–623, 1921.
81. Howes, EL and Harvey, SC: The age factor in the velocity of the growth of fibroblasts in the healing wound. J Exp Med 55:577–590, 1932.
82. Chvapil, M and Koopmann, CF, Jr: Age and other factors regulating wound healing. Otolaryngol Clin N Am 15:259–270, 1982.
83. DuNouy, PL: Cicatrization of wounds. III. The relation between the age of the patient, the area of the wound and the index of cicatrization. J Exp Med 24:461–470, 1916.
84. Billingham, RE and Russel, PS: Studies on wound healing, with special reference to the phenomenon of contracture in experimental wounds in rabbit's skin. Ann Surg 144:961–981, 1956.
85. Deitch, EA, Clothier, J: Burns in the elderly: An early surgical approach. J Trauma 23:891–894, 1983.
86. Housinger, T, et al: Conservative approach to the elderly patient with burns. Am J Surg 148:817–820, 1984.
87. Doberaurer, W: Zum einfluss des lebensalters auf die heilung kunstlicher hautdefekte. Klin Med (Wien) 18:199–204, 1963.
88. Schmitt, W and Beneke, G: Untersuchungen der bindegewebsproliferation in verschiedenen levensaltern. Virchows Arch Abt B Zellpath 5:351–364, 1970.
89. Longaker, MT and Adzick, NS: The biology of fetal wound healing: A review. Plast Reconstr Surg 87:788–798, 1991.
90. Carrel, A and Hartmann, A: Cicatrization of wounds. I. The relation between the size of the wound and the rate of contraction. J Exp Med 24:429–450, 1916.
91. Nelson, CA and Dennis, C: Technical factors in the gain of strength in sutured abdominal wall wound in rabbits. Surg Gynecol Obstet 93:461–467, 1951.
92. Smith, M and Enquist, IF: A quantitative study of impaired healing resulting from infection. Surg Gynecol Obstet 125:965–973, 1967.
93. Madden, JE, et al: Studies in the management of the contaminated wound. IV. Am J Surg 119:222–224, 1970.
94. Irvin, TT: Collagen metabolism in infected colonic anastomoses. Surg Gynecol Obstet 143:220–224, 1976.
95. Bucknall, TE: The effect of local infection upon wound healing. Br J Surg 67:851–855, 1980.
96. Tenorio, A, et al: Accelerated healing in infected wounds. Surg Gynecol Obstet 142:537–543, 1976.
97. Raju, DR, et al: A study of the critical inoculum to cause a stimulus to wound healing. Surg Gynecol Obstet 144:347–350, 1977.
98. KanGruber, D, et al: Acceleration of wound healing by a strain of *Staphylococcus aureus*. Surg Forum 31:232–234, 1980.
99. KanGruber, D, et al: Acceleration of wound healing by *Staphylococcus aureus*. Surg Forum 32:76–78, 1981.
100. Levenson, SM, et al: Wound healing accelerated by *Staphylococcus aureus*. Arch Surg 118:310–320, 1983.
101. Laato, M, Niinikoski, J, and Gerdin, B: The effects of *Staphylococcus aureus* bacteria and its products on wound healing. In Wadstrom, T, Eliasson, I, Holder, I, and Ljungh, A (eds): Pathogenesis of Wound and Biomaterial-Associated Infections. Springer-Verlag, London, 1990, pp 25–34.
102. DeHaan, BB, Ellis, H, and Wilks, M: The role of infection on wound healing. Surg Gynecol Obstet 138:693–700, 1974.
103. Hogstrom, H, et al: Influence of intraperitoneal *Escherichia coli* with septicemia on healing of colonic anastomoses and skin wounds. Eur Surg Res 17:128–132, 1985.
104. Freihoffer, U, et al: The effect of bacterial endotoxin on connective tissue growth and wound tensile strength. Surg Forum 11:293–295, 1969.
105. Jacob, R and Houck, JC: A chemical description of inflammation and repair. Surg Gynecol Obstet 109:85–88, 1959.
106. Houck, JC and Jacob, R: Connective tissue. II. Distant dermal response to local inflammation. Proc Soc Exp Biol Med 106:145–147, 1961.
107. Greenhalgh, DG and Gamelli, RL: Is impaired wound healing caused by infection or nutritional depletion? Surgery 102:306–312, 1987.
108. Rhoads, JE, Fliegelman, MT, and Panzer, LM: The mechanism of delayed wound healing in the presence of hypoproteinemia. JAMA 118:21–25, 1942.
109. Daly, JM, Vars, HM, and Dudvich, SJ: Effects of protein depletion on strength of colonic anastomoses. Surg Gynecol Obstet 134:15–21, 1972.
110. Steiger, E, et al: Postoperative intravenous nutrition: Effects on body weight, protein regeneration, wound healing and liver morphology. Surgery 73:686–691, 1973.
111. Irvin, TT: Effects of malnutrition and hyperalimentation on wound healing. Surg Gynecol Obstet 146:33–37, 1978.
112. Temple, WJ, et al: Effect of nutrition, diet and suture material on long-term wound healing. Ann Surg 182:93–97, 1975.

113. Moss, G, et al: Postoperative metabolic patterns following immediate total nutritional support: Hormone levels, DNA synthesis, nitrogen balance and accelerated wound healing. J Surg Res 21:383–393, 1976.
114. Mochizuki, H, et al: Mechanism of prevention of postburn hypermetabolism and catabolism by early enteral feeding. Ann Surg 200:297–310, 1984.
115. Moore, EE and Jones, TN: Benefits of immediate jejunostomy feeding after major abdominal trauma: A prospective randomized study. J Trauma 26:874–881, 1986.
116. Bozetti, F, Terno, G, and Longoni, C: Parental hyperalimentation and wound healing. Surg Gynecol Obstet 141:712–714, 1975.
117. Peacock, EE, Jr: Wound Repair, ed 3. WB Saunders, Philadelphia, 1984, pp 120, 163.
118. Ehrlich, HP and Hunt, TK: Effects of cortisone and vitamin A on wound healing. Ann Surg 167:324–328, 1968.
119. Levenson, SM, et al: Supplemental vitamin A prevents the acute radiation-induced defect in wound healing. Ann Surg 200:494–512, 1984.
120. Winsey, K, et al: Effect of supplemental vitamin A on colon anastomotic healing in rats given preoperative radiation. Am J Surg 153:153–156, 1987.
121. Niu, XT, et al: Effect of dietary supplementation with vitamin A on arterial healing in rats. J Surg Res 42:61–65, 1987.
122. Demetriou, AA, et al: Vitamin A and retinoic acid: Induced fibroblast differentiation in vitro. Surgery 98:931–934, 1985.
123. Smith, KP, Zardiackas, LD, and Didlake, RH: Cortisone, vitamin A, and wound healing: The importance of measuring wound surface area. J Surg Res 40:120–125, 1986.
124. Ehrlich, HP, Tarver, H, and Hunt TK: Inhibitory effects of vitamin E on collagen synthesis and wound repair. Ann Surg 175:235–240, 1972.
125. Kagoma, P, et al: The effect of vitamin E on experimentally induced peritoneal adhesions in mice. Arch Surg 120:949–951, 1985.
126. Greenwald, DP, et al: Zone II flexor tendon repair: Effects of vitamins A, E, β-carotene. J Surg Res 49:98–102, 1990.
127. Alvarez, OM and Gilbreath, RL: Thiamine influence on collagen during the granulation of skin wounds. J Surg Res 32:24–31, 1982.
128. Grenier, JF, et al: Pantothenic acid (vitamin B_5) efficiency on wound healing. Acta Vitaminol Enzymol 4:81–85, 1982.
129. Vallee, BL and Falchuk, KH: Zinc and gene expression. Phil Trans R Soc Lond B 294:185–197, 1981.
130. Peacock, EE, Jr: Wound Repair, ed 3. WB Saunders, Philadelphia, 1984, pp 120, 127.
131. Pories, WJ, et al: Acceleration of wound healing in man with zinc sulfate given by mouth. Lancet 1:121–124, 1967.
132. Pories, WJ, et al: Acceleration of healing with zinc sulfate. Ann Surg 165:432–436, 1967.
133. Serjeant, GR, Galloway, RE, and Gueri, MC: Oral zinc sulfate and sickle cell ulcers. Lancet 2:891–892, 1970.
134. Greaves, MW and Ive, FA: Double-blind trial of zinc sulfate in the treatment of chronic venous leg ulceration. Br J Dermatol 87:632–634, 1972.
135. Haley, JV: Zinc sulfate and wound healing. J Surg Res 27:168–174, 1979.
136. Agren, MS, Chvapil, M and Franzen, L: Enhancement of re-epithelialization with topical zinc oxide in porcine partial-thickness wounds. J Surg Res 50:101–105, 1991.
137. Pinnell, SR and Martin, GR: The crosslinking of collagen and elastin. Proc Natl Acad Sci USA 61:708–714, 1968.
138. Siegel, RC, Pinnell, SR, and Martin, GR: The crosslinking of collagen and elastin. Properties of lysyl oxidase. Biochemistry 9:4486–4492, 1970.
139. Peacock, EE, Jr: Wound Repair, ed 3. WB Saunders, Philadelphia, 1984, pp 88, 120.
140. Leach, RM, Jr, Muenster, AM, and Wein, EM: Studies on the role of manganese in bone formation. II. Effect upon chondroitin sulfate synthesis in chick epiphyseal cartilage. Arch Biochem Biophys 133:22–28, 1969.
141. LaVan, FB and Hunt, TK: Oxygen and wound healing. Clin Plast Surg 17:463–472, 1990.
142. Hunt, TK and Pai, MP: The effect of varying ambient oxygen tensions on wound metabolism and collagen synthesis. Surg Gynecol Obstet 135:561–567, 1972.
143. Juva, K, et al: Hydroxylation of proline and the intracellular accumulation of a polypeptide precursor of collagen. Science (USA) 152:92–94, 1966.
144. Niinikoski, J: Effect of oxygen supply on wound healing and formation of experimental granulation tissue. Acta Physiol Scand 34(suppl):1–72, 1969.
145. Niinikoski, J: Oxygen and wound healing. Clin Plast Surg 4:361–374, 1977.
146. Hunt, TK, et al: Tissue oximetry: An interim report. World J Surg 11:126–132, 1987.
147. Hall, A, et al: Response of ischemic leg ulcers in hyperbaric oxygen. In Brown, IW, Jr, and Cox, BG (eds): Proceedings of the Third International Conference on Hyperbaric Medicine. Natl Acad Sci–Natl Res Council, 1966, pp 625–630.

148. Slack, WI, Thomas, DA, and Perrins, D: Hyperbaric oxygenation in chronic osteomyelitis. Lancet 1:1093–1094, 1965.
149. Bleser, F, Sztuka, JC, and Muller, JP: Effects of hyperbaric oxygen, THAM and antibiotics on experimental burns in rats. Eur Surg Res 3:409, 1971.
150. Fischer, BH: Topical hyperbaric oxygen treatment of pressure sores and skin ulcers. Lancet 2:405–409, 1969.
151. Hart, GB, et al: Treatment of burns with hyperbaric oxygen. Surg Gynecol Obstet 139:693–696, 1974.
152. Slack, WI, Thomas, DA, and DeJode, LRJ: Hyperbaric oxygen treatment of trauma, ischemic diseases of limbs and varicose ulceration. In Brown, IW, Jr and Cox, BG (eds): Proceedings of the Third International Conference on Hyperbaric Medicine. Natl Acad Sci–Natl Res Council, 1966, pp 621–624.
153. Kernahan, DA, Zingg, W, and Kay, CW: The effect of hyperbaric oxygen on the survival of experimental skin flaps. Plast Reconstr Surg 36:19–25, 1965.
154. Gruber, RP, et al: Hyperbaric oxygenation of pedicle flaps without oxygen toxicity. Plast Reconstr Surg 46:477–480, 1970.
155. Marzella, L, et al: Mechanisms of impaired cutaneous wound healing in obese diabetic (db/db) mice. Wounds 2:135–147, 1990.
156. White, MJ and Heckler, FR: Oxygen free radicals and wound healing. Clin Plast Surg 17:473–484, 1990.
157. Finer, NN, et al: Vitamin E and retrolental fibroplasia prevention of serious ocular sequelae. CIBA Found Symp 101:147, 1983.
158. Catanzaro-Guimaraes, SA: Histometric determination of collagen fibers in granulating wounds of alloxan diabetic rats. Experentia 24:1168–1169, 1968.
159. Goodson, WH, III and Hunt, TK: Studies of wound healing in experimental diabetes mellitus. J Surg Res 22:221–227, 1977.
160. Goodson, WH, III and Hunt, TK: Wound healing and the diabetic patient. Surg Gynecol Obstet 149:600–608, 1979.
161. Goodson, WH, III and Hunt, TK: Deficient collagen formation by obese mice in a standard wound model. Am J Surg 138:692–694, 1979.
162. Seifter, E, et al: Impaired wound healing in streptozotocin diabetes. Prevention by supplemental vitamin A. Ann Surg 194:42–50, 1981.
163. Gottrup, F and Andreassen, TT: Healing of incisional wounds in stomach and duodenum: The influence of experimental diabetes. J Surg Res 31:61–68, 1981.
164. Goodson, WH, III and Hunt, TK: Wound collagen accumulation in obese hyperglycemic mice. Diabetes 35:491–495, 1986.
165. Yue, DK, et al: Effects of experimental diabetes, uremia, and malnutrition on wound healing. Diabetes 36:295–299, 1987.
166. Greenhaulgh, DG, et al: PDGF and FGF stimulate healing in the genetically diabetic mouse. Am J Pathol 136:1235–1246, 1990.
167. Levin, ME and O'Neal, LW: Peripheral vascular disease. In Ellenberg, M and Rifkin, H: Diabetes Mellitus. Theory and Practice, ed 3. Medical Examination Publishing, New Hyde Park, NY, 1983, pp 803–828.
168. Black, CT, et al: Protein glycosylation and collagen metabolism in normal and diabetic rats. J Surg Res 47:200–202, 1989.
169. McMurry, JF, Jr: Wound healing with diabetes mellitus. Better glucose control for better wound healing in diabetes. Surg Clin N Am 64:769–778, 1984.
170. Grotendorst, GR, et al: Stimulation of granulation tissue formation by platelet-derived growth factor in normal and diabetic rats. J Clin Invest 76:2323–2329, 1985.
171. Broadley, KN, et al: The diabetic rat as an impaired wound healing model: Stimulatory effects of transforming growth factor-beta and basic fibroblast growth factor. Biotechnol Therapeut 1:55–68, 1989.
172. Hennessey, PJ, Black, CT, and Andrassy, RJ: Epidermal growth factor and insulin act synergistically during diabetic healing. Arch Surg 125:926–929, 1990.
173. Tsuboi, R and Rifkin, DB: Recombinant basic fibroblast growth factor stimulates wound healing in healing-impaired db/db mice. J Exp Med 172:245–251, 1990.
174. Devereux, DF, et al: Effects of tumor bearing and protein depletion on wound breaking strengths in the rat. J Surg Res 27:233–238, 1979.
175. Weinzweig, J, et al: Supplemental vitamin A prevents the tumor-induced defect in wound healing. Ann Surg 211:269–276, 1990.
176. Peacock, EE, Jr: Wound Repair, ed 3. WB Saunders, Philadelphia, 1984, pp 128–133.
177. Howes, EL, et al: Retardation of wound healing by cortisone. Surgery 28:177–181, 1950.
178. Sandberg, N: Time relationship between administration of cortisone and wound healing in rats. Acta Chir Scand 127:446–455, 1964.
179. Woost, PG, et al: Effect of growth factors with dexamethasone on the healing of rabbit corneal stromal incisions. Exp Eye Res 40:47–60, 1985.

180. Pierce, GF, et al: Transforming growth factor β reverses the glucocorticoid-induced wound healing deficit in rats: Possible regulation in macrophages by platelet-derived growth factor. Proc Natl Acad Sci USA 86:2229–2233, 1989.
181. Laato, M, et al: Epidermal growth factor (EGF) prevents methylprednisolone-induced inhibition of wound healing. J Surg Res 47:354–359, 1989.
182. Bland KI, et al: Experimental and clinical observations of the effects of cytotoxic chemotherapeutic drugs on wound healing. Ann Surg 199:782–790, 1984.
183. Cohen, SC, et al: Effects of cyclophosphamide and adriamycin on the healing of surgical wounds in mice. Cancer 36:1277–1281, 1975.
184. Devereux, DF, et al: The quantitative and qualitative impairment of wound healing by adriamycin. Cancer 43:932–938, 1979.
185. Devereux, DF, Kent, H, and Brennen, MF: Time dependent effects of adriamycin and x-ray therapy on wound healing in the rat. Cancer 45:2805–2810, 1980.
186. Ferguson, MK: The effects of antineoplastic agents on wound healing. Surg Gynecol Obstet 154:421–429, 1982.
187. Falcone, RE and Napp, JF: Chemotherapy and wound healing. Surg Clin N Am 64:779–795, 1984.
188. Greenhalgh, DG and Gamelli, RL: Do nutritional alterations contribute to adriamycin-induced impaired wound healing? J Surg Res 45:261–265, 1988.
189. Lawrence, WT, et al: The reversal of an adriamycin induced healing impairment with chemoattractants and growth factors. Ann Surg 203:142–147, 1986.
190. DeCunzo, LP, et al: The effect of interleukin-2 administration on wound healing in adriamycin-treated rats. J Surg Res 49:419–427, 1990.
191. Reinisch, JF and Puckett, CL: Management of radiation wounds. Surg Clin N Am 64:795–802, 1984.
192. Luce, EA: The irradiated wound. Surg Clin N Am 64:821–829, 1984.
193. Mustoe, TA, et al: Reversal of impaired wound healing in irradiated rats by platelet-derived growth factor-BB. Am J Surg 158:345–350, 1989.
194. Fischel, RS, et al: Cyclosporine A impairs wound healing in rats. J Surg Res 34:572–575, 1983.
195. Nemlander, A, et al: Effect of cyclosporine on wound healing. An analysis with viscous cellulose sponges. Transplantation 36:1–6, 1983.
196. Black, KS, et al: Cyclosporine-induced long-term allograft survival and its potential in posttrauma tissue replacement. J Burn Care Rehabil 8:531–535, 1987.
197. Barbul, A, et al: Interleukin 2 enhances wound healing in rats. J Surg Res 40:315–319, 1986.
198. Steenfos, HH, et al: Selective effects of tumor necrosis factor-alpha on wound healing in rats. Surgery 106:171–176, 1989.
199. Mooney, DP, O'Reilly, M, and Gamelli, RL: Tumor necrosis factor and wound healing. Ann Surg 211:124–129, 1990.
200. Lynch, SE, Colvin, RB, and Antoniades, HN: Growth factors in wound healing. Single and synergistic effects on partial thickness porcine wounds. J Clin Invest 84:640–646, 1989.
201. Pierce, GF, et al: Platelet-derived growth factor and transforming growth factor-β enhance tissue repair by unique mechanisms. J Cell Biol 109:429–440, 1989.
202. Schultz, GS, et al: Epithelial wound healing enhanced by transforming growth factor-α and vaccinia growth factor. Science 235:350–352, 1987.
203. Pierce, GF, et al: In vivo incisional wound healing augmented by platelet-derived growth factor and recombinant c-sis gene homodimeric proteins. J Exp Med 167:974–987, 1988.
204. McGee, GS, et al: Recombinant basic fibroblast growth factor accelerates wound healing. J Surg Res 45:145–153, 1988.
205. Brown, GL, et al: Enhancement of epidermal regeneration by synthetic epidermal growth factor. J Exp Med 163:1319–1324, 1986.
206. Sprugel, KH, et al: Effects of growth factors in vivo. I. Cell ingrowth into porous subcutaneous chambers. Am J Pathol 129:601–613, 1987.
207. Knighton, DR, et al: Classification and treatment of chronic nonhealing wounds. Successful treatment with autologous platelet-derived wound healing factors (PDWHF). Ann Surg 204:322–330, 1986.
208. Carter, DM, et al: Clinical experience with crude preparations of growth factors in healing of chronic wounds in human subjects. In Barbul, A, Pines, E, Caldwell, M and Hunt, TK (eds): Growth Factors and Other Aspects of Wound Healing: Biologic and Clinical Implications. Alan R. Liss, New York, 1988, pp 303–317.
209. Robson, MC, et al: Clinical studies on growth factors in pressure sores: Preliminary report. Prog Clin Biol Res 365:95–102, 1991.
210. Brown, GL, et al: Enhancement of wound healing by topical treatment with epidermal growth factor. New Engl J Med 163:1319–1324, 1989.
211. Cohen, IK, et al: Topical application of epidermal growth factor does not enhance re-epithelialization of partial thickness wounds in human volunteers. Presented at the First Annual Scientific Meeting of the Wound Healing Society, Abstract 8, 1991.

SECTION II

The Care

"And what is as important as knowledge?" asked the mind.
"Caring and seeing with the heart," answered the soul.

Flavia

CHAPTER 6

Triage and Resuscitation of the Burn Patient

Sidney F. Miller, MD, FACS
Reginald L. Richard, MS, PT
Marlys J. Staley, MS, PT

The initial screening and resuscitative management of the burn patient establishes the basis for the patient's entire hospitalization and may affect the final outcome of the patient's care. Many medical decisions made during the first few hours after injury have long-term effects on the functional and cosmetic results of the patient. The purpose of this chapter is to present critical issues addressed during the early period of hospitalization so that therapists can better understand how the consequences of burn injury can affect the patient's treatment program. The therapist's role during the resuscitative phase is to evaluate the patient and begin planning for the patient's rehabilitation course of treatment.

PATHOPHYSIOLOGY

The primary goals in the initial management of the burn patient are to treat the effects of burn wound shock and to assess the extent of the injury and any other associated injuries that might have occurred at the time of the burn.[1] Depending on the temperature of the agent causing the injury and the duration of the exposure, as discussed in Chapter 3, the burn injury produces a central area of wound necrosis surrounded by a zone of altered and sluggish blood flow or stasis and a more peripheral region of increased blood flow or hyperemia.[2] In the area of burn wound necrosis, cellular damage leads to the release of a variety of toxic substances and electrolytes into the general circulation. Fluid and serum proteins are lost from the circulation, leading to hypovolemia and hypotension.[1-3] In the burn region of stasis, the relatively decreased blood flow produces cellular hypoxia and a corresponding acidosis that leads to further hypotension. The area of tissue hyperemia is characterized by increased blood flow with a diversion of additional plasma volume away from the central circulation. Those tissues that are only partially damaged depend for their survival on the capillary circulation for a prolonged period; if circulation remains poor or is lost for any reason, additional tissue death will occur. If tissue ischemia and necrosis develop in the area of stasis, then the original central area of necrosis will expand. Therefore, the goals of the resuscitation phase are to treat the patient's overall hypovolemia and specifically to maintain the capillary circulation to the remaining viable tissues and internal organs.

COMPLETE TRAUMA ASSESSMENT

The process of the initial assessment of the burn patient is the same as for any other trauma patient. A complete trauma assessment of the patient is performed and includes a primary and secondary survey. The burn wounds attract the most attention upon the patient's admission, but initially the wounds only need to be covered and protected from further damage. However, the patient needs a quick but thorough examination so that any associated injuries are detected and treated immediately.[1]

Mechanism of Injury

The manner in which the burn injury occurred determines the approach to the overall evaluation and resuscitation of the patient in the emergency room. For example, if the patient was burned in a closed space and the possibility of an inhalation injury exists,[1] immediate decisions regarding the patient's breathing status must be made. If the patient was burned in an automobile accident or factory explosion, associated fractures or a closed head injury must be considered. Scald burns from hot liquids are viewed differently depending upon the agent causing the burn. Boiling water that quickly runs off the patient tends not to burn as deeply as hot grease, which adheres to the person's skin and continues to burn until it cools or is removed. In addition, there are differences between electrical and chemical burns that are discussed separately in this chapter.

Primary Survey

The primary patient survey is confined to the ABCs: *a*irway, *b*reathing, and *c*irculation.[1] First and foremost, the patient's airway must be established. The trachea must be patent and the patient must be breathing independently. If an inhalation injury has occurred, a bronchoscopy of the patient is performed to assess the status of the airway[2] and, if needed, an endotracheal tube (ET) is inserted.[1] If there is a delay in establishing the airway until the patient is wheezing or in severe respiratory distress, a tracheostomy usually will have to be performed under more complicated conditions.[2] Experience has shown that early placement of an ET may avoid a very difficult surgical tracheostomy later. By placing an ET early, the consequences of a

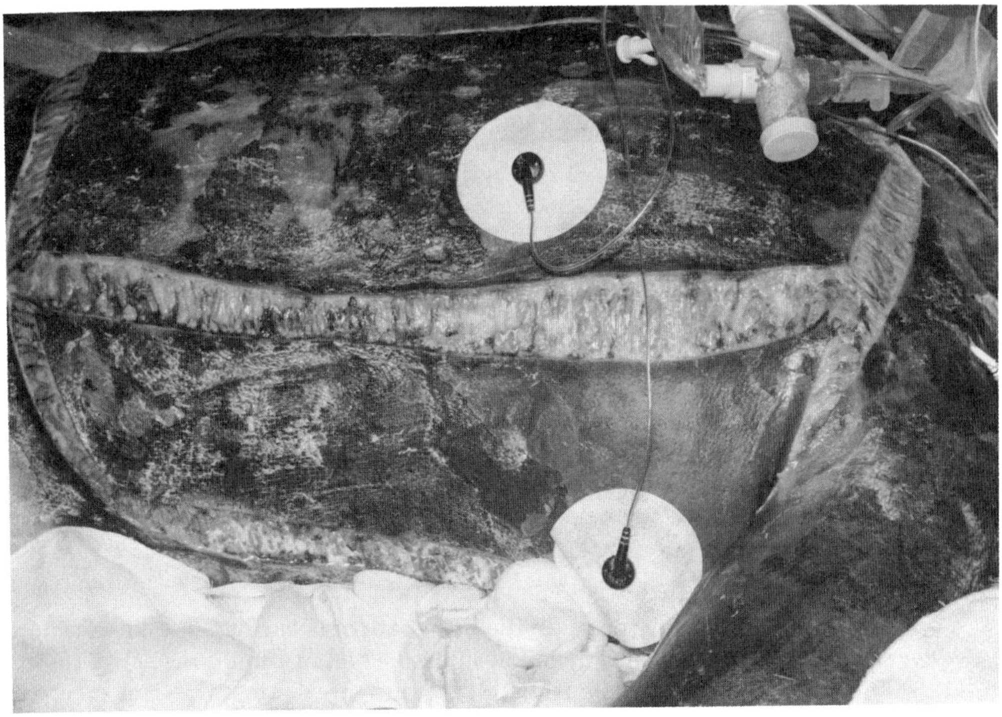

FIGURE 6–1. Escharotomy of thorax to allow for normal chest wall excursion during breathing. Note the extent of the incision gap created by ventilation.

delayed tracheostomy, such as pneumonia, are avoided. Pneumonia is more common in the patient who has a tracheostomy as the protection provided by the upper airway is lost.

Once the airway has been established, attention is turned to the patient's breathing. The lungs must be inflating and expanding as the patient breathes. Occasionally, a leathery full-thickness burn encircling the chest may limit mechanical excursion of the chest wall.[1,3] This condition impairs full expansion of the lungs just as a balloon cannot be inflated in a box. If there is inadequate excursion of the chest wall noted by the physician, an escharotomy of chest tissue may be performed to allow for chest wall expansion[2] (Fig. 6–1). In addition, the patient should be examined for a pneumothorax and a decision should be made regarding the need for a ventilator.

Lastly, circulation is assessed. Any uncontrolled bleeding must be identified and managed. Circulation is supported by appropriate administration of intravenous (IV) fluids. The amount is based on the burn size estimate, which will be described later. Two large-bore 16-gauge needles are used to deliver fluids intravenously. The IVs should be placed in the most readily accessible locations[1] while trying to avoid insertion through any burn area[2,3] or areas that will interfere with joint range of motion or other rehabilitation activities. The patient with a major burn will usually have an indwelling Foley catheter inserted in the urinary bladder so that the adequacy of the fluid resuscitation can be monitored.[3,4]

The primary survey should require approximately 3 to 5 minutes to complete. Once the airway is patent, the patient is breathing adequately, and access to and support of the circulation is established, the secondary survey is performed.

Secondary Survey

The secondary survey encompasses a complete evaluation of the patient. After all of the immediate life-threatening problems have been managed at the time of the primary survey, a complete history and physical examination can be performed.[1]

PATIENT HISTORY

A detailed patient history is necessary. The date of the patient's most recent tetanus immunization should be determined. When the patient last ate also must be determined because if the patient requires immediate surgery, aspiration of the stomach contents can be avoided by the placement of a nasogastric (NG) tube. Additionally, a nasogastric tube is frequently inserted to treat a gastric ileus and avoid the risk of aspirating gastric contents into the lungs with resultant pneumonia. Gastric ileus usually disappears within 24 to 48 hours.

ASSOCIATED INJURIES

The primary cause of early death in the burn patient is attributed to one or more associated injuries, in particular, inhalation injury.[2] The burn injury itself will rarely produce a dangerous level of hypotension or other life-threatening problems except in extreme circumstances. Undetected hemorrhage or internal injuries, such as rupture of the spleen, further contribute to hypotension and shock. Long bone, rib, and neck fractures also can result from major trauma and must be thoroughly sought out.

Therapists may contribute to identifying associated patient injuries through their own initial evaluation. The therapist's knowledge of musculoskeletal function, normal joint range of motion, and gait parameters assist in the early detection of pathologic conditions, the discovery of which might otherwise be delayed.[5]

ASSOCIATED ILLNESSES

Associated illnesses play a significant role in the care of already physiologically compromised patients. The patient with pre-existing cardiac or renal disease may have additional difficulties with heart function or urinary output. One of the most challenging burn patients to manage is someone who required dialysis for kidney failure prior to the burn injury. Assessing the adequacy of fluid resuscitation in these patients is most difficult.

The patient with diabetes or the patient who is chronically on corticosteroids is more prone to infections than nondiabetics or patients not on steroids. Many other diseases or conditions compound the effect of the burn injury, but the four mentioned account for the majority of associated medical problems, particularly in the older population.

To reiterate, associated medical problems may have a significant impact on the burn patient. Diabetic and cardiac patients are at an increased risk for complications and death than patients with a similar-size burn injury but who do not have such complications. The referring physician and the burn physician must actively seek information about pre-existing illnesses and medications and consider these factors when caring for the burn patient.

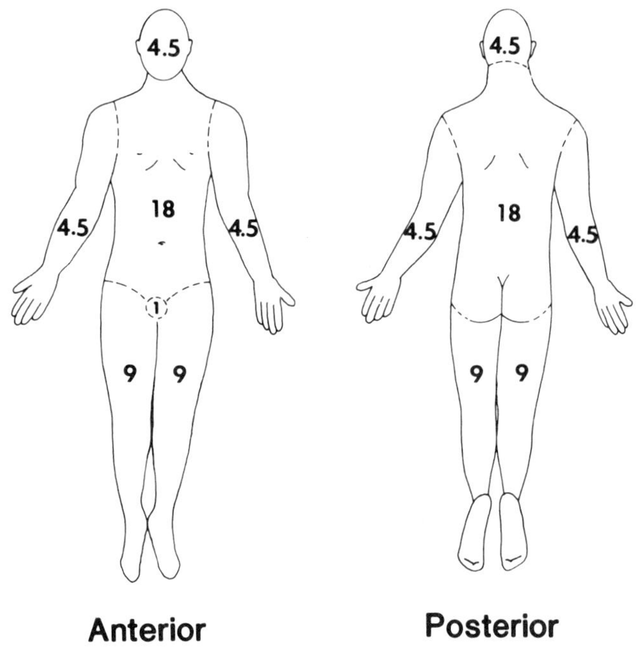

FIGURE 6–2. Rule of 9s to estimate extent of burn injury by percentage.

Burn Size Estimate

Following the primary and secondary survey, the next priority is to assess the burn wound. A body diagram and chart are used to estimate burn size. Commonly, the *Rule of 9s* is used because it is easy to remember.[1-4] The body surface of an adult is divided into 11 segments of 9 percent, or multiples of 9 percent, with 1 percent reserved for the perineum (Fig. 6–2). An alternative method is to use the palm of the patient's hand, which represents approximately 1 percent of the patient's body surface. Small areas can be estimated by using the relative size of the patient's hand as a reference.[4]

Frequently, a modified chart, devised by Lund and Browder,[6] is used to estimate burn size in children because this chart may be more accurate[2,3] (Table 6–1). Many clinicians also use it for estimating burn size in adults. During the first year of life, a child's head is approximately twice as large as an adult's in proportion to the total

TABLE 6–1. Child Burn Size Estimation Table (Percent Total Body Surface Area)

	Age (years)				
Burn Area	**1**	**1–4**	**5–9**	**10–14**	**15**
Head	19	17	13	11	9
Neck	2	2	2	2	2
Anterior trunk	13	13	13	13	13
Posterior trunk	18	18	18	18	18
Genitalia	1	1	1	1	1
Upper extremity (each)	9	9	9	9	9
Lower extremity (each)	14.5	15.5	17.5	18.5	19.5

body surface area. When using the Rule of 9s in children, 9 percent is taken from the legs and added to the head for a child up to 1 year of age. Each subsequent year, 1 percent is returned to the legs until, at approximately age 9, the child's head is in proportion to that of an adult's. A recent study[7] reported that the use of these two methods was just about evenly divided among burn units and suggests that there is not a standard for use of either the Rule of 9s or Lund and Browder, except by facility preference.

Calculated burn sizes are only estimates.[4] Superficial areas of burn that are pink or red, such as a sunburn, are not used in the estimate. Only partial- and full-thickness areas of burn are used in estimating the extent of burn.[4]

Many decisions regarding care, both during and after hospitalization, are based on these "estimates" and therefore should be recorded as accurately as possible and performed by staff who are skilled in this evaluation. Many hospitals base their staffing on the average burn size of the patients admitted to the unit.[9] Some insurance companies determine the amount of reimbursement according to the burn size and depth.[9-11] There is a need for better and more objective methods of estimating burn size and depth and much research is being performed in this area.

Burn Depth Estimate

An equally important aspect of the resuscitation phase is to estimate the burn depth.[4] Burns are divided into three classes by depth of injury: superficial, partial thickness, and full thickness. This classification is based on a subjective estimate of the amount of remaining epithelial-lined skin appendages that can re-epithelialize the wound. However, only an actual biopsy of the skin can objectively assess the state of the deep dermal structures. If a number of hair follicles and sweat glands have survived, the wound is classified as a partial-thickness burn. If these skin appendages are destroyed, the injury is considered to be a full-thickness burn that will require skin grafting to heal. These skin appendages must have their capillary blood supply maintained during the resuscitation phase of care. If this blood supply is lost, the surviving appendages will die. Infection also will lead to a loss of skin appendages and the conversion of a partial-thickness to a full-thickness burn.

Pain associated with a burn injury is a cardinal sign of a partial-thickness burn because the dermally contained nerve endings remain intact. These burns usually are red and blanch when pressure is applied because the capillary blood flow is present. Serum is lost from the capillaries and the wounds become edematous and exhibit a wet surface.

Some partial-thickness burns may require skin grafting. Large areas of deep partial-thickness burn, partial-thickness burns that become infected and convert to full-thickness burns, and those in locations where cosmesis is important may need to be skin-grafted. Frequently the healed partial-thickness burn of the head and neck and hand has a much poorer cosmetic result than when these same areas are grafted. The decision to graft these areas depends on the amount of donor sites available and the amount of additional burn requiring grafting. With larger burns and limited donor sites, grafting of these areas may have to take a lower priority. With very extensive burns, later reconstruction and resurfacing of these healed partial-thickness burns may be required.

Full-thickness burns are painless, do not blanch with pressure, and are dry and leathery in appearance. Most burns are a combination of full- and partial-thickness burns and therefore are difficult to evaluate.

INTRAVENOUS FLUID NEEDS

The primary objectives of resuscitation are to maintain capillary circulation to the viable skin appendages and general circulation to vital organs.[1] Because of the damage to the capillaries, skin, and subcutaneous tissues, a large amount of plasma escapes from the general circulation into the damaged tissues and needs to be replaced.[1,3] Burn size estimates are used in the fluid resuscitation of the burn patient to calculate the patient's intravenous fluid needs. The initial fluid used is lactated Ringer's solution, which closely resembles the fluid and electrolyte composition of serum.[2,3,12] The most commonly used formula today to determine the amount of fluid replacement is referred to as the Parkland or Baxter formula.[13] This formula estimates the intravenous fluid needs during the first 24 hours after the burn injury as follows:

2–4 ml lactated Ringer's × % body surface area burned × weight in kg

There are other formulas that have been suggested as guidelines for the fluid needs of the burn patient. Currently, interest is being focused on the use of hypertonic saline solutions.[2,14] These solutions contain three to six times as much sodium chloride (NaCl) as Ringer's lactate. The advocates of these solutions suggest that the same effect as obtained with lactated Ringer's solution can be obtained with smaller total volumes of fluid administered. There are very strong advocates on both sides of this controversial issue.

ASSESSMENT OF THE ADEQUACY OF RESUSCITATION

Fluid formulas only are guides to the fluid resuscitation of the burn patient.[2] They represent a level to initiate fluid replacement, but close monitoring of the patient is required to fully determine the adequacy of the resuscitation.[3] As stated earlier, the goal of resuscitation is to establish satisfactory perfusion of vital organs. The two most important vital organs are the brain and the kidney. The patient should be alert and oriented and produce an acceptable urine output. The rate of urine flow is a measure of the blood flow to the kidneys. If the blood flow is satisfactory, the adult patient should produce 30 to 50 ml of urine an hour and children should produce 0.5 to 1 ml/kg/hour.[1] Fluids rates must be adjusted to maintain the urine output at this rate. Less output than this suggests that the blood flow to the kidneys is inadequate and more IV fluids are needed. Urine output of greater than 50 ml/hour in an adult suggests that the patient is receiving too much fluid. Fluid overload can lead to cerebral or pulmonary edema or heart failure and can be as detrimental to the patient as insufficient amounts of fluid.[1,3] Careful monitoring of the patient is necessary to ensure an adequate fluid volume while avoiding an overload of the patient's vascular system.

Special monitoring lines are needed sometimes to assess the adequacy of fluid resuscitation. The Swan-Ganz catheter provides information about cardiac function

TABLE 6–2. Normal Laboratory Blood Values

	Males	Females
Red blood cell count	4.3–5.8 × $10^6/\mu L$	4.0–5.25 × $10^6/\mu L$
White blood cell count	4.7–11.4 × $10^3/\mu L$	4.7–11.4 × $10^3/\mu L$
Hemoglobin	13.0–17.0 g/dl	11.5–15.5 g/dl
Hematocrit	39.0–50.0%	36.0–48.5%

TABLE 6–3. Normal Values for Common Laboratory Tests

Sodium	134–149 mEq/liter
Potassium	3.5–5.3 mEq/liter
Calcium	8.4–10.2 mg/dl
Albumin	3.4–5.0 g/dl
Glucose	70–115 mg/dl
Transferrin	252–429 mg/dl
Prothrombin time (PT)	10.6–12.3 sec
Partial thromboplastin time (PTT)	21.3–31.0 sec

better than the central venous pressure (CVP) line.[1,2] However, during the early resuscitation phase, either method can be used to monitor the patient for fluid overload.[1]

Therapists may be concerned as to whether range of motion and transfers are permitted with patients with central and peripheral fluid lines. The catheter tips used several years ago were rigid and the potential existed for the end to break. Present-day catheters have flexible tips that accommodate movement and lessen the risk of an embolus. The more prominent risk of moving or performing exercises on patients with resuscitation lines is that the lines may be extracted from their insertion sites. As long as precautions are taken to prevent this occurrence, exercising or transferring patients is permissible. If readings on the patient's monitor becomes distorted, repositioning the limb usually will correct the interference.

Several laboratory tests are also obtained on patients in the early resuscitation phase (Tables 6–2 and 6–3).[1] The primary tests are the hematocrit, serum osmolality, and serum sodium. These three tests are additional indicators of the adequacy of fluid resuscitation. Ideally, the hematocrit should be less than 55 percent, the osmolality less than 350 mosm, and the serum sodium less than 155 mEq/liter. If the results of these tests are higher than the suggested levels, more fluid is required to increase the fluid volume of the blood to decrease their concentration. By maintaining the appropriate electrolyte levels and urine output, one is assured of adequate fluid resuscitation for the burn patient and fluid overload can be avoided.

ESCHAROTOMY

During the shock phase of recovery from the burn injury, peripheral vasoconstriction occurs in the body to shunt blood from the peripheral to the central circulation. The extremities may appear pale, feel cool, and exhibit poor capillary refill.[3] The normal physiologic response of burn wound shock is corrected once the patient is properly resuscitated, has adequate circulation, and is in a properly heated environment.[1,2]

However, a significant problem can occur that must be addressed in the early postburn period. As previously described, the full-thickness burn is characteristically leathery and rigid. As edema fluid accumulates in the injured tissues, particularly after fluid resuscitation has begun, the overlying and unyielding circumferential full-thickness burn eschar may act as a tourniquet causing a severely decreased blood flow to the extremity. If this condition is allowed to continue, ischemic gangrene of the digits or extremity will occur, requiring amputation.

An assessment of selected peripheral pulses is important during the early resuscitative period to confirm the adequacy of the peripheral circulation, particularly in patients with circumferential burns of the extremities. The easiest method of assessing the circulation to the extremity is to monitor the pulse in the ankle, foot, or wrist by palpation. The pulse also can be evaluated in an extremity by using a Doppler ultrasound device. This instrument assesses blood flow on the basis of sound waves generated by the passage of blood through the vessels.[2,3] One also can observe capillary refill in the patient's nail beds. By compressing on the nail bed and releasing, the nail bed should become pink in about 2 seconds or the time needed to say "capillary refill." If refilling is delayed or does not occur, severe vascular compromise in the extremity may be occurring. If a therapist detects a vascular impairment when treating a patient, the therapist should notify the physician immediately so that he or she can determine the necessity for an escharotomy (Fig. 6–3).

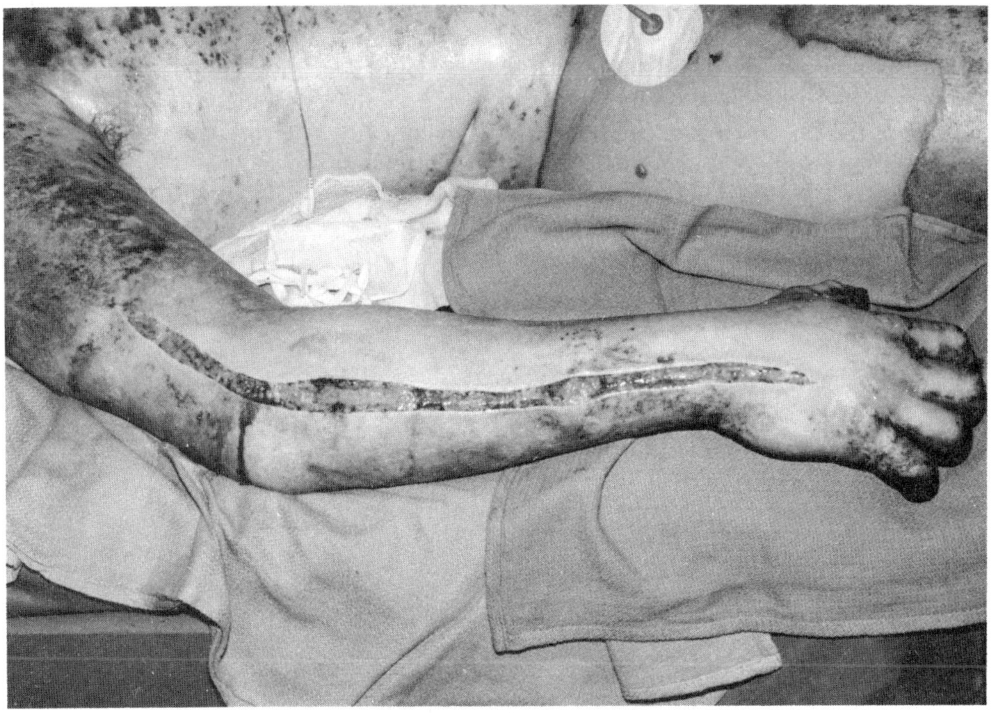

FIGURE 6–3. Escharotomy of limb to relieve constricting pressure to permit distal circulation to the extremity. Note the width of the incision line caused by the underlying tissue pressure.

An escharotomy is a longitudinal incision through the full-thickness burn to the layer of subcutaneous fat of an extremity. This incision allows the overlying rigid burned tissue to expand and release the constricting pressure on the underlying blood vessels.[1,2] The incision, performed with a scalpel or by electrocautery,[15] theoretically should be a painless procedure because the nerve endings have been destroyed by the burn.[1] However, caution to avoid pain is advised in areas of questionable mixed burn depth. Frequently there may be brisk venous bleeding associated with the incision that can be managed with a bulky dressing and elevation of the extremity.[1,2] Distal pulses and capillary refill should return after the escharotomy.

The therapist should be aware of when escharotomies have been performed and the location of these incisions. However, once hemostasis of the area has been achieved, usual exercises are permitted as part of the treatment program.[16]

INDICATIONS FOR HOSPITALIZATION

A consideration in the early postburn period is whether the patient needs hospitalization.[4] One guideline for hospitalizing patients is the "5–10–20 rule" established by the American Burn Association.[17] Usually, any patient with a burn involving greater than 20 percent of the total body surface should be hospitalized. Because the very young and old are less tolerant of burn injuries than other patients, a total body burn of 10 percent warrants hospitalization. In addition, a patient with a 5 percent or greater full-thickness burn should be hospitalized.

Other indications for hospitalization include any major associated injuries that could compound the effects of the burns or medical conditions that could complicate management of the burn[4] (Table 6–4). Patients with burns involving the perineum, hands, feet, and face should be considered for hospitalization even though the percentage of the body surface involved may be relatively small (Fig. 6–4). Due to their functional importance, burns of the hands and feet are extremely critical and their management should take place in a burn center where personnel have experience in caring for these injuries. For cosmetic and psychologic reasons, burns to the face require specialized care that is best provided in the hospital setting.

TABLE 6–4. Criteria for Hospitalization of Burn Patient

20% or greater total body burn
10% or greater burn of child or older adult
5% or greater full-thickness injury
Burns to the hands, feet, face, perineum
Burns of the eyes or ears
Any suspected inhalation injury
All electrical and chemical burns
Patients with pre-existing illness
Patients with associated injuries

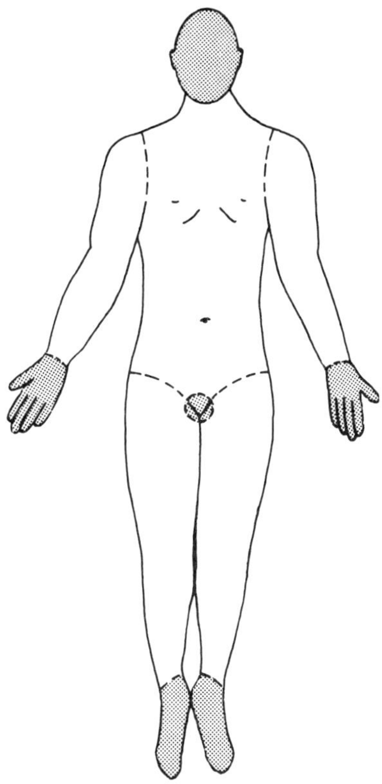

FIGURE 6–4. Schematic diagram of body with shading to highlight special areas that require hospitalization.

SPECIFIC SITES OF CONCERN

There are several body areas that, if burned, require special consideration. Involvement of the eye with any type of burn should always be evaluated by an ophthalmologist in the hospital. The nose and the ears have very thin skin layers over cartilage and therefore are very susceptible to further injury. Placing excessive pressure on these areas, by nasogastric and endotracheal tubes through and near the nose and pillows against the ears, can further damage cartilage tissue. These areas must be protected as much as possible to avoid poor cosmetic results that are difficult to reconstruct. The therapist plays an integral role in the management of these special areas as discussed in the chapter related to positioning.

OTHER BURN INJURIES

The previous information dealt with thermal burns that make up the majority of burn injuries. In addition, burns also occur from electricity and chemicals (see Chapter 21). Although they occur less frequently, these injuries present unique problems that warrant discussion.

Electrical Injuries

Electrical injuries are probably the most significant injuries encountered in burn care. Frequently, there will be tissue damage from the passage of the electric current and from fire if clothing is ignited by the electricity. The major problem of the electrical injury is the initially undetermined internal injury. Electrical energy enters and passes through the body until a point of grounding is reached. The current can travel throughout the entire body or for just a short distance. This passage of electrical current has multiple, extensive biochemical effects. Electric current can cause contraction and fibrillation of both skeletal and cardiac muscle,[1,18] destruction of cell membranes, thrombosis of blood vessels, and necrosis and coagulation of tissues.[1,2] The violent contraction of the muscles with the passage of the current can produce fractures that may go undetected in the early resuscitation period.[5] The injured muscles release electrolytes and myoglobin into the bloodstream, and these have the potential to produce further damage. Potassium released from these tissues can cause cardiac damage so that the patient will need to be monitored.

Myoglobin released from the damaged muscle mechanically can plug the renal tubules and can lead to renal failure.[1,2,3] In patients who have a significant myoglobinuria, a higher-than-usual urine output is desired. Those patients who have a "port wine"-colored urine in the emergency department usually will have their intravenous fluids administered at a rate to produce a urine output of 100 to 150 ml/hour until the urine grossly clears of myoglobin. Additionally, an osmotic diuretic may be given to increase the urine output and flushing of the myoglobin from the kidneys.

Injured muscle can swell and increase the pressure in the compartments of the muscle. Patients with such injury frequently need a fasciotomy,[3] an incision of the overlying fascia, to release the pressure in the muscular compartments. Damaged muscle tissue needs to be fully debrided as soon as possible following injury to reduce the source for rapid growth of bacteria that will lead to further necrosis, abscess, and sepsis. Extensive muscle loss in electrical injuries frequently has a significant effect on the patient's rehabilitation. Amputations are often an adverse sequela to an electrical burn. Electrical injuries present challenges to therapists as the exercise program may be complicated by the presence of amputations or the loss of large amounts of muscle mass.

Chemical Injuries

Chemical injuries are another special type of burn. These injuries usually involve just the skin, similar to thermal burns. The major difference between chemical and thermal injuries is that chemical injuries are initially treated with massive dilution by continuous showering frequently for a prolonged period after the injury.[2] Attempts to chemically neutralize the burn can have an adverse effect. For example, the mixture of a strong acid, such as hydrochloric acid (HCl), with a strong base, such as sodium hydroxide (NaOH), produces an exothermic reaction. This resultant heat can cause additional damage to the skin.[1]

Because there are many different chemicals used at home and in the workplace, neutralizing a chemical injury may be near impossible. Knowing the actual chemical producing the injury is most important, because some chemicals require specific treatments and others can be absorbed through the skin causing systemic effects.[2] Hydrogen fluoride (HF) is a commonly used agent in glass and metal etching. With HF injuries, the chemical becomes bonded to the subcutaneous tissues and continues to produce damage until neutralized with calcium gluconate. The employer usually can provide the name of the chemicals involved, but education of the public must be directed to encourage family members to bring the container of the chemical with the patient to the emergency room.

SUMMARY

The resuscitation phase of recovery from a burn injury provides a basis for patient survival and the entire course of hospitalization and care. Procedures and assessment made during this period will have a far-reaching effect on the resultant disability or function that the patient might experience.

The burn patient must first be evaluated the same as other trauma patients with a complete body assessment. This evaluation includes the ABCs (airway, breathing, circulation) of resuscitation in addition to recognition of any associated life-threatening injuries. A medical history of past patient illnesses that might complicate the healing of the burn wound should be obtained. Attention is then given to the burn injury itself, where the burn depth and extent are estimated for determining the course of treatment. Intravenous fluid replacement needs are calculated from the estimate of burn severity and necessitates close monitoring to ensure correct perfusion levels.

Hospitalization usually is necessary for burns of the young and aged, and when the hands, feet, face, and perineum are involved. Electrical and chemical burns present unique problems that require special attention for an optimal outcome.

REFERENCES

1. Dimick, AR: Emergency care. In Hummel, RP (ed): Clinical Burn Therapy, John Wright PSG, Boston, 1982, pp 7–24.
2. Demling, RH and LaLonde, C: Burn Trauma, Thieme Medical Publishers, New York, 1989.
3. MacMillan, BG: Initial replacement therapy. In Hummel, RP (ed): Clinical Burn Therapy. John Wright PSG, Boston, 1982, pp 51–83.
4. Hummel, RP: Triage and transfer procedures. In Hummel, RP (ed): Clinical Burn Therapy. John Wright PSG, Boston, 1982, pp 25–34.
5. Slater, RR, Jr, and Peterson, HD: Bilateral femoral neck fractures after electrical injury: A case report and literature review. J Burn Care Rehabil 11:240–243, 1990.
6. Lund, CC and Browder, NC: The estimation of areas of burns. Surg Gynecol Obstet 79:352, 1944.
7. Miller, SF, et al: Burn size estimate reliability: a study. J Burn Care Rehabil 12:546–559, 1991.
8. Stachowski, M and Kondela-Cebulski, P: Physical therapists in burn care. Phys Ther 63:1091–1095, 1983.
9. Warden, GD, Saffle, JR, and Kravitz, M: Potential DRG reimbursement vs. actual cost for burn care. I. Patients with less than 25% TBSA. J Burn Care Rehabil 7:45–48, 1986.
10. Hunt, JL and Purdue, GF: Cost containment/cost reduction: The economic impact of burn DRGs. J Burn Care Rehabil 7:417–421, 1986.
11. Rees, JM and Dimick, AJ: Washington Burn Watch. J Burn Care Rehabil 10:354–355, 1989.
12. Baxter, CR and Shires, T: Physiological response to crystalloid resuscitation of severe burns. Ann NY Acad Sci 150:874–894, 1968.
13. Baxter, CR: Fluid volume and electrolyte changes in the early post burn period. Clin Plast Surg 1:693–709, 1974.

14. Monafo, WW, Chuntrasekul, C, and Ayvazian, VH: Hypertonic sodium solutions in the treatment of burn shock. Am J Surg 126:778–783, 1973.
15. Feller, I and Archambeault, C: Nursing the burned patient. Institute for Burn Medicine Press of Braun-Brumfield, 1973, p 128.
16. Nothdurft, D, Smith, PS, and LeMaster, JE: Exercise and treatment modalities. In Fisher, SV and Helm, PA (eds): Comprehensive Rehabilitation of Burns. Williams & Wilkins, Baltimore, 1984, p 98.
17. Resources for optimal care of patients with burn injury. In Resources for optimal care of the injured patient. American College of Surgeons Committee on Trauma, 1990.
18. Richard, RL, Miller, SF, and Finley, RK, Jr: Restoration of normal function involving herniated quadricep muscles following electric burn injury. J Burn Care Rehabil 6:347–349, 1985.

CHAPTER 7

Burn Wound Care

Jeffrey R. Saffle, MD, FACS
W. Andrew Schnebly, PT

Proper care of burn wounds is fundamental to successful burn treatment. Every member of the burn team must understand thoroughly the principles that underlie rational wound management and be proficient in a variety of wound care techniques. The history of burn treatment essentially has been the history of wound care[1,2] and this continues to remain so today. The recent development of early burn wound excision and immediate skin grafting has obviated the need for much of the prolonged, painful debridement and gradual development of granulation tissue that was the standard of therapy only 30 years ago. However, this development did not remove the need for meticulous wound care and has led to many new innovations in wound management that present new challenges to the wound care provider.

This chapter will present the principles of wound care, describe various wound care techniques currently in practice, and discuss the applications of those systems to specific problems in burn wound management. Proficiency in burn care requires familiarity with burn wounds. Therapists should take every opportunity to examine each burn wound they care for on a regular basis.

PHYSIOLOGIC PRINCIPLES OF WOUND CARE

Wound healing is a complex process that begins immediately after injury and ends many months later. Because wound healing is reviewed in Chapter 5, this chapter reviews only those components of healing that are essential for understanding of all wound care techniques. Knowledge of these concepts will help the therapist to understand the many variations in management that exist for burn wounds, to evaluate new techniques and procedures rationally, and to avoid dependence on rigid protocols that are all too common in burn care. Important principles of wound management are outlined in Table 7–1.

TABLE 7–1. Principles of Wound Management

Principle	Description	Practical Application
Oxygen availability	All phases of wound healing require oxygen. Hypoxia retards healing, favors infection. Oxygen delivery to tissues can be impaired by reduced circulation, edema, or the presence of necrotic debris on the wound surface.	Assure circulation: avoid constricting casts and wraps; elevate affected extremities. Avoid edema: elevate affected extremities; begin range of motion and ambulation early. Remove necrotic debris.
Debridement	Burns develop necrotic tissue on the wound surface that supports bacteria, encourages infection, and prolongs inflammation and healing. Debridement is the practice of removing dead tissue from a wound. This includes blisters, dead skin, and accumulated topical creams and ointments.	*Careful washing and debridement of burn wounds is the mainstay of burn treatment!* Eschar separates gradually; repeated gentle debridement is more successful than a single overly aggressive approach. Too vigorous debridement removes healing skin and damages new blood vessels and may retard wound closure.
Granulation tissue	Granulation tissue is formed by the growth of new capillaries, encourages eschar separation, and forms a vascular bed that can be readily grafted. Granulation tissue is not necessary for graft adherence.	Meticulous debridement encourages capillary growth by removing overlying eschar and reducing infection. Debriding dressings, such as wet-to-moist dressings, help granulation tissue form.
Epithelialization	Epithelial "buds" originate from skin appendages and grow outward to resurface partial-thickness burns. Wounds which "separate" and show epidermal growth within 14 days of injury can be permitted to heal spontaneously; deeper injuries require excision and skin grafting.	Careful, gentle debridement helps eschar separate and helps epidermis regenerate. Once wounds "bud," they should be washed even more gently. Superficial wounds can be treated with protective dressings that speed epidermal growth, but must be watched closely for infection.
Contraction	All open wounds contract. Infection favors this process because it deepens injury and prolongs healing. Necrotic debris prolongs inflammation and favors contraction.	Wound cleansing is necessary to help wounds heal rapidly, which minimizes contraction. Ambulation and range of motion should begin early and continue throughout all phases of wound healing.

Preservation of Circulation and Oxygen Delivery

All phases of wound healing require a continuous supply of oxygen to proceed normally. If blood supply to the wound is reduced, then oxygenation is impaired, capillary growth and wound remodeling are impeded, and the "cleaning up" of foreign material is slowed.[3–6] Reduced tissue oxygenation greatly favors infection because bacteria require less oxygen than defending cells and consume available oxygen.[7] As bacteria proliferate, they generate an advancing margin of hypoxia that favors their spread and blocks local defenses. The result is a wound that heals poorly, if at all, and stimulates inflammation and scarring.[8] As a corollary, treatment with hyperbaric oxygen can be used to combat some types of anaerobic infections, to improve survival of ischemic flaps and grafts, and to promote healing of problem wounds.[9] Hyperbaric oxygen has been used in some burn centers to assist wound healing. Good results have been reported, although this technique has not been widely utilized.[10,11]

Though vascular disease, anemia, shock, and other systemic disorders impede wound oxygen delivery, burn patients are also at risk of developing poor perfusion as a consequence of edema and impaired circulation. Edema is an inevitable consequence of burn injury and is exacerbated by dependent positioning and disuse. Therapists can effectively treat these problems by observing the following guidelines: (1) removal or replacement of constricting casts and bandages that can reduce capillary blood flow and venous return; (2) regular changing of dressings to remove bacterial innoculum and debris, permit air to reach the wound, and stimulate blood flow; (3) institution o. early and continuous motion of affected areas throughout care; (4) limitation of the use of crutches and wheelchairs, and immediate ambulation whenever possible; (5) elevation of affected extremities when patients rest. Enforcing these principles is a major task for therapists and must be done tirelessly if wounds are to heal without complications.

Debridement of Necrotic Tissue

Burn injury results in necrosis of skin and subcutaneous tissue. This burned tissue, called *eschar,* releases powerful chemical mediators that stimulate leukocytes to digest debris but also damage capillaries and skin elements.[8] The presence of necrotic tissue within a wound prolongs inflammation and retards healing and epidermal coverage.

Debridement is the removal of dead material within a wound to enhance normal healing. Historically, debridement was first widely practiced during World War I. Battlefield surgeons discovered that regular excision of dead tissue from wounds reduced the incidence of infection and greatly accelerated healing.[12] This principle is now widely recognized by surgeons as a fundamental concept in wound management, particularly in burn care. *The meticulous and regular performance of debridement is the cornerstone of successful burn wound management!*

An extension of the concept of debridement has been the development of burn wound excision with immediate skin grafting. There is confusion in some burn centers, however, where "debridement" ends and "excision" begins. Though they are both applications of the same principle, their practical definitions dictate where, how, and by whom they are performed. In this chapter, *debridement* is defined to mean the gentle, gradual removal of loose necrotic eschar and debris performed by the therapist or nurse at the bedside or in the hydrotherapy tank. In contrast, *excision* consists of the surgical removal of eschar and, inevitably, some viable tissue.

Formation of Granulation Tissue

As any deep burn wound heals, capillary buds multiply, extend into the wound, and proliferate into a network of new blood vessels called *granulation tissue.* For many years, granulation tissue was considered the goal of wound care because its appearance meant that dead tissue had been removed, and because this tissue readily accepted skin grafts.[13] Wound care consisted of repeated painful debridement of eschar, often for weeks, until granulation tissue appeared. Waiting prolonged periods for granulation tissue to develop often permitted deep partial-thickness burns to heal with unacceptable scarring and poor quality skin coverage. However, granulation tissue is not essential for good graft adherence. Clinicians now realize that early burn wound excision and skin grafting can be performed before deep eschar separates, thereby reducing hospitalization, infection, and metabolic stress. Other disadvantages of granulation tissue[14-19] include prolonged inflammation encouraging the growth of dense scar and impaired epidermal migration.[8] Despite an encouraging appearance, the irregular surface of granulation tissue contains exudate and debris that is colonized by bacteria that can destroy skin grafts or serve as a focus for sepsis. In some problem wounds such as those with exposed fascia, tendons, or bone, some infected wounds, or wounds with poor circulation, waiting for granulation tissue may be the only way to achieve graft coverage (Fig. 7–1). Even these wounds often are excised to reduce infection and to speed the growth of granulations.[14] Meticulous debridement, avoidance of infection, and encouragement of circulation all aid in the formation of granulation tissue and subsequent graft adherence.

Epithelialization

Even the most superficial burn damages epidermis. Conversely, burns often are said to be "healed" when they are covered with new epidermis. In fact, healing continues for several months after epithelialization. However, coverage of the burn with viable skin is a major goal of treatment for all members of the burn team.

As eschar separates, skin "buds" emerge from the sites of epidermal appendages.[13] These tiny islands of new epidermis proliferate over the surface of the wound (Fig. 7–2). Epidermal growth is aided by eschar separation, which, in turn, is aided by meticulous debridement. The decision to perform skin grafting often depends on the rate at which eschar separation and epidermal coverage occur, because this interval coincides with the depth of the injury and the amount of scar which eventually forms.[20] Infection is a major enemy of epidermal growth. Infected partial-thickness burns or donor sites may "convert" to full-thickness injuries with destruction of epidermal appendages. Such wounds often require skin grafting.

New epidermis is extremely fragile and can be disrupted by even minor mechanical trauma. Epidermal growth proceeds best in a moist, protected environment. The

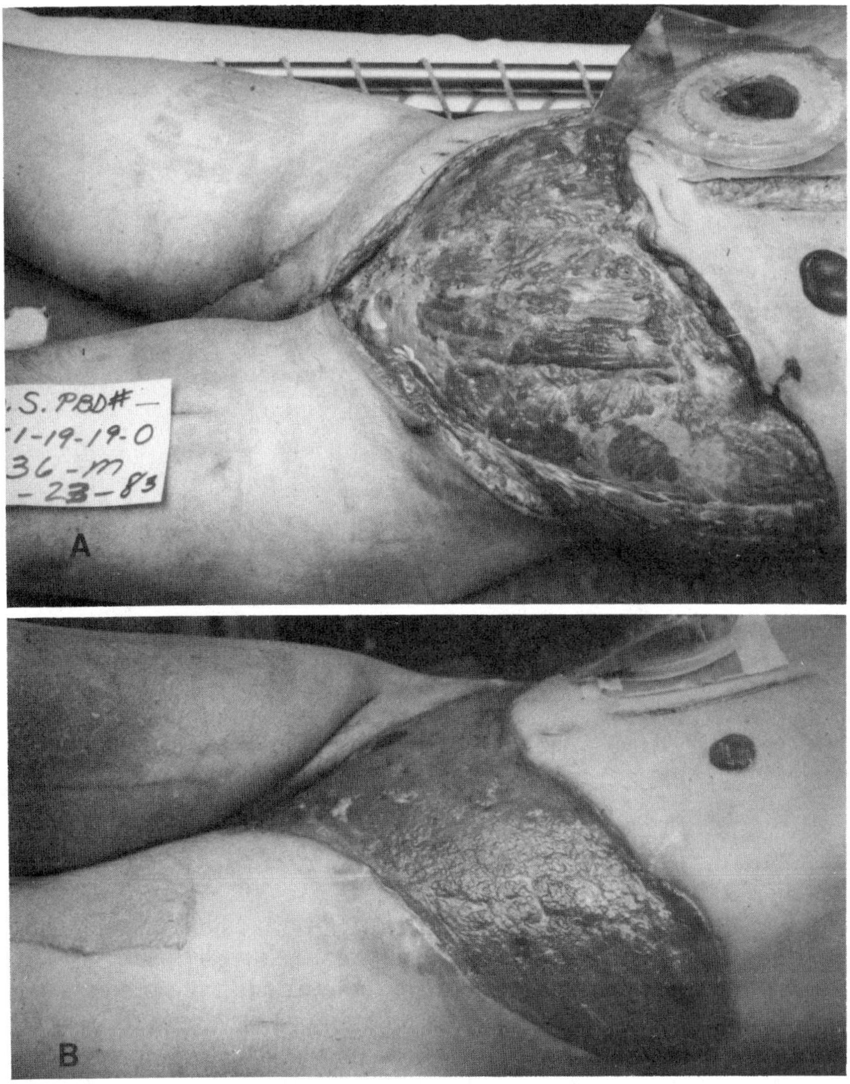

FIGURE 7–1. Granulation tissue. (*A*) Wound resulting from massive soft-tissue infection, which necessitated full-thickness excision of the abdominal wall to the level of the muscle, as well as placement of a colostomy due to perineal necrosis. The wound was dressed with antibiotic wet-to-moist dressings to provide further debridement, and encourage the growth of granulation tissue. (*B*) The same wound 3 weeks later, covered with granulation tissue and ready for autograft coverage.

so-called open technique, and other techniques that permit exposure of burns to the air, lead to formation of dessicated eschar, essentially a scab, that retards epidermal migration and slows healing. Wet-to-dry dressings and vigorous debridement also disrupt epidermis. In recent years, a number of synthetic, "occlusive and semi-occlusive" dressings have been advocated for use on superficial burns and donor sites because they protect fragile epidermis during the early phases of healing and provide a moist environment. In experiments and clinical trials, superficial wounds healed more quickly when covered with such dressings.[21-27]

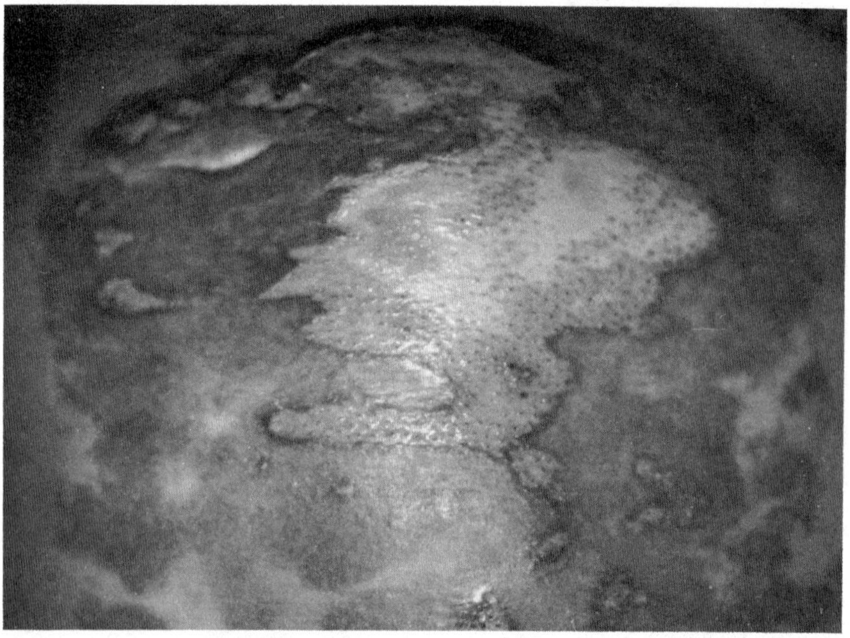

FIGURE 7–2. Skin buds. This small wound of the abdominal wall is approximately 10 days old. The margins of the wound have epithelialized completely; centrally, a regular pattern of raised epithelial buds can be seen growing through the remaining eschar. Wounds with this appearance do not require skin grafting, though continued daily debridement will be required until the wound is entirely healed.

Wound Contraction

Wound contraction is a normal and necessary aspect of healing. As inflammation subsides in a healing wound and new collagen remodels and "matures," contraction subsides, but this process may require many months and may produce disastrous consequences for the patient in the process. The extent of wound contraction varies in response to depth of injury and to the adequacy of coverage. Wounds left open will continue to contract until closed or covered, and this includes healed deep burns covered only by epidermis and areas of poor skin graft adherence. Skin grafting reduces contraction[8,28] and the more completely grafts adhere, the less contraction occurs. Grafted wounds require meticulous care to prevent infection, motion, and bleeding, which contribute to graft loss and increased contraction. Because infection deepens the burn wound, destroys residual dermis, and increases the inflammation that produces scarring, every effort should be made to prevent this occurrence.

METHODS OF WOUND CARE

There are probably as many ways to manage wounds as there are physicians, nurses, and therapists caring for them. However, all wound management techniques fall into categories based on the physiology behind the technique. This section is divided into two parts, the first dealing with general techniques of wound care, and the second outlining protocols for wound management.

General Techniques of Wound Care

WOUND EVALUATION

The degree of involvement of therapists in burn wound care varies among facilities. In some facilities, therapists provide primary wound care themselves; in others, wound care is provided mainly by nurses. Regardless of the circumstances, however, the therapist should not treat the burn patient without knowing the status of the wounds under the dressings. Therefore, the therapist should be informed of each patient's wound status. Therapists often spend a great deal of time with patients, which gives them a unique opportunity to answer questions concerning all phases of treatment. Therapists must understand all aspects of burn wound management, even if they do not provide this care themselves.

The use of a burn wound evaluation form is helpful to record the observations of various staff members, and to forward this information on to other team members. Figure 7–3 is an example of such a form, which contains space for a detailed drawing of the burn wound, as well as subjective and objective observations, assessment, and goals of treatment. All aspects of the wound should be noted during the dressing change, including appearance of the dressing; color of the wound; appearance of the surrounding skin; presence or amount of edema; and the amount, consistency, and odor of any drainage. Any significant changes should be noted and communicated to the physician. Such a form may be filled out only on admission, although for large or complex wounds, periodic or even daily completion of this form may help staff members communicate the progress a wound is making. This type of form also is useful in formulating care plans and in quality assurance.

CLEAN AND STERILE TECHNIQUE

During wound care, precautions are taken to protect not only the patient but also the care provider from the transmission of disease. Recent concerns over transmission of the human immunosuppressive virus (HIV) in either direction has underscored the need for meticulous use of precautions in performing wound care. Familiarity with universal precautions as well as protocols for both clean and sterile (or aseptic) technique is mandatory for all burn care providers.

Immediately following burn injury, the skin surface is sterile, because cutaneous bacteria are destroyed by the burn.[13,29] Within 24 to 48 hours, however, the wound is colonized by bacteria that originate primarily from the patient: *Staphylococcus* and *Streptococcus* initially, followed in a few days by enteric flora including *Klebsiella, Enterobacter,* and others. Only later does colonization with "burn unit" flora, *Pseudomonas,* methicillin-resistant *Staphylococcus,* and other pathogens usually occur. Because burn wounds usually are not sterile, they often can be handled with clean technique to isolate the patient from the provider and prevent the introduction of exogenous bacteria to the wound. Clean technique is used in treating burns on outpatients because it provides satisfactory cleansing and protection of the wound and because sterile technique is difficult to teach to patients and families. Sterile technique is reserved for conditions in which the wound must be protected as much as possible from contamination from exogenous bacteria. Even though the wound itself usually is not sterile, the dressings that touch it should be. Examples of this situation

BURN WOUND EVALUATION FORM

Date__________ Time __________ Post Injury Day __________ Date of Injury __________

Name ______________________________ Age __________ Sex __________

Diagnosis ______________________________

Burn Size: Total __________ Full-thickness __________ Allergies __________

Evaluation done by______________________________

Diagram the wound and note significant findings/abnormalities/changes in management

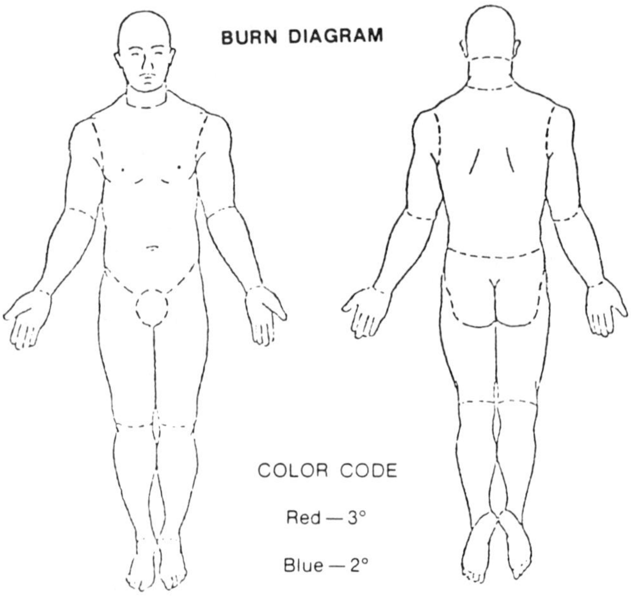

BODY AREA	APPEARANCE	TREATMENT	COMMENTS

SUMMARY/RECOMMENDATIONS: ______________________________

FIGURE 7–3. Typical form used for periodic wound evaluation. This form is completed to document wound status and record wound care techniques on various areas.

include the application of topical creams or ointments to freshly washed wounds, dressing changes on fresh skin grafts, or the performance of invasive procedures.

The components of clean and sterile techniques are reviewed in Appendix 7-1. Frequent hand washing is the single most important mechanism for limiting cross-contamination between patients and is the mainstay of clean technique. However, the use of gloves alone now has been supplanted by widespread adoption of protocols requiring disposable gowns, hats, masks, and glasses or goggles as well, to protect care providers as completely as possible from inadvertent transmission of bacterial or viral diseases.

HYDROTHERAPY

Many of the goals of daily wound cleansing can be facilitated by "hydrotherapy," a term that encompasses many methods of washing the burn wound or the entire patient. Bathing patients permits thorough washing of all areas, promotes general hygiene, and contributes to the patient's feeling of well-being.[30-33] In addition, gentle active range-of-motion exercises often can be performed during hydrotherapy without damaging injured extremities or fragile skin grafts.

In recent years, the concept of hydrotherapy has been challenged. Some authors feel that bathing in a common tank or tub increases cross-contamination between patients, can be dangerous and stressful, and may be contraindicated in very sick patients.[34-36] In addition, routine hydrotherapy often requires a team of nurses and therapists and is very consumptive of time and resources. For these reasons, some facilities now use disposable plastic liners that help prevent cross-contamination between patients, or restrict washing to a shower or spray.[33-34] Some clinicians advocate isolating patients as completely as possible to prevent exchange of bacteria and use only "bed baths" for washing and debridement of burns. In a recent survey of American burn centers, Thomson et al.[37] found that 92 percent of facilities reported that they continue to use some form of hydrotherapy in wound care, although the type (shower versus tub) and frequency of this treatment varied among facilities.[37] Sixty-four percent of responding centers had hydrotherapy facilities located within the burn center.

A variety of hydrotherapy techniques can be adapted for use with particular patients. Partial immersion in a Hubbard tank is used for nonambulatory patients or those with extensive injuries as shown in Figure 7-4. After removal of old dressings, the patient is placed on a tank stretcher and suspended above the tank by an electric hoist. The patient is gently washed to remove remaining creams and ointments and residual eschar. He or she is partially immersed briefly for bathing and further debridement, then resuspended above the tank for rinsing with a hand-held shower. Next, the patient is covered with dry blankets and is dried thoroughly. New dressings are applied to one body area at a time, while keeping the others covered. The Hubbard tank permits access to the patient from every side, which allows a team of nurses and therapists to complete the procedure quickly. This approach limits time in the tub, which can be stressful and uncomfortable, streamlines the process, and permits more patients to be treated. Although some critically ill patients are too unstable to undergo hydrotherapy, it is possible to "tank" patients on ventilators if a nurse is available to assist.

Ambulatory patients with more limited wounds can be bathed in a smaller tub. Some tanks have chairs that can be raised and lowered to facilitate access and egress

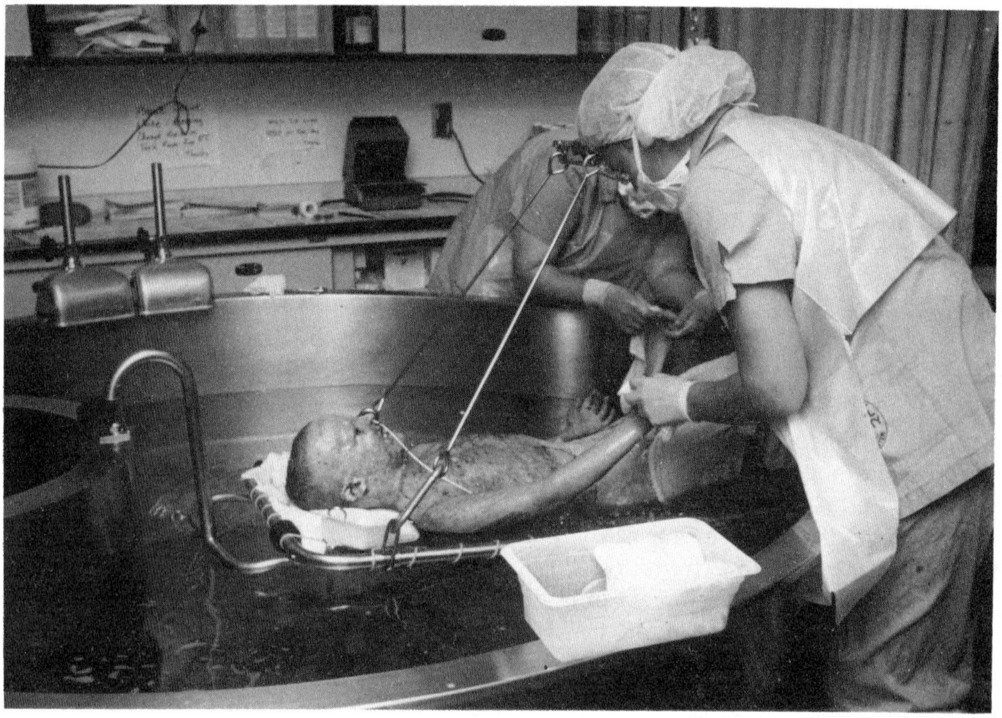

FIGURE 7–4. Wound cleansing and debridement is performed in the Hubbard tank on a routine basis. Note that care providers are wearing plastic gowns, hats, masks, and gloves as part of routine body substance precautions.

from the tank.[31-37] As an alternative, a shower stall (with a chair) can be used to provide total body cleansing for ambulatory patients. Patients with small burns can wash the affected area in a basin or sink. Therapists should make every effort to use the least complicated method of wound care, and patients should be encouraged to perform as much of their own dressing change as possible. These actions encourage activity and minimize dependence, and are helpful in preparing patients for discharge.

Hydrotherapy can be utilized successfully with children, if performed carefully.[37,40] Many children tolerate bathing well and can be distracted with toys while wounds are washed and debrided. A variety of antibacterial solutions and detergents can be added to tank water to aid in cleansing and help prevent the transfer of organisms by hydrotherapy. Thomson et al.[37] found that sodium hypochlorite (bleach), povidone-iodine, and chlorhexidine gluconate (Hibiclens) were the most frequently used additives. A variety of other commercial soaps and detergents also were used frequently. The properties of various additives have been reviewed in several publications.[36,38,39]

PRINCIPLES OF BANDAGE APPLICATION

Many wound care techniques require the application of bandages or wrappings to hold dressings or topical antibacterial medications in place, provide physical protection for the wound, and prevent venous stasis. In many circumstances, the technique used to apply the wrap can determine its effectiveness. Principles of bandage application are outlined in Appendix 7–2.

Wound Care Protocols

DRESSING SELECTION

The overall function of a wound dressing is to provide an optimal healing environment. Carr et al.[41] have outlined the characteristics of an ideal wound covering, and these are listed in Table 7–2. In the protocols that follow, no single wound care regimen incorporates all these characteristics fully. For the therapist, selection of a particular approach is based on the priorities presented by the patient and the wound, personal experience with particular techniques, and staff experience. In many cases more than one regimen will be applicable to a particular wound. Although the clinician does not need to master all the techniques presented, every therapist should be competent in at least one method of treatment for each type of burn wound encountered in practice.

INITIAL ASSESSMENT AND CARE OF BURN WOUNDS

The initial care of the burn patient represents a unique opportunity for both evaluation and treatment. Burn depth often can be assessed most accurately during initial debridement.[42] A determination of the extent of injury is made at this time. This estimation will dictate many aspects of early care, including fluid and nutritional requirements, choice of dressings, and approach to occupational and physical therapy. In addition, initial wound care is often the first time to meet, comfort, and reassure an apprehensive patient, while beginning to teach the principles of wound care that will continue throughout hospitalization and after discharge. For all these

TABLE 7–2. Characteristics of the Ideal Dressing

1. Protects surrounding skin from maceration/infection
2. Removes necrotic debris
3. Minimizes bacterial growth
4. Promotes the formulation of granulation tissue
5. Encourages re-epithelialization
6. Avoids dehydration and maintains body temperature
7. Prevents further contamination
8. Manages exudate
9. Minimizes disruption of the wound bed
10. Controls odor
11. Relieves pain
12. Stays in place
13. Easy to apply and remove
14. Saves time
15. Is cost effective

Adapted from Carr, R, et al: Comparative study of occlusive wound dressings on full thickness wounds in domestic pigs. Wounds 1:53, 1989.

reasons, the therapist should take every opportunity to be present and participate in initial wound management.

Initial Patient Assessment

The first priority in caring for the burn patient is not the wound itself. Assessment of airway, breathing, and circulation; placement of intravenous lines; beginning fluid resuscitation; detection and treatment of associated injuries; and assuring that the patient is as warm and comfortable as possible should take precedence over debridement.[43] To minimize confusion that could compromise patient safety, all burn team members should delay wound care until resuscitation is under way.

Initial Debridement

Initial debridement can be performed in the emergency room before moving the patient to the burn center, in the hydrotherapy department, or even at bedside. The rules for debridement are the same, regardless of where initial debridement is performed. Encircling objects such as watches, bracelets, rings, and other jewelry may act as tourniquets, causing constriction and ischemia, and should be removed.[44]

Assessment of Wounds

Although some approximation of burn extent and depth may be made during initial assessment, a second detailed evaluation of all burn injuries should be performed as soon as the patient is stabilized and resuscitation is underway. As each body area is cleansed and debrided, burn depth and extent are calculated and diagrammed carefully.[45] Characteristics of burns of various depths are outlined in Chapter 3 and illustrated in Figures 7-5 to 7-7.[44]

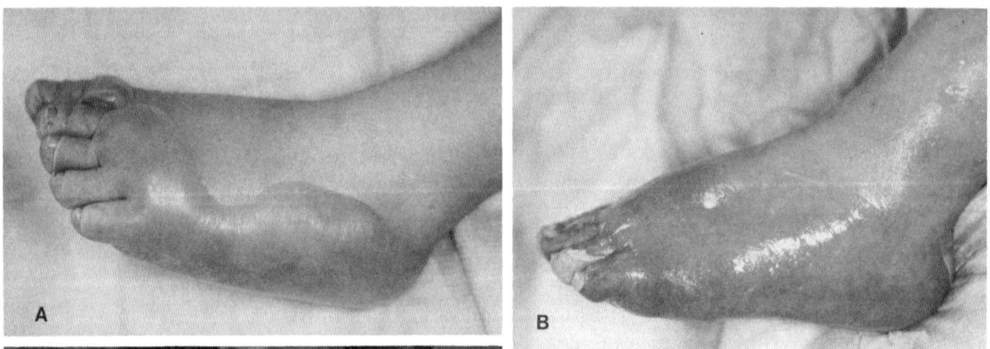

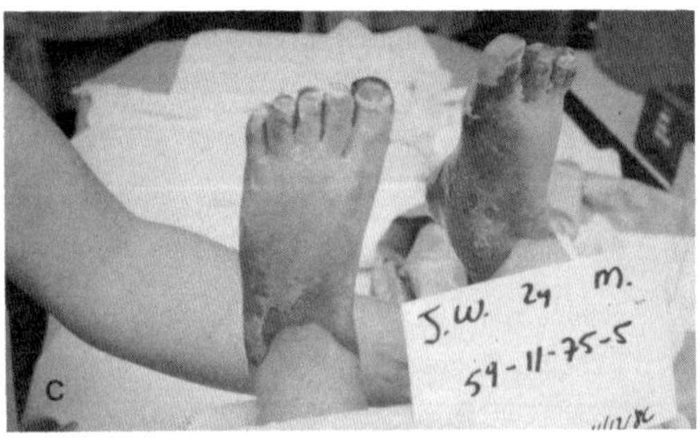

FIGURE 7-5. (*A*) This child was burned when his mother placed him into the bathtub without checking the water temperature. The dorsal foot and toes are covered with tense, fluid-filled blisters typical of superficial partial-thickness burns. (*B*) The same foot following debridement of blisters. The wound was dressed with Bacitracin ointment, Adaptic gauze, and gauze wraps. (*C*) A similar wound after 4 days. The thin layer of eschar covering the wound will continue to require debridement at least daily for several more days.

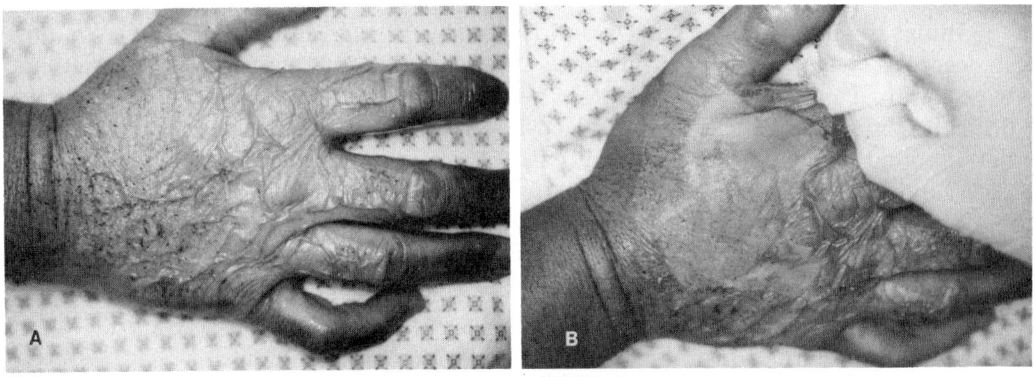

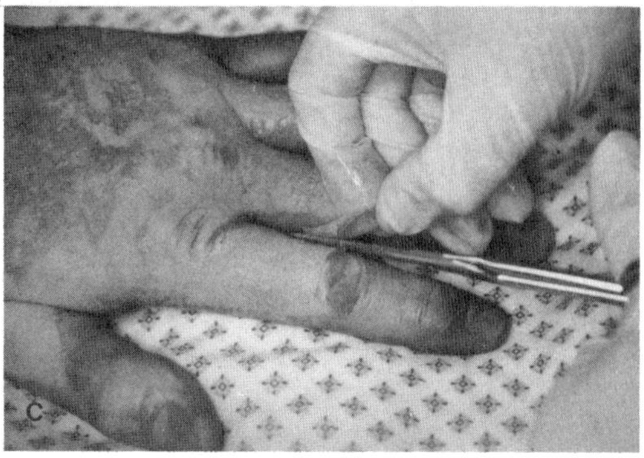

FIGURE 7–6. (*A*) This man sustained a deep partial-thickness burn from hot grease. The blistered skin contains little fluid, and the wound is relatively painless. (*B*) Debridement of the wound reveals a pale, dry, relatively anesthetic wound. (*C*) Scissors are used to trim the edges of the blistered skin of the fingers. This wound was dressed with silver sulfadiazine and gauze wraps and eventually healed.

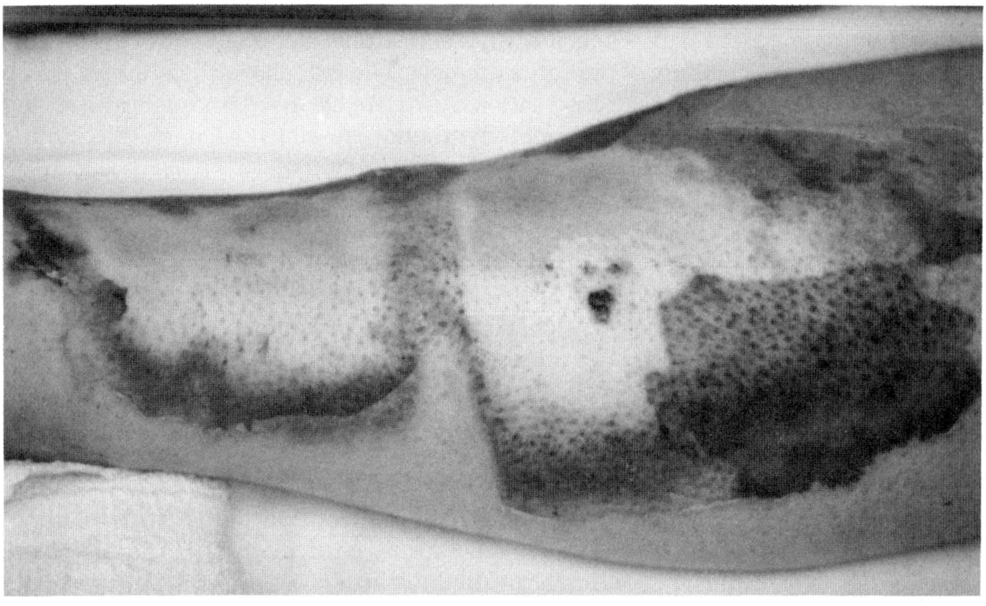

FIGURE 7–7. A full-thickness burn caused by flaming gasoline. This wound already has been debrided, revealing a dry, contracted appearance, ranging in color from white to dark brown. This wound was dressed with silver sulfadiazine and gauze wraps. Two days following injury, the wound was excised and skin grafted.

Initial treatment of all burn wounds usually is very similar. In many circumstances, the location of the burn dictates the type of treatment to be used more than burn depth. Distinguishing accurately between partial- and full-thickness burns is difficult, and many injuries are of mixed depth. Often the "true" depth of a burn is not apparent for many days after injury. For these reasons, therapists must examine all wounds frequently and assess them repeatedly.

WOUND CLEANSING AND DEBRIDEMENT

The principle of debridement is the mainstay of care for any open wound. Therapists who treat burns must be proficient in debridement techniques.

Rationale

Debridement consists of removing dead tissue as it loosens. This procedure expedites wound healing and prevents infection by mechanically removing bacteria. Gentle, frequent (several times daily) washing and debridement also improve circulation, remove old antibiotic creams and ointments, and facilitate range of motion, giving the patient a feeling of cleanliness and well-being.

Choice of Wounds

All burn wounds are washed and debrided. For superficial partial-thickness wounds, formal debridement may be needed only once or twice; deeper burns require wound care for weeks, or until the wound is excised surgically. Even after surgery, grafted wounds and donor sites are bathed and debrided as necessary.

Technique

All burns are debrided when initially seen. Initial debridement of fresh burns may need to be particularly thorough to remove blisters, shave the wound, and remove soil and necrotic debris.[46] Thereafter, burns are cleansed and debrided at least every 12 hours, unless covered with synthetic dressings such as Biobrane or Duoderm.

Warm water or saline to which a small amount of mild soap (Hibiclens, Joy, or Ivory liquid) has been added is used to wash wounds. Cutaneous wounds can be washed with clean tapwater, and sterile water is not needed for washing. The wound is washed gently with a washcloth or gauze pad, which removes bits of topical ointment, dead skin, and separating eschar. Blistered skin is grasped with a dry gauze pad and gently removed (Figs. 7–8 and 7–9); blunt scissors are used to trim the edges of blisters or eschar (see Fig. 7–7). Repeated gentle washing with fresh cloths will help loosen tenacious debris. Wounds should be rubbed sufficiently hard to remove loose debris, but not hard enough to cause bleeding. This principle should be taught to family members.

Following debridement, hair should be shaved from burned areas, including a 1- to 2-inch margin of unburned skin. Some burns, particularly on the scalp, can be obscured by hair, and the assessment of the burn extent is facilitated by shaving all burned areas. In addition, hair left on burns traps debris and old topical agents, favors bacterial overgrowth, and serves as a source of pain during subsequent care.[47,48] As a last step, the affected area should be washed with tepid water, then patted dry and dressed. The dressing technique may determine the frequency of

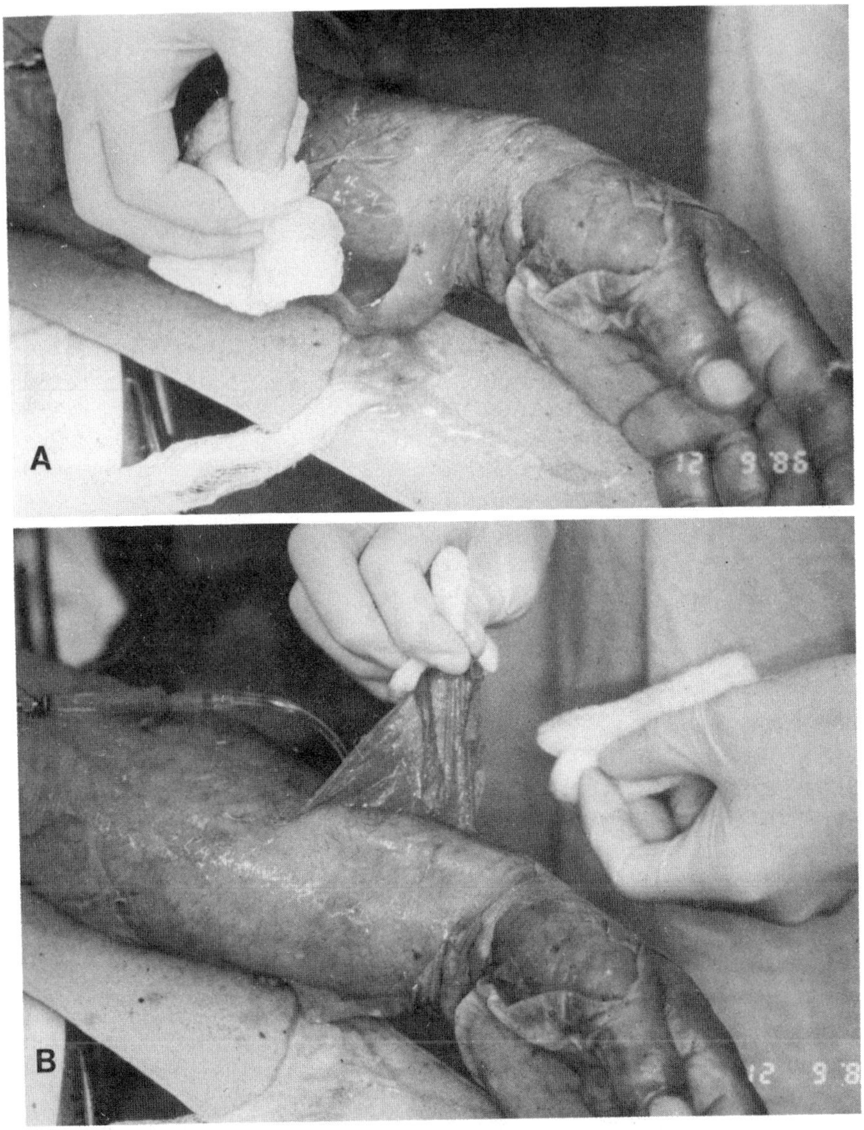

FIGURE 7–8. (*A*) Initial management of an intact blister includes removing the nonviable skin with a gauze pad. Note the gelatinous nature of the blister fluid. (*B*) Debridement continues until all nonviable tissue is removed. Debridement will continue onto the hand, and scissors will be used to trim blister edges on the palm and fingers.

dressing changes, but wounds are cleaned and debrided the same way regardless of the dressing employed. Several additional guidelines should be followed in all wound care procedures.

The Patient Should Be Kept Warm

One of the skin's major functions is temperature regulation, which is disrupted following burn injury, as heat loss from evaporation and convection increase significantly. Burn patients become cold very quickly, have increased sensitivity to cold, and have a difficult time warming up again.[47] A popular misconception is that ice water or

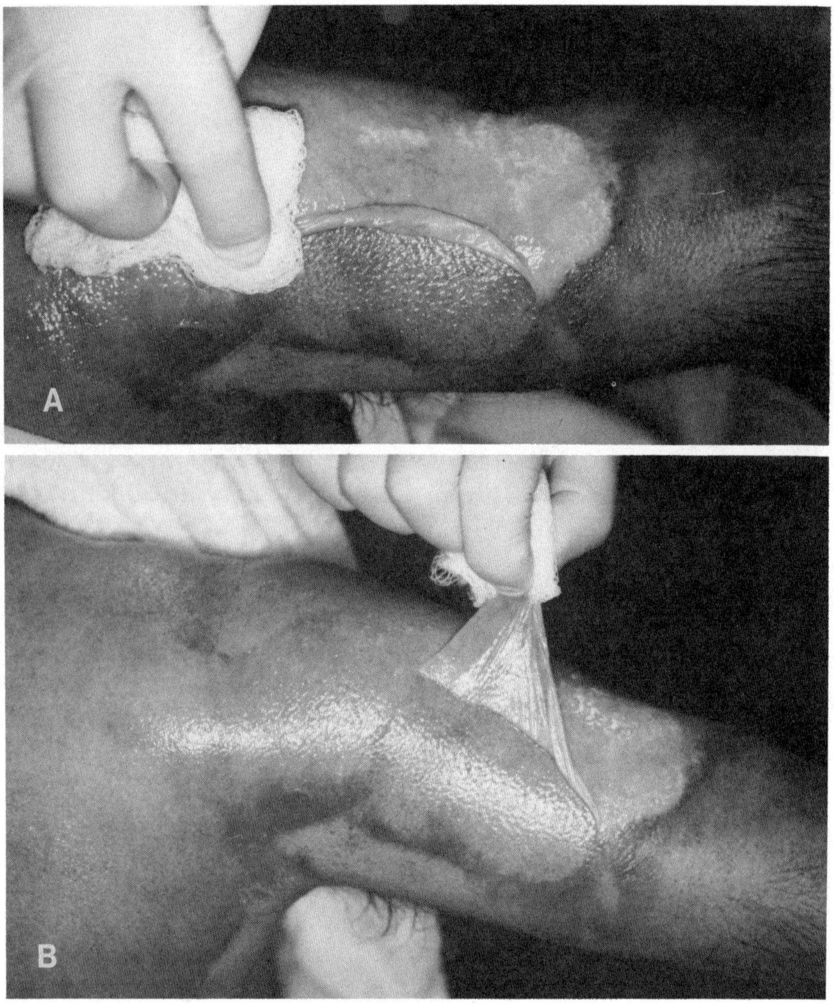

FIGURE 7–9. (*A*) Superficial partial-thickness burn, on postburn day 3 displays a layer of exudate and debris which is gently removed during wound care. (*B*) Loosened eschar can be grasped with a gauze pad and removed.

cold, wet towels should be left on wounds following burns. Cold water may limit burn depth if used immediately after injury; however, it should be used for only a few minutes.[49] Hypothermia, or even frostbite, can result if ice is used in initial burn treatment.[50]

Patients should be bathed or showered in water which is approximately 100°F. Washing is restricted to 20 minutes or less to minimize heat and electrolyte loss, stress, and discomfort, particularly for patients with large wounds. A team approach will expedite wound cleansing. As stated previously, patients should be covered and dried with warm blankets and towels immediately following cleansing and one area should be redressed at a time while other areas are kept covered. Room temperature should be kept at least 85°F in the hydrotherapy area at all times, and supplemented as needed with heat lamps or shields.

The Patient Should Be Kept Comfortable

Debridement is uncomfortable for the patient and should be performed as gently as possible. Even simple bathing can be stressful and frightening. Relieving all discomfort may be impossible, but if patients perceive that the team is mindful of their discomfort, this empathy will reduce anxiety and help them cooperate with wound care. General anesthesia rarely is needed if debridement is performed gently and analgesics are used. In general, narcotics, sedative agents, or nitrous oxide should be used with caution and not administered unless nursing or physician staff is available to monitor patient response. Wound exposure to the air is painful. Wounds should be left uncovered as little as possible, debrided quickly, and redressed as soon as debridement is completed. Granting the patient some control over the wound care process when possible, and permitting "time-out" periods, provided they are short, can greatly reduce anxiety and help the patient tolerate debridement better.[51] Some burn centers also have reported success with the use of hypnosis during wound care.[48]

Management of Blisters

All blisters should be opened and debrided. Although an intact blister is theoretically sterile, few blisters are substantial enough to remain intact for long. Blister fluid will "set" into a gelatinous film if debridement is delayed. This film is the beginning of eschar, and is an ideal culture medium for bacteria. Rockwell and Ehrlich[52] have outlined further reasons for evacuating blisters. Blister fluid impairs normal function of neutrophils and lymphocytes, which reduces the effectiveness of local immunity. Blister fluid also contains arachidonic acid metabolites that increase the inflammatory response and retard the fibrinolytic process that maintains dermal vascular patency.[52] All of these effects delay healing of the burn wound.

Wound Surveillance

Each area of the burn should be washed and debrided carefully with each dressing change. All old creams and ointments must be removed, and the lack or presence of remaining residue is sometimes a useful indicator of the thoroughness of cleansing. Eschar separates and loosens gradually. An area that is firmly adherent initially may be easily removed later. Wounds should be inspected daily for evidence of infection and to assess healing. Deep partial-thickness burns that show no eschar separation after 10 to 14 days of debridement may benefit from excision and skin grafting.[50]

Enzymatic Debridement

In addition to mechanical debridement performed when wounds are washed and dressings changed, topical enzymatic agents are available for wound debridement. Enzymatic products include Elase and Travase (Sutilains)[54] ointments (Appendix 7-3). When applied to burn wounds, these preparations "digest" necrotic tissue, cause early separation of eschar, and promote healing. Enzymatic debridement can be used to provide a "chemical escharotomy," to delineate the depth of burn injury, or to prepare a wound for early skin grafting.

The enzymatic ointment is applied three to four times daily, often in conjunction with a topical antimicrobial such as silver sulfadiazine. When the wound is washed, old ointment and any debris that has developed also is removed and a new layer of ointment reapplied. Pain and bleeding can be complications of this form of therapy. In addition, the film that develops on the wound surface with the use of enzymatic debridement may resemble the purulent exudate that forms on infected wounds. Some experience may be necessary to distinguish normal by-products of enzymatic debridement from wound infection.

"OPEN" TECHNIQUE

The open technique consists simply of leaving wounds exposed to the air, or using minimal dressings.[55,56] This technique is the "natural" way for wounds to heal and often works very well, though the reasons are poorly understood.

Rationale

Burn wounds that are left open to air rapidly will develop a layer of eschar consisting of dead skin elements, serum, and other fluids that have oozed through the skin and dried. In superficial wounds eschar is composed primarily of serum that dries into a scab and is in many ways a satisfactory dressing. This eschar is tough, adherent, and protective; it retards evaporative losses, reduces pain, and protects the wound from bacterial invasion; and eventually separates as new epidermis grows beneath it. However, as wounds become deeper or larger, open treatment is less satisfactory. Bacteria proliferate more readily within thick eschar, which takes a long time to separate, often exposing granulation tissue. This process can be accelerated by excising eschar, but unless the wound is covered to prevent exposure and dessication, the exposed tissue again dies and a new layer of eschar forms. Even in relatively superficial wounds, the presence of a dessicated scab retards epithelial migration.

Another major drawback of the open technique is that patients find such wounds uncomfortable and unsightly. The use of topical agents and other dressings is often comforting to patients, as they are perceived as more "therapeutic" than the open technique.

Choice of Wounds

A scab can be a trouble-free dressing for small burns, especially if they are superficial and located away from joints. Wounds of the face, ears, and scalp do well if treated with a modification of the open technique, in which a thin layer of transparent ointment is applied to the wound surface. Some fresh skin grafts can be treated in this manner.

The open technique is not well suited for use on wounds that cross joints because the scabs that form continually crack, bleed, and hurt. As wounds become large or deep, the need for more vigorous debridement and aggressive topical antibiotics also increases, and these wounds are harder to manage with the open technique. A modification of the open technique often is used on fresh donor sites by covering them with dry or impregnated gauze, which serves as a wick to transport blood and serum to the gauze surface, where it dries, facilitating scab formation.[57] Donor sites are easy to treat in this manner, but relatively uncomfortable for the patient.

Technique

Wounds treated by the open technique should be washed once or twice daily, patted dry, and either left dry or covered with a thin layer of ointment (Appendix A).

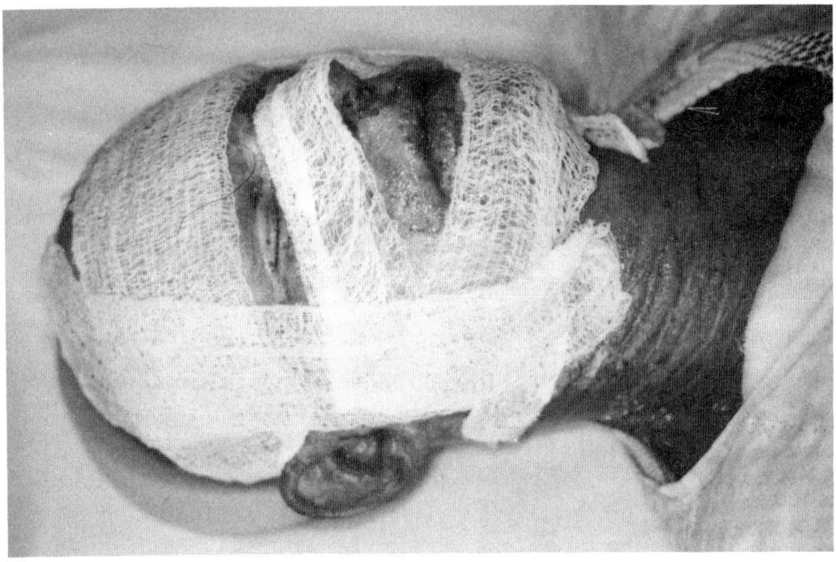

FIGURE 7–10. Debridement of partial-thickness burn of the face using "wet-to-moist" dressing technique. Note the gauze "doughnut" instead of a pillow, which keeps the patient's ears from touching the bedclothes.

Formed scabs that are adherent and dry should not be soaked off, but loose, moist, or purulent debris should be removed gently with washing. Facial burns are often treated with the open technique, with the addition of intermittent wet-to-moist dressings for debridement (Fig. 7–10).

Wound Surveillance

Open wounds become infected easily, especially if they are not kept clean. Scabs should be inspected frequently to be sure they are dry and adherent. Pus found beneath a scab should be soaked off or gently unroofed, and the wound treated with topical antibiotics. Infection can be difficult to detect beneath a large eschar, which is a major disadvantage to the open technique, so these wounds must be watched carefully. Whenever eschar separates from an open wound and the underlying tissue is not healed, the wound should be dressed with antibiotic cream or ointment dressings.

TOPICAL ANTIBIOTICS

For the past 20 years, the use of antibiotic creams and ointments has been the standard treatment for burn wounds (see Appendix A).[29] By reducing the incidence of burn wound infections, these agents have significantly reduced mortality in burn patients.

Rationale

As mentioned previously, the surface of a fresh burn is usually sterile for 24 to 48 hours after injury. Bacterial colonization of an open wound invariably occurs, however, and bacteria invade the necrotic eschar. As bacteria proliferate, they become more effective in overwhelming local defenses and creating an advancing margin of tissue necrosis and vascular invasion that is termed *burn wound sepsis.*

There are only two ways to reduce bacterial counts effectively. One is removal of necrotic debris and bacteria through debridement or excision. The other is the use of antibiotics. Because burn eschar has no blood supply, topical antibiotics (those applied to the wound itself) are necessary to kill bacteria directly.

A number of topical antibiotic agents now are available for burn care and are reviewed in Appendix 7–3.[29,58–63] Foremost among these agents are silver sulfadiazine (Silvadene, Thermazene) and mafenide acetate (Sulfamylon).

Choice of Wounds

Topical antibiotics can be used on any burn wound. Most frequently, however, they are used on large or deep injuries where there is a significant amount of eschar. Very deep or infected wounds are usually dressed with silver sulfadiazine or mafenide acetate. A variety of other agents, including Bacitracin, Neosporin, and Furacin can be used on more superficial burns, donor sites, and healing skin grafts. In addition to their antibacterial qualities, topical agents maintain a moist environment; provide a soothing, comfortable covering for wounds; reduce the stiffness often experienced in dry wounds; and reduce evaporative losses.

Technique

The antibiotic action of some topical creams and ointments lasts for only 8 to 12 hours after application and must be reapplied at regular intervals. In addition, the regular replacement of these agents, combined with debridement, cleanses the wound and reduces the risk of infection. In some cases, a significant advantage of antibiotic creams is that they provide something to wash off the patient and require that washing be done frequently.

Prior to the reapplication of topical antibiotics, dressings are removed, the wound is washed with all traces of old cream or ointment removed completely, and the wound is patted dry (Fig. 7–11). Topicals are reapplied using a sterile glove, tongue blade, or cotton swab to the manufacturer's recommended thickness. Topical creams are applied thickly enough that they cannot be seen through. Ointments should be applied much more thinly, but at least thick enough to give the entire wound a glistening appearance. Once in place, topicals can be left open, though they tend to dry quickly and come off on every surface they contact. To prevent this occurrence, topical creams or ointments are usually covered with dry gauze and elastic bandages (Ace wraps, Tubigrip, or Surginet; see Appendix 7–2). If the topical is sufficiently aqueous (silver sulfadiazine is 70 percent water), the gauze dressing will not stick to the burn if changed at least twice daily. A layer of nonadherent or petrolatum gauze is useful over ointments to prevent dressings from sticking to the wound (Fig. 7–12). Nonadherent gauze sheets should be placed so that they extend $\frac{1}{2}$-inch beyond the margin of the wound and overlap slightly. Occlusive dressings should not be used with topicals, as they favor bacterial proliferation.

As wound healing progresses, topical antibiotic use must be re-evaluated regularly and changes in care made as needed. The more powerful antibiotics may slow separation of eschar and tissue re-epithelialization.[63] As the size of unhealed burn decreases below 20 percent, using a bland topical in place of sulfadiazine or mafenide often is possible, thus encouraging healing and in a far less expensive manner.

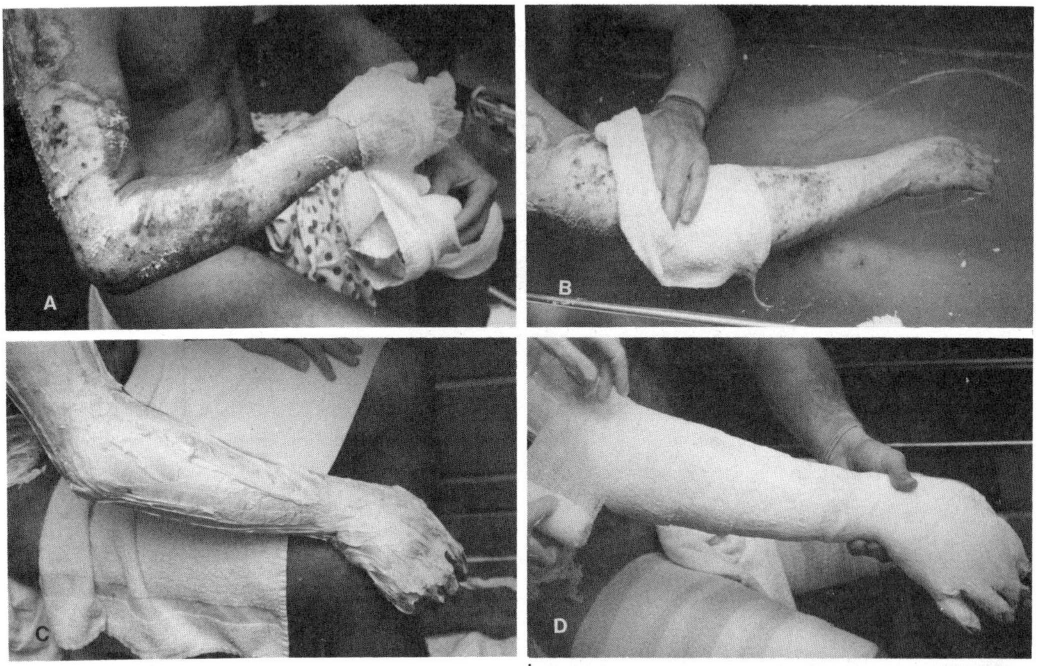

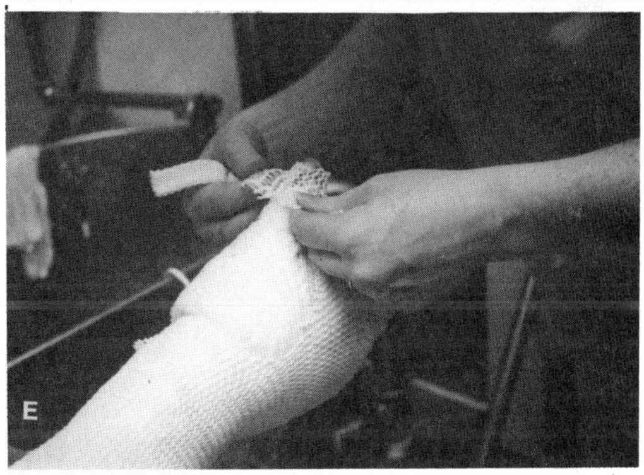

FIGURE 7–11. Dressing change with silver sulfadiazine. (*A*) Patient with deep partial and full-thickness burns to the right arm, shoulder and back, removing old dressings prior to washing and debridement. (*B*) In the hydrotherapy tank, the patient washes his wounds to remove old antibiotic cream and perform gentle debridement. (*C*) Application of a uniform layer of silver sulfadiazine over the entire wound. The cream should be just thick enough that it cannot be seen through. (*D*) Fingers are wrapped individually, and gauze wraps are applied from distal (fingers) to proximal (shoulder). (*E*) Gauze is held in place with elastic netting.

Wound Surveillance

Topical creams and ointments tend to soften eschar and speed its separation, so thorough debridement must be used at least once daily as part of this technique. As the wound separates, the need for powerful antibiotic creams also diminishes. Granulation tissue requires much less debridement if it is kept moistened with ointment to prevent bleeding and scab formation. Burn wound sepsis often is heralded by erythema at the wound margins, increased pain, purulent exudate from beneath eschar, or dramatic black or green discoloration of the wounds. The therapist must alert the physician immediately if these are seen.

Topical agents have specific side effects. Silver sulfadiazine and mafenide acetate are sulfa drugs, to which some people are allergic. Sulfadiazine may cause leukopenia, though there is controversy over whether this mandates discontinuing the agent.[63,64] Mafenide acetate is a carbonic anhydrase inhibitor; prolonged or extensive use can cause significant metabolic acidemia that may require a change in topical medication.[63]

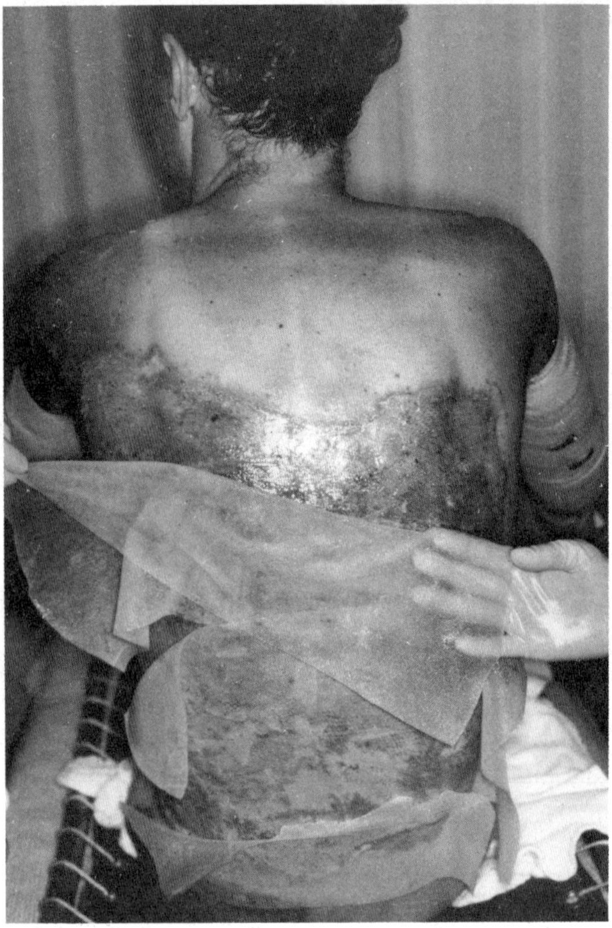

FIGURE 7–12. Ointment dressings. Postoperative day 10 following excision and skin grafting of burns of the back. Wounds are covered with a thin layer of Bacitracin ointment and Adaptic gauze, shown here, before wrapping with gauze rolls and elastic netting.

BIOLOGIC DRESSINGS

A variety of natural or "biologic" substances are available for wound treatment. Though the opinions of burn surgeons vary greatly as to their usefulness, they all accomplish roughly the same goals. Often, the decision to use a biologic dressing, and which dressing to use, is based on risks, availability, and costs, as well as efficacy. This section discusses only those dressing materials that are directly derived from living organisms and are thus truly "biologic." Synthetic occlusive and semiocclusive dressings are described in the next section.

Rationale

The ideal covering of the body is skin itself. Dressings that cover wounds should resemble skin as closely as possible and perform several important functions (see Table 7–2). The functions include pain relief, reduction of evaporative fluid and heat loss, adherence, flexibility, protection from infection, reduction of bacterial colonization, and stimulation of local blood flow. Dressings that could become vascularized like autologous skin and not be rejected could eventually eliminate the need for autografting. In efforts to develop such an ideal wound cover, several naturally occurring substances have been used.[65,66] Currently available biologic dressings include human homograft skin (fresh or frozen), xenograft pigskin (fresh, frozen, or lyophylized), and fresh human amniotic membrane.

Choice of Wounds

Biologic dressings have been advocated in several circumstances: (1) Immediate coverage of superficial partial-thickness wounds; (2) coverage of granulation tissue to "clean up" the wound; (3) as a "test" of graft adherence; (4) or as a skin substitute on excised wounds for which no autograft skin is available.[65] In recent years, biologic dressings have been used less frequently on superficial wounds because of the high costs, unpredictable availability, and risks (i.e., disease transmission) of some biologic agents. Probably the widest use of biologic dressings today is in the temporary coverage of excised large burn wounds. For this purpose, fresh, cadaver homograft is the agent of choice. In patients with major burns, the general immunosuppression that accompanies the burn injury assists in homograft adherence and vascularization for weeks to months. Homograft skin also can be used over widely meshed autografts to protect the grafts while epithelialization of the mesh interstices takes place. Biologic dressings are not routinely used on donor sites.

Technique

Biologic dressings can be applied and treated in a manner identical to autografts. They can be secured with staples, sutures, or compressive dressings, and treated with ointment, synthetic covering, or antibiotic soaks.

Wound Surveillance

Biologic dressings are susceptible to all the factors that cause autograft loss, including bleeding, infection, motion, and an inadequate graft bed. Infection can develop readily beneath opaque biologic dressings that can be hard to detect. In addition, rejection of these foreign substances can occur and cause suppuration, detachment, or even dissolution of the agent. In cases of severe rejection, redness, swelling, and pain surrounding the dressing makes this process difficult to distinguish from infection.

SYNTHETIC (OCCLUSIVE AND SEMIOCCLUSIVE) DRESSINGS

In recent years, a number of products have been marketed as "miracle" dressings for burns and other wounds. Most of these products actually are occlusive or semiocclusive dressings that function in a few simple ways.

Rationale

Exposure to the air is a mixed blessing for burn wounds. Exposed wounds invariably become colonized with bacteria, though free circulation of air over wounds also promotes healing and may minimize bacterial penetration. Exposure to the air also is painful, particularly for superficial injuries. Finally, open wounds invariably develop a layer of dessicated eschar that retards epithelial migration and often requires debridement, which further damages regenerating skin elements and prolongs healing time.[67,68]

A variety of synthetic products now are available that are classified as occlusive or semiocclusive dressings. These dressings include plastic films, hydrocolloids, hydrogels, collagen-impregnated dressings, and others (Appendix B). Appendix 7–4 reviews a number of common products, their main uses, and advantages and disadvantages. Synthetic dressings act by "sealing off" the wound and providing physical protection and a moist environment that favors epidermal growth.[21-27,67,68] These dressings also provide pain relief, retard evaporative loss, and permit more comfortable motion. While bacterial invasion through the dressing is retarded,[69] proliferation of bacteria that already exist beneath the dressing may be enhanced by the "greenhouse" environment produced by the dressing. Similarly, if necrotic debris is trapped beneath such a dressing, it more easily liquefies and suppurates.

Choice of Wounds

Most occlusive and semiocclusive dressings are used primarily on fresh partial-thickness burn wounds or donor sites. Patients with superficial wounds may benefit greatly from the pain relief afforded by these dressings. Such wounds have little necrotic debris and often demonstrate brisk epidermal growth when protected by synthetic dressings. Deeper burns, old burns, and infected wounds should be treated by active debridement and topical antibiotics, though some small deep wounds can be treated with a hydrocolloid, especially those over finger joints or elbows.

Occlusive and semiocclusive dressings are widely used on fresh skin grafts. Unna's boot dressings can be used successfully over grafts, particularly on the lower extremities, where the dressing applies uniform pressure to the wound, permitting early ambulation.[27] In addition, because Unna's boot can remain in place for several days without being changed, this dressing is ideal for outpatient care. Biobrane is also useful for covering fresh skin grafts.[27] Biobrane is elastic and durable and provides significant mechanical protection for grafts placed on the trunk, especially the back, if it is stretched tightly over the graft and stapled into position (Fig. 7-13). No other dressing is necessary except loose gauze pads to absorb any moisture that leaks through the Biobrane. Biobrane also can be used on freshly excised wounds while

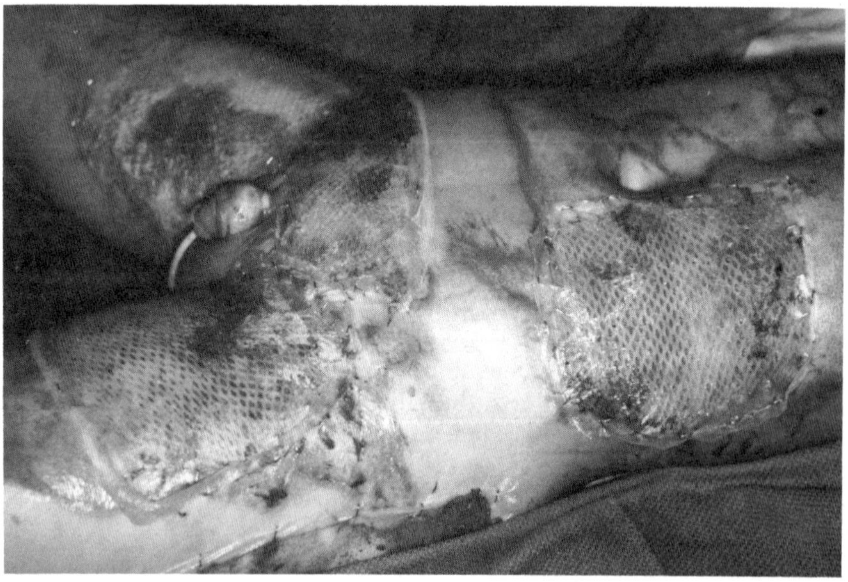

FIGURE 7-13. Two days following excision and skin grafting of the thighs and anterior trunk. Biobrane is stapled over the grafts, holding them securely in position. This type of dressing also has been used on the donor sites visible on the posterior thigh.

awaiting autografting, much like a biologic dressing. Biobrane's collagen-impregnated structure adheres to the fresh wound, providing temporary coverage.

Technique

Wounds selected for treatment with occlusive or semiocclusive dressings should be clean and dry. Blisters, loose skin, and any loose eschar should be gently debrided, and the wound washed and patted dry. Some dressings (Duoderm, Op-Site) require a margin of unburned skin to which the dressing can adhere, and adherence can be enhanced by the use of an adhesive such as tincture of benzoin. Biobrane usually is stapled in place, and the staples left for several days until the dressing is adherent. Once in place, the dressing should be covered with a protective gauze wrap.

Wound Surveillance

These types of dressings can be valuable if used carefully, but disaster may ensue if they are neglected. The major risk of occlusive and semiocclusive dressings is infection, which can develop very insidiously beneath the dressing, particularly if it is opaque. Recent evidence, however, suggests that wounds under occlusive dressings may become infected less frequently than open wounds.[69] Though judicious use of these dressings may eliminate the pain of frequent dressing changes, clinicians should not ignore them or delay too long in removing them. Dressings should be inspected regularly, even if no dressing change is planned. Loosening of the dressing, or collection of cloudy fluid beneath the dressing, may indicate infection, in which case the dressing should be changed and the wound inspected carefully. Films like Op-Site may wrinkle and adhere poorly when used over joints. Fluid collecting under the film can be gently aspirated with a syringe, but if fluid accumulations occur repeatedly, the film should be removed and the wound dressed with an antibiotic ointment or cream.

DEBRIDING DRESSINGS

Topical antibiotics may cause eschar to loosen, but a separate procedure is sometimes required for debridement. Using a type of dressing that itself provides significant debridement of eschar is possible.

Rationale

The action of debriding dressings is mechanical, though these dressings can be combined with topical antibiotics under some circumstances. When wet dressings are applied to wounds, they soften the uppermost layer of eschar. As the wound begins to dry, the eschar sticks to the dressing and, when the dressing is removed, the eschar is removed as well. In essence, these dressings "strip" the wound when they are changed.

Choice of Wounds

Dressings that debride work best on wounds covered with softened eschar, since scabs are often too dry to slough without applying undue force. Conversely, wounds covered thickly with topicals do not dry sufficiently for the dressing to remove much eschar. Once the majority of eschar has separated and been removed, debriding dressings are no longer needed. These dressings tend to stick excessively to granulation tissue (unless kept very moist), and they can damage existing epithelium and delay epithelial regeneration. In addition, these dressings can be painful to remove. For these reasons, they should be used only when needed for their cleansing action, and discontinued once the majority of eschar has been removed.

Technique

Debriding dressings are often called "wet-to-dry" dressings,[68] but this term should be abandoned, because the dressing is not necessarily completely dry before being removed. Such a procedure is extremely painful and excessively abrasive, causing significant bleeding in some cases and damaging normal tissue. For that reason, the term "wet-to-moist" should be used for these dressings. Debriding dressings should be applied following regular washing and debridement of wounds. Gauze pads or rolls are soaked in saline solution, Ringer's lactate, or antibiotic solutions; wrung out lightly; and packed loosely into the wound and covered with dry gauze and elastic wraps. Because of the tendency of these dressings to dessicate, they should not be left in place longer than 6 to 8 hours without being changed. Even then, they may be excessively dry when removal is attempted, and may necessitate moistening before completing their removal. For facial burns, small gauze pads ("four by eights") moistened with saline can be opened and spread over the face for 20 to 30 minutes as a short debriding dressing between applications of ointment (see Fig. 7-10). For badly infected wounds, wet-to-moist dressings can be modified into "wet-to-wet" antibiotic soaks.

Wound Surveillance

Excessive bleeding may be encountered when dried dressings are removed. If bleeding occurs, the interval between dressings should be shortened, or the dressings moistened lightly before removal. As necrotic debris gradually is removed from the wound, clean granulation tissue or even healed epidermis will be seen. At this point, debriding dressings will produce excessive bleeding and may retard healing. A gentler dressing, usually an antibiotic ointment or cream, should be used at this time.

ANTIBIOTIC WET DRESSINGS

Dressings that are kept intentionally wet have three uses: to keep the wound moist, to improve the adherence of fresh skin grafts, and to effectively deliver concentrated antibiotic solutions by softening the eschar.

Rationale

Antibiotic soaks are used for fresh meshed skin grafts, as well as heavily infected wounds. Meshed grafts have interstices that are essentially small open wounds. If allowed to dry, these interstices form a collection of tiny scabs, and the resulting dessication may reduce the adherence of the graft lattice and impede epithelialization of the mesh openings. By keeping the entire wound moist, antibiotic soaks create an environment that is optimal for epidermal growth. In addition, wet dressings conform closely to the graft surface, help provide uniform pressure that prevents graft motion and fluid collection, and improves graft adherence and vascularization. Soaks also can be used to deliver antibiotics in severely infected wounds. Mafenide acetate soaks have been advocated for use in invasive infections,[70] because the agent penetrates deeply through eschar or grafts.

Choice of Wounds

Antibiotic soak dressings have been used primarily in two circumstances: to dress fresh meshed skin grafts, particularly on the extremities where they can be tightly secured with wraps, and to reduce bacterial contamination of infected wounds.

Technique

Initially, fresh skin grafts are dressed with a single layer of fine mesh gauze, Xeroform or Adaptic gauze.[71] This dressing is covered with two layers of wet gauze dressings soaked in antibiotic solution, between which are placed multiple perforated rubber catheters. The dressing is then wrapped with gauze and elastic wraps and splinted if necessary (Fig. 7–14). Wet soaks placed on skin grafts on the trunk require circumferential elastic wraps, or they can be covered with large gauze pads stapled into position.

Following application of the dressing, the wounds are moistened every 2 hours, either by pouring antibiotic solution directly over the dressing or by injecting 50 to 100 mL of antibiotic solution into each rubber catheter (see Appendix 7–3 for composition of some standard antibiotic solutions). The first dressing change following skin grafting is performed at 48 to 72 hours. At that time, a "dry" dressing of antibiotic ointment, nonadherent gauze, and bulky gauze wraps can be applied. Wet dressings placed on infected wounds are changed as needed for further debridement or inspection.[57]

Wound Surveillance

Wet dressings must be applied and secured meticulously on fresh skin grafts. Uncooperative patients, especially children, may disrupt the dressings or pull out the

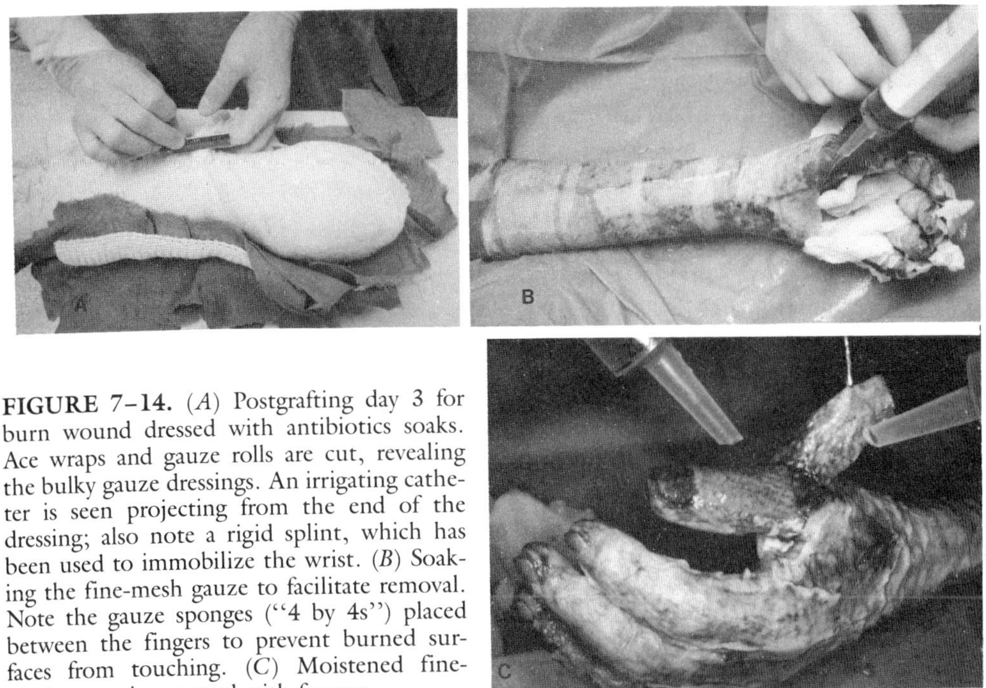

FIGURE 7–14. (*A*) Postgrafting day 3 for burn wound dressed with antibiotics soaks. Ace wraps and gauze rolls are cut, revealing the bulky gauze dressings. An irrigating catheter is seen projecting from the end of the dressing; also note a rigid splint, which has been used to immobilize the wrist. (*B*) Soaking the fine-mesh gauze to facilitate removal. Note the gauze sponges ("4 by 4s") placed between the fingers to prevent burned surfaces from touching. (*C*) Moistened fine-mesh gauze is removed with forceps.

rubber catheters. Dressings that are still reasonably intact should be left in place and moistened directly with a syringe. Antibiotic solutions must be warmed at least to room temperature before use, as continued soaking with cold solutions can produce maceration, graft loss, and a "trench-foot" injury, in addition to being very uncomfortable for the patient. Finally, wet dressings, even when used carefully, will macerate surrounding tissue and should not be used for longer than four days.

DAILY WOUND CARE

All wound care techniques require planned regular dressing changes, although the interval between inspections may vary. As a general rule, larger, deeper, and more contaminated wounds should be examined and redressed more frequently. Some topical agents (antibiotic soaks, for example, especially silver nitrate) have short durations of effectiveness once applied to wounds, and must be changed when that effectiveness expires. Other topicals may remain effective for longer periods (sulfadiazine, mafenide), but even when they are used, regular dressing changes and debridements are required to remove debris and bacteria. Wounds dressed with silver sulfadiazine or mafenide, and wounds in wet-to-moist dressings, are generally changed two to three times daily, while wounds dressed with other topical ointments are changed twice daily, including skin grafts and donor sites. Wounds dressed with more occlusive biologic and synthetic dressings may not require complete changing for several days, but these wounds should be inspected at least daily to look for evidence of infection. Occlusive and semi-occlusive dressings must remain intact and "sealed" to the wound to provide a barrier against infection. For that reason, such dressings should not be partially removed unless the entire dressing is removed and replaced. Partial removal nullifies many of the advantages of such dressings, and should be done only if infection is seriously suspected.

Burn wounds are very dynamic. Therapists who observe burn wounds regularly must be alert to the signs of infection, as even a burn that is healing well can develop significant infection within a few hours. Findings should be documented and brought to the attention of other burn team members if infection is suspected.

Management of Special Care Areas

The previous information is a guide to general burn wound care. Several body areas, however, require specific care as follows.

FACE

Facial burns are particularly distressing to patients, families, and burn team members alike. Injuries in this area may compromise vision. Many types of soap, including Hibiclens, are harmful to the eyes, and should not be used in washing the face. Shur-Clens, a nonirritating skin wound cleanser, is very effective in removing dirt and debris from wound surfaces without damaging the eyes.[72] Facial burns often reveal a discolored epidermis that does not blister; therefore, gentle rubbing of all discolored areas is necessary to remove damaged skin. Particular care and gentleness should be used around the nose, mouth, and eyes to avoid allowing fluid or debris to enter these orifices.

fragile and because there is no egress of blood through interstices in the graft, as occurs in meshed grafts.

Hematomas must be evacuated when found. Surprisingly, a graft will recover well following drainage of a hematoma and the restoration of a solid interface between the graft and its nutrient supply. Though most hematomas are easily detected, care should be taken to inspect all surfaces of the graft for irregularities or "blisters" that can indicate fluid collections. If the fluid collection is small and near the graft margin, the fluid can be expressed using a cotton-tipped swab to gently "roll" the fluid out from under the edge of the graft. As an alternative, the fluid can be aspirated with a syringe, or one or more small openings can be cut in the graft to allow expression of the fluid. Gentle pressure usually will remove serous fluid easily, but clotted blood can be much more tenacious. Blood that does not express easily can be irrigated free, using a flexible intravenous catheter and half-strength hydrogen peroxide. Care must be taken not to inject the peroxide into viable tissue. Once the hematoma is removed, the wound should be irrigated with saline to remove the peroxide and debris. Following evacuation of fluid, the graft should be redressed using a gentle wrap. A very large hematoma may require restapling the graft in position. The manipulations to remove fluid collections beneath fresh grafts usually are performed by physicians, although small fluid collections can be removed safely by experienced therapists under a physician's direction.

Skin Graft Infection

Infection often results in complete graft loss and is thus the most feared complication of skin grafting. All grafts should be inspected for infection at each dressing change, and the dressing immediately changed on any grafted wound suspected of harboring infection. Infection may be heralded by a musty or sweetish odor coming from the wound, by coloration of the dressing (*Pseudomonas* infection classically produces a bright green drainage) or the graft itself (blackish, pale), or by excessive or purulent exudate. Sometimes the only evidence of graft infection is disappearance of the graft, caused by bacterial digestion of the grafted skin.

If infection of a graft is suspected, the physician should be notified immediately. Suspicious-looking dressings should be saved for the physician to inspect. If the skin graft is still in place, every effort should be made to salvage the graft, which often is possible despite the presence of infection. Occlusive dressings are removed immediately, and the graft washed gently with dilute Hibiclens or other detergent solution. Infected grafts often heal well if left open to the air to dry, or if dressed only with a thin layer of ointment over the graft. As an alternative, infected grafts can be dressed in wet soaks with antibiotic irrigation. Mafenide acetate soaks are particularly effective against *Pseudomonas* and yeast; acetic acid or sodium hypochlorite (Dakin's solution) can be used as well. Dressings on infected grafts should be changed frequently to remove bacterial innoculum, refresh the antibacterials used, and permit further inspection of the graft.

DONOR SITES

Skin grafting requires the harvesting of autologous skin from donor sites. Donor sites are significant wounds and often require as much or more attention than the burn itself for the first few days following the skin harvest. Split-thickness donor sites are harvested at varying depths, but are physiologically similar to partial-thickness burns and can be treated in similar ways.

The treatment of donor sites is based on several considerations. The dressings for donor sites should provide significant pain relief, enhance epithelial regeneration, and prevent infection. A once popular donor site dressing was dry fine mesh or Scarlet Red gauze, applied directly over the donor site and permitted to dry, forming a scab (Fig. 7–16). The dressing was left in place until the underlying skin was healed.[57] Although still used in many burn centers, dry gauze dressings are far from ideal. The scab formed by such a dressing is prone to crack and bleed. They are very uncomfortable, especially when hair grows into the gauze, and take a long time to separate from the wound. Infection that develops beneath such a large scab can be difficult to detect. For these reasons, donor sites are now more frequently treated with either topical antibiotic medications or synthetic dressings. Biobrane, Op-site, Duoderm, and other synthetic occlusive and semiocclusive dressings can be applied to donor sites, and these dressings are well suited for this purpose.[27,78] Biobrane can be stapled over donor sites and remain in place until the wound heals (see Fig. 7–16). Op-site and other plastic films must adhere to the normal skin surrounding the donor site and require a margin of normal skin for this purpose. For this reason use of such materials is restricted to moderately small donor sites. Hydrocolloid dressings, like Duoderm, also can be used to dress donor sites and may offer significant improvements in the speed of healing.[24] Alternatively, donor sites can be treated with antibiotic creams or ointments in a manner identical to that of partial-thickness burns. Any donor site suspected of being infected should have the dressing removed immediately and redressed with silver sulfadiazine or other topical antibiotic for several days.

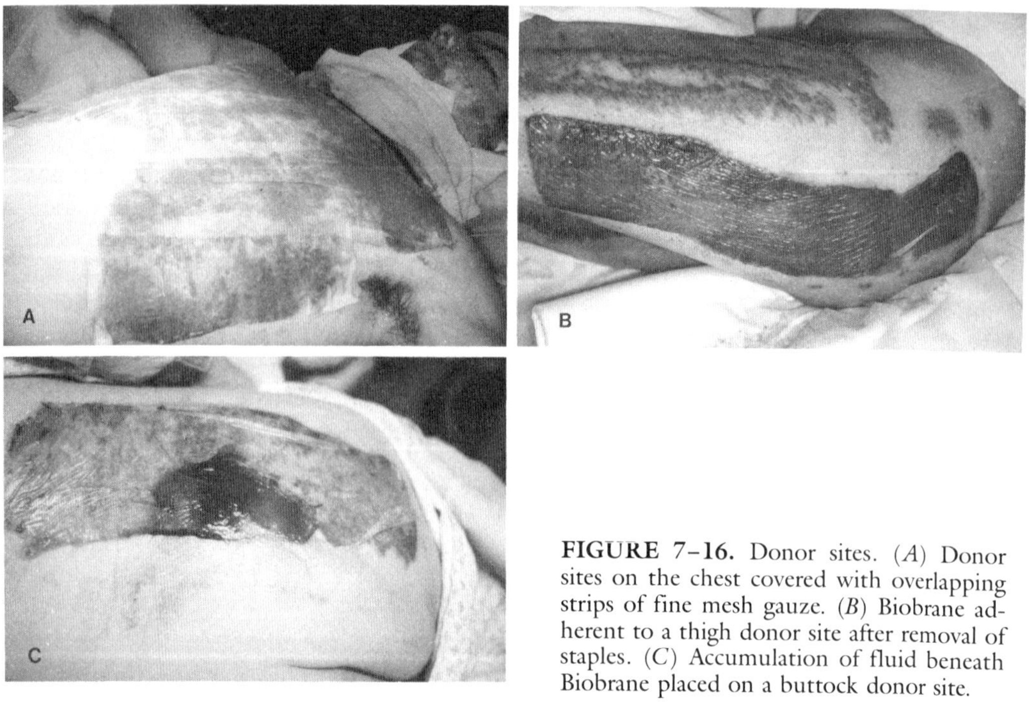

FIGURE 7–16. Donor sites. (*A*) Donor sites on the chest covered with overlapping strips of fine mesh gauze. (*B*) Biobrane adherent to a thigh donor site after removal of staples. (*C*) Accumulation of fluid beneath Biobrane placed on a buttock donor site.

MANAGEMENT OF HEALED WOUNDS

All burn wounds, including skin grafts and donor sites, are said to be "healed" when they have achieved epithelial coverage. At that time, dressings are no longer needed, but skin care must continue. Epithelialized wounds usually are dry and flaky, and may itch from lack of normal skin oils. Partial-thickness wounds and donor sites will regain normal oil production in time, but many grafted wounds do not. These healed burn wounds should be treated routinely with topical moisturizers at least twice daily until flakiness and itching resolves. Many patients find they must use these agents more frequently. A variety of topical moisturizers available commercially are included in Appendix C. The ideal moisturizer should be gentle, hypoallergenic, and devoid of perfumes or alcohol. Patients may need to experiment with different agents to find one which is not irritating with long-term use. Topical or systemic antipruritic medications (Benadryl, Vistaril, Atarax) may be needed as well, although reliance on them can be reduced if moisturizers are used frequently and liberally.

Healed burn wounds are susceptible to hyperpigmentation when exposed to the sun. Patients should be advised to avoid sun exposure on all burned areas for 12 months following injury, or until any redness or dark coloration has resolved.

Management of Other Burn-Related Wounds

The previous section presented techniques used for treatment of typical or "standard" burn injuries. However, burn wounds often are not typical and a host of management techniques may be needed to treat wounds of exceptional depth, or wounds complicated by infection or graft loss. This section describes protocols for management of some problem wounds.

EXPOSED TENDONS

In several areas of the body, tendons are located just beneath the skin with relatively little subcutaneous fat to protect them from injury. The extensor tendons of the hands and feet, the Achilles tendon at the ankle, and the triceps tendon at the elbow are particularly susceptible to injury from deep burns. Tendons have little blood supply, and once exposed they will not support a skin graft. In addition, exposed tendons quickly become dessicated and dissolve from the action of surrounding leukocytes and bacteria, resulting in loss of function and mobility.

The most frequently exposed tendons are the dorsal extensor mechanisms of the fingers, particularly over the metacarpophalangeal (MCP) or interphalangeal (IP) joints (Fig. 7-17). In all but the most severe cases, wounds with areas of exposed tendons are treated initially with skin grafting, because small areas of tendon exposure may attain satisfactory graft coverage from surrounding areas of vascularized tissue. Even if healing fails to occur, some graft adherence around the edges of exposed tendons greatly simplifies their care.

Exposed tendons must be kept moist at all times to prevent dessication. Wet dressings or biologic dressings can be used for this purpose. In less severe cases, the exposed tendon will become covered with granulation tissue gradually and can be regrafted, or simply will heal. Areas with exposed tendons should be immobilized as

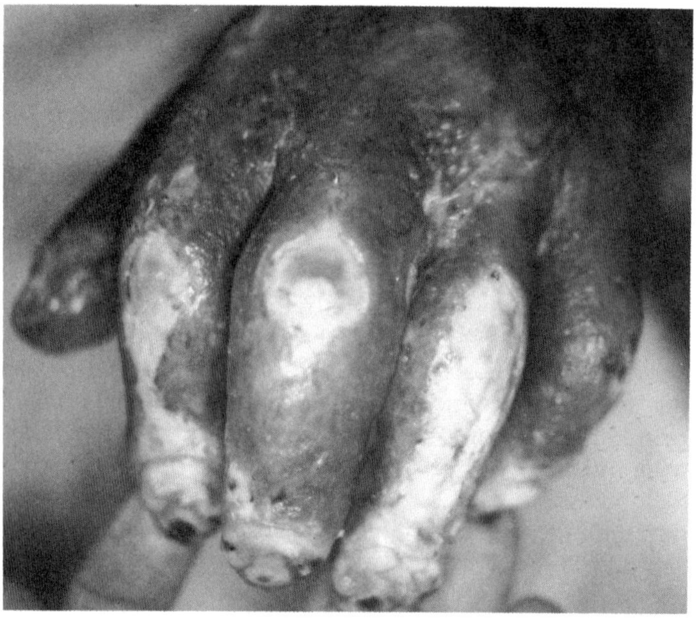

FIGURE 7–17. Exposed extensor tendons of the index, long, and ring fingers. Graft take is evident along the sides of the fingers. The joints are immobilized with wires.

much as possible because it is difficult for granulation tissue to cover a sliding tendon. Immobilization can be accomplished by splinting the joint, wrapping it in a bulky dressing, or pinning the joint (see Fig 7–17).

Many dressing materials available today will provide a moist wound environment for exposed tendons. Hydrocolloids and gels have the best potential to keep exposed tendons moist, but these dressings also may permit infection beneath them and have been used relatively little for this purpose. A "wet-to-moist" antibiotic dressing, changed at least three times daily, is useful to protect a tendon from dessication, while providing some gentle debridement, and enhancing growth of granulation tissue. When applying this dressing, the moist gauze should be packed gently into all areas of the wound using a cotton swab. If the use of wet-to-moist dressings is prolonged, care must be taken that moisture does not macerate and destroy surrounding healthy skin or skin grafts. To prevent maceration, the surrounding tissue should be protected with an ointment. Antibiotic creams can be used over exposed tendons. Their high water content helps keep exposed tendons moist. Ointment dressings also can be used and help prevent dessication of exposed tendons.

Severe burns of the volar wrist or ankle, usually from electrical injuries, can cause extensive exposure of tendons that will lead to a functionless hand or foot unless the exposed tendons are covered quickly with viable tissue (Fig. 7–18). Local rotational flaps, pedicle flaps, or, more recently, free tissue transfers have been used with success to cover these large injuries.[79,80]

EXPOSED BONE

Bone that is left exposed invariably dessicates and dies, leading to a nonhealing wound and the potential for chronic infection. Areas of cortical bone should be kept clean through frequent debridement and application of topical antibiotics. Wet dress-

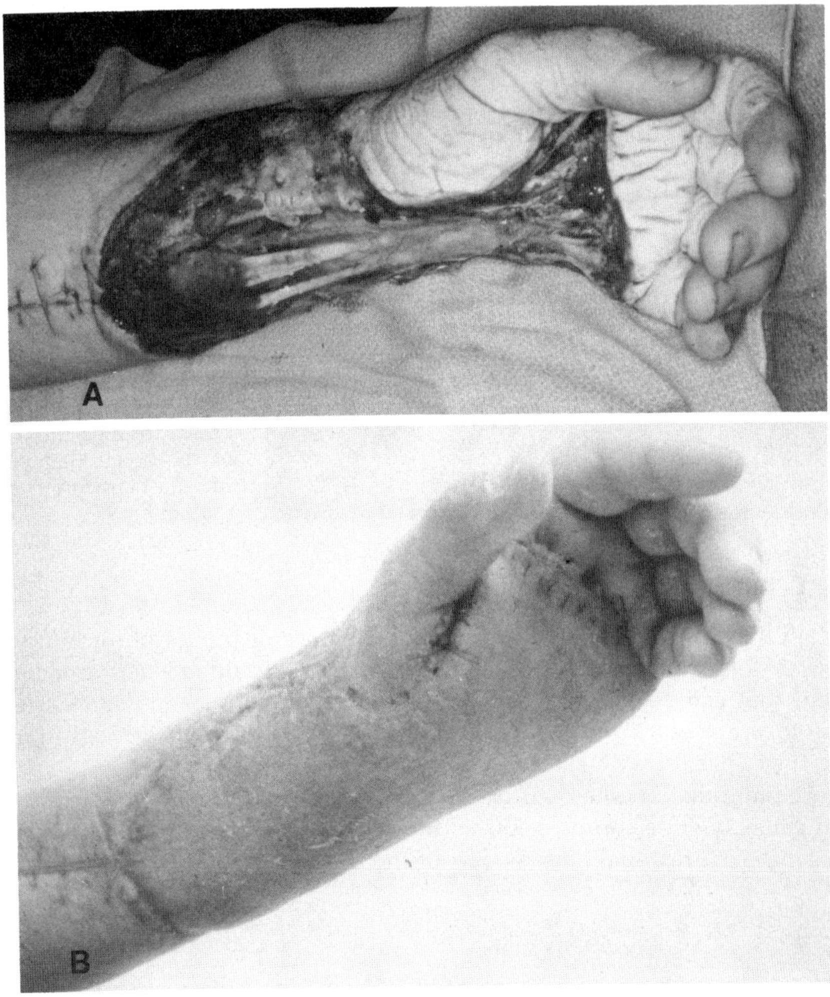

FIGURE 7–18. (*A*) Exposed tendons of the hand and wrist following surgical excision of a high-voltage electrical injury. (*B*) The same hand following coverage with an abdominal pedicle flap. The tendons were completely covered and range of motion was preserved.

ings also can be used to keep the wound moist and provide gentle debridement. One method of treating exposed bone is to drill a number of small holes through the outer table of the bone into the marrow cavity, permitting outgrowth of granulation tissue through the holes, that eventually covers the bone (Fig. 7–19). This practice is time-consuming and often complicated by infection or bony sequestration (sloughing of bits of dead bone). Skin grafts placed directly over bone often heal poorly and remain fragile. In addition, bone is weakened significantly by drilling and can be predisposed to fractures. A more efficient alternative, when available, is early coverage of exposed bone with pedicle or free flaps.

Exposure of joints frequently requires amputation of the extremity, especially if the joint is dessicated or infected. If exposed joints can be kept free of infection and reasonably moist, they can sometimes obtain coverage from granulation tissue. Antibiotic soak dressings, homograft, and hydrocolloid dressings all can be used for these purposes. Immobilizing the joint by means of pins or splints also helps in this process.

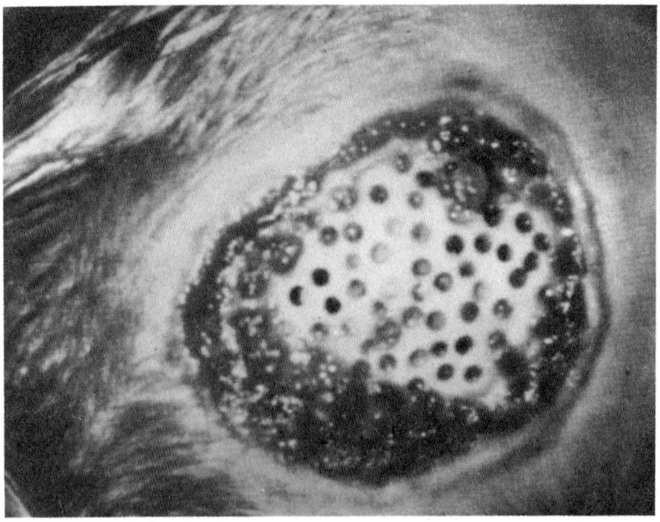

FIGURE 7–19. Treatment of a high-voltage injury to the cranium, resulting in exposed calvarium. Holes have been drilled through the outer table of the bone. Granulation tissue can be seen growing from the holes.

AMPUTATIONS

Certain burn injuries require amputation because of the depth of injury, severe infection, or loss of function. Ideally, amputations should be performed through intact skin that can be sutured. In this case, amputation care is similar to suture line care. In other cases, however, amputations are performed through open burn wounds, then covered with skin grafts.

Sutured amputation sites can be dressed with a thin film of ointment and non-adherent gauze. Gentle compression with elastic wraps will reduce limb edema and begin to shape the residual limb as part of the preprosthetic training.

PIN SITES

Patients who have sustained orthopedic trauma in addition to burn injury may have Steinman pins inserted through viable tissue as part of an external fixation apparatus. In other patients, pins may be placed to aid in immobilizing joints or suspending extremities above the bed. Pin sites should be washed with a cleansing solution, dried, and covered with antibiotic ointment. Pin track sites rarely become infected; however, they must be inspected regularly for drainage or surrounding erythema. If bony infection develops, the pin often will loosen. If a loose pin is detected, the physician should be notified immediately. The pin almost certainly will require removal.

SUTURED WOUNDS

The simplest surgical treatment for a wound is excision and closure with sutures. Although primary closure of a wound is not possible when treating large burn injuries, it can sometimes be accomplished with small burns. In addition to acute burns, a number of reconstructive procedures performed on burn wounds, including Z-, Y-, and W-plasties, and other procedures, produce suture lines.

Within a few hours, any sutured wound should "seal" with a thin layer of fibrin, which closes off the inner wound from the surface. This fibrin seal gradually is strengthened by fibroblasts and collagen deposition. Within 10 to 14 days, the wound should be strong enough to permit suture removal. Suturing a deep wound closes its surface. Usually, immediate closure is beneficial, protecting the wound from contamination and producing prompt healing by approximation, but it can prove harmful if infection is sequestered beneath the surface. For that reason, sutured wounds should be inspected daily for evidence of erythema, swelling, or drainage, and the physician notified immediately if infection is suspected.

Suture lines are dressed with a thin film of ointment, nonadherent gauze, and an elastic bandage. After the first 48 hours, the wound should be dry and sealed over, and a dressing is no longer needed. However, sutured wounds should continue to be dressed daily with dry gauze to protect the wound from trauma, including having suture ends snag in clothing. Sutured wounds may require immobilization with a splint or bulky dressing, particularly if the wound is a reconstructive procedure performed to release a contracture. Suture care is continued for 10 to 14 days, at which time sutures are removed. Gentle range-of-motion exercises can be started within a few days of closure in some cases, but should await suture removal in others.

Management of Special Patients

Although debridement, daily wound care, and selection of topical antimicrobials is similar for all patients, a number of patient groups require special wound care considerations to meet special needs. Various factors are known to affect wound healing and may warrant modifications in burn wound management.[81] Several of these factors are common enough to merit specific mention.

AGE

Infants and Toddlers

Small children are frightened easily and will resist dressing changes. Every effort should be made to explain wound care to children, although this does not always ensure cooperation. Wound care should be performed gently and calmly and as quickly as possible. If a child's parents will be providing outpatient care, they should be involved in the process gradually to be sure they will understand and cooperate with wound care. Sometimes the child will tolerate the dressing less well if a parent is present, and the parent should be asked to leave the dressing area. Once children realize that the dressing change will proceed regardless of their behavior, they usually become more compliant and cooperative and their parents can be allowed back into the area. Following completion of the dressing, time should be spent comforting and playing with the child.

The selection of an appropriate wound care technique should be made with the child's age in mind. Because children often are unable to cooperate with debridement and other painful procedures, debriding "wet-to-moist" dressings may need to be used more frequently to remove eschar. Cooperation with meticulous dressings, such as ointment and nonadherent gauze dressings for individual fingers, may be impossible, and silver sulfadiazine, which can be applied more quickly and easily, may be required. Removal of staples or sutures may prove difficult in small children who cannot cooperate. For this procedure, as well as for initial debridement, which must be particularly thorough, anesthesia may be necessary. The therapist should inform the physician if it appears that the child will require anesthesia for a particular procedure.

The small size of children makes the application of dressings difficult, and they often will actively try to remove dressings, which can be a challenge to the therapist's creativity. As a general rule, dressings on the hands and arms should extend above the elbow, and may need to include the chest to prevent children from pulling their hands out of the wrap. Dressings on the feet should extend above the knee. Even when these techniques are used, dressings may need to be replaced frequently. A simple trick for home dressings is to cover the dressed extremity with a clean sock, which can be safety-pinned to the inside of the child's shirt sleeve. Perineal or buttock burns in very small children are impossible to protect from soilage by feces or urine. A convenient dressing consisting of a layer of sulfadiazine or ointment applied to the inner surface of a disposable diaper makes a clean "one-piece" dressing that can be changed as often as needed.

The Elderly

Because the dermis atrophies with age, elderly patients resemble children in that they often sustain surprisingly severe injuries from relatively minor insults and may require grafting for wounds that would heal on younger adults. Elderly patients are "burn prone" because of diminished sensation, alertness, and judgment, and they often require hospitalization for minor injuries because of physical infirmity as well as limited family or financial support.[82]

Several special considerations must be kept in mind when caring for elderly burn patients. Wound healing may be prolonged by vascular disease or general infirmity, and burn wounds are more susceptible to infection in the elderly. Debridement of burn wounds should be less aggressive than in younger adults to avoid damaging fragile healing epidermis. Antibiotic creams may be needed for longer periods while eschar gradually separates. A frail elderly patient can be incapacitated by even a small burn and may require placement in an extended care facility for wound care.

PATIENTS WITH DIABETES

Wounds heal poorly in diabetics and easily are infected. As a result, wound care must be meticulous, may be prolonged, and grafting frequently is required for relatively trivial injuries. Topical antibiotics should be used with these patients, and wounds closely followed for evidence of infection until completely healed. Diabetic vascular disease can be severe, particularly in the feet. Even a minor burn to the feet can produce a wound that will heal with great difficulty and even require amputation. To prevent these injuries, therapists should take every opportunity to teach meticulous foot care to diabetic patients.

PATIENTS WITH NEUROLOGIC DISORDERS

Patients with seizures, paralysis, disorders of sensation, or spasticity, and the mentally ill are prone to household accidents or even self-inflicted burn wounds.[83] These patients incur full-thickness burns more frequently than other patients because their impairments often prevent them from perceiving injuries or escaping from them.

Wound care in patients with neurologic impairments often requires special consideration to the patient's ability to perceive and cooperate with treatment. Though some patients may have little or no sensation, which in some ways makes wound care easier to perform, these patients also are unable to protect their wounds from further injury, including pressure necrosis from prolonged sitting or lying. The ability to perform wound care and activities of daily living can be compromised severely in a neurologically impaired patient, even with a small burn injury. Therefore, recruiting a responsible family member or friend to assist with these activities may be necessary. A number of disease-specific considerations also should be kept in mind. Paralyzed patients must be reminded to be extremely careful when bathing to avoid further injury from hot water. The symptoms of multiple sclerosis can be exacerbated by bathing in hot water, and patients with this disorder may experience a flare-up of their disease if bathed repeatedly. In such patients, wound care may need to be performed without bathing. Many paraplegic patients with burns over anesthetic areas experience reflex spasticity or autonomic symptoms (hypertension, tachycardia) when wounds are dressed, so dressing changes must be performed gently to prevent the occurrence of these symptoms.

Outpatient Wound Management

Patients who require outpatient burn wound management fall into three groups: patients who never require admission and can be followed as an outpatient from the time of injury; patients admitted for a few days and then followed as outpatients; and patients initially admitted for extensive burn care (possibly grafting), and then followed after discharge.[46]

GROUP 1: "STRICT" OUTPATIENTS

Patients who never require inpatient care typically have small or superficial burns and must be competent to care for themselves and their wound. In making this determination, therapists must assess the patient's psychologic, social, and physical resources as well as the injury itself.

During the initial outpatient visit, the wound is evaluated and debrided carefully and dressed with topical agents or biosynthetic dressings. The patient should be given a written handout that explains anticipated problems and contains a telephone number to call for questions or problems. Wound care should not be taught on the first visit, when patients are stressed and anxious. Instead, patients should return the following day with someone who can learn wound care and dressing application. At that time the wound should be reassessed and cleaned, and the caregiver instructed in wound management, as well as range-of-motion exercises and ambulation. In addition, sufficient supplies are dispensed for wound care until the next appointment. The patient may need to return several times until all parties are comfortable with the outpatient management of the burn injury. At each follow-up visit, the adequacy of wound management, functional assessment, and range of motion are evaluated. The interval between subsequent appointments depends on the progress of the wound, as well as the patient's ability to comply with the dressing change protocol. This frequency should be at least weekly. As the wound heals, subsequent visits are scheduled for scar evaluation and therapy as needed.

GROUP 2: "TEMPORARY" INPATIENTS

Many patients with minor or moderate-sized injuries require temporary inpatient care for fluid management, pain control, or associated medical problems; to learn wound care; to assure adequate social resources; or for other reasons. Once these problems are solved and the patient is ready for outpatient management, the patient is asked to designate a caregiver to assist with wound care. As an alternative, a home health agency can be contacted and asked to participate in home wound care. In either case, however, the clinician should know that the patient has adequate resources for wound care, meals, housekeeping, and transportation. Designating one caregiver to be the wound care "specialist" usually works better than trying to teach a host of different people, none of whom are likely to master wound care.

Instruction in wound care may be facilitated by having the patient and caregiver review a video tape or other materials on wound care and dressing applications. Next, the caregiver should watch at least one dressing change performed by a staff member. Because the visual impact of burn wounds can be a shock to the uninitiated, the therapist needs to watch the caregiver closely during the initial dressing. Several dressing changes may be needed before the caregiver feels ready to assume responsibility for wound care.

When demonstrating wound care, the staff member uses the same "clean" technique that will be used at home. Clean technique includes hand washing, use of clean gloves, a clean surface for dressings, and a clean tub or shower area. When the caregiver feels comfortable, he or she may assist with the dressing change process, gradually increasing the involvement in wound care until he or she is able to complete the entire dressing change. Additional opportunities are provided until the caregiver, the therapist, and the patient are confident that discharging the patient will not jeopardize the progress of wound healing, nor put undo stress on the caregiver or patient.

In teaching wound care, patients and families are reminded that discharge will not be planned until the caregiver is comfortable with the entire wound care process, and the patient is able to cooperate with all phases of care, including therapy. Successful outpatient management requires a number of components in addition to wound care, and benefits from input from the entire burn team. Table 7–3 is a list of criteria that patients must meet before discharge.[46]

GROUP 3: OUTPATIENT CARE FOLLOWING DEFINITIVE TREATMENT

This group compromises patients with large burns or those who have had skin grafting. For these patients who may have been in the hospital for an extended period, discharge may seem both exciting and frightening. Patients must work gradually toward discharge and not be released until they are comfortable with wound management and therapy.

The process of discharge planning is identical to that used in group 2. A designated caregiver is appointed to learn wound care. The patient may be using some type of compression garment, and the caregiver and patient will have to demonstrate their skill in applying these supports, as well as providing wound care. Initially, patients are seen daily following discharge, and the interval between visits gradually

TABLE 7–3. Criteria for Discharge from the Burn Center

Patient criteria (to be assessed by physician and nurses)
- No impending medical problems
- Adequate intake of fluids and nutrition
- Adequate pain control on oral medications
- Cooperative with wound care and therapy
- Understands and demonstrates compliance with therapy program

Family/caregiver criteria (to be assessed by therapist)
- Demonstrates willingness and ability to perform wound care
- Understands the therapy program
- No aversion to the burn wound

Social criteria (to be assessed by social worker)
- Transportation available for follow-up appointments
- Available place to stay with heat, water, bathing facilities
- Finances for meals, pharmacy supplies, transportation

is lengthened as patients demonstrate satisfactory progress with wound care, therapy, and daily living.

ADDITIONAL OUTPATIENT FOLLOW-UP

In all patients, compliance with outpatient follow-up is critical. Return appointments are used not only to evaluate wounds but to answer questions, reassure patients and family, and ascertain the success of treatment. Patients should be questioned about pain, compliance with wound care and therapy, oral intake, and general health. Changes in wound care, decisions regarding surgery, and other aspects of wound management are accomplished at this time as well. Patients may "fail" outpatient management and require readmission for fluid support, pain control, or closer instruction with wound care. Therapists should be alert to problems in any area of treatment and notify the physician if a patient is unable to manage outpatient care. At the end of each outpatient visit, the therapist should make sure that the patient has all adequate supplies and medications to last until the next appointment.

SUMMARY

Therapists who provide care for burn wounds must do so in accordance with established principles of wound healing. A continuous supply of oxygen and circulation to healing wounds must be assured at all times. Debridement to remove necrotic material as well as old topical agents should be performed regularly to reduce the risk of infection and encourage the separation of eschar and growth of granulation tissue. Growth of new epithelium can be enhanced by appropriate debridement and choice of dressings. Wound contraction should be prevented by the prompt and continuous use of range-of-motion exercises and other therapy.

Regardless of the type of wound care employed, therapists must be adept at the initial assessment of burn injuries as well as the repeated evaluation of wounds for infection and proper healing. The principles of clean and sterile technique are employed in all wound care procedures and are taught to patients and caregivers for outpatient treatment. Other important techniques for therapists include the use of hydrotherapy in burn wound management and the proper procedure for bandage application.

Therapists need not be familiar with every technique for burn wound care, but every therapist should know the types of wound care techniques available, and their place in the armamentarium of burn wound management. The initial assessment and debridement of a burn wound, and the selection of a proper wound care technique, is essential to the success of any wound care regimen. The therapist can choose among a wide array of wound care protocols, including enzymatic debridement, "open" technique, various topical antibiotics and biologic dressings, debriding dressings, antibiotic wet dressings, and a rapidly growing selection of occlusive and semiocclusive dressings. The success of any of these methods requires understanding of the rationale for the method chosen, appropriate selection of patients and wounds, meticulous technique, and careful surveillance of the wound.

Burn wounds are very dynamic, and the therapist must be able to keep up with changes that occur in the burn wound. By repeatedly observing and assessing wounds, these changes can be detected and lead to appropriate modification of wound management techniques. Modifications of standard wound care techniques are required for management of burns that involve the face, eyes, ears, hands, feet, and perineum.

In addition to burn injuries, therapists often are required to care for skin grafts and donor sites. The techniques used to manage burn wounds can be successfully adapted to these circumstances as well. Burn wounds that are unusually deep, extensive, or infected require specialized care. Exposed tendon and bone, amputations, pin sites, and suture lines are examples of wounds that require modification of wound care regimens.

Just as some wounds require modification of wound care techniques, some patients require special treatment as well. Special attention should be directed toward patients at the extremes of age, the very young and very old, patients with diabetes, and patients with neurologic impairment.

In addition to providing burn wound care to hospitalized patients, therapists frequently are involved in evaluating and treating burn wounds in outpatients and in teaching wound care to patients' families or friends. A variety of different circumstances are encountered in working with outpatients, including patients with small injuries who never require hospitalization, patients with moderate injuries who are hospitalized for a short time, and patients who are treated on an outpatient basis following conclusion of hospital care for major burn injuries.

CASE STUDY

HISTORY

The patient was a 27-month-old girl who was burned on her head, face, neck, trunk, and arms when she pulled a pot of boiling water off the stove. On admission to the burn center, her wounds were blistered, with a small amount of fluid beneath the blisters. Initial debridement was performed by washing the burned areas with dilute Hibiclens solution and gently removing blistered skin.

The wounds were noted to be pale to dark red in color, relatively dry, and blanched poorly. Total burn size was 21 percent of the body surface area, most of which appeared to be a superficial partial-thickness to deep partial-thickness injury.

On the second postburn day, the face and trunk appeared pale pink to white in color with areas of brighter pink around the edges, characteristic of deep partial-thickness or "indeterminate" depth wounds (Fig. 7-20A).

On postburn day 4, the formation of solid eschar over the central chest and abdomen was noted (Fig. 7-20B). Areas of new epidermis were visible at the edges of the wound, particularly on the shoulders.

On postburn day 18, areas of solid eschar were seen on the upper chest bilaterally and the center of the abdomen (Fig. 7-20C). In contrast, the burns of the shoulders, arms, and the edges of the trunk wound were largely epithelialized. The lower face also had epithelialized but the forehead remained unhealed.

On postburn days 19 and 20, the burns of the forehead, chest, and abdomen were excised and then skin grafted. Donor sites were harvested from her back and buttocks.

PROBLEM LIST

Acute burn wounds of varying depths
Burn wounds to multiple body surface areas
Wound care following surgical excision
Wound care for skin grafts
Wound care for donor sites
Healed burn wound care

GOALS

Re-epithelialization of all superficial partial-thickness wounds
Prevent conversion of partial-thickness wounds to full-thickness wounds
Prevent wound sepsis
Prevent skin graft loss
Prevent conversion of donor site to full-thickness wound

INTERVENTIONS

Initially, the wounds of the trunk and arms were dressed with silver sulfadiazine cream and light gauze wraps. The face was treated with Bacitracin ointment. Because the depth of injury was indeterminate, the wounds were followed for several days before a decision regarding the need for skin grafting was made. Wound care consisted of twice-daily washings with application of silver sulfadiazine to the chest, abdomen, and arms. The face was placed in wet-to-moist debriding dressings for 20 minutes twice daily, then coated with a thin layer of Bacitracin.

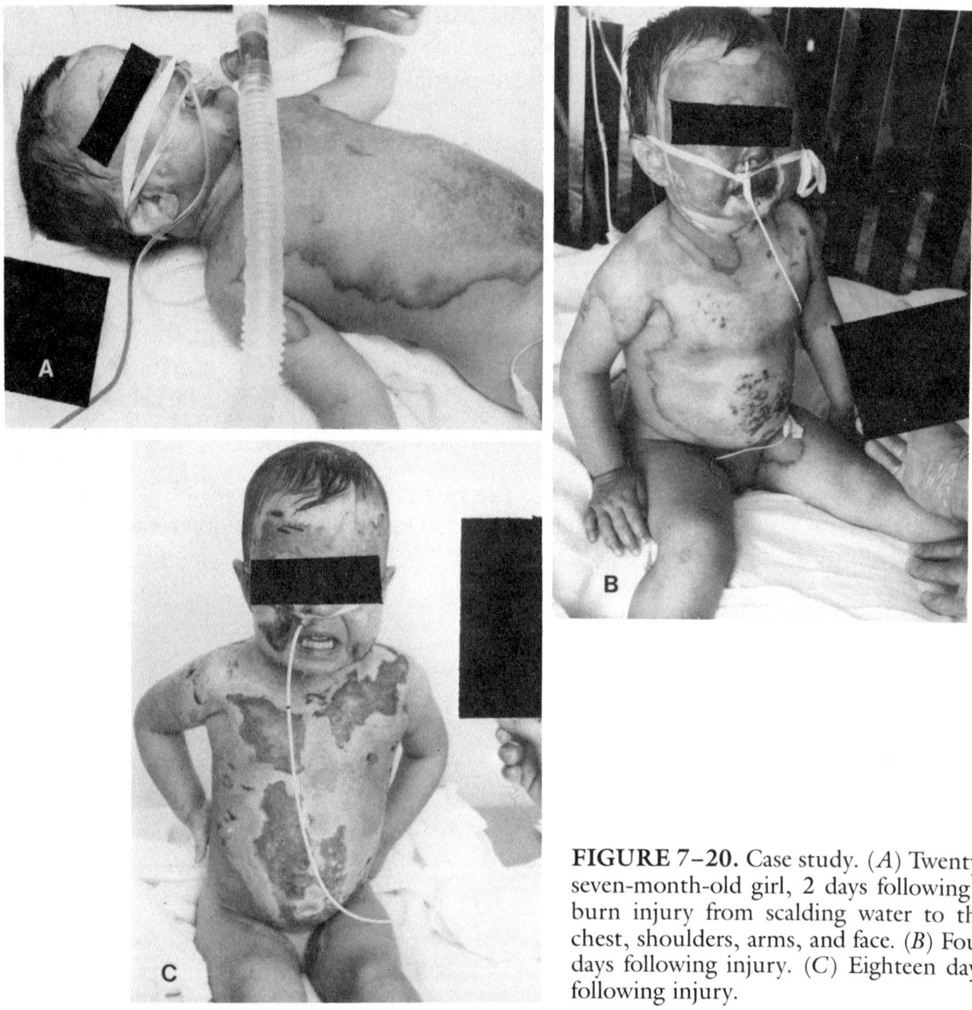

FIGURE 7–20. Case study. (*A*) Twenty-seven-month-old girl, 2 days following a burn injury from scalding water to the chest, shoulders, arms, and face. (*B*) Four days following injury. (*C*) Eighteen days following injury.

With regular washing and gentle debridement, the eschar that had formed over the central chest and abdomen began to separate at the edges. As the eschar became more solid on the upper chest and center of the abdomen, and the shoulders and arms began to re-epithelialize, the wound care regimen gradually was modified so that the silver sulfadiazine was placed only on the areas of solid eschar.

As the eschar separated over the shoulders and trunk, areas of skin buds were exposed that were dressed with Bacitracin and Adaptic gauze. As these areas filled in with solid epidermal coverage, dressings were left off. Instead, the epithelialized areas were treated with a moisturizing cream, applied sparingly, and rubbed into the skin until it disappeared.

Following excision of the forehead, chest, and abdomen, the wounds were dressed in wet soaks consisting of bulky gauze wraps and irrigating catheters. The excised wounds of the trunk were kept moist by injecting 50 mL of Sulfamylon solution through each catheter every 2 hours, while the forehead dressing was moistened with saline in a similar fashion.

The following day, the patient returned to surgery. The forehead was covered with a sheet graft, which was sutured into position and dressed only with a light coating of Bacitracin ointment. The excised wounds of the chest and abdomen also were sheet grafted and dressed with Biobrane, which was stretched tightly over the fresh grafts and stapled into place. The Biobrane dressings remained dry and intact for the next several days. Donor sites on her back and buttocks were dressed with Biobrane, which was stapled into position.

RATIONALE

Twice-a-day wound cleansing and gentle debridement followed by the application of a topical antibiotic and gauze bandage assists to prevent burn wound invasion. On indeterminate-depth wounds, silver sulfadiazine is usually the topical agent of choice. However, a bland ointment generally is used on the face regardless of depth. Wet-to-moist dressings on the face also assist with debridement. As wounds re-epithelialize, the topical antibiotic should be a bland ointment and silver sulfadiazine then should be restricted to areas of eschar to soften it and minimize microbial growth.

Following excision of the burn wound, the tissue should be kept moist to prevent desiccation in preparation for skin grafting. Donor sites and skin grafts can be treated in a variety of ways. Donor sites are treated as partial-thickness burns and skin grafts are dressed so as to minimize movement. Following healing of the burn wound and donor site and adherence of the skin graft, a moisturizing cream helps keep the areas lubricated and pliable.

REFERENCES

1. Artz, CP: History of burns. In Artz, CP, Moncrief, JA, and Pruitt, BA (eds): Burns: A Team Approach. WB Saunders, Philadelphia, 1979, pp 3–17.
2. Haynes, BW: The history of burn care. In Boswick, J (ed): The Art and Science of Burn Care. Aspen, Rockville, Maryland, 1987, p 201.
3. Hunt, TK: Physiology of wound healing. In Clowes GHA (ed): Trauma, Sepsis, and Shock: The Physiological Basis of Therapy. Marcel Dekker, New York, 1988, pp 443–471.
4. Knighton, DR, et al: Oxygen tension regulates the expression of angiogenesis factor by macrophages. Science 221:1283–1285, 1983.
5. Knighton, DR, et al: Regulation of wound healing angiogenesis—Effect of oxygen gradients and inspired oxygen concentration. Surgery 90:262–270, 1981.
6. Hunt, TK and Pai, MP: Effect of varying ambient oxygen tensions on wound metabolism and collagen synthesis. Surg Gynecol Obstet 135:561, 1972.
7. Hohn, DC, et al: The effect of O_2 tension on the microbial function of leukocytes in wounds and in vitro. Surg Forum 27:18–20, 1976.
8. Orgill, D and Demling, RH: Current concepts and approaches to wound healing. Crit Care Med 16:899–908, 1988.
9. Brim, PS, et al: Hyperbric oxygen therapy. JAMA 263:2216–2220, 1990.
10. Cianci, P, et al: Adjunctive hyperbaric oxygen reduces the need for surgery in 40–80% burns. J Hyperbar Med 3:97–101, 1988.
11. Wiseman, DH and Grossman, AR: Hyperbaric oxygen in the treatment of burns. Crit Care Clin 1:129–145, 1985.
12. Davis, JH: History of trauma. In Mattox, KL, Moore, EE, Feliciano, DV (eds): Trauma. Appleton and Lange, Norwalk, 1988, p 14.
13. Teplitz, C: The pathology of burns and the fundamentals of burn wound sepsis. In Artz, CP, Moncrief, JA, and Pruitt, BA (eds): Burns: A Team Approach. WB Saunders, Philadelphia, 1979, pp 45–94.
14. Baxter, CR: Early surgical excision and immediate grafting. In Artz, CP, Moncrief, JA, and Pruitt, BA (eds): Burns: A Team Approach. WB Saunders, Philadelphia, 1979, pp 224–234.

15. Desai, H, et al: Early burn wound excision significantly reduces blood loss. Ann Surg 211:753–762, 1990.
16. Demling, RH and LaLonde, C: Early burn excision attenuates the postburn lung and systemic response to endotoxin. Surgery 108:28–35, 1990.
17. Tompkins, RG, et al: Significant reductions in mortality for children with burn injuries through the use of prompt eschar excision. Ann Surg 208:577–585, 1988.
18. Demling, RH: Improved survival after massive burns. J Trauma 23:179–183, 1983.
19. Janzekovic, Z: A new concept of skin grafting of burns. J Trauma 10:1103–1108, 1970.
20. Deitch, EA, et al: Hypertrophic burn scars: Analysis of variables. J Trauma 23:895–901, 1983.
21. Bayley, EW: Wound healing in the patient with burns. Nursing Clin North Am 25:205–220, 1990.
22. Hansbrough, JF, et al: Clinical experience with Biobrane biosynthetic dressing in the treatment of partial thickness burns. Burns 10:415–418, 1984.
23. Hermans, MHE and Hermans, RP: Preliminary report on the use of a new hydrocolloid dressing in the treatment of burns. Burns 11:125–130, 1984.
24. Feldman, DL, Rogers, A, and Karpinski, RHS: A prospective trial comparing Biobrane, Duoderm, and Xeroform for skin graft donor sites. Surg Gynecol Obstet 173:1–5, 1991.
25. Davis, SC, Mertz, PM, and Eaglstein, WH: Second degree burn healing: The effect of occlusive dressings and a cream. J Surg Res 48:245–251, 1990.
26. Alvarez, OM, Hefton, JM, and Eaglstein, WH: Healing wounds: Occlusion or exposure. Inf Surg 1:173–181, 1984.
27. Heimbach, DM and Engrav, LH: Surgical Management of the Burn Wound. Raven Press, New York, 1984.
28. Stone, PA and Madden, JW: Effect of primary and delayed split skin grafting on wound contraction. Surg Forum 25:41, 1974.
29. Monafo, WW and Ayvazian, VH: Topical therapy. Surg Clin North Am 58:1157–1171, 1978.
30. Edlich, RF, et al: Bioengineering principles of hydrotherapy. J Burn Care Rehabil 8:580–584, 1987.
31. Edlich, RF, et al: Design of hydrotherapy exercise pools. J Burn Care Rehabil 9:505–506, 1989.
32. Roberts, ML and Pruitt, BA: Nursing care and psychological considerations. In Artz, CP, Moncrief, JA, and Pruitt, BA (eds): Burns: A Team Approach. WB Saunders, Philadelphia, 1979, p 371.
33. Konop, DJ: General local treatment. In Trofino, RB (ed): Nursing Care of the Burn-Injured Patient. FA Davis, Philadelphia, 1991, pp 50–52.
34. Neville, C and Dimick, AR: The trauma table as an alternative to the Hubbard tank in burn care. J Burn Care Rehabil 8:574–575, 1987.
35. Richard, RL, et al: Autocontamination of the burn patient by hydrotherapy. Bull Clin Rev Burn Injury 1:40, 1984.
36. Edlich, RF, et al: Water treatment of hydrotherapy exercise pools. J Burn Care Rehabil 9:510–515, 1988.
37. Thomson, PD, et al: A survey of burn hydrotherapy in the United States. J Burn Care Rehabil 11:151–155, 1990.
38. Richard, RL: The use of chlorine bleach as a disinfectant and antiseptic in whirlpools. Phys Ther Forum 7:7–8, 1988.
39. Richard, R: P. T. topics. Phys Ther Forum 9:6, 1990.
40. Gordon, MD: Nursing care of the burned child. In Artz, CP, Moncrief, JA, and Pruitt, BA (eds): Burns: A Team Approach. WB Saunders, Philadelphia, 1979, pp 390–409.
41. Carr, R, et al: Comparative study of occlusive wound dressings on full thickness wounds in domestic pigs. Wounds 1:53–61, 1989.
42. Moylan, JA: First aid and transportation of burned patients. In Artz, CP, Moncrief, JA, and Pruitt, BA (eds): Burns: A Team Approach. WB Saunders, Philadelphia, 1979, pp 151–158.
43. Nebraska Burn Institute, Initial assessment and management, Chapter 1. In Manual of Advanced Burn Life Support. Lincoln, Nebraska, 1987.
44. Nebraska Burn Institute, Wound Management, Chapter 4. In Manual of Advanced Burn Life Support. Lincoln, Nebraska, 1987.
45. Lund, CC and Browder, NC: Estimation of area of burns. Surg Gynecol Obstet 79:352–358, 1944.
46. Rockwell, WB and Ehrlich, HP: Should burn blister fluid be evacuated? J Burn Care Rehabil 11:93–95, 1990.
47. Wilmore, DW, Long, JM, and Mason, AD: Catecholamines: Mediator of the hypermetabolic response to burn injury. Ann Surg 189:653–670, 1984.
48. West, DA and Shuck, JM: Emotional problems of the severely burned patient. Surg Clin North Am 58:1189–1204, 1978.
49. Demling, RH, Mazess, RB, and Wolbert, W: The effect of immediate and delayed cold immersion on burn edema formation and resorption. J Trauma 19:56–62, 1979.
50. Warden, GD: Outpatient care of thermal injuries. Surg Clin North Am 67:147–158, 1987.
51. Beckmeyer, D, et al: Time-outs take a new twist. Proc Am Burn Assoc, 23:176, 1991.
52. Rockwell, WB and Ehrlich, HP: Fibrinolysis inhibition in human burn blister fluid. J Burn Care Rehabil 11:1–6, 1990.
53. Shuck, JM: Outpatient management of the burned patient. Surg Clin North Am 58:1107–1117, 1978.

54. Pennisi, VR, et al: Travase, an effective enzyme for burn debridement. Plast Reconstruct Surg 51:371-376, 1973.
55. Muir, IFK, Barclay, TL, and Settle, JAD (eds): Burns and Their Treatment. Butterworths, London, 1987, pp 63-94.
56. Hummell, RP: Care of the burn wound. In Hummel, RP (ed): Clinical Burn Treatment. John Wright, Boston, 1982, pp 85-110.
57. MacMillan, BG and Lang, D: Nursing care in the operating room. In Artz, CP, Moncrief, JA, and Pruitt, BA (eds): Burns: A Team Approach. WB Saunders, Philadelphia, 1979, pp 411-452.
58. Fox, CL: Silver sulfadiazine—A new topical therapy for *Pseudomonas* in burns. Arch Surg 96:184, 1968.
59. Moncrief, JA: Topical antibacterial therapy for the burn wound. Clin Plast Surg 1:563-579, 1974.
60. McEvoy, GK (ed): AHFS Drug Formulary 91. Bethesda, Maryland, American Society Hospital Pharmacy, 1991.
61. Mangus, DJ, Morgan, LR, and Gilchrest, D: The selection of topical solutions in antibacterial burn wound therapy. Burns 3:257-260, 1977.
62. Konop, DJ: General local treatment. In Trofino, RB (ed): Nursing Care of the Burn-Injured Patient. FA Davis, Philadelphia, 1991, pp 43-67.
63. Monafo, WW and Freedman, B: Topical Therapy for Burns. Surg Clin North Am 67:133-145, 1987.
64. Chan, CK, Janett, F, and Moylan, JA: Acute leukopenia as an allergic reaction to silver sulfadiazine in burn patients. J Trauma 16:395-396, 1976.
65. Luterman, A, Kraft, E, and Bookless, S: Biologic dressings: An appraisal of current practices. J Burn Care Rehabil 1:18-22, 1980.
66. Tavis, MJ, Thornton, J, and Danet, R: Current status of skin substitutes. Surg Clin North Am 58:1233-1248, 1978.
67. Alvarez, O, et al: Moist environment for healing: Matching the dressing to the wound. Wounds 1:35-51, 1989.
68. Feedar, JA and Kloth, LC: Conservative management of chronic wounds. In Koth, LC, McCulloch, JM, and Feedar, JA (eds): Wound Healing: Alternatives in Management. FA Davis, Philadelphia, 1990, pp 133-176.
69. Hutchinson, JJ and McGuckin, M: Occlusive dressings: A microbiologic and clinical review. Am J Infect Control 18:257-268, 1990.
70. Lee, JJ, et al: Use of 5% sulfamylon (mafenide) solution after excision and grafting of burns. J Burn Care Rehabil 9:602-605, 1988.
71. Warden, GD, Saffle, JR, and Kravitz, M: A two-stage technique for excision and grafting following thermal injury. J Trauma 22:98-103, 1982.
72. Rodeheaver, GT, et al: Pluronic F-68: A promising new skin-wound cleanser. Ann Emerg Med 9:572-576, 1980.
73. Miller, RA: Burns of the face. In Artz, CP, Moncrief, JA, and Pruitt, BA (eds): Burns: A Team Approach. WB Saunders, Philadelphia, 1979, pp 411-452.
74. Saffle, JR, Zeluff, GR, and Warden, GD: Intramuscular pressure in the burned arm: Measurement and response to escharotomy. Am J Surg 140:825-831, 1981.
75. Schnebly, WA, et al: A nonsplinting approach to the care of the thermally injured patient. J Burn Care Rehabil 10:263-266, 1989.
76. Warden, GD, Saffle, JR, Schnebly, A, and Kravitz, M: Excisional therapy of facial burns. J Burn Care Rehabil 7:24-30, 1986.
77. Harnar, T, Engrav, L, and Marvin, J, et al: Dr Paul Unna's boot and early ambulation after skin grafting of the leg. Plast Reconstr Surg 69:359-360, 1982.
78. Heimbach, DM: Early burn excision and grafting. Surg Clin North Am 67:93-107, 1987.
79. Hunt, JL, Sato, RM, and Baxter, CR: Acute electric burns: Current diagnostic and therapeutic approaches to management. Arch Surg 115:434-438, 1980.
80. Slater, H, et al: Free flaps in selected burn patients. J Burn Care Rehabil 7:385-387, 1986.
81. Harding, KG: Wound care: Putting theory into clinical practice. Wounds 2:21-32, 1990.
82. Saffle, JR, et al: The continuing challenge of burn care in the elderly. Surgery 108:534-543, 1990.
83. Larson, CM, et al: Complications of Burn Care in Patients with Neurologic Disorders. J Burn Care Rehabil 10:17-26, 1989.

APPENDIX 7-1: PRINCIPLES OF CLEAN/STERILE TECHNIQUE

CLEAN TECHNIQUE

Clean technique is intended to prevent cross-contamination between patients and care providers and provides physical cleanliness, but does not produce or protect a sterile environment.

Indications

Dressing changes on small burns, outpatient wounds, "healed" (epithelialized or partly epithelialized) skin grafts and donor sites. In dressing large open burn wounds, sterile technique often is used to apply topical antibiotics and fresh bandages, but clean technique is used to remove old dressings.

Technique

1. Rules for body substance precautions are observed and followed.
2. If isolation technique is warranted, precautions must be observed thoroughly. There is no such thing as "almost" isolation technique.
3. Areas that are considered clean (a counter where clean equipment is placed) must be distinguished from those that are considered dirty (a sink), and not interchanged.
4. All necessary supplies and topical ointments or creams should be opened before beginning wound care. Dressings should be kept sterile if possible until used. Dressings can be opened onto a sterile drape or into a sterile basin. A clean container is acceptable provided that it is not used for any other patient. As an alternative, an assistant can open dressings as they are needed.
5. Clean gloves are worn to remove old dressings and topical antibiotics and to wash and debride the wound.
6. Materials that have touched the patient's wound should not be permitted to touch the therapist's skin or clothing. Disposable gowns or aprons as well as gloves are worn to prevent such contact.
7. Soiled materials should be placed immediately in a covered container.
8. Tapwater can be used for washing the patient's wound when used with appropriate soap or detergent.
9. Following washing and debridement, gloves should be changed before applying new topical antibiotics.
10. Individually wrapped dressings can be obtained from a common source for each dressing change. Reusable supplies (e.g., jars of ointment that have been opened or basins used for washing) should be kept separate for each patient and not used for other patients.

11. Any item dropped on the floor must be discarded immediately or returned for cleaning. Soiled linen should be placed directly into closed hampers and not touch the floor.

STERILE TECHNIQUE

Sterile technique is used only in the hospital, as its effective use requires practice, and it usually is indicated in circumstances where breaks in techniques cannot be permitted. It is intended to protect the patient from "cross-contamination" from others as well as to guard against contamination with the patient's own bacteria. Although burn wounds themselves are almost never sterile, the use of sterile technique prevents introduction of exogenous bacteria to the wound, by permitting the wound to contact only sterile dressings.

Indications

Sterile technique is used routinely in the performance of surgical procedures and also may be used for invasive "bedside" procedures (e.g., central line placement) in the burn unit. In wound care, sterile technique may be used following debridement and washing, for the application of topical antibiotics and dressings under circumstances that are as free from contamination as possible. Fresh skin grafts also may be treated with sterile technique.

Technique

1. The rules for body substance precautions should be followed at all times.
2. Before the therapist begins the dressing change, a sterile field should be set up using a sterile drape or basin. All sterile dressings and topicals are opened onto this field. As an alternative, an assistant wearing clean gloves may open dressings as needed provided the dressings are not touched.
3. The outer inch of a sterile field is not considered sterile.
4. Reaching over a sterile field or coughing or sneezing near a sterile field causes contamination of the field.
5. The only object that can touch a sterile object and remain sterile is another sterile object.
6. If there is any doubt that an object is sterile, consider it not sterile.
7. Any object held below the waist is considered contaminated.
8. Instruments soaked in disinfectants should not be considered sterile. Only dry, formally sterilized instruments should be considered sterile.
9. Any object that will pierce or penetrate below the skin surface must be sterile. Any dressing covering a broken skin surface must be sterile.
10. Tapwater should not be used on sterile dressings or fresh grafts. Sterile water or saline should be used.
11. Following debridement and cleansing, the therapist can put on sterile gloves before applying topical antibiotics or dressings. Clean gloves also can be used,

but should be changed following removal of old dressings, before applying new topical antibiotics.

BODY SUBSTANCE PRECAUTIONS

1. Hands should be washed before and after each patient contact, and after touching any contaminated dressings or surfaces.
2. Gloves should be worn for contact with all secretions, excretions, blood, and body fluids, or dressings that have been in contact with patients. This includes contact with any open wound.
3. During dressing changes, a gown or apron should be worn over clothing to prevent soiling of clothing and should be changed at the end of the dressing.
4. A mask and goggles or protective glasses should be worn if splashing is likely.

APPENDIX 7–2: PRINCIPLES AND PRECAUTIONS FOR BANDAGE APPLICATION

1. Soiled dressings should be disposed of properly in a closed or disposable container. A soiled bandage never should be reused.
2. Sterile bandages should be kept on a sterile field prior to being applied.
3. Dressings should be kept as light as possible to avoid interfering with range-of-motion exercises and activities of daily living.
4. Fingers and toes should be wrapped individually to prevent development of syndactyly and tissue maceration between the digits.
5. Rolled gauze bandages or elastic wraps should be handled so they will unroll from the bottom of the roll and will unroll around the body part as it is applied.
6. The wrap should be applied from distal (fingers, toes) to proximal (shoulder, hip).
7. Greater pressure should be applied distally than proximally and the wrap's pressure diminished from beginning to end.
8. A bandage should not be applied in a circular fashion around an extremity, but rather in a spiral, diagonal direction.
9. Major joints should be wrapped in a "figure-of-8" pattern.
10. An inelastic bandage should not be applied too snug.
11. Tape should not be applied circumferentially around an extremity.
12. Tape should not be applied to newly healed skin to hold bandages in place.
13. Elastic bandage clips should be covered with tape, especially if used on a pediatric patient.
14. Limbs that have dressings secured by tubular netting should be monitored. It often is necessary to use a size larger than recommended by the manufacturer. Netting should not be allowed to roll down and create a "garter" effect.

APPENDIX 7–3: TOPICAL AGENTS FOR BURN WOUND CARE[a,b]

Agent[c]	Uses	Advantages	Disadvantages	Comments[d]
		Creams		
Silver sulfadiazine 1% cream (Silvadene, SSD, Thermazene)	Partial- and full-thickness burns, infected burns and donor sites.	Wide antibacterial spectrum, including *Pseudomonas*; comfortable, easy to apply; deeply penetrating; moderate absorbance; softens eschar.	Sulfa allergy; transient leukopenia seen, especially in patients with major burns; regular cleansing and debridement is essential.	Introduced in 1968 as an anti-pseudomonal agent; the most widely used topical in America, and probably the agent of choice for treating most large/deep burns.
Mafenide acetate 0.5% cream (Sulfamylon)	Deep or infected injuries, as alternative to sulfadiazine.	Very wide antibacterial spectrum, including *Pseudomonas* and yeast; very deeply penetrating into eschar.	Sulfa allergy; carbonic anhydrase inhibitor causes hyperventilation; painful following application.	A powerful and effective alternative to sulfadiazine; use on large areas should be monitored; also available as solution for wet dressings (see below).
Nitrofurazone 0.2% compound (Furacin cream and impregnated gauze)	Routine treatment of partial- and full-thickness burns. Can be used as "dry" dressing for grafts and donor sites.	Wide antibacterial spectrum but less effective against *Pseudomonas*. Comfortable, soothing.	Hypersensitivity/dermatitis; superinfection and development of resistant organisms. Less effective against yeast.	Widely used product for routine burn care; less effective for complicated (very deep or infected) wounds.
Nystatin 100,000 units/g (Mycostatin, Nilstat)	Burn wounds, grafts, or donor sites colonized with yeast; can be combined with other topicals for mixed infections.	Activity restricted to yeast, especially *Candida*. Also available as ointment.	Infrequent hypersensitivity.	Good product for yeast infections; also available as ointment or powder for soaks.

Ointments				
Gentamycin 0.1% Ointment (Garamycin)	Smaller partial- and full-thickness burns. Useful as a general ointment for donor sites and skin grafts.	Effective against gram-negatives, some *Pseudomonas*; most *Staphylococci* and *Streptococci*.	Hypersensitivity; nephro/ototoxic in large volumes; resistance is common with prolonged use. Ineffective against yeast.	Use is probably best restricted to small/superficial burns; routine use may promote emergence of resistant strains.
Bacitracin Ointment, 50 U/g (plus Neomycin, 0.5% and polymyxin B, 5000 U/g)	Partial and full-thickness outpatient burns, healing wounds, donor sites.	Effective against gram-positive organisms; soothing and comfortable.	Hypersensitivity/rashes; not a powerful antibiotic; superinfection with yeast; ineffective for gram-negative bacteria.	Good general burn ointment; prolonged use, especially on healed skin, can lead to rash or skin breakdown; available as solution for soaks; a variety of formulations available.
Povidone-iodine ointment (Betadine)	Partial- and full-thickness burns; some skin grafts.	Wide-spectrum antiseptic.	Dermatitis; tends to harden eschar; metabolic acidosis reported; retards healing.	Not indicated for large injuries because of systemic toxicity.
Enzymes (Travase, Elase)	Enzymatic debridement of deep partial- and full-thickness burns.	Speeds eschar removal, prepares wound for grafting without excision (in theory).	Liquefies eschar producing a film that must be cleansed and debrided; bleeding can be a problem; infections are hard to detect; painful on application.	Controversial substance with unique action; advocates claim "chemical excision" is quick, preserves tissue; critics claim normal tissue may be damaged; graft adherence is poor; infections frequent.

(Continued on next page)

APPENDIX 7–3 *(Continued)*

Solutions				
Silver nitrate 0.5% solution	Wet dressings for partial- and full-thickness burns, applied as "soaks" to gauze dressings at 2–3 hr intervals; poor penetration limits use in very large burns.	Wide spectrum of antibiotic activity; less effective against *Pseudomonas* or yeast.	Painful on application; stains wounds, dressings, bedding dark brown; hypotonic solution that "leaches" sodium and chloride; not available commercially, must be made by pharmacy.	"Old-fashioned" burn dressing, now largely replaced by more powerful creams (sulfadiazene, mafenide); serious electrolyte problems result from prolonged use, especially on large burns.
Acetic acid 0.5% solution	Fresh grafts or infected wounds.	Excellent activity against *Pseudomonas*.	Acidosis results from prolonged use on large wounds; not effective against all organisms.	Effective antipseudomonal, probably best restricted to small wounds.
Sodium hypochlorite (Dakin's solution)	Dilute chlorine bleach for soaking fresh grafts; infected wounds.	General bactericidal; cleans and dries infected wounds.	Painful following application; can cause bleeding; acidosis; must be made in hospital.	Probably best used on small wounds.
Mafenide acetate 0.5% solution	See under "creams" for general description. Mafenide "soaks" are very effective in treating infected burns, contaminated grafts, and for "wet-to-moist" dressings for untidy wounds. Mafenide solution is not available commercially and must be made by the hospital pharmacy from powder. Can be combined with Nystatin powder for use in mixed fungal infections.			
Bacitracin/Neomycin/ Polymyxin	See under "ointments" for general description. Formulated as "triple antibiotic solution" (TAB). This is excellent as a soak for fresh grafts and in wet-to-moist dressings for infected wounds. Must be prepared by hospital pharmacy. Can be combined with Nystatin powder in mixed fungal infections.			

[a]See Refs. 56–62.

[b]Note: This table is restricted to antibiotic agents that are used commonly in burn treatment (agents used primarily for moisturizing are not included). Liquid formulations [mafenide acetate, silver nitrate, acetic acid] are not available commercially. See appendices for lists of manufacturers of specific products and for instructions for preparing specific formulations.

[c]Agents are listed by their proper name; their usual formulation, and commonly used brand name.

[d]Comments reflect the opinions of the authors, particularly with regard to the relative usefulness of various agents.

APPENDIX 7–4: COMMONLY USED SYNTHETIC BURN DRESSINGS[a]

Product[b]	Description	Uses[c]	Advantages	Disadvantages
		Collagen-Impregnated Gauze		
Biobrane	Nylon fabric impregnated with collagen bonded to silicon membrane. Once applied, collagen enhances adherence to wound; perforations permit egress of fluid; permeable to air.	A, C, D	Tough and elastic; provides mechanical protection for fresh skin grafts in any location; available as gloves, squares, strips, and sheets.	Dries to form a "scab" which is uncomfortable; softens when wet, permitting ingress of bacteria; relatively expensive.
		Ointment-Impregnated Gauze		
Adaptic, Vaseline	Gauze fabric impregnated with various compounds designed to make the dressing nonadherent.	B, C, D	These dressings can be used alone, or with ointments on fresh burns or grafts, or used alone on donor sites.	Dries to form a "scab" if left on more than 12 hr. Should not be used directly on deep or infected burns.
		Other Gauze Dressings		
Scarlet Red, fine mesh	Fine-mesh gauze is a fabric for use on donor sites, skin grafts, or partial-thickness burns. Scarlet Red is similar to fine mesh gauze, but is impregnated with aniline dye which enhances epidermal growth.	C, D	For open treatment of donor sites. Can also be used as the first layer of antibiotic wet dressings (see text).	These dressings dry to form a "scab" that is uncomfortable, cracks, and bleeds. Infection is hard to detect beneath these dressings.
		Hydrocolloid Dressings		
DuoDerm, Intrasite, J & J ulcer dressing, etc.	Hydrophyllic colloid that absorbs wound moisture, forming a soft suspension and "sealing" the wound; though "occlusive," these are permeable to oxygen.	A, D	Soothing and comfortable; surface is dry; can be left on for up to 7 days; available as individual sheets. May be useful on small deep or infected wounds.	Opaque; gel forms a film that can resemble pus; requires a margin of normal skin for adherence; limited use on infected wounds; when placed on irregular surfaces, it tends to crack and lift off. Maceration may occur beneath dressing.

(Continued on next page)

APPENDIX 7–4 (*Continued*)

		Hydrogels		
Vigilon, Elastogel	Lattice work of polymers which absorbs fluid, similar to hydrocolloid.	A, D	Cool and soothing on application; can be left on for days.	Adheres poorly and must be held in place by a secondary dressing; absorbs slowly and can leak; may macerate tissues over time.
		Films		
Op-Site, Tegaderm	Thin, transparent polyurethane film; does not stick to wounds; permeable to oxygen and water vapor. [*Note:* Similar products include polyvinylidine (Saran Wrap) and polyethylene (Glad Wrap)]	A, D	Transparent; comfortable; available as adhesive-backed sheets of various sizes; epidermal growth is rapid under these films.	Requires a margin of normal skin to adhere; frequently comes loose; fluid can "blister" beneath film or leak; limited to small wounds. Cannot be used over infected wounds or wounds that contain eschar.
		Other Dressings		
N-terface	Nonstick fabric which is nonabsorbent and permeable to fluid and air.	A, C, D	Translucent; available in sheets or rolls; does not adhere to grafts.	Does not adhere to or "seal" wounds; useful as a nonstick dressing; must be held in place with other wraps.
Hydron	Spray-on plastic (poly [2-hydroxyethylmethacrylate]) dressing can be applied over topical antibiotics.	B, E	Provides wound protection with antibiotic creams and ointments.	Difficult to apply; toxic to eyes; expensive; opaque, may conceal infection.
Unna boot	Gauze wrap containing lanolin and zinc oxide; dries to a stiff "cast-like" dressing. Very comfortable; protective; can be left on for days without changing; somewhat permeable to air.	C	Provides gentle, uniform pressure and mechanical protection to fresh grafts; permits early ambulation and discharge.	Covers wounds completely; bleeding, infection cannot be seen. Use is limited to fresh skin grafts.

[a] Refs. 21–27, 29, 39, 54, 61, 65, 67, 75. This table lists a number of products with which the authors have no personal experience. See the text for more detailed discussion of the use of each product. No endorsement of a particular product is implied here. Similarly, this table primarily lists products by class; no attempt has been made to include every brand name.

[b] A complete list of products and solutions used in wound care is included in Appendix A.

[c] Uses: (A) Fresh, superficial partial-thickness burns of trunk and extremities; (B) superficial burns—all locations; (C) fresh skin grafts; (D) donor sites; (E) Deep partial- and full-thickness burns.

CHAPTER 8

Surgical Management of the Burn Patient

Sidney F. Miller, MD, FACS
Marlys J. Staley, MS, PT
Reginald L. Richard, MS, PT

The depth and size of a burn injury determine whether surgical intervention will be necessary for the burn patient. The use of anesthesia creates a risk for the patient. Therefore, surgical procedures should be well planned and kept to a minimum. Therapists should be included as part of the operating room team[1,2] as their input can assist the physician in decisions regarding skin grafting priorities, pinning of joints, postoperative positioning and splinting, and timing of scar band releases. The ultimate goal of surgical management is to achieve a functional, durable, and cosmetically acceptable skin surface. The purpose of this chapter is to provide information regarding the various phases of burn surgery, burn wound excision and coverage with skin grafts or temporary coverings, and several reconstructive surgery techniques to enable the therapist to plan a patient's postoperative positioning, splinting, and exercise program.

PHASES OF BURN SURGERY

The timing of surgical procedures for the burn patient can be divided into three phases: resuscitative, wound coverage, and reconstructive. The procedures performed during the resuscitative phase usually are designed to save the life or limb of the patient. After the patient is medically stable, the burned tissue is removed, followed by coverage of the area with a skin graft. Several methods of wound coverage are available. Functional and cosmetic repairs of deformities and contractures are performed in the reconstructive phase and may require several months to years following the initial injury to accomplish.

Resuscitative Phase

When a patient is admitted to the hospital, an airway may need to be established and escharotomies or fasciotomies to restore circulation to an extremity may be required (see Chapter 6). Emergency operations for any related internal injuries are performed in the first few hours after the burn. Fractures, intra-abdominal injuries, and other associated life-threatening chest, intracranial, or extremity injuries must be managed in the immediate postburn period. With some electrical injuries, early amputation is the appropriate treatment for an injured limb. Amputating the necrotic limb immediately may be better than attempting to salvage the limb segment, because the segment serves as a source of rapid colonization of bacteria, which can lead to sepsis. In addition, damaged muscle tissue releases myoglobin into the general circulation that can occlude the renal tubules and lead to kidney failure. After life-threatening injuries have been addressed, attention should be given to covering the burn wound.

Wound Coverage Phase

Until the last 15 to 20 years, the method of care for burn patients was to treat the burn wound with a topical antibiotic until the eschar separated from the underlying subcutaneous tissue. This separation resulted from infection below the eschar due to the action of proteolytic enzymes produced by the bacteria. In approximately 3 to 4 weeks following the burn, the eschar loosened and was debrided. Another 1 to 2 weeks was required to prepare the wound for skin grafting. With the development of more advanced topical antibiotics in the 1960s, burn surgeons noticed a change in the time frame for separation of the burn eschar. Because the antibiotics penetrated the eschar so well, the growth of subeschar bacteria with subsequent separation of the eschar was delayed as long as 6 to 8 weeks. Dead skin, with a poor or absent blood supply, is prone to infection. Thus, the burn patient was allowed to remain with an undrained abscess of bacteria growing below the eschar. Delayed eschar separation resulted in lengthened patient hospitalization and recovery and patient mortality from sepsis was high.

BURN WOUND EXCISION

Excision means to cut out or remove. Primary excision is the removal of nonviable tissue in the operating room while the patient is under anesthesia, rather than allowing time for the eschar to separate. The goal of early burn eschar excision is to totally remove all nonviable burned skin using a dermatome (an instrument that cuts thin slices of tissue), free-hand knife, scalpel, or electrocautery (Fig. 8–1). The main types of excision are tangential (sequential) and full-thickness. Tangential excision, performed on deep partial-thickness burns, is the removal of tissue in sequential layers to a base of viable dermis and is usually an excision to the deeper layers of the dermis (Fig. 8–2). A knife or dermatome, set at a thickness of 0.025 to 0.030 inches, is used. Multiple passes of the instrument across the burn wound are made until there is good capillary bleeding in the excised area. Full-thickness excision is removal of necrotic tissue down to viable subcutaneous fat or fascia. This excision is performed

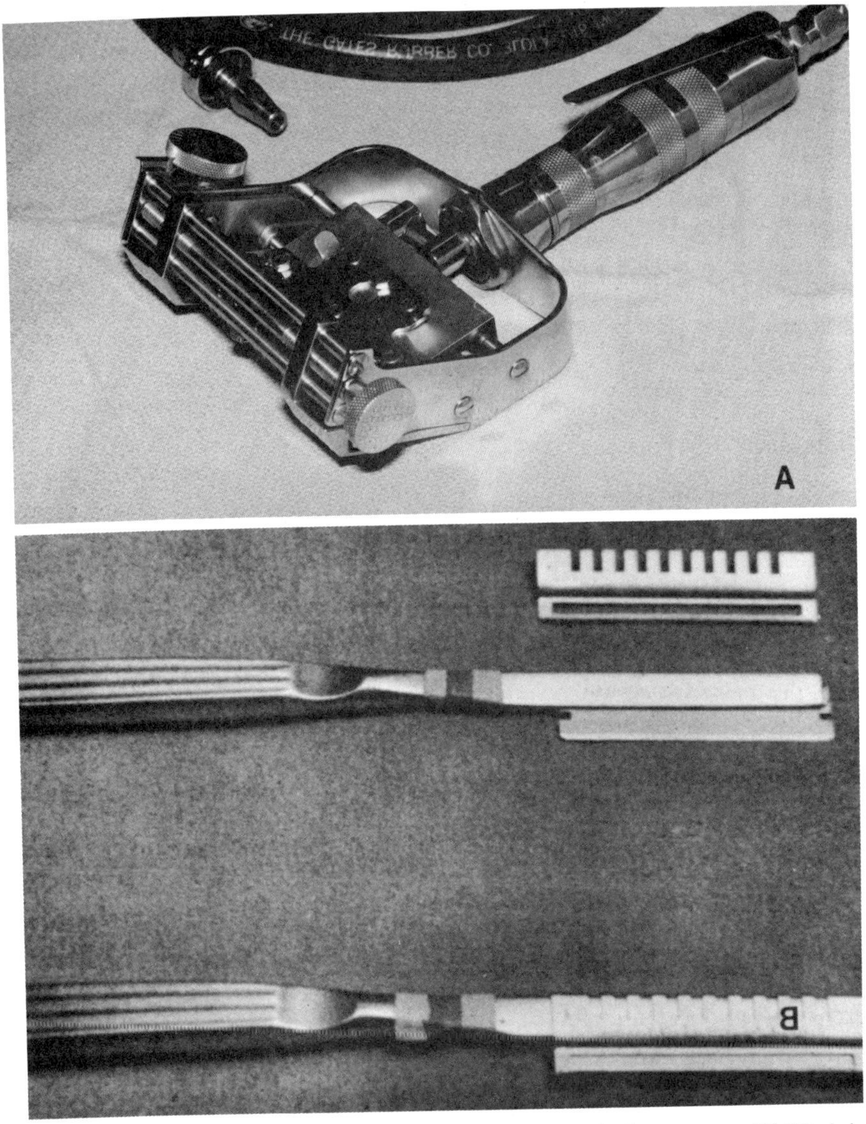

FIGURE 8–1. Instruments used for excision. (*A*) Brown air dermatome, (*B*) Weck knife.

by making an incision at the interface between normal skin and the eschar. The incision is carried into viable tissue under the eschar, to remove all of the eschar. There is some controversy as to whether this excision should be performed down to the subcutaneous fat or fascial layer. Either method is acceptable and will lead to good healing of the skin graft. However, having some subcutaneous tissue remaining for scar mobility and improved cosmesis of the scar is preferable.

Some advantages of surgical excision include the rapid removal of eschar, decreased likelihood of wound sepsis, decreased number of painful mechanical debridements, decreased length of hospital stay, and early initiation of less painful motion. Some disadvantages are the potential for massive blood loss, possible complications associated with anesthesia, and difficulty differentiating between viable

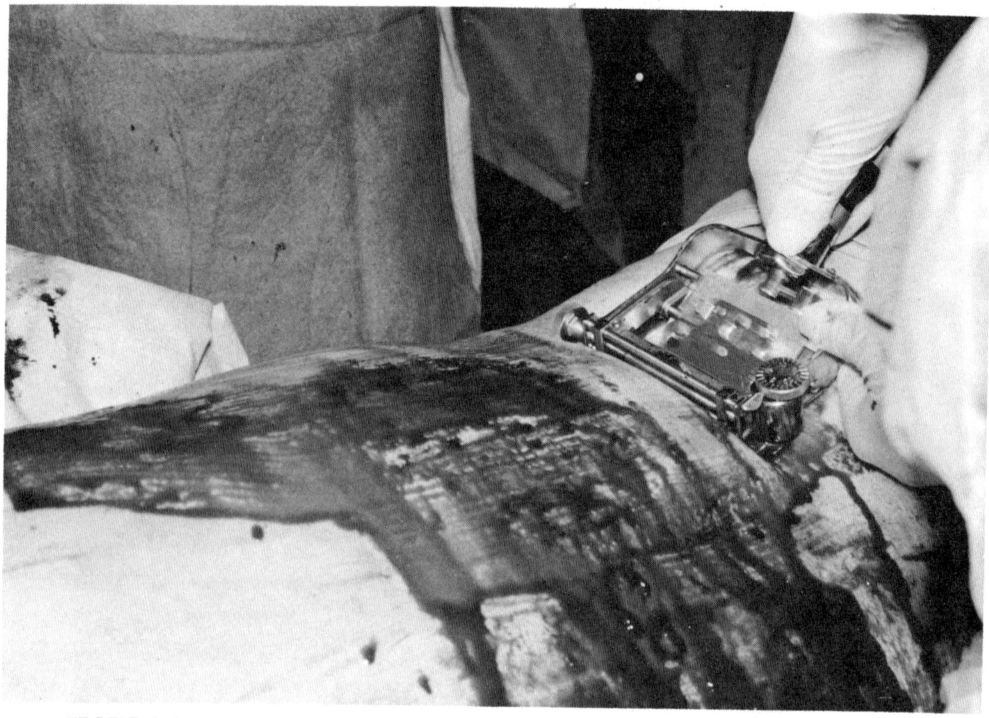

FIGURE 8–2. Tangential excision with dermatome until bleeding base is achieved.

and nonviable tissue. Additional disadvantages associated with fascial excision include greater cosmetic defect and risk of distal edema, nerve damage and exposing joints and tendons.[3-5]

One of the major advances related to the surgical management of the burn patient during the last several years has been the transition to early excision and skin grafting. In 1970, Dr. Janzekovic[6] published a report on a series of patients she treated with early excision of eschar. Her idea seemed so simple and practical that many burn surgeons immediately began programs of early excision. The rationale was that the earlier the dead skin was removed, the faster the wound would heal. If the excision was done within the first 3 to 4 days, skin graft survival was high and the patient's length of hospitalization was similar to that of a patient admitted for elective surgery. A debate over which approach was most beneficial ensued for several years, but currently early excision is being performed on all age groups by a majority of burn surgeons.[3-5,7-9] If a burn wound remains uncovered by skin, colonization with bacteria will occur and maintaining full movement of a joint will become difficult.[10] Therefore, the goal is to excise the full-thickness burn before the wound is colonized and motion lost.

To be a candidate for early excision the patient must be medically stable and able to withstand the stress associated with anesthesia and blood loss. If the patient enters the burn unit late or with burn wounds already heavily infected, the wounds require thorough daily cleansing and debridement with the application of topical antimicrobial agents to the infected tissue. Skin grafting at this time will result in loss of the skin graft and should be postponed until the bacteria count is acceptable (organism count less than 10^5).

The decision whether to perform a tangential or full-thickness excision resides with the surgeon and challenges his or her ability to clinically determine the depth of the burn wound. In large burn wounds with mixed deep partial- and full-thickness injury, partial-thickness burns that might heal without skin grafting should not be excised. On the other hand, tangential excision may not remove all of the nonviable dermis that may prevent a successful skin graft. Currently, there is no test available that can determine accurately burn depth, which makes the excision of eschar somewhat of an art rather than a science.

If the patient's wound is not grafted immediately following excision, the positioning, splinting, and exercise program should be resumed. However, dressings should be monitored closely during exercise to ensure that uncontrolled bleeding does not occur. The patient is given usually additional medicine to control pain following surgical excision, and exercise will be more successful when timed with the patient's medication schedule.

SKIN GRAFTING

Once the eschar is removed, the next important stage of surgical management of a burn patient is wound coverage. There are several alternatives to achieve wound closure. The most efficient method is to excise the burn wound and suture the skin closed. This is a very acceptable method for some small burns and frequently is overlooked. Small burns managed in this fashion usually heal with minimal scarring and can be performed on an outpatient basis.

When a larger full-thickness injury occurs or a deep partial-thickness injury takes longer than 3 weeks to heal, autografting usually is required. An autograft, commonly referred to as a skin graft, consists of removing skin from a donor site and placing it on a recipient wound site of the same patient. While a patient is in the operating room, the therapist can evaluate a patient's joint range and perform stretching and range-of-motion exercises prior to application of the skin graft.[1,11-13] These procedures can be accomplished while other surgical team members are preparing the donor sites and harvesting donor skin.

Skin grafts initially adhere to the recipient bed by the surface tension of the serum from the recipient site. Later, a fibrin matrix forms and acts as a biologic glue to hold the graft on the wound bed. After approximately 48 hours, blood vessels in the wound anastomose with vessels in the graft to establish a permanent circulatory system and give the graft a pink color.[10,14]

For the circulatory connection to form, a graft must remain immobile on its bed. Skin grafts are stapled or sutured in place then either left open or covered with dry or wet dressings, depending on the physician's preference (see Chapter 7). The therapist develops a postoperative positioning program for the patient so that grafted areas remain elongated and immobilized until revascularization occurs. This program may require the patient to be placed on a pressure-relieving mattress or to have the therapist splint the patient in the operating or recovery room. Restraints, slings, or other positioning devices may be needed and all patients should be re-evaluated postoperatively for any changes in the treatment program. Most grafts will have adhered by the second to fifth postoperative day, after which time staple removal can begin (Fig. 8–3). Some common reasons for skin graft failure include hematoma or seroma formation beneath the graft, excessive bacteria on the recipient site, mobility of the graft on its bed, or inadequate excision of the wound to a healthy recipient bed.

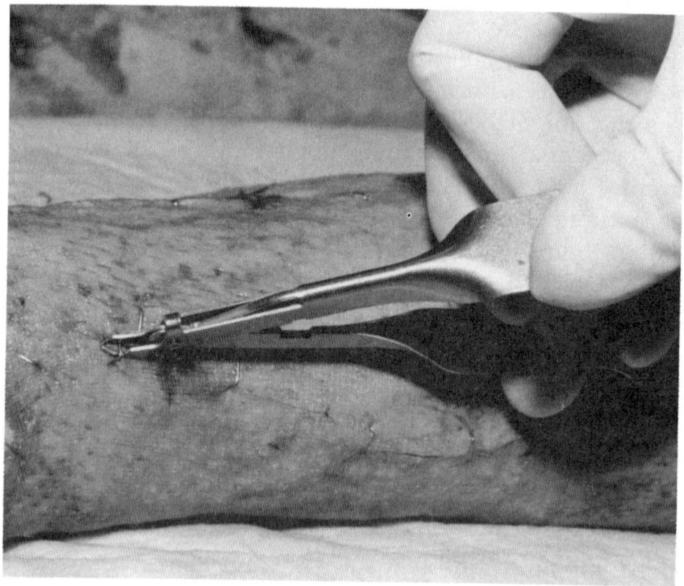

FIGURE 8–3. Staple removal from adhered mesh skin graft.

Skin grafting of burned areas follows certain priorities. Patient survival is the first priority. The wound is closed as quickly as possible to decrease the chance of sepsis. Wound closure usually involves grafting large, flat surfaces such as the chest and anterior upper and lower extremities. With early excision and good skin graft adherence, the total burn size can be decreased to a small, nonlethal size. If survival is not an issue, function and cosmesis are the next priorities. The hands and arms, face, feet, and joint surfaces are frequently the first areas grafted.

Split-Thickness Skin Graft

For patients with large body surface area burns, the most common method of wound coverage is the split-thickness skin graft (STSG). With this method, a skin graft is harvested from an unburned area on a patient (Fig. 8–4). Skin grafts are generally 0.007 to 0.016 inches in thickness, which leaves sufficient dermis so the donor site will heal in 10 to 14 days. Coverage of the burn wound with a STSG depends on the extent and location of the wound and the amount of donor skin available.

Split-thickness skin grafts can be applied as "sheet" grafts, whereby a strip of skin is removed from a donor site and transferred without alteration to the burned area (Fig. 8–5). Sheet grafts are durable, which is particularly beneficial for coverage of areas exposed to shearing forces (e.g., palms of hands and soles of feet).[15] Sheet grafts also limit wound contraction and are preferred in locations where contraction will compromise function.[15,16] Sheet grafts, when applied to a wound, cover the area with a more continuous layer of dermis than does a meshed graft because of its interstices.[17,18] Therefore, a sheet-graft should be considered when grafting the neck and joint surfaces of growing children.[15] Sheet grafts routinely are used on the face and neck and preferably on the hands because they give an excellent cosmetic result, especially when attention is paid to matching skin color of the donor and recipient sites. Also, hyperpigmentation is less likely to occur.[15] One of the disadvantages of sheet grafts is that blood, serous drainage, or bacteria may collect underneath a graft,

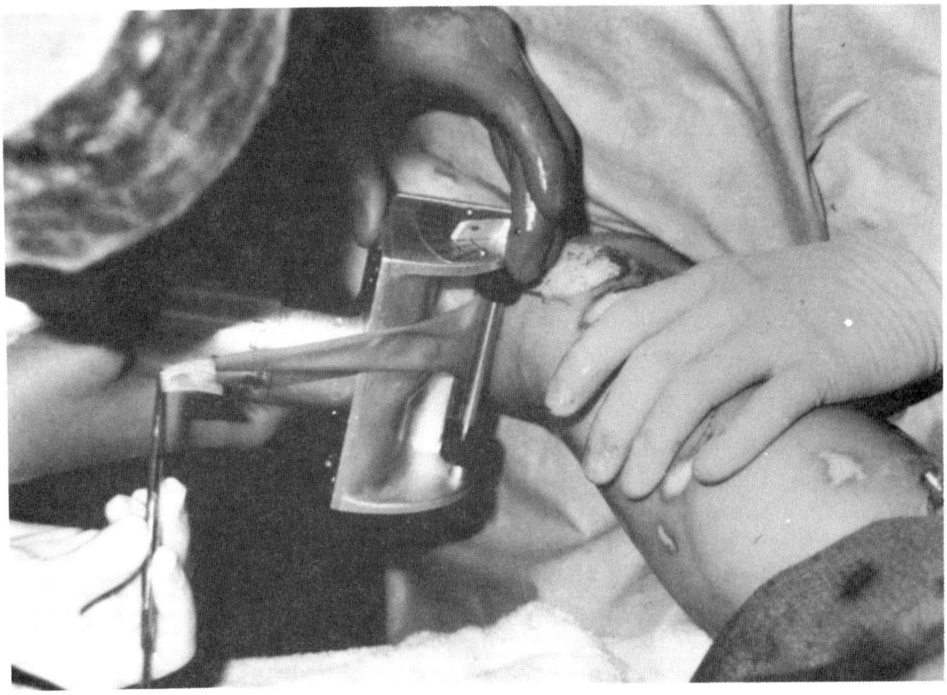

FIGURE 8-4. Harvesting of STSG from donor site using a dermatome.

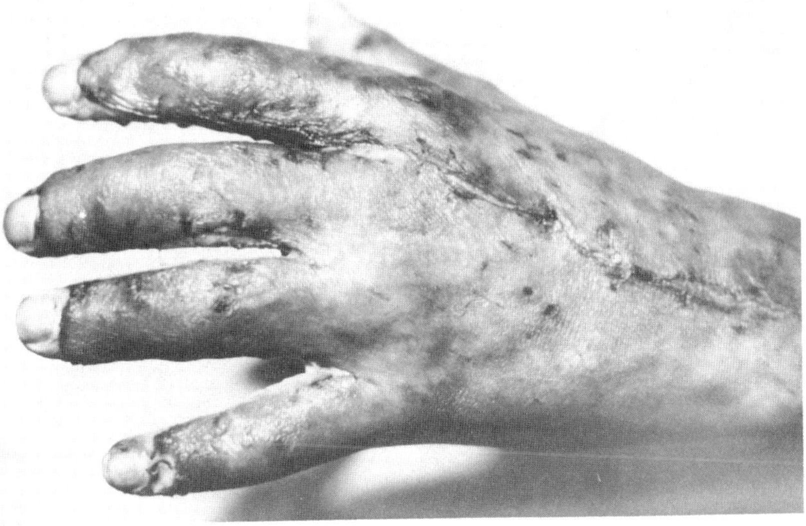

FIGURE 8-5. Sheet graft on hand, postoperative day 7.

causing a graft to become separated from the wound bed and lost. Therefore, a sheet graft should be placed on an infection-free recipient bed where hemostasis has been achieved. These grafts must be fixed securely to the surrounding skin, by staples, steristrips, or sutures, and require a considerable amount of care during the first few days if they are treated with the open method (see Chapter 7). The therapist or nurse may use a cotton applicator to gently roll any collected fluid from under the graft to its edges during the first 24 to 48 hours. The amount of area that sheet grafts cover is limited to the actual dimensions of the donor site; therefore some method to expand the donor skin to cover a larger area frequently is necessary.

An early attempt to expand the amount of available skin was through the use of "pinch" grafts.[19] With this method, hundreds of fingertip size grafts were used to cover the burn wound. Later, a variety of dermatomes have been developed that made harvesting of skin grafts easier and their thickness more consistent than the previously used freehand method of sheet or pinch grafts. Not until 1964, when Tanner[20] described his mesher, did the first truly effective method of expanding the amount of donor skin to cover the burn wound become available.

Following the harvesting of a skin graft, the skin is placed on a plastic template and fed through the meshing apparatus. The mesher uses a cutting bar that passes over angled grooves of a template (Fig. 8–6). The angle of the grooves determines the amount of expansion. The mesher can expand available skin from $1\frac{1}{2}$ up to 9 times its original size (Fig. 8–7). The 9:1 expansion is very difficult to work with and used rarely. The pattern of the meshed skin graft will remain when the graft heals; therefore, every effort should be made to avoid use of meshed grafts on the face, neck, and

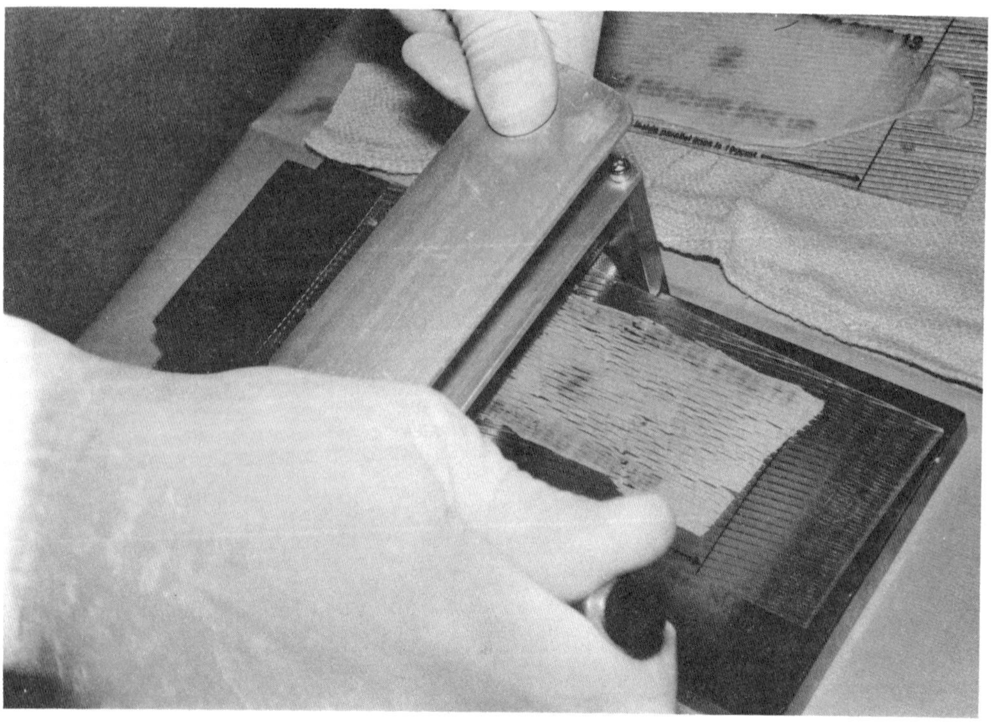

FIGURE 8–6. Harvested skin is placed on template and then fed through mesher to expand the tissue.

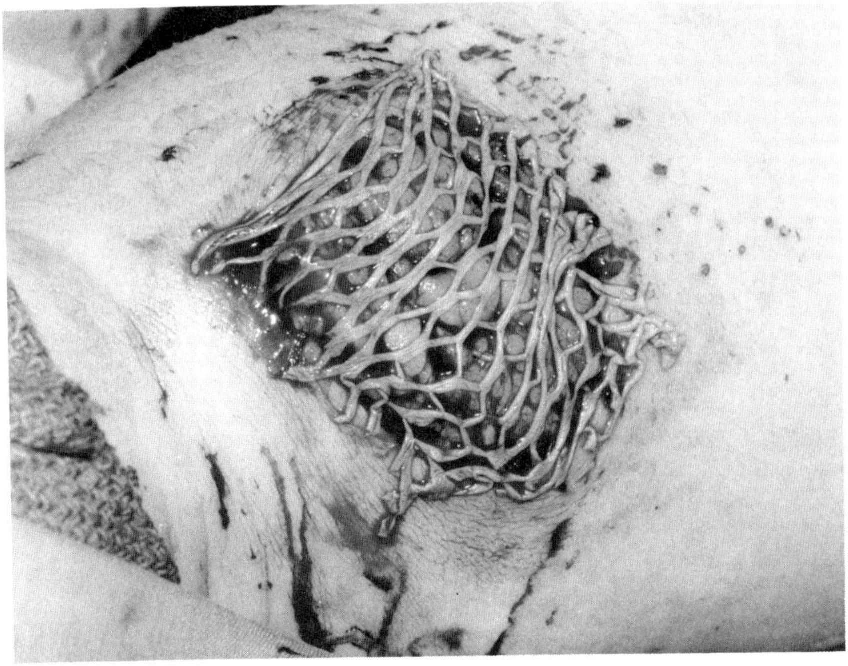

FIGURE 8–7. Skin expanded 3:1 and placed on excised wound.

hands. Meshed skin grafts are useful when donor site size must be restricted and on wounds with irregular contours or contaminated beds, since they drape well and allow for passage of exudate through the interstices in the graft.[15] They are, however, less durable than sheet grafts and tend to contract more[6] (Fig. 8–8).

Full-Thickness Skin Graft

Full-thickness skin grafts (FTSG) are harvested surgically by excising the entire thickness of the skin down to, but not including, subcutaneous tissue. These grafts are generally 0.025 to 0.030 inches in thickness. Full-thickness grafts are more durable and tend to contract less than STSGs.[21] For these reasons they are especially useful on the palms of the hands.[22,23] FTSGs are used frequently in reconstructive surgery, over pressure points, or anywhere extra skin thickness, protection or less shrinkage is preferable.

Donor Site

The split-thickness donor site is similar to a superficial partial-thickness injury and only epithelialization is required for healing to occur. Epidermal appendages are left intact; therefore, hair, sweat glands, sebaceous glands, and nerves will regenerate. If the donor site is in an area of a bony prominence or loose skin, a saline solution is injected subcutaneously to elevate the skin, creating an even surface for the dermatome to glide over. Split-thickness donor sites generally heal in 10 to 14 days and can be reharvested three to four times. The donor site created from a FTSG can be closed primarily if relatively small or will require a skin STSG if the site is large.

The burn surgeon may have little choice as to donor site selection, but if possible the donor skin should match the recipient site in texture and color as much as pos-

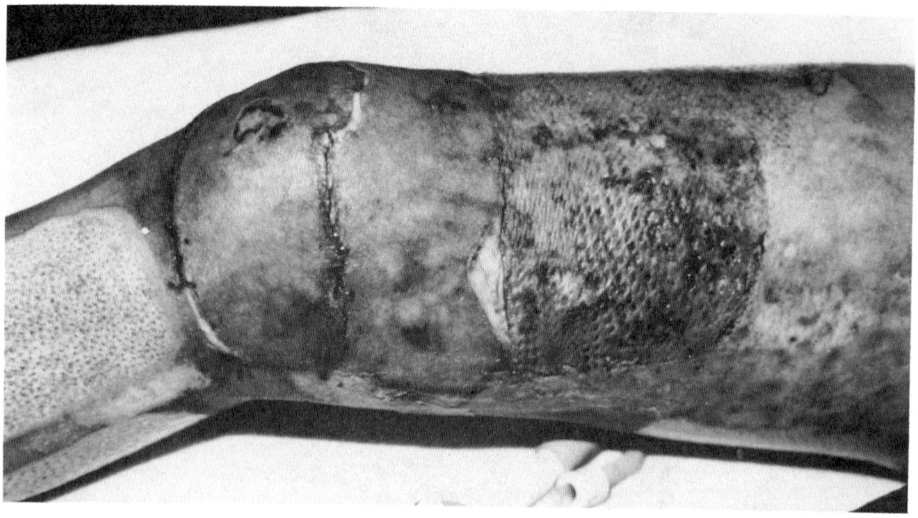

FIGURE 8–8. Right lower extremity of burn patient with (left to right) donor site, sheet graft and mesh graft in place.

sible. The skin color above the clavicles is different from that below the clavicles, and should be considered when selecting a donor site. When large amounts of skin are needed, the thighs or back generally are used because large skin surfaces are available. Most areas of the body, including the scalp, can serve as a donor site.

Because donor sites resemble partial-thickness burns, they are usually painful for the patient. Nonetheless, exercises should be performed in the presence of donor sites the same as they are with areas of partial-thickness burn. Generally, donor sites do not cross or involve joint skin creases and are fairly superficial in depth. Therefore, they are at minimal risk for the development of contractures. However, in patients who are reluctant to move, skin tightness and posterior axillary fold banding may develop. This tightness has been noted in patients with upper back donor sites who do not exercise their shoulders. Donor sites that have been harvested repeatedly are at greater risk for hypertrophic scar development.

Cultured Skin Substitutes

Patients with large total body surface area (TBSA) burns (>50 percent) may not have enough donor skin available to provide complete wound coverage following primary excision. Consequently, donor sites must be harvested repeatedly and healing time is prolonged with each subsequent harvest. Ideally, if a patient's own skin could be grown in a laboratory, wound coverage would be expedited. The risk of infection and time of patient immobilization would be decreased and rejection, which occurs with other biologic coverings, would not occur. For these reasons, much attention has been directed recently toward "growing skin" in a laboratory for use on patients with large burns.

Cultured skin substitutes restore the essential functions of the skin, provide a barrier to the environment, and control evaporative water loss.[24] Currently, there are three different models of cultured skin being investigated; however, there is a wide variety of techniques used for each model. Cultured skin substitutes are very expensive and experience with them still is quite limited. The reader is directed to the references for further details.

The first model is the use of *cultured keratinocytes,* referred to as cultured epidermal autografts (CEA).[25,26] A small biopsy of unburned skin from the patient is used to supply the epidermal cells for the cultures. The CEAs then are grown into sheets from the keratinocytes. After 2 to 3 weeks of growth, the epidermal cells are separated from the substrate on which they were grown by chemical lysis of the intercellular bonds. The epidermal cells then are applied to a carrier material for placement on the patient. Recently a commercial laboratory began manufacturing cultured skin autografts and can supply 200 3 × 3-inch pieces of cultured skin 3 weeks after a skin biopsy has been delivered to them.[26] Additional CEAs can be provided every 2 to 3 weeks thereafter as needed. Although cultured keratinocytes provide more material to cover the patient's wounds, they have less durability than skin grafts because there is no dermis present. Also, because an epidermal cell to connective tissue attachment must occur, which may require weeks to months, blisters and skin breakdown become a frequent problem (Fig. 8–9).

The second model is the use of *composite skin,* which contains both dermis and epidermis.[27–32] The addition of a viable dermis imparts durability and strength to the tissue. A collagen gel, made a variety of ways by different researchers, is populated with fibroblasts from the patient and allowed to grow. At the same time, keratino-

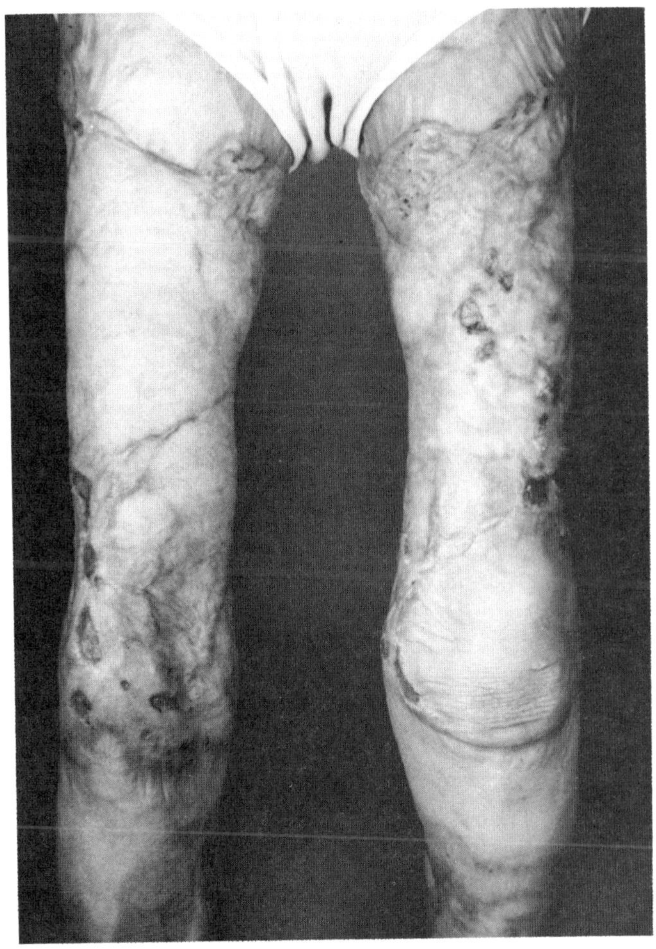

FIGURE 8–9. Skin breakdown on patient's anterior thighs where cultured epidermal cells were applied $1\frac{1}{2}$ years earlier.

cytes from the patient are grown separately. After a period of 2 to 3 weeks, the keratinocytes are placed onto the collagen matrix. The bilayer material then is placed on a patient's vascularized, infection-free recipient bed. The new material does not have a vascular plexus and is at great risk for microbial overgrowth during the non-vascular, non-nourished time period.[33] Clinically, this lack of a vascular plexus delays the initiation of exercise following placement of the cultured skin graft. Vascularization of the composite skin requires ingrowth of the blood vessels from the recipient site. Five to seven days or longer may be required for this to occur and during that time the skin should remain immobile on its bed.

A third model for cultured skin involves the use of *allogeneic (cadaver) skin.*[34–36] A biopsy is obtained from the patient and keratinocytes are cultured. Allogeneic skin is applied to the patient's wound and the epidermis is removed by dermabrasion. The patient's own cultured epithelium then is placed on the exposed allogeneic dermis. This type of cultured skin substitute is not rejected by the patient because the epidermis contains the elements that cause rejection, not the dermis. To improve the chance of adherence, decrease the risk of infection, and minimize the length of time until movement can be initiated, fresh allograft, with its vascular plexus, is superior to frozen allograft.

TEMPORARY WOUND COVERAGE

The only acceptable permanent coverage for a burn wound is a patient's own skin. However, some other forms of temporary wound coverage often are required for a patient with a large body surface area burn. Temporary wound coverings provide a protective barrier for the patient while donor sites heal for future harvesting.

Biologic Coverings

For patients who do not have adequate donor sites, a number of biologic wound coverings, usually applied in the operating room, are available. Homograft, heterograft and amnion are types of biologic dressings available for use with burn patients. A *homograft,* also called an *allograft,* is skin from another human, and originally was somewhat difficult to obtain. An example of a homograft is skin from a cadaver. With the increased interest in organ procurement and the more common existence of community tissue banks, cadaver skin is now readily available to most burn units. The original interest in cadaver skin was to use it as a permanent skin covering. This procedure has been accomplished, on a very limited basis, with the use of immunosuppressive drugs.[37,38] The body reacts to the application of homograft with the normal antigen-antibody response and rejection usually occurs after approximately 2 to 3 weeks. The length of time a homograft can remain on the wound can be extended with the use of immunosuppressive agents, but in most instances, all of the homograft will need to be replaced.[39] Homograft application provides wound coverage while donor sites heal and additional autografts become available (Fig. 8–10). Additional uses of cadaver skin are to cover an excised wound until cultured skin becomes available or to protect autografts placed on an excised wound. Cadaver skin coverage of meshed grafts protects them during the crucial early days of graft revascularization. The 6:1 and 9:1 meshed autografts are very fragile and covering the autografts for 3 to 5 days with homograft improves skin graft adherence. The homograft must be removed before it becomes attached to the wound so that the underlying skin graft is not removed when the homograft is removed.

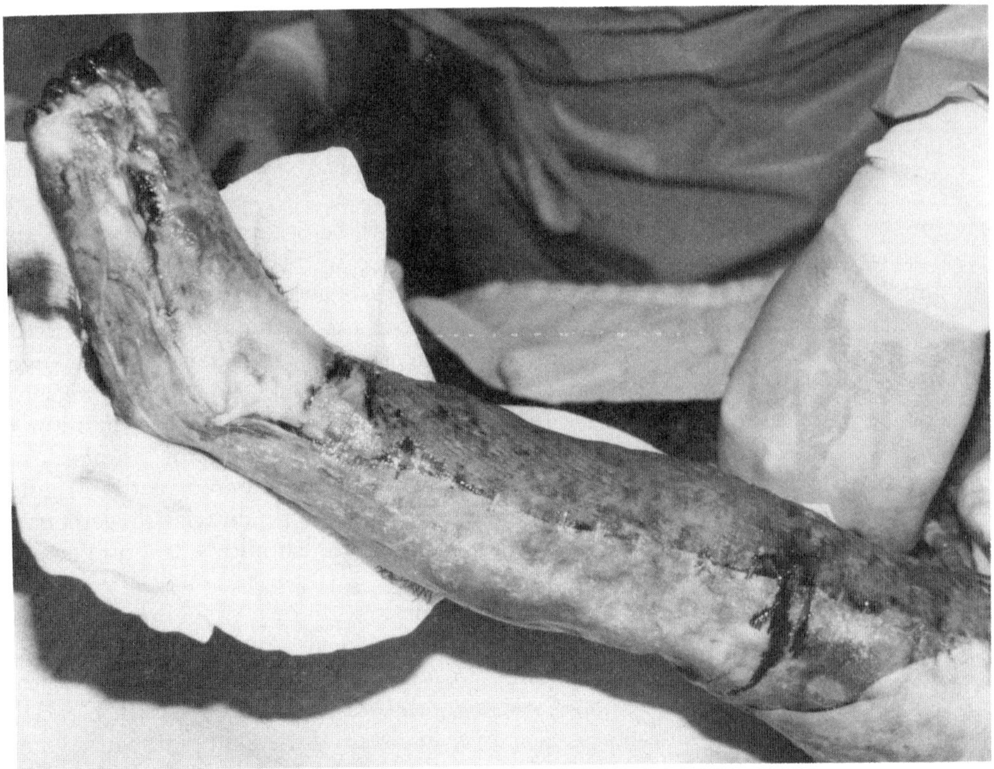

FIGURE 8–10. Homograft on patient's left lateral leg and foot. Note autograft on anterior aspect of leg.

A *heterograft* or *xenograft* is skin from a different species such as a pig. The skin from a pig closely resembles human skin and is the most widely used heterograft. Pigskin is available in a fresh or frozen state. Some pigskin is impregnated with silver nitrate to help reduce the risk of infection. In addition to the physiologic properties of providing a barrier to the environment and body water conservation, a heterograft can act like a mechanical debrider as it is removed, taking with it necrotic tissue that has adhered to the underside.

Amnion, the membrane of the placenta, is obtained fresh following childbirth and is an excellent biologic dressing for partial- and full-thickness burns. Amnion is separated from the placenta at the time of delivery and kept refrigerated or frozen. The amnion only needs to be washed and then stored in a physiologic solution. However, because of the high percentage of drug users among pregnant patients in large urban hospitals, there are concerns of placental/amnion transfer of AIDS or hepatitis. Therefore, the use of amnion is very limited.

Synthetic Coverings

During the last several years a number of synthetic coverings, which have many characteristics of biologic coverings, became available for use with burn patients (see Chapter 7 and Appendix B). These dressings are used to aid healing of partial-thickness burns, cover skin grafts, and provide temporary coverage for excised wounds and donor sites. Biobrane, a silastic membrane bonded to a bovine collagen sheet with a nylon backing, was the first of these dressings to be developed and is widely used. Synthetic coverings produce a relatively painless donor site that allows the burn patient to move more comfortably.

PINNING OF JOINTS

Immobilizing the digits of the fingers or toes can be accomplished through the use of Kirschner wires (K-wires). K-wires are inserted into the osseous tissue while the patient is anesthetized. The number of K-wires inserted, as well as the joints immobilized, should be documented specifically. If the tip of the K-wire extends beyond the surface of the tip of the digit, a plastic or rubber cap or cork is placed over the exposed metal to protect the patient and the care provider. As with any invasive procedure, there is a potential for infection and the pin site should be monitored routinely for signs of infection.[12] When the K-wires are removed, the number and location from where the wires were removed should be compared to the original documented location. If the patient exhibits undue anxiety or pain with movement of a particular joint that was previously pinned, a radiograph should be taken to ensure that all K-wires were removed.

K-wires are used to splint a joint and limit motion, thereby providing additional protection to exposed tendons and joints of the fingers and toes prior to skin graft coverage. Following skin grafting, K-wires are used to immobilize a joint until the graft has adhered sufficiently to allow assistive range-of-motion exercises (Fig. 8–11). K-wires used to prevent contractures remain in place until the skin graft can tolerate exercise and/or splinting. For example, following skin grafting to the dorsal foot and toes, K-wires are inserted to position the toes in neutral extension. When passive toe flexion and the use of a dorsal foot splint can be initiated without compromising the integrity of the skin graft, the K-wires can be removed. If a tendon is ruptured or if there is extensive joint damage, the joint may need to be fused. In this instance, the K-wire remains in place a minimum of 6 weeks. During the reconstructive phase, K-wires can help to correct a deformity by maintaining an optimal alignment of a joint following the release of the soft tissues.

Reconstructive Phase

A number of reconstructive operative procedures may be required for the burn patient. Pediatric patients may require multiple reconstructive procedures because scars do not elongate as children grow. Brou and colleagues[40] have developed an inventory form to assist the burn team in identifying and tracking the functional and esthetic limitations of patients that allows them to prioritize and plan reconstructive surgical procedures. The most common procedure is the release of scar contractures. Contractures usually occur across joints when the scar shortens and pulls a joint into a position of deformity. Also, contractures develop at the commissures of the mouth and occasionally at the lower eyelids. The correction of a contracture usually involves dividing the tense scar band and the application of a skin graft. During the first year after injury, burn scars undergo a maturation process whereby they soften and lengthen. Usually, unless the scar is impairing function, the surgical release of contractures is performed after the scars have matured. Most recently, however, revision of immature scars in children has been successful.[41]

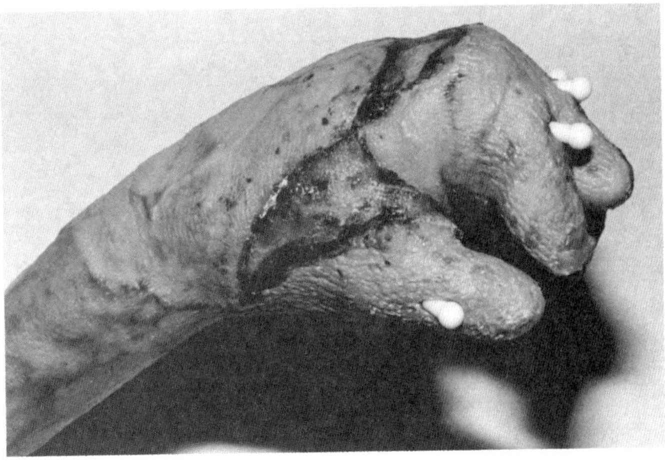

FIGURE 8–11. K-wire pinning of left hand to maintain thumb and metacarpophalangeal joints in optimal position while skin grafts heal.

SCAR REVISION

Scar revision can be accomplished in a number of ways.[42,43] Small hypertrophic scars can be excised and the site closed primarily by sutures. Segmental scar reduction can be accomplished by excising a central portion of the scar and suturing the edges. Every several months additional scar is excised until all of the scar is removed. Scars can be excised completely and covered by a split-thickness or full-thickness skin graft. Dermabrasion, a surgical procedure where the epidermis is mechanically sanded, is used to smooth the skin and enhance the appearance of meshed skin grafts.

Another commonly encountered scar tissue problem involves the developing breast in the female patient who experienced chest burns at an early age. The inelastic scar tissue of the chest may not allow for proper development of the breasts and the skin overlying the developing breast may need to be released or expanded.

SKIN FLAPS

A skin flap is a full-thickness portion of the skin that includes subcutaneous fat and occasionally portions of muscle. Flaps are used to cover excised or debrided burn wounds. Three common types of flaps are *rotational, local advancement,* and *free flaps.*[44–47] The main advantages of flaps are that they have sensation and, more importantly, the thickness of these flaps provides a protective covering to areas where the skin is very thin and subject to shear or pressure.

A simple form of rotational flap is the Z-plasty. *Plasty* is a suffix that means molding, shaping, or the result of a surgical procedure.[48] The term is used in conjunction with various prefixes to denote the appearance of the incision made during surgical release of scar bands when skin grafting is not necessary. There should be adjacent normal skin to interpose into the line of scar tension. The Z-plasty and Y-V-plasty are two common procedures used to release small scar bands on the hands, face, axilla, and antecubital and popliteal regions.[43] Z-plasties are useful for mild contractures or when the contracture is a linear band, as the Z breaks up the line of tension. The scar is lengthened by introducing normal tissue from each side into the central scar band (Fig. 8–12). A Y-V-plasty also can break up a scar band and is useful where normal tissue is available from only one side of a scar (Fig. 8–13). After the

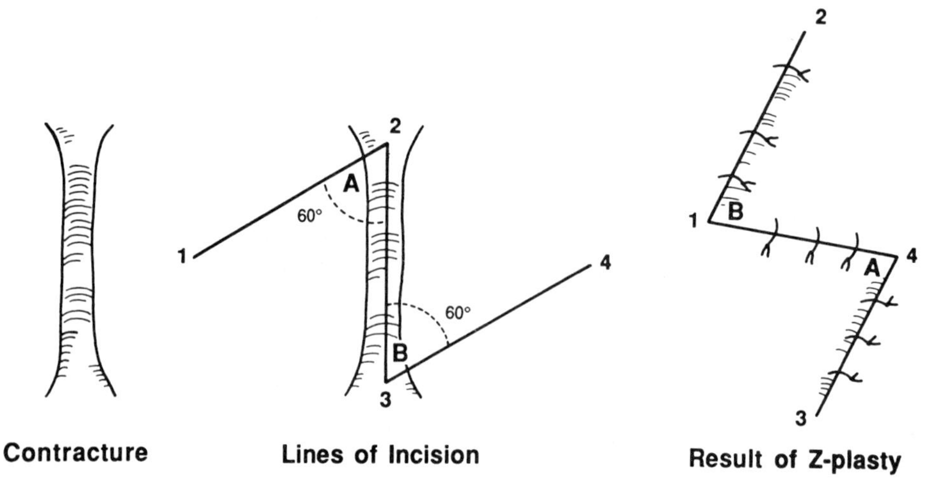

FIGURE 8–12. Diagram depicting stages of Z-plasty revision of scar contracture. (Courtesy of D. Greenhalgh, 1991.)

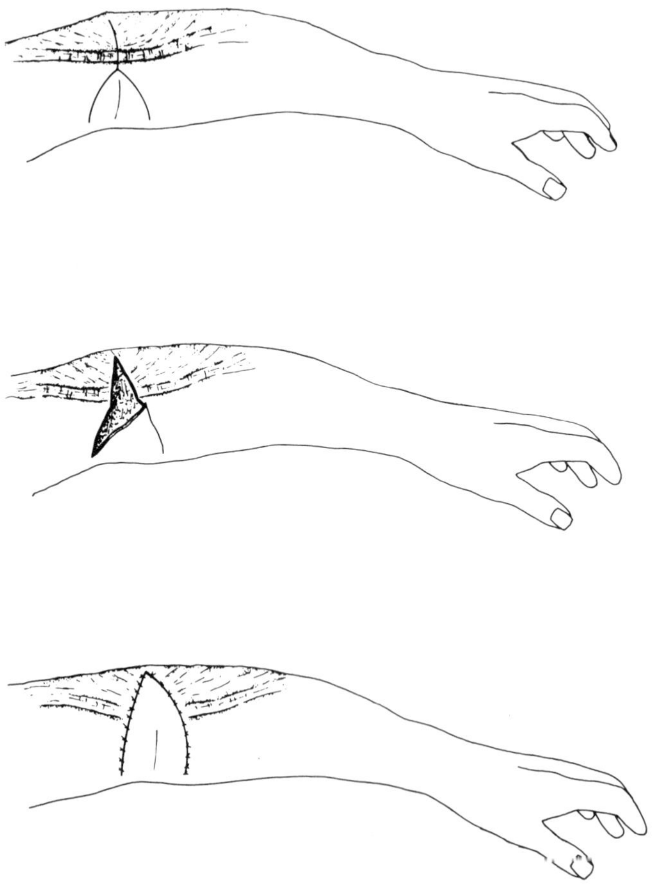

FIGURE 8–13. Diagram depicting Y-V-plasty technique for correction of scar band. (*Top*) Inverted Y incision is made through normal and scarred tissue. (*Middle*) Normal tissue is lifted and scar band separates. (*Bottom*) Normal tissue is advanced into area of scar and sutured in place to make a V.

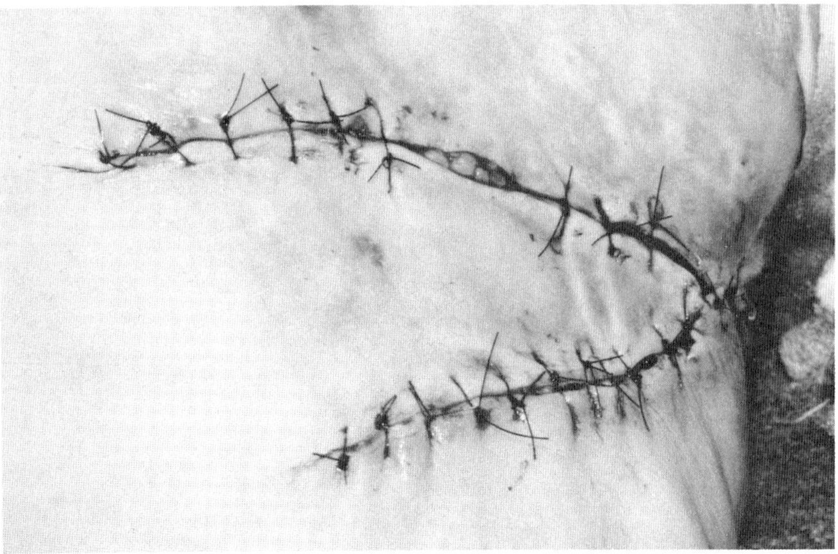

FIGURE 8–14. After scar excision, normal skin is advanced to fill the defect and sutured in place.

folds are interposed, they are sutured in place. The sutures remain in place for 10 to 14 days depending on the location and physician preference. During this time, patients can perform active movements, providing tension is not applied to the suture line. Stretching exercises and massage are initiated following healing of the wound edges and removal of the sutures. Compression therapy for scar control generally is not indicated following these procedures.

Local advancement or rotational flaps are used to cover nearby or adjacent wounds and are created in such a fashion that their blood supply is maintained. The site from which the rotational flap is taken will need a split-thickness skin graft, but with advancement flaps, no grafting is necessary (Fig. 8–14).

Free flaps are harvested from a remote site and a microvascular anastomosis is required to re-establish the blood supply to this flap at the recipient site. The donor site will require skin grafting. Free flaps have limited use but are most beneficial to reconstruct the hands and face[49] (Fig. 8–15). Therapists may need to fabricate splints to maintain a limb in a sometimes awkward position (e.g., the forearm against the nose) during the time of flap vascularization. Similar to Z-plasties, advancement, rotational and free flaps seldom require compression therapy.

TISSUE EXPANDERS

By using tissue expansion, a scar can be replaced by adjacent tissue with nearly normal color, texture, sensation and hair-bearing qualities for that area.[50] Expanders are polymeric silicone balloons with a valve for injecting saline.[51] They are surgically placed either above the muscle fascia deep in the subcutaneous fat or under muscle.[50] Tissue expanders are used primarily to reduce alopecia (loss of hair), when there is a shortage of tissue, to create a flap with skin and functioning muscle, or to revise scars adjacent to normal skin[51] (Fig. 8–16). With the use of tissue expanders, the skin is initially thinned. However, the depth of the tissue returns to normal after approximately 2 years.[52] Complications of this procedure include pain when the expander is

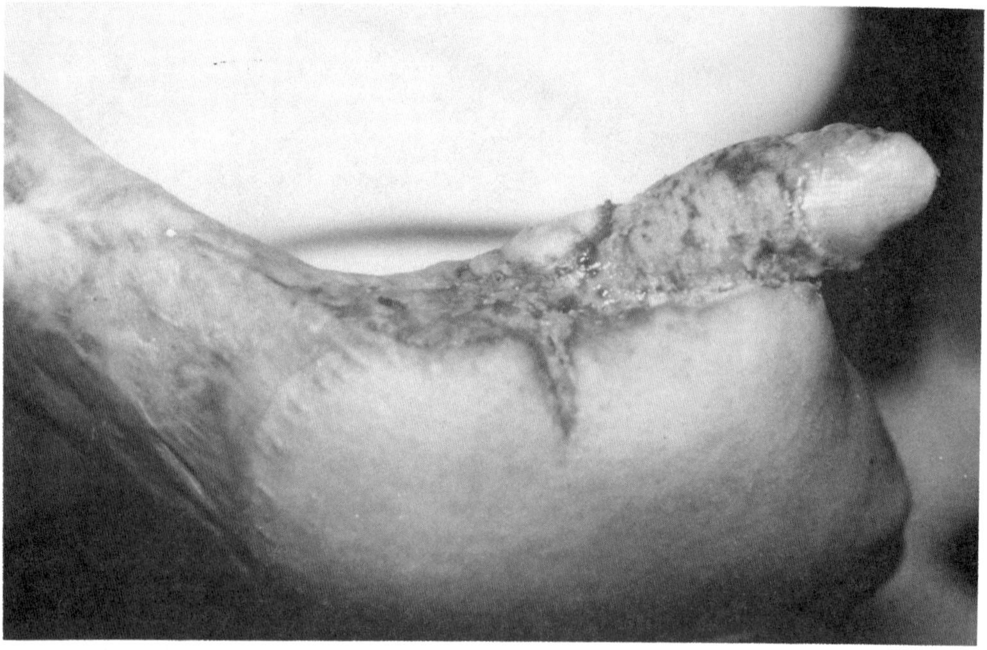

FIGURE 8–15. Free flap transfer of toe to replace amputated right thumb.

injected, seroma or hematoma formation, infection, and ischemia of the tissue with expansion.[53] After the surgical site heals, the sutures are removed and saline is injected into the expander. The amount of saline that is injected is determined by the tolerance of the tissue and the patient. When the area is palpated it should be firm and the patient should experience only minimal pain or tenderness. The balloon is serially injected weekly with saline. Once the overlying skin has been successfully stretched to a predetermined size, the expander is removed and the skin may be used for a flap or skin grafting.

SUMMARY

Surgery plays an integral part in the management of the patient with burns. The therapist is involved to maintain maximal range of motion without jeopardizing the skin grafts. A variety of surgical procedures can be used. By being familiar with the different types of procedures, the therapist can develop a treatment plan that will be of maximum benefit to the patient to accomplish the goal of full recovery and function.

Emergent life-saving procedures occasionally are necessary during the first few hours after the burn injury. Most of the surgical procedures during this time period will be performed to manage associated injuries. Next, the removal of the eschar and the application of skin grafts becomes a primary concern. The goal is to remove all the burned skin and to cover the wound with skin grafts in one or two operations. However, donor sites may be limited and a number of methods may be used to expand the available skin so that a maximum amount of burned area can be covered.

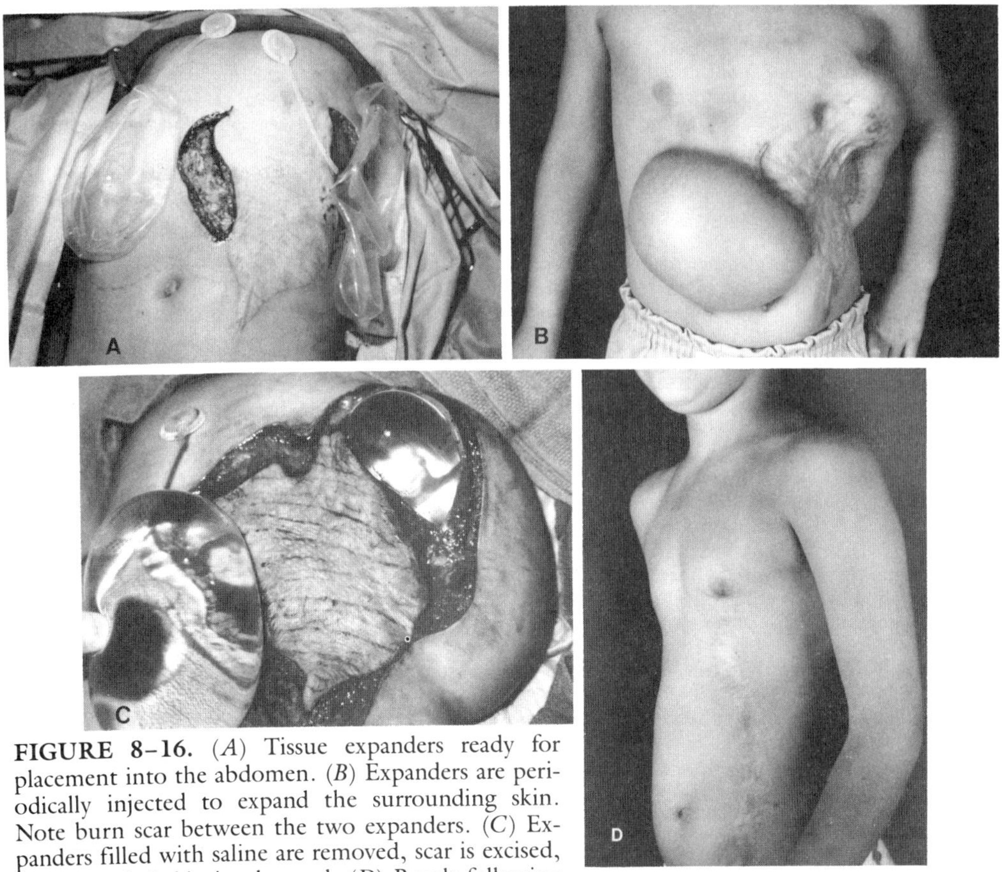

FIGURE 8–16. (*A*) Tissue expanders ready for placement into the abdomen. (*B*) Expanders are periodically injected to expand the surrounding skin. Note burn scar between the two expanders. (*C*) Expanders filled with saline are removed, scar is excised, and expanded skin is advanced. (*D*) Result following tissue expansion.

Biologic and synthetic coverings are used temporarily to protect the burn wound surface from contamination when there is not enough skin to cover the area.

Prior to surgery, postoperative positioning, splints that may be used to immobilize the graft site, and commencement of exercise should all be discussed with the patient in order to encourage compliance and minimize fear. Additionally, the therapist's interventions include range of motion under anesthesia, postoperative positioning and splinting programs, and initiation of exercise programs without interfering with skin graft adherence.

REFERENCES

1. Petro, JA and Khan, M: Operative management of the burned patient. In Nicosia, JE and Petro, JA (eds): Manual of Burn Care. Raven Press, New York, 1983, pp 89–98.
2. Hammond, J and Ward, CG: Surgical fixation of skin grafts. J Burn Care Rehabil 9:516–517, 1988.
3. Heimbach, DM: Early burn wound excision and grafting. In Boswick, JA (ed): The Art and Science of Burn Care. Aspen, Rockville, Maryland, 1987, pp 65–72.
4. Demling, RH and Lalonde, C: Burn Trauma. Thieme Medical Publishers, New York, 1989, pp 118–145.
5. Heimbach, DM and Engrav, LH: Surgical Management of the Burn Wound. Raven Press, New York, 1984, pp 13–49.
6. Janzekovic, Z: A new concept of the early excision and immediate grafting of burn. J Trauma 10:1103–1108, 1970.

7. Baxter, CR: Early surgical excision and immediate grafting. In Artz, CP, Moncrief, JA, and Pruitt, BA (eds): Burns, A Team Approach. WB Saunders, Philadelphia, 1979, pp 224–233.
8. Burke, JF, Quinby, WC, and Bondoc, CC: Primary excision and prompt grafting as routine therapy for the treatment of thermal burns in children. Surg Clin North Am 56:477–494, 1976.
9. Slater, AL, Slater, H, and Goldfarb, IW: Effect of aggressive surgical treatment in older patients with burns. J Burn Care Rehabil 10:527–530, 1989.
10. Hartford, CE: Surgical management. In Fisher, SV and Helm, PA (eds): Comprehensive Rehabilitation of Burns. Williams & Wilkins, Baltimore, 1984, pp 28–63.
11. Koepke, GH: The role of physical medicine in the treatment of burns. Surg Clin North Am 50:1385–1399, 1970.
12. Johnson, CL, O'Shaughnessy, EJ, and Ostergren, G: Burn Management. Raven Press, New York, 1981, pp 91–103.
13. Blassingame, WM, et al: Range of motion of the shoulder performed while patient is anesthetized. J Burn Care Rehabil 10:539–542, 1989.
14. Bryant, MW: Wound Healing Clinical Symposia. CIBA Pharmaceutical Company, New Jersey, 1977.
15. Pensler, JM and Mulliken, JB: Skin grafts: To mesh or not to mesh. Contemp Surg 32:45–49, 1988.
16. Petry, JJ and Wortham, KA: Contraction of wounds covered by meshed and non-meshed split thickness graft. Br J Plast Surg 39:478–482, 1986.
17. Rudolph, R, et al: The life cycle of the myofibroblasts. Surg Gynecol Obstet 145:389–392, 1977.
18. Rudolph, R, et al: Contractile fibroblasts by skin grafts. Surg Forum, 28:524, 1977.
19. Shedd, DP: Surgical History. Surgery, 43:1024–1036, 1958.
20. Tanner, JC, et al: The mesh skin graft. Plast Reconstr Surg 34:287–292, 1964.
21. Fidler, JP: Debridement and grafting of full-thickness burns. In Hummel, RP (ed): Clinical Burn Therapy. John Wright & Sons, Great Britain, 1982, pp 118–137.
22. Schwanholt, C, Greenhalgh, DG, and Warden, GD: A comparison of full thickness vs. partial thickness autografts for the coverage of deep palm burns in the very young pediatric patient. Proc American Burn Association 23:66, 1991.
23. Merrill, SW, et al: Full-thickness skin grafting for contact burns of the palm in children. J Burn Care Rehabil 6:501–507, 1986.
24. Boyce, ST, et al: Skin wound closure in athymic mice with cultured human cells, biopolymers, and growth factors. Surgery 110:866–876, 1991.
25. Gallico, GG, et al: Permanent coverage of large burn wounds with autologous cultured epithelium. N Engl J Med 311:448–451, 1984.
26. Biosurface Technology, Cambridge, Massachusetts, 1990.
27. Boyce, ST and Hansbrough, JF: Biologic attachment, growth and differentiation of cultured human epidermal keratinocytes on a graftable collagen and chondroitin-6-sulfate substrate. Surgery 103:421–431, 1988.
28. Bell, E, et al: A living tissue formed in vitro and accepted as a full thickness skin equivalent. Science 211:1042–1054, 1981.
29. Hull, BE, Finley, RK, and Miller, SF: Coverage of full-thickness burns with bilayered skin equivalents: A preliminary clinical trial. Surgery 107:496–502, 1990.
30. Hansbrough, JF, et al: Burn wound closure with cultured autologous keratinocytes and fibroblasts attached to a collagen-glycosaminoglycan substrate. JAMA 262:2125–2130, 1989.
31. Heimbach, DM, et al: Artificial dermis for major burns; a multi-center randomized clinical trial. Ann Surg 208:313–320, 1988.
32. Nanchahal, J, et al: Cultured composite skin grafts: Biological skin equivalents permitting massive expansion. Lancet 11:191–193, 1989.
33. Boyce, ST: Personal communication, December, 1991.
34. Cuono, CB, et al: Composite-autologous-allogeneic skin replacement: development and clinical application. Plast Reconstr Surg 80:626–635, 1987.
35. Heck, EL, Bergstrasser, PR, and Baxter, CR: Composite skin graft: frozen dermal allografts support the engraftment and expansion of autologous epidermis. J Trauma 25:106–112, 1985.
36. Fang, CH, et al: Observations on stability and contraction of composite skin grafts: Xenodermis or allodermis with an isograft overlay. J Burn Care Rehabil 11:538–542, 1990.
37. Grossman, AR, Brones, M, and Fishman, G: Permanent skin coverage of critical burns using cadaver skin and cyclosporine. Proc American Burn Association 22:69, 1990.
38. Hewitt, CW, et al: Reconstructive allotransplantation: Considerations regarding integumentary/musculoskeletal grafts, cyclosporine, wound coverage in thermal injury, and the immune response. J Burn Care Rehabil 11:74–85, 1990.
39. Sakabu, SA, et al: Cyclosporine A for prolonging allograft survival in patients with massive burns. J Burn Care Rehabil, 11:410–418, 1990.
40. Brou, JA, et al: Inventory of potential reconstructive needs in the patient with burns. J Burn Care Rehabil 10:555–560, 1989.
41. Greenhalgh, DG, Gaboury, T, and Warden, GD: The early release of axillary contractures in pediatric patients with burns. J Burn Care Rehabil 14:39–42, 1993.

42. Feller, I and Grabb, WC (ed): Reconstruction and Rehabilitation of the Burned Patient. Thomson-Shore, Dexter, Michigan, 1979.
43. Engrav, LH, et al: Partial excision of residual burn lesions. J Burn Care Rehabil 5:398–402, 1987.
44. Hallock, GG: Local random fasciocutaneous flaps for repair of the burned elbow. J Burn Care Rehabil 12:26–32, 1991.
45. Maruyama, Y: Ascending scapular flap and its use for the treatment of axillary burn scar contracture. Br J Plast Surg 44:97–101, 1991.
46. Hayashi, A and Maruyama, Y: Subclavicular approach in head and neck reconstruction with the latissimus dorsi musculocutanoeus flap. Br J Plast Surg 44:71–74, 1991.
47. Ohkubo, E, et al: Restoration of the anterior neck surface in the burned patient by free groin flap. Plast Reconstr Surg 87:276–284, 1991.
48. Stedman's Medical Dictionary, 23rd ed. Williams & Wilkins, Baltimore, 1976.
49. Hallock, GG: The radial forearm flap in burn reconstruction. J Burn Care Rehabil 4:318–322, 1986.
50. Sasaki, GH: Tissue expansion: guidelines and case analysis. Dow Corning Wright, Arlington, Tennessee, 1986.
51. Cohen, M, et al: The role of tissue expansion in the reconstruction of secondary burn defects. J Burn Care Rehabil 10:220, 1989.
52. Pasyk, KA, Argenta, LC, and Austad, ED: Histopathology of human expanded tissue. Clin Plast Surg 14:435–445, 1987.
53. Manders, EK, et al: Soft-tissue expansion: Concepts and complications. Plast Reconstr Surg 74:493–507, 1984.

SECTION III

The Rehabilitation

Therefore, strengthen the hands that are weak and the knees that are feeble, and make straight paths beneath their feet, so that the limb which is lame may not be put out of joint, but rather be healed.

Hebrews 12:12

CHAPTER 9

Burn Patient Evaluation and Treatment Planning

Reginald L. Richard, MS, PT
Marlys J. Staley, MS, PT

A major burn is a physical injury of extreme proportions that ravages the body, beyond the surface of the skin, to affect all body systems of the patient. As such, therapists logically should be involved in the care and treatment of patients with this type of injury.

The mortality rate for patients with large total body surface area burns continues to decline.[1,2] As a result, the need for therapeutic and rehabilitative intervention is rising and assuming an increasingly important role in the overall and eventual recovery of the burn patient.

The ultimate goal of burn rehabilitation always has been to return patients back into society in as near to their normal functional capacity as what existed prior to the burn injury.[3] In the past, scar tissue contractures and deformities were an expected part of even small burn injuries.[4-7] Today, therapists are progressively treating burn patients in an attempt to prevent these complications from occurring.

Evaluating a burn patient and planning a course of treatment is an ongoing process requiring daily modification.[8,9] This chapter describes evaluation and treatment planning for a patient having an acute major burn injury. Using this information, each therapist will need to decide upon the appropriate depth of detail to be recorded about patients with lesser burns for quality assurance, reimbursement needs, or research purposes. Additionally, although the role of therapists in burn care can vary with each facility, the information provided will focus on the therapist's involvement to rehabilitate the patient rather than as a provider of wound care.

PATIENT EVALUATION

During the first 48 to 72 hours after the patient is admitted to the hospital, there can be a great deal of commotion due to the many needs of the patient.[10] A therapist should perform the initial evaluation as soon as possible following the patient's hospitalization, even though the activity surrounding the patient during this time may encumber the process.[3,8-11]

Compared to other patient diagnoses treated by therapists, the burn injury itself can provoke anxiety in several ways. The immense amount of pain patients experience, the odors associated with burned skin, and the sometimes hysterical reaction of the family to what has occurred all can produce stress for even a veteran therapist. In addition, there may be an accumulation of edema causing distortion of the patient's physical features and the appearance of the wounds may create a situation that can overwhelm the patient and therapist.

Regardless of the distracting features associated with the burn trauma and associated pathophysiology, the patient undergoes a physical evaluation similar to any other patient, with a few exceptions and additions. Except in the cases of electrical injury, concomitant injury, or a known pre-existing physical deficit, the therapist's evaluation initially can be performed in a cursory manner. At first, most burn patient limitations are due to secondary complications of the burn injury. For example, common causes of early limitation in motion are pain, edema, and constricting eschar or a combination of these.[9,12] Subsequently, as edema subsides and the eschar is removed, a patient's range of motion should improve, provided that extenuating circumstances of scar contracture formation or strength loss are prevented. As these limiting complications begin to resolve, a more specific recording of joint range of motion is necessary to follow the patient's progress and the efficacy of treatment.

There are instances when a more in-depth and comprehensive initial evaluation is performed on burn patients. Specifically, patients experiencing an electrical injury should be tested for sensation and muscle strength. These two tests are important to gain added information about the extent of injury. Because much of the damage caused by the passage of electric current through the body occurs subcutaneously (see Chapter 21), testing of the intact skin for sensory deficits and muscles for strength loss due to suspected neurologic involvement can aid the surgeon in making decisions about possible surgical interventions.

The initial evaluation may be performed at the time of admission in the emergency room, during the initial wound care session, at bedside, or at the first wound dressing change. The areas to be addressed in a comprehensive patient initial evaluation are listed in Table 9-1. Depending on the patient's previous state of health or comorbid condition, an extensive evaluation of all categories listed may not be necessary at the time of admission. Since burn patients undergo many predictive physical changes, such as edema reduction, time may be better utilized reducing rather than measuring the edema. In addition, therapists should remember that in most instances, just prior to the burn injury, the patient was functioning at a normal level.[10]

COMPONENTS OF AN EVALUATION

Patient Demographic Information and History

The initial patient evaluation should begin by determining the patient's physical condition prior to the injury. This information can be obtained from the admitting history and physical by the physician, a family member, or the patient, if he or she is physically and mentally alert and oriented. Factors that may interfere with obtaining a

TABLE 9–1. Contents of a Comprehensive Burn Patient Evaluation

1. Patient name	21. Sensation
2. Diagnosis	22. Range of motion
3. Referring physician	23. Strength
4. Medical record number	24. Flexibility
5. Room number	25. Mobility
6. Insurance coverage	26. Transfer status
7. Admission date	27. Ambulation status
8. Burn date	28. Posture
9. Date of evaluation	29. Neurologic status
10. Cause of burn	30. Developmental level
11. Associated injuries	31. Psychologic status
12. Past medical history	32. Behavior and emotional status
13. Vision/hearing	33. Social support
14. Age	34. Affect of patient
15. Gender	35. Pain tolerance
16. Distribution of burn	36. Functional activities
17. Burn wound assessment	37. Hand dominance
18. Respiratory status	38. Activities of daily living
19. Endurance	39. Occupation/school grade
20. Edema/limb circumference	40. Leisure activities

history directly from the patient include endotracheal intubation, loss of consciousness, delirium, narcotic interference with sensorium, age (with children), or any previous psychologic problems. The patient's past medical history including vision and hearing acuity, balance and co-ordination, and neuromuscular or skeletal deficits, particularly in the elderly, are basic information items to be obtained. Any previous deficiencies in these areas can impact goal setting and treatment plans for the patient.

Evaluation items 1 through 6 in Table 9–1 include administrative and insurance information. The patient's insurance source can help the therapist to decide what resources are available. The dates of burn occurrence and admission to the facility, compared to the initial evaluation date, must be known. The latter also is important for quality assurance purposes. The time interval between the burn injury and when the therapist first sees the patient can influence the success of the initial contact. A delay between when the burn occurred and the initial evaluation can make the initial contact less than optimal. The initial evaluation may be delayed when the patient: (1) failed to seek admission to the hospital because the extent or depth of the burn was underestimated, (2) had little understanding of the healing process and the subsequent effects of poor healing, (3) maintained the burned limb in a comfortable position to ease pain, thereby facilitating limitations in range of motion,[4,13] or (4) obtained treatment at a facility that lacked early rehabilitation intervention and was subsequently transferred for more definitive burn care.

In any instance, a lapse in time before treatment is initiated may make the initial evaluation of range of motion and functional movement difficult and painful. In addition, a patient who received therapy at a facility unfamiliar with treating burn patients may not readily accept a burn therapist's treatment approach. The outcome may include voiced objections by the patient to the different approach, especially if the approach is perceived as more uncomfortable.

Whenever possible, the therapist should attempt to speak with the patient in a calm setting before the evaluation to explain the reasons for burn rehabilitation, express an understanding of the patient's situation, and gain the patient's commitment to the burn program. This interaction enables the patient to view the therapist as an ally rather than just another staff member who will cause more pain.[9,10]

The depth of the patient's wounds can be anticipated by knowing the agent that caused the burn.[2] Hot liquids, which flowed off the patient, cause more superficial burns than those of abuse cases where a child was held immersed in scalding bath water for an extended period of time. Similarly, flame burns tend to produce a deep injury while true electrical burns may cause extensive tissue damage.

When a patient complains of pain at sites other than the burn areas, or when the description of the pain is different than is typically experienced by the burn patient, then an associated injury should be suspected. For example, a patient admitted with partial-thickness burns to the anterior trunk, shoulder area and arms from an explosion, who experiences a "catching-type" pain at 80° of shoulder abduction, warrants further investigation of a possible shoulder joint injury. Confirmation of an additional injury should be made based on other physical findings during the evaluation.[14]

Burn Severity Index

In 1980, Tobiasen and colleagues[15,16] devised a formula to predict burn patient survival and published a revised version in 1982. The results of the original study highlighted seven variables that are associated with increased burn patient mortality. The seven variables included: (1) age, (2) gender, (3) percentage of body surface burned, (4) percentage of partial-thickness burn, (5) percentage of full-thickness burn, (6) number of critical sites, and (7) the presence of inhalation injury. These variables correspond to items 14 to 18 in Table 9-1 and are key indicators to project the amount of therapeutic intervention that may be required for each patient.

AGE

Burns of the very young and aged are associated with a high mortality rate.[2] Likewise, burn injuries to these extreme age populations have a high rate of morbidity. Children are more susceptible to scar contracture development than adults.[7,17,18] Bowden[19] demonstrated a negative relationship between age and return to work. This finding may be due to the older patient's decreased ability to recover from burn injuries when compared to younger patients.

GENDER

Burn injuries disproportionately occur more frequently in males than females.[20] Occupationally and socially, men and boys, respectively, have a greater exposure to burn-causing agents.[14] However, Tobiasen et al.[15,16] have indicated that women are at greater risk to die from their burn injury than men for reasons not explained. Bowden[19] also reported that women required more time to return to work than men for the same extent of burn. This gender difference may be due to factors associated with the burn injury, such as cosmetic concerns.

BURN WOUND ASSESSMENT

A primary component of a burn patient evaluation is the burn wound. The wound assessment should include estimating the total percent of the body surface burned, the differentiation between partial- and full-thickness injury, and the location of these wounds. Usually, this information is recorded on a burn assessment form containing an outline of the body that graphically depicts the location and depth of the burns and a segmental percentage breakdown of the total body surface area (see Chapter 6).

Extent of Burn Injury

The total amount of the body surface area burned has a significant effect on the development of scar contractures. Kraemer and co-workers[21] and others[18,22] have described a direct relationship between the percent of body burn and the resultant number of contractures developed (Fig. 9-1). The percent total body burn is important information for patient resuscitation and survival statistics and also for therapists to project the amount of time needed for patient treatment.

Depth of Burn Wound

The eventual treatment interventions used by the therapist are based on the burn wound depth. Superficial partial-thickness burn wounds usually heal without scar contracture formation or hypertrophy. Typically, these wounds heal within a few days to 2 weeks. Therapeutic interventions involve preservation of the patient's mobility and functional status primarily by preventing loss of strength and endurance during hospitalization. Also, the therapist may need to manage the pain experienced by these patients during treatment.

Deep partial-thickness burns present a major challenge to the therapist due to the resultant scar tissue produced to heal these wounds. In their classic study, Dobbs and Curreri[23] demonstrated an 18 percent incidence of lost motion with partial-thickness burns. Full-thickness burn injuries further compounded the patient's outcome. An increased incidence of lost motion and scar contracture development was noted if the overlying area was a full-thickness burn.[23]

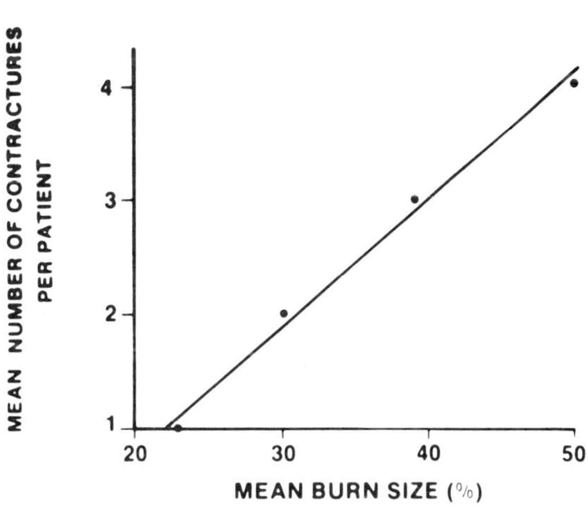

FIGURE 9-1. Graph demonstrating the direct relationship between the percent total body burn and resultant number of burn scar tissue contractures. (From Kraemer et al,[22] p 262, with permission.)

TABLE 9–2. Common Anatomic Sites of Burn Scar Contracture

Eyelid
Commissures or perioral area of mouth
Anterior neck
Anterior axillary fold
Posterior axillary fold
Antecubital space
Forearm
Wrist flexion crease
Dorsal hand and finger surface
Palmar hand and finger surface
Lateral trunk
Perineum
Popliteal space
Achilles tendon area
Dorsal foot surface and toes
Plantar foot surface and toes

Location of Burn

The anatomic location and distribution of the burn wounds are extremely important considerations for the therapist to anticipate contracture development and to appropriately focus the treatment.[21,23–26] Any burn that involves a skin crease overlying the surface of a joint is susceptible to the development of a scar tissue contracture. However, there are particular surface areas of the body and joint movements that are at particular risk as noted in Table 9–2. It appears that some patients tend to develop scar contractures due to various associated burn conditions.[27] Eight parameters have been observed to influence the development of scar tissue contractures (Table 9–3). Patients in an intensive care unit may be prone to contracture development because of their immobility. Dobbs and Curreri[23] documented a 2.6 percent incidence of motion lost in areas without any overlying burn.

RESPIRATORY STATUS

The Burn Severity Index associates inhalation injury with a high mortality. Frequently, a patient may be admitted to the hospital with only the complication of

TABLE 9–3. Parameters Contributing to Scar Contracture Formation

1. Length of hospitalization
2. Ventilator dependence
3. Intensive care length of stay
4. Percent of hospitalization spent in intensive care
5. Number of skin graft operations
6. Number of joint surface areas requiring skin grafting
7. Septic or bacteremia bouts
8. Number of anatomic areas splinted

smoke inhalation following a house fire. This type of injury may or may not necessitate involvement of the burn therapist, depending on the physician's discretion and hospital policy. However, a severe burn compounded by an inhalation injury should alert the therapist to anticipate additional physical problems. Patients suffering an inhalation injury pose greater challenges for therapists because the injury may affect the patient's eventual endurance capacity.[28,29] Patients with extensive burns who require ventilatory support generally are confined to bed, or are less mobile, due to the seriousness of the injury.

Edema and Limb Circumference

During the evaluation of a burn patient, the amount of tissue edema may be worthwhile to note. Edema formation usually limits itself by 30 hours after injury and with proper intervention continues to diminish throughout the period of wound healing.[2] Initially, specific limb circumferences usually are not recorded but edema can be rated grossly as minimal to severe. Once edema development has stabilized, specific measurements can be taken periodically to evaluate the effectiveness of techniques designed to reduce edema.[30,31] Measuring edema in a patient with an acute burn injury using the water displacement method may be difficult. This measurement technique requires the patient to place the limb in a dependent position that may be painful because of vascular compromise. However, selected tape measure circumferences can be used as an objective means to record changes in edema.

What appears as noncompromising edema soon after admission may progress to a critical level later. A notable increase in limb size, along with other signs of circulatory compromise, necessitates physician notification for possible decompression.

Sensation

Unless the patient was injured by electrocution or sustained a possible spinal cord injury resulting from an auto accident or fall while escaping the fire, an extensive sensory evaluation probably is not warranted. Testing of cutaneous sensation by pin-prick can be used to help determine the depth of burn injury rather than for neurologic reasons.

Joint Range of Motion

The standard indicator for burn patient progress or regression is goniometric measurement of joint range of motion. However, only in very extreme cases does a burn injury directly involve a joint. Upon initial evaluation, a limitation in joint range of motion is commonly due to pain, edema, or inelastic eschar.[9,32,33] As pain and edema resolve and eschar is removed, range of motion should increase, provided proper therapy has been employed.

Limitations in motion are noted more for treatment planning purposes rather than for diagnosing a pathologic state. Uninvolved joint areas are grossly evaluated. If an abnormal range in any joint is detected, a more indepth evaluation is warranted.

Muscle Strength

If a burn patient functioned at a normal level prior to the burn, a specific manual muscle test may not be necessary. A manual muscle test should be considered in cases of electric injury, severe edema, or if a particular injury is suspected.[10] Edema, pain, and anxiety of the patient may cause a nonphysiologic decrease in strength that usually is inconsequential at the time of admission.[10] However, the patient must be assessed if he or she can actively move all extremities so that a baseline for future active motion can be established.

Flexibility

The combination of joint range of motion and muscle balance, or flexibility, should be noted in the initial evaluation.[34] With a burn injury, patient hyperflexibility ("double-jointed") can be an asset since the patient begins with a "bonus" of movement that is an advantage for preventing scar contractures. However, this extra motion means there is additional movement to be regained should a deficit in range of motion occur.

Patients with hypermobile or hypomobile movement usually recognize this condition in themselves. If a patient is unable to communicate the extent of his or her flexibility, it usually can be detected when evaluating joint range of motion or positioning the patient's limb.

Conversely, any initial lack of flexibility must be noted. One cannot simply assume that a deficit is due to pain, edema, or tight eschar. A patient may have a history of arthritis or previous injury to a particular joint that should be determined before attempting to increase a patient's range of motion.

Mobility and Ambulation

MOBILITY

The degree to which a patient is able to move about freely in bed or during transfers is initially a matter of level of consciousness, burn location, pain, and preference in medical management whether the patient may be out of bed. In general, patients are hesitant to move due to pain and fear of causing more damage. Edema and bandages also may interfere with movement. Burns to the hands, especially the palms, can limit grasp and adversely affect bed mobility and transfers.

One area often overlooked by therapists is the need for patient mobility in bed. The skin integrity of the patient is already compromised in many areas due to the burn injury and patients confined to bed are at risk for additional tissue damage. Patients need to be instructed and the staff should be reminded of the importance for the patient to frequently change position in bed. Changing bed positions will assist in preventing further tissue damage and preserve the integrity of the remaining intact skin.

How, and to what extent, the burn patient is able to move or transfer should be noted on the initial evaluation. In addition, the activities of rolling side-to-side during dressing changes, pelvic elevation for bedpan placement, and transferring to a chair should be noted. This information can aid in determining the amount of assistance the burn staff will need to lend the patient during activities and allow the therapist to begin problem solving to help the patient overcome any limitation in mobility.

AMBULATION

Permission for a patient to ambulate is a medical decision. Currently, the tendency is to begin ambulation earlier in the patient's hospitalization course as discussed in Chapter 13. Upon arising, dependent pain and associated hypotension, due to lower extremity burns, are major obstacles that may interfere with ambulation. Location of the burn may inhibit ambulation especially when the plantar aspect of the foot, Achilles tendon area or popliteal space is involved. Deviations in gait patterns are related primarily to pain. Patients tend to walk without bearing weight on the burned extremity due to pain. If the posterior surface of the lower extremity is involved, patients assume the position of ankle plantarflexion with either extreme knee flexion or knee extension and trunk flexion. True pathologic gait deviations from burn scar contractures can develop, but usually in the later stages of recovery.

Posture

An upright, relaxed posture is seldom seen in the burn patient early in hospitalization. With anterior trunk burns or as a general response to pain, shoulder elevation and protraction, combined with forward head and trunk flexion may be apparent at the initial evaluation. If the patient has lower extremity burns, hip and knee flexion with toe walking may predominate. With lateral trunk or unilateral extremity burns, side bending to the side of the burn secondary to pain may be the posture noted.

An antalgic gait can be a cause for poor posture in burn patients if they assume a mass flexed trunk position.[35] Both gait and posture improve as the patient's wounds heal if proper therapy intervention to prevent permanent scar contracture formation has been performed. Patient education should emphasize the consequences of continued improper posture and should provide encouragement and instruction for proper body alignment to avoid improper posture from becoming a habit.

ENDURANCE

Cardiovascular endurance of the burn patient is limited more from the overall systemic and catabolic effects of the burn injury than from a particular pathologic condition unless an inhalation injury is present. The initial distance the patient ambulates is noted more for patient feedback and motivation than for diagnostic purposes. A patient's aerobic capacity is affected by consequences of the burn injury, such as bed rest and immobilization, rather than as a direct result of the injury.[36-41]

Neurologic and Psychologic Factors

The patient's neurologic status usually is intact unless a specific neurologic injury resulted from the burn, as in the case of electric injuries. However, a gross evaluation of all major motor nerves is recommended. The need for this cursory evaluation is especially important of those nerves that are common sites of peripheral nerve injury (see Chapter 10, Table 10–1). This baseline information acts as a reference with which to compare the patient's status if a deficit is noted later.

Infants should be screened to determine their developmental level for purposes of treatment planning. Infants dominated by age-appropriate postures or reflexes will require evaluation of the governing positions of the trunk and limbs in relationship to the location of the burn wounds. Burn scar contractures tend to develop across skin creases, especially on flexor surfaces.[4] Treatment intervention should concentrate on offsetting the infant's neurologic bias to assume a fetal position that predisposes them to develop flexion contractures.

The patient's behavioral, mental, and emotional status should be noted for several reasons. The past and ongoing behavior of children and adults may indicate future compliance with the rehabilitation program.[42] Rebellious or strongly independent individuals may demonstrate control issues over therapy decisions. Conversely, many patients become overly dependent on the therapist and the nursing staff for simple needs and refuse to self-initiate tasks. They may attempt to manipulate the medical staff and cause conflict between personnel.[43] In either case, the therapist should attempt to establish a working relationship with the patient to accomplish the goals of therapy and make the patient feel part of the "burn team."

The affect, or outward appearance and reaction to situational circumstances, of the patient can provide insight to his or her emotional state. Patients with a major burn injury who appear in total control of their emotions may be subconsciously expressing denial of their situation.[10] Early in the course of their hospitalization, these patients mistakenly may be given too much responsibility for their own rehabilitation. When this happens, and the patient stops being "the ideal patient model," patient and therapist alike have difficulty changing the course of treatment.

Therapists need to constantly re-evaluate the patient's progress and maintain control of the direction the therapy program moves so that contractures and other burn sequelae do not reach the point of becoming uncontrollable. At the same time, the patient should be involved in the treatment program to the extent that they have a sense of ownership of their recovery and investment in the future.

The emotional support a patient receives from family, friends, or co-workers can be a great resource when provided in a positive manner.[9] Determining whether this support is an asset or a liability to the patient and the rehabilitation program will help the therapist determine the amount of assistance the patient may receive outside of the formal treatment setting.

The patient's ability to tolerate pain is paramount to the success of the rehabilitation program.[10] Asking patients about their pain level tolerance may be beneficial by committing the patient to a level of behavior. A visual analog or number scale from 1 to 10 can be used for this purpose. If a patient states that he or she has a high pain tolerance that equates to a 7 on a pain scale, then the therapist can use this pain indicator as a guide during rehabilitation interventions. If the patient is unable to give a verbal statement, asking family members how they would classify the patient's pain tolerance is helpful. Either way, the therapist soon discovers the patient's pain tolerance to physical intervention and this information should be used when treating the patient.

Functional Activities

The patient's ability to perform functional activities can be predicted based on the evaluation factors discussed thus far. If a deficit exists in any of the evaluation parameters that have been described, then a patient's functional level will be compromised.

Hand dominance should be recorded for functional and patient self-assistive purposes. Most people use their dominant hand to perform tasks, and if a burn involves a single upper extremity, then it usually involves the dominant hand. If a burn injury involves the patient's nondominant hand, the patient will tend to avoid using this nondominant hand more than usual and rely on the dominant hand for most activities. Patients need to be encouraged to use the involved hand for activities to assist in the rehabilitation of that involved area.

Knowing the patient's previous daily routine is helpful to plan appropriate treatments as hospitalization progresses. Work, leisure, completed school level and personal interests should be incorporated into the treatment program wherever appropriate and feasible. The accomplishment of basic tasks such as feeding, grooming, and personal hygiene add to the patient's feeling of progress and self-worth. Assistive devices may be required to accomplish these activities.[9,44]

PRINCIPLES OF TREATMENT PLANNING

Plans for a burn patient treatment program are derived from the information recorded during the initial evaluation (Table 9–4). After the evaluation information has been collected, a logical, problem-solving sequence can be used to determine the treatment approach. Two fundamental tenets affecting burn patient rehabilitation should be kept in mind. First, the major factor interfering with burn rehabilitation is the development of burn scar contractures and second, burn scar contractures are preventable. Therefore, the majority of rehabilitation approaches and treatment time should be concentrated to support these tenets.

Patient Goals

At the time of the patient's admission, the short-term goal is to preserve the patient's range of motion and functional ability or, at least, to prevent a further loss of motion if hindered by edema or tight eschar. The long-term goal for all patients is for them to return to their preburn functional state.[10]

Goals will vary depending on the patient's physical status and phase of recovery.[3] For example, during the acute stage of recovery, if edema interferes with grasp, then one goal is to decrease hand and finger edema. Similarly, if contractures develop during the patient's hospitalization, then the goal is to regain lost movement. Remembering the ultimate short- and long-term goals for the patient aids the therapist and patient in establishing interim goals.

Focus of Treatment

From a physical perspective, the potentially most formidable consequence of any burn injury is the development of burn scar contractures and hypertrophy. Normal skin covering the body essentially is one continuous sheet of tissue without interruption. Skin is a highly elastic and mobile tissue that permits movement. In theory,

TABLE 9–4. Treatment Plan Considerations

Precautions/contraindications
Type of treatment
Depth/location of wounds
Pre/post skin grafting
Focus of treatment
Edema control
Positioning recommendations
Splint recommendations
Types of exercise
Treatment location
Treatment time of day
Frequency of treatment
Duration of treatment
Intensity of treatment
Short-term goals
Long-term goals

inelastic scar tissue can cause a limitation in motion anywhere in the body depending on the extent of skin it replaces and the direction of the desired movement. In general, contractures tend to develop on the flexor surfaces of the body and involve the upper trunk and extremities more than the lower extremities.

When establishing a treatment program for a burn patient, the therapist must first focus on the areas prone to scar contracture development.[10] Treatment emphasis should include implementing a comprehensive treatment plan using positioning, splinting, heat or electrotherapeutic modalities, and exercise.[9,10] The specific interventions used depend upon the location of the burn and the patient's need. However, the goal is to preserve trunk and limb range of motion by counteracting the contractile nature of the scar tissue.

Scar tissue contracts until encountering an opposing force. Its contractile nature continues 24 hours a day until the tissue is fully mature, which can take up to 3 years following injury.[9] Physical measures should be directed toward minimizing this ongoing process. Areas of scar tissue should be continually elongated by proper positioning, splinting, range of motion, massage, and compression therapy until the contractile process is controlled and range of motion is easily maintained. When a patient's range of motion is easily attained, greater emphasis can be placed on other physical needs of the patient such as muscle strengthening and endurance training.[9]

Theoretically, scar contractures are preventable; in reality, scar contractures can develop. Therefore, as the extent of burn increases, minimizing the number and severity of contractures assumes a greater emphasis in the treatment process.

The therapist needs to optimize the amount of time that is spent with each patient to minimize the deleterious effects of contracture formation. Allocating time for treatment priorities is based on the location of the burns and the functional importance of the structures involved. For example, if a burn injury involves the hands, lower extremities proximal to the midcalf, and abdomen, the priority for treatment is in the sequence that the areas are listed.

Often, therapists have difficulty balancing the sometimes overwhelming patient challenges they encounter with the desire to meet every need of the patient. What often happens is that all areas of need receive a little treatment time and the area needing the most focused treatment time receives relatively little. Eventually, if all priority areas receive the time they deserve, and the initial goal of full range of motion of an area is achieved, time will become available for more secondary areas of concern like cardiovascular fitness. As an example, hand function should have overwhelming priority over endurance activities.

Daily Treatment

LOCATION AND SCHEDULE

The therapist should survey the patient's wounds during dressing changes as frequently as possible until the wounds are healed.[9] Range-of-motion treatments can be given during the time that dressings are changed so the wounds can be inspected and also to observe the impact movement has on the wound. The therapist can determine if tight eschar limits motion, if superficial tendons become apparent when motion occurs, or if tissue begins to separate with movement.

Treating patients during their dressing change has the advantage of allowing greater freedom of movement from restricting bulky bandages or painfully adherent dressings.[9] Conversely, performing range of motion during this time can cause more pain for patients because exposed and sensitive nerve endings lie unprotected and become irritated when handled.[9] Additionally, denuded tissue tends to desiccate when left exposed, which makes moving more painful. A lengthy exposure time also may cause an increase in metabolism for the patient in response to the "cooler feeling" environment. Treatment during this time should be scheduled in advance with the personnel who change the dressings so adequate time is allowed in the dressing change schedule.[9,10]

Anytime the patient has had surgery for excision and skin grafting, the first post-operative therapy treatment should be done during a dressing change. This dressing time allows the therapist to reassess the patient for donor site and skin graft location, condition of the skin graft, and possible exposure of tendons from debridement. Therapists also can gain an indirect assessment of the patient's range-of-motion status by assisting with the dressing change if they avail themselves of the chance to help move or support the patient's limbs while the wounds are washed and dressed.

Bedside treatments offer several advantages. A therapist may have an easier time scheduling a specific time to treat the patient at bedside rather than trying to treat a particular patient during a dressing change. If the dressings are not adherent to the wounds, the dressings act as padding for the therapist's hand placement while performing passive or active-assistive exercises. When the patient lies supine, the bed acts as a stabilizing station for the patient's trunk and allows the patient to relax. The therapists can assume a position that is in good biomechanical alignment with the patient for an effective treatment session.[45,46] Some equipment, such as a trapeze and pulleys, may be available for bedside treatment sessions, but patient rooms generally lack the space and equipment variety that is available in the rehabilitation department.

Transporting patients to the rehabilitation department for treatment depends on hospital policy and the design of the burn facility (whether self-contained or open). Patients treated outside of their rooms may feel a sense of progress since they are no longer confined to their "sick room." For some patients, treatment in the department removes them from the protective environment of the burn unit and encourages interaction with unfamiliar individuals such as other staff members or patients. At times, burn patients perceive other patients as being in worse condition than themselves and that can add a positive influence to their recovery.

In addition to the treatment location, the time of day that the patient is treated requires consideration. Early morning treatment times at bedside often are the most difficult for patients. They have been inactive throughout the night and generally are "stiff." After being splinted or positioned correctly through the night, beginning movement in the morning may be uncomfortable. However, treatments administered early in the morning are of benefit to patients. The therapist is able to assist the patient with range of motion that leads to more independent functions such as eating breakfast. Also, this early morning treatment permits subsequent movement to occur with optimum tissue length to reinforce scar remodeling.

Whenever possible, a patient's therapy schedule should coincide with the administration of pain medication.[9] Analgesics and intramuscular narcotics require approximately 20 to 30 minutes to begin to act so therapy treatments should be scheduled when patients will benefit most from their pain medication. Patients frequently are given more potent pain medication before having their dressings changed. However, performing therapy during dressing changes may not be optimal, particularly if the patient is highly anxious. A therapy treatment at this time can exacerbate a patient's perception of pain. The use of sedatives or bedside anesthetics, however, may diminish the patient's pain to the point that a therapy treatment during the dressing change may be opportune.

Another optimal time to perform therapy is late in the afternoon. At this time, the patient very often is physically fatigued from previous activities during the day and frequently is simply too tired to offer much resistance to treatment. In many instances, the patient will even sleep through an exercise session that earlier would have been painful. Regardless of when the therapy session occurs, informing the patient of the therapy schedule in advance helps alleviate anxiety. This preliminary notice gives patients the opportunity to mentally prepare themselves for the treatment and allows them time to plan their day so that their personal affairs do not interfere with the therapy session.[9]

FREQUENCY

In addition to splinting and proper positioning, the frequency a burn patient needs a formal treatment session to prevent the formation of burn scar contractures is unknown. In the literature, the recommended number of treatment sessions varies from "frequently"[23,47-49] to four times daily.[17] As previously stated, the primary indicator of patient progress is range of motion. If a patient's range of motion decreases between sessions, then the frequency of therapy should be increased. On the other hand, if a patient exhibits satisfactory improvement, then the frequency of therapy can be considered acceptable. If patient progress is without undue physical stress, the frequency of treatment may be increased to include more advanced treatments such as muscle strengthening or endurance training.

The number of days per week that burn patients are treated varies among facilities from 5 to 7.[50] This treatment range does not mean that treatment 5 days per week is sufficient nor does it mean that therapy 7 days per week is necessary. The weekly frequency of patient treatment appears to be dictated by policy and staffing in each facility.

DURATION

The length of each formal therapy session is highly variable. This parameter depends upon the extent, depth, and location of the burn and the number of adjacent joint surfaces involved, patient pain tolerance, stage of recovery, and wound healing.

Ideally, the treatment session should last as long as necessary to accomplish the short-term goals of the treatment session. Complete range of motion of all involved areas should be included.[10] Isolated joint movement should be achieved and, more importantly, combined range-of-motion patterns involving adjacent wound sites should be accomplished. Frequently, a patient is able to demonstrate complete range of motion of an isolated joint area but will exhibit a deficit in function when attempting to combine these separate motions at an extreme range of movement.

Treatment time may include instruction of exercises to be performed at bedside by patients and family members. Independent exercises are performed to reinforce range of motion or to treat areas that do not require the presence of the therapist, such as simple active or isometric exercises.

INTENSITY

A third component of treatment is the intensity of the program including quantity, length, and speed at which the exercises should be performed. Generally, this exercise parameter is governed by the patient's pain tolerance and previous work habits. Patients in the intensive care unit can be evaluated as to their response to treatment using a physiologic monitor.[51] The therapist can physically monitor a patient's response to the exercise intensity by palpation of heart pulse rate, counting the respiration rate, and blood pressure auscultation.[9]

The intensity level of the exercise program should be kept low during early hospitalization due to the catabolic state that patients undergo with a major burn.[10] Patients who experience severe pain should be allotted more time to perform stretching exercises or for ambulation. However, an agreement needs to be made between the therapist and patient regarding the amount of time the patient is allowed to perform requested activities.

Some patients possess a higher threshold for pain and can tolerate greater physical demands. Becoming personally familiar with each patient and adjusting the treatment program to accommodate individual differences is a vital component of successful burn rehabilitation. Balancing treatment intensity often reflects the therapist's abilities rather than the patient's capabilities.

Clinical Guidelines

Treatment of burn patients may be relatively unfamiliar to therapists. Many of the principles related to current burn rehabilitation resulted from the experience of clinicians.[52] Consequently, there remains much to learn and substantiate regarding the basis for clinical practice when treating the patient with a burn injury. The adages

TABLE 9–5. Common Burn Treatment Adages

Mornings are always the worst.
Range of motion *first.*
Burn scar contracture is a lack of tissue to go around.
Stretch opposite the burn.
The sum of the parts does not always equal the whole.
If it's white–it's tight.
Pinching pain *or* stretching pain?

listed in Table 9–5 are empirical guidelines that are helpful in the treatment of burn patients.

One perplexing situation that occasionally arises concerns the initiation and continuation of therapy with patients who have, according to statistics, suffered a mortal burn.[10] As the survival rate for patients with major burn injuries continue to rise, therapy should proceed until the patient's demise is certain. Reports of patients surviving extensive burn injury have become more frequent and, as the extent of injury increases, so does the need for rehabilitation services.

Scar tissue contractures occur in predictable areas of the body that limit motion in specific directions. When treating burn patients, the treatment emphasis is placed on movements in the direction opposite to that of anticipated deformity.[23] For example, a burn to the antecubital space can cause the elbow to assume a flexed position. Therefore, the elbow needs to be positioned, splinted, and exercised in the direction of elbow extension.

Patients with a major burn injury may have involvement of multiple joint skin creases. Treatment emphasis should be placed on achieving complete range of motion of all affected areas in a combined fashion even though individual areas have full isolated movement. There may be enough scar tissue length to complete a single movement, but insufficient length is available when the soft tissue is required to elongate over multiple joint areas (Fig. 9–2).

Resumption of exercise to areas involving skin grafts depends on the protocol of the treatment facility. However, exercise of areas not involved in the surgery should be continued.[9] Donor sites usually do not need to be exercised because donor sites rarely cross skin creases or result in permanent loss of motion. Forcing a patient to move with a painful donor site only causes more pain. Nonetheless, the sooner the patient is allowed to move, the less time the patient has to experience the negative effects of bedrest and immobility.

Immature scar tissue will change from a pink or red color to white, or blanch, with the application of a stretching force if the scar tissue is tight. Hence, if the scar tissue turns white with elongation, then the tissue is tight and needs to be treated. When treating burn patients, scar tissue should be elongated until it blanches and this stretch is then sustained for a prolonged period of time.[9,10,53] The optimal duration of time to elongate scar tissue remains undefined but generally the longer the stretch is maintained, the better the outcome. An elongating force should be maintained until the tissue color returns or the tissue becomes more pliable to palpation.

When a burn patient experiences a limitation in motion due to pain during an exercise session, the therapist needs to ask, "Is it stretching pain or pinching pain?" Stretching pain results from the attempted elongation of tissue to gain range of mo-

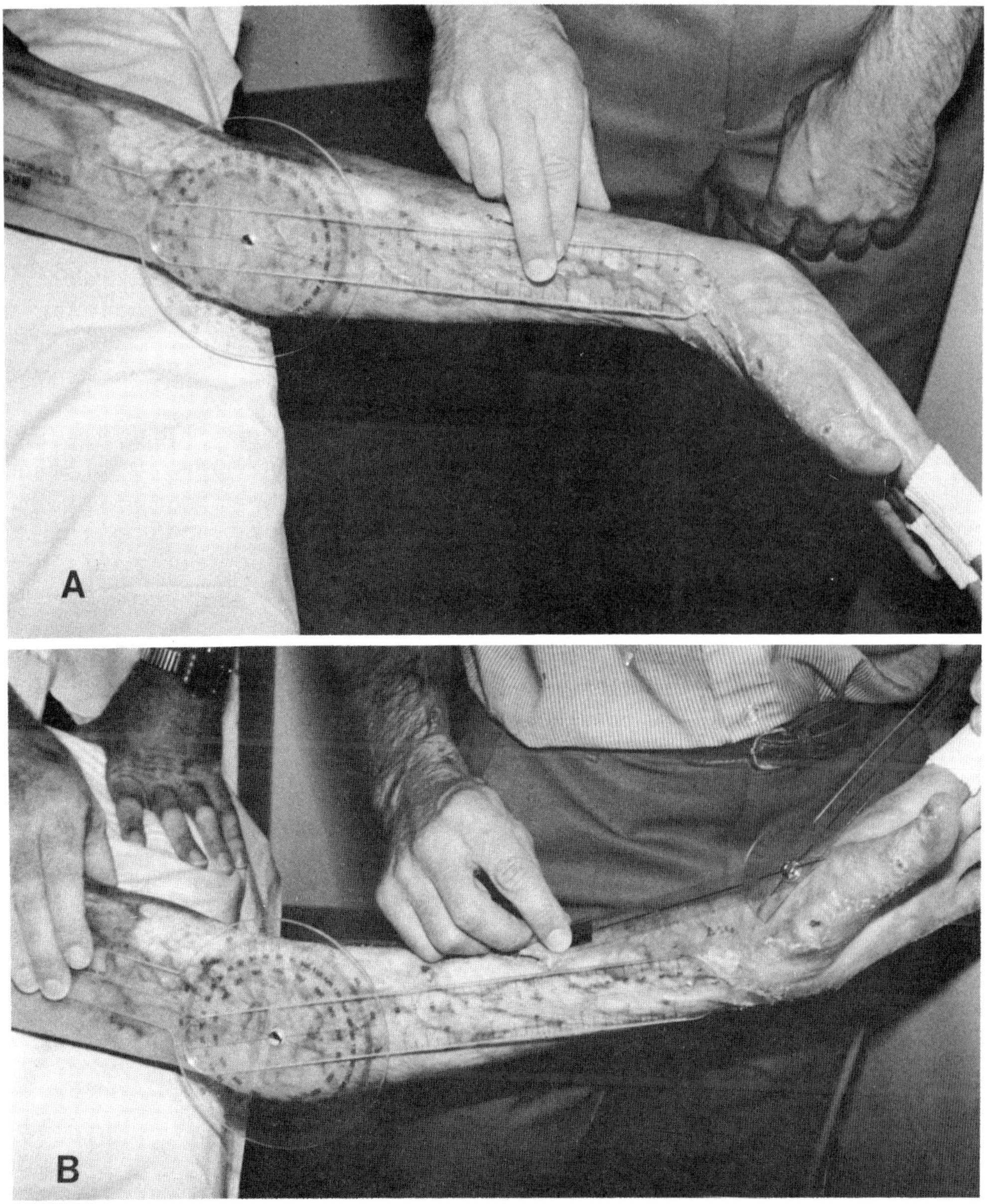

FIGURE 9–2. (*A*) Patient displaying approximately −10° of active left elbow extension without regard for the position of the wrist. (*B*) The patient's limitation in elbow extension is increased to −25° when the wrist is actively extended 30°. Note in both figures the scar tissue blanching that occurs with tissue elongation.

tion of an involved area. This "stretching pain" is located in the focused area of the treatment and is difficult to avoid when treating burn patients. Frequently, when treating an area involving circumferential burns, pain that limits motion occurs on the surface opposite of that being stretched. In this instance, the tender tissue may be folding upon itself and causes a "pinching pain." Continuation of the treatment in that particular direction may be a source of unnecessary discomfort to the patient and should be avoided.[54]

SUMMARY

A patient who has sustained a major burn injury requires a thorough evaluation by a therapist. While a gross estimate of strength and range of motion usually suffice initially, key factors that should be noted include past medical history, associated injuries, baseline active movement, extent, depth and location of burns, presence of edema, and patient's pain tolerance.

The treatment program for a patient with an acute burn begins with goal setting. The establishment of short- and long-term goals provides the therapist with a framework for the rehabilitation program. The all-encompassing long-term goal is to return the patient into society in an optimum physical and psychologic condition. This requires focusing the treatment on the prevention of scar tissue deformities. Other physical manifestations of the burn injury, such as deconditioning from hospitalization, are secondary to the primary focus of preventing scar contractures and hypertrophy. Through frequent re-evaluation and treatment modification, short-term goals are set and accomplished. Treatment includes daily exercise as well as a conscientious effort on the part of all burn team members to adhere to a proper positioning and strict splinting schedule for the burn patient.

REFERENCES

1. Feller, I and Archambeault, C: Nursing the Burned Patient. Institute for Burn Medicine, Braun-Brumfield Press, Ann Arbor, 1974, p 10.
2. Demling, RH and LaLonde, C: Burn Trauma. Thieme Medical Publishers, New York, 1989.
3. Nothdurft, D, Smith, PS, and LeMaster, JE: Exercise and treatment modalities. In Fisher, SV and Helm, PA (eds): Comprehensive Rehabilitation of Burns. Williams & Wilkins, Baltimore, 1984, pp 96–147.
4. Evans, EB, Larson, DL, and Yates, S: Preservation and restoration of joint function in patients with severe burns. JAMA 204:843–848, 1968.
5. Koepke, GH: The role of physical medicine in the treatment of burns. Surg Clin North Am 50:1385–1399, 1970.
6. Larson, DL, et al: Contracture and scar formation in the burn patient. Clin Plast Surg 1:653–666, 1974.
7. Bartlett, RH, et al: Rehabilitation following burn injury. Sur Clin North Am 58:1249–1262, 1978.
8. Johnson, CL, O'Shaughnessy, EJ, and Ostergren, G: Burn Management. Raven Press, New York, 1981, p 42.
9. Giuliani, CA and Perry, GA: Factors to consider in the rehabilitation aspect of burn care. Phys Ther 65:619–623, 1985.
10. Wright, PC: Fundamentals of acute burn care and physical therapy management. Phys Ther 64:1217–1231, 1984.
11. Adams, RB, et al: Cardiovascular rehabilitation of patients with burns. J Burn Care Rehabil 11:246–255, 1990.
12. Moncrief, JA: Third degree burns of the dorsum of the hand. Am J Surg 96:535–544, 1958.
13. Willis, BA, Larson, DL, and Abston, S: Positioning and splinting the burned patient. Heart Lung 2:696–700, 1973.

14. Slater, RR and Peterson, HD: Bilateral femoral neck fractures after electrical injury: A case report and literature review. J Burn Care Rehabil 11:240–243, 1990.
15. Tobiasen, J, et al: A graded risk index of burn severity. J Burn Care Rehabil 1:31–35, 1980.
16. Tobiasen, J, Hiebert, JM, and Edlich, RF: A practical burn severity index. J Burn Care Rehabil 3:229–232, 1982.
17. Larson, DL, et al: Techniques for decreasing scar formation and contractures in the burned patient. J Trauma 11:807–823, 1971.
18. Ward, RS: Pressure therapy for the control of hypertrophic scar formation after burn injury. J Burn Care Rehabil 12:257–262, 1991.
19. Bowden, ML, Thompson, PD, and Prasad, JK: Factors influencing return to employment after a burn injury. Arch Phys Med Rehabil 70:772–774, 1989.
20. Hummel, RP: Clinical Burn Therapy. John Wright PSG, Boston, 1982, p 4.
21. Kraemer, MD, Jones, T, and Deitch, EA: Burn contractures: Incidence, predisposing factors, and results of surgical therapy. J Burn Care Rehabil 9:261–265, 1988.
22. Stern, PJ, Benedict, FE, and MacMillan, BG: Surgical treatment of elbow contractures in postburn children. Plast Reconstr Surg 76:441–446, 1985.
23. Dobbs, ER and Curreri, PW: Burns: Analysis of results of physical therapy in 681 patients. J Trauma 12:242–248, 1972.
24. Chang, FC and Herzog, B: Burn morbidity: A follow-up study of physical and psychological disability. Ann Surg 183:34, 1976.
25. Huang, TT, Blackwell, SJ, and Lewis, SR: Ten years of experience in managing patients with burn contractures of axilla, elbow, wrist, and knee joints. Plast Reconstr Surg 61:70–76, 1978.
26. Bartlett, RH, et al: Rehabilitation following burn injury. Surg Clin North Am 58:1249–1262, 1978.
27. Richard, R: Unpublished material, 1989.
28. Mlcak, RP, et al: Cardiopulmonary stress testing in children convalescing from thermal injury. Proc American Burn Association Annual, Baltimore, 23:161, 1991.
29. McElroy, K, et al: Cardiovascular adaptation: Exercise stress-testing the pediatric burn patient, a continuation. Proc American Burn Association Annual, Salt Lake City, 24:92, 1992.
30. Salisbury, RE, et al: Postburn edema of the upper extremity: Evaluation of present treatment. J Trauma 13:857–862, 1973.
31. Richard, RL, Ause-Ellias, KL, Miller, SF, and Finley, Jr, RK: The effect of mechanical compression on post burn healing hand edema: A preliminary report. Proc American Burn Association Annual, Salt Lake City, 24:155, 1992.
32. Dimick, AR: Pathophysiology. In Fisher, SV and Helm, PA (eds): Comprehensive Rehabilitation of Burns. Williams & Wilkins, Baltimore, 1984, pp 16–27.
33. Dimick, AR: Emergency care. In Hummel, RP: Clinical Burn Therapy. John Wright PSG, Boston, 1982, pp 7–24.
34. Sharkey, BJ: Physiology of Fitness. Human Kinetics Publishers, Champaign, Ill., 1979, p 72.
35. Khalili, AA, Betts, HB, and Stone, NH: Rehabilitation medicine in the prevention and management of burn deformities; Organization and techniques. In Stone, NH (ed): Profiles of Burn Management. Industrial Medicine Publishing Company, Miami, 1969, p 48.
36. Wilmore, DW: The Metabolic Management of the Critically Ill. Plenum Medical Book Company, New York, 1977.
37. Saltin, B, et al: Response to exercise after bed rest and after training. Circulation 38:VII-1-77, 1968.
38. Halar, EM and Bell, KR: Contracture and other deleterious effects of immobility. In DeLisa, JA (ed): Rehabilitation Medicine Principles and Practice, JB Lippincott, Philadelphia, 1988, pp 448–462.
39. Halar, EM and Bell, KB: Rehabilitation's relationship to inactivity. In Kottke, FJ and Lehmann, JF (eds): Krusen's Handbook of Physical Medicine and Rehabilitation, ed 4. WB Saunders, Philadelphia, 1990, pp 1113–1133.
40. Cisar, C, Staley, M, and Hiruska, R: Physical fitness adaptations of the severe burn patient following discharge. Proc American Burn Association Annual, Chicago, 18:23, 1986.
41. Black, S, et al: Oxygen consumption for lower extremity exercises in normal subjects and burned patients. Phys Ther 60:1255–1258, 1980.
42. Questad, KA, et al: Relating mental health and physical function at discharge to rehabilitation status at three months postburn. J Burn Care Rehabil 9:87–89, 1988.
43. Andreasen, NJC, et al: Management of emotional reactions in seriously burned adults. N Engl J Med 286:65–69, 1972.
44. White, RW: Motivation reconsidered: The concept of competence. Psychoanal Rev 66:297–333, 1959.
45. Richard, RL: OASIS positioning: A respite for therapists. J Burn Care Rehabil 11:552–553, 1990.
46. Richard, RL and Shanesy, CP: Arm-cradle technique. Clin Management 11:57–58, 1991.
47. Boswick, JA: Comprehensive rehabilitation after burn injury. Surg Clin North Am 67:159–166, 1987.
48. Moncrief, JA: Burns of specific areas. J Trauma 5:278–291, 1965.
49. Yeakel, MH, Gronley, JK and Tumbusch, WT: A fiberglass positioning device for the burned hand. J Trauma 4:57–70, 1964.

50. Stachowski, M and Kondela-Cebulski, P: Physical therapists in burn care. Phys Ther 63:1091–1095, 1983.
51. Richard, RL, Staley, MJ, and Miller, SF: The physiologic effects of range of motion exercise on critically-ill patients. Publication pending.
52. Johnson, CL and Trotter, MJ: Survey of burn education in entry-level physical therapy programs. Phys Ther 68:530–533, 1988.
53. Helm, PA, et al: Burn injury: Rehabilitation management in 1982. Arch Phys Med Rehabil 63:6–16, 1982.
54. Richard, RL: Approaches to circumvent pain when exercising the burned patient. Phys Ther Forum 4:1–4, 1985.

CHAPTER 10

Approaches to Positioning the Burn Patient

Lois M. Apfel, OTR
Christy P. Irwin, OTR
Marlys J. Staley, MS, PT
Reginald L. Richard, MS, PT

Proper positioning is one of the fundamental tenets necessary for successful burn patient rehabilitation. A burn patient's positioning program is designed to minimize edema formation, prevent tissue destruction and maintain soft tissues in an elongated state to facilitate functional recovery. Burn scar contractures can be anticipated by the location, extent of the body involved, and the depth of the burn wound. Positioning the burn patient should be implemented to the extent that contractures are averted without compromising mobility and function. The purpose of this chapter is to educate therapists about the unique positioning requirements of burn patients so that a successful strategy can be developed to assist with minimizing contracture formation in this patient population.

Total body and specific site positioning techniques are used to minimize pathophysiologic effects from the burn, enable optimal wound care and prevent localized neuropathies[1] (Table 10–1). In addition to positioning, the use of fluidized air and pillow beds and special mattresses provides pressure reduction for the patient with a large burn without a vigorous turning schedule. These beds are equipped with adaptations that allow the patient to be positioned as needed to minimize contracture formation (Appendix D).

A positioning program is developed to meet each individual patient's needs and should be modified throughout hospitalization. Patients are positioned supine, side-lying and prone for 2- to 4-hour periods. Adjustments in the alignment of the extremities are made when altering the patient's position in bed.[2] If possible, the patient also should sit in a chair twice a day. Daily monitoring of the patient's medical status, range of motion, and skin condition will assist the therapist in deciding how

TABLE 10–1. Common Nerve Lesions

Nerve	Cause
Occipital cutaneous	Pressure from head donut pillow
Cervical radiculopathy	Electric injury sequelae
Suprascapular	Hyperprotraction and excessive forward rotation of shoulder
Brachial plexus	Prolonged side lying Prolonged prone position Pressure from dressings Prolonged, excessive abduction of shoulder
Median	Excessive sustained stretch of wrist in flexion/extension
Ulnar	Prolonged pressure on flexed elbows in prone position, prolonged elbow flexion, or prolonged pressure along medial epicondyle
Radial	Direct injections Pressure in axilla
Hand digital	Hard pressure between fingers
Peroneal	Frog-lying position Pressure from dressings
Foot digital	Hyperextension and subluxation of toes

Adapted from Helm et al,[1] p 420, with permission.

long positions are to be maintained and what other modifications are necessary in a positioning program. For example, if a patient is having difficulty maintaining range of motion between exercise sessions, a patient-specific positioning program may need to be followed at all times except for dressing changes and exercise. If the patient's range of motion and skin condition remain acceptable, positioning may be necessary only at night.

Specific positions are used to align individually the extremities, neck and trunk and are considered to be "anticontracture" positions. The popular adage "the position of comfort (fetal position) is the position of contracture" appears well-founded. In general, the patient should be positioned in the opposite direction of comfort, that is, opposite the location of the burn wound and impending contracture. This approach is especially true of burns that involve joint or flexor surfaces of the body. Table 10–2 outlines and Figure 10–1 illustrates the most commonly used anticontracture positions.

EDEMA CONTROL

Initially, a positioning program focuses on reducing edema through elevation of the extremities. Edema develops within 8 to 12 hours after burn injury and peaks at approximately 36 hours. Failure to reduce edema in the first 48 to 72 hours can result in organized edema components creating a fixed deformity.[2] Furthermore, improper elevation during the initial period of edema may lead to calcification and increased bone density, especially in the elbow.[1] Elevation of an extremity above heart level can be accomplished using common items such as pillows, bath blankets, towels, foam

TABLE 10–2. Burn Patient Positioning

Body Area	Contracture Predisposition	Preventive Positioning
Neck	Flexion	Extension Hyperextension
Anterior axilla	Shoulder adduction	Shoulder abduction
Posterior axilla	Shoulder extension	Shoulder flexion
Antecubital space	Elbow flexion	Elbow extension
Forearm	Pronation	Supination
Wrist	Flexion	Extension
Dorsal hand/finger	MCP hyperextension IP flexion Thumb adduction	MCP flexion IP extension Thumb palmar abduction or opposition
Palmar hand/finger	Finger flexion Thumb opposition	Finger extension Thumb radial abduction
Hip	Flexion Adduction External rotation	Extension Abduction Neutral rotation
Knee	Flexion	Extension
Ankle	Plantarflexion	Dorsiflexion
Dorsal toes	Hyperextension	Flexion
Plantar toes	Flexion	Extension

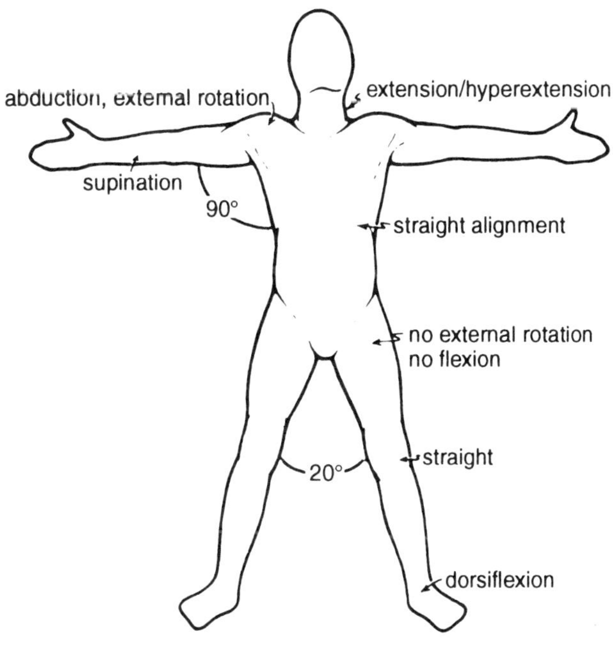

FIGURE 10–1. General body positioning for prevention of contractures.

wedges, bedside tables, and stockinette. If the head of the bed position is changed, the position of the extremities will need to be changed accordingly to maintain proper elevation. In addition, elevation of the upper extremities must be maintained while the patient is lying, sitting, or ambulating. Lower extremities should be elevated when the patient is sitting by placing them on a footstool.

POSITIONING OF THE VARIOUS BODY PARTS

Head and Neck

Patients who have sustained head burns that include the ears should not be allowed use of a pillow in order to avoid a development of chondritis of the ear. A foam or gel-filled donut is useful to elevate the ears from the bed (Fig. 10–2) (Appendix E). A partially filled intravenous (IV) bag is an alternate method. If a patient's head needs elevation for eating or drinking, raising the head of the bed rather than using a pillow is the preferred method.

Anterior or circumferential neck burns predispose patients to neck flexion contractures. Contracture of the anterior neck is the most common contracture requiring surgical release.[3] To minimize this problem, the use of pillows is contraindicated and the neck should be placed in extension or hyperextension, as feasible, without compromising the patient's respiratory status.[4]

Several options for neck positioning can be used to achieve extension. An easy and quick method is a towel roll placed under the patient's shoulders or between the scapulae. A foam cervical collar or donut around the patient's neck is useful to prevent neck flexion when lying in bed and during upright activities. The use of hyperextension or staggered mattresses also encourages neck extension (Fig. 10–3). A towel roll or pillow can be placed under the head if the top mattress is too high. If the

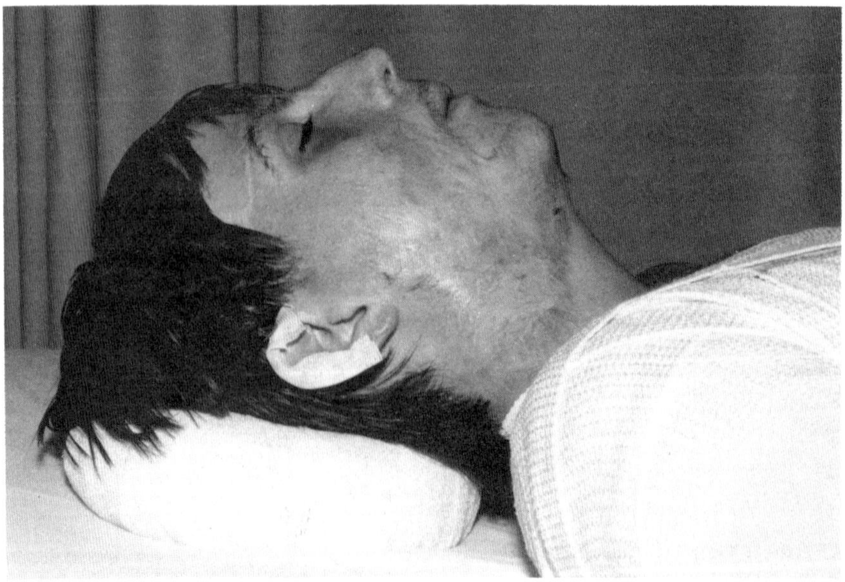

FIGURE 10–2. A donut under the head protects the cartilage of the ear from pressure.

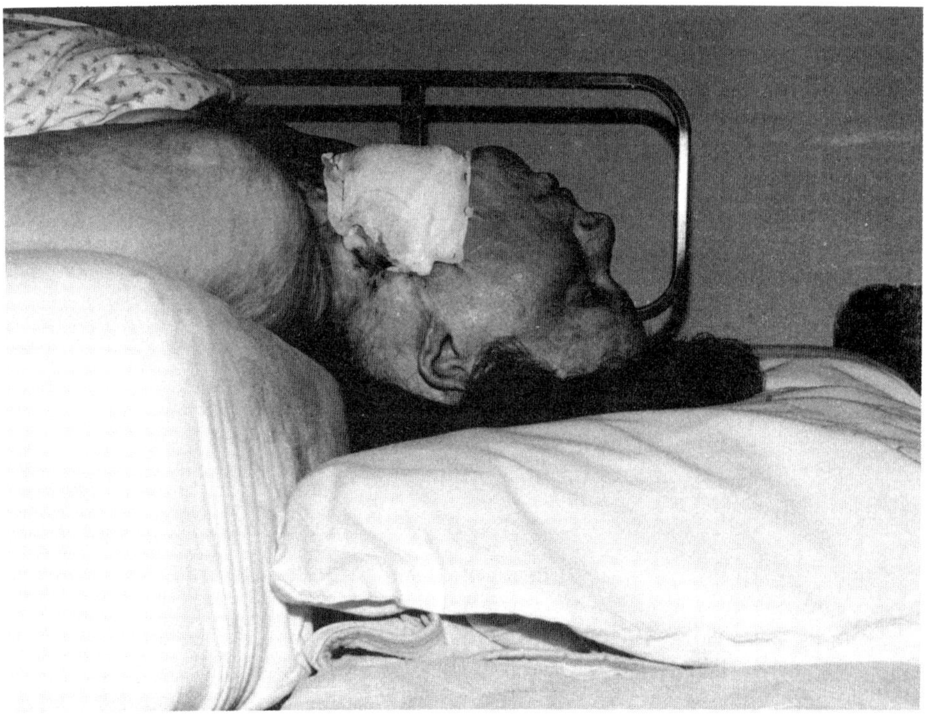

FIGURE 10–3. A short mattress placed over a standard mattress allows gravity to pull the neck into hyperextension. Bath blankets or towel rolls under the head can grade the amount of hyperextension desired.

patient is on a pillow-type air bed, several "pillows" or cells of air can be deflated under the patient's head to encourage neck extension.

If a neck burn is asymmetrical, a lateral flexion contracture toward the side of the burn can be expected. This can cause muscle imbalance and ultimately lead to a postural deformity. The neck should be positioned so that the head is held in midline. Towel rolls, wedges, IV bags, or sand bags placed lateral to the head, on the same side as the burn, minimizes lateral tightness. Positioning environmental stimuli such as televisions, toys, bed trays, and visitors on the nonaffected side will encourage the patient to turn and stretch the neck. Lying prone with the head rotated away from the side of the burn also may be utilized to stretch the neck. When a neck burn is posterior and the ears are not involved, a pillow may be used to elevate the head and lengthen the posterior tissues.

Trunk

Deformities of the trunk may include shoulder girdle protraction with glenohumeral adduction if the burn involves the clavicular and/or pectoral region. Burns extending from the pectoral region to an area below the umbilicus may cause a kyphosis. Burns of the lower back may lead to a lordosis, while a lateral trunk burn may cause a scoliosis with the concavity toward the burned side. In addition to these postural deformities, improper trunk alignment might impair chest expansion required for good ventilation.[3]

When the chest is burned, the shoulder girdles should be positioned in retraction. Positioning for chest burns may include placing a square towel or bath blanket between the scapulae and extending caudally as far as comfortable. Alternatively, the patient can lie supine with hands clasped behind the head with elbows resting on the bed. A figure-of-eight elastic wrap to pull the shoulders into retraction, cervical fracture braces, and clavicular straps can be used when skin integrity allows (see Chapter 11).

Lateral trunk burns require the trunk to be maintained straight to prevent scoliosis of the spine. Towel rolls, blankets, sand bags, and foam wedges can be utilized to maintain trunk alignment while in bed by placing them on the side of the trunk where the burn is located.

Shoulder

A patient with burns of the anterior axilla will tend to posture in shoulder adduction and internal rotation. Therefore, shoulder abduction and external rotation is the position of choice to prevent deformity. If the axilla is spared, but the anterior chest, superior aspect of the arm or lateral posterior trunk is burned, the anterior or posterior axillary folds may develop contractures preventing shoulder abduction and flexion, respectively.

The recommended position for the shoulder when the axilla is burned is 90° of abduction with 15° to 20° of horizontal adduction to avoid stretching and compression of the brachial plexus.[5,6] Some therapists believe the shoulder can be positioned in approximately 130° to 150° of flexion and externally rotated without damaging the brachial plexus, if done for short periods of time or intermittently, such as with a shoulder continuous passive motion (CPM) machine. However, abduction past 90°, especially in elderly patients, for even short time periods may cause pain[2] and adversely affect the brachial plexus. When the burn involves the elbow and the shoulder, elbow extension must be maintained during shoulder positioning.

Many options are available to hold a patient in the positions just described. Murphy slings, made from stockinette and attached to an IV pole or an overhead ceiling tract, are especially helpful in the early stage of positioning to achieve elevation along with shoulder abduction (Fig. 10–4). A soft restraint at the wrist, which is tied to the headboard, maintains shoulder abduction and external rotation with the elbow flexed. Alternately, a wrist cuff, with or without the use of a splint, can be fastened to a positioning screen to afford various angles of shoulder and elbow positioning[7] (Fig. 10–5). Foam wedges, towel rolls, pillows, and bath blankets placed between the axilla and trunk are convenient positioning devices. In addition to abduction, these objects can be layered and placed under the arm to achieve shoulder flexion. For the compliant patient, overbed or bedside tables can be used to place the forearms while the patient is lying in bed with the shoulders abducted and elbows extended. To assist in maintaining this position in the less-compliant patient, slings made of synthetic lambswool and yarn can be placed around the arm and secured to the head of the bed.

A foam wedge can be secured to the trunk and upper extremity using Velcro or foam straps inserted through slits in the wedge. This device can be used for posi-

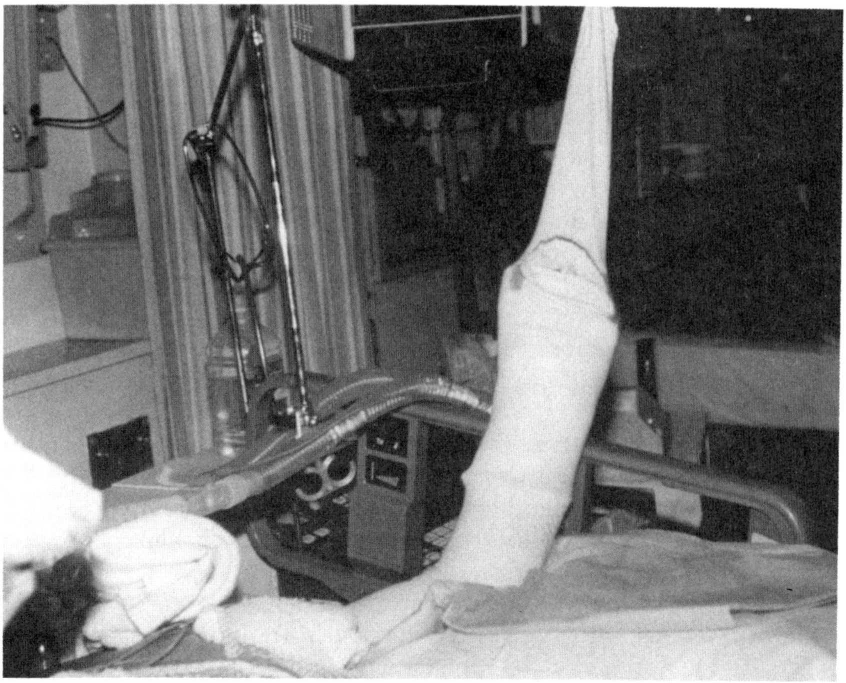

FIGURE 10–4. Murphy slings are utilized for shoulder and elbow positioning and hand elevation depending on the directional pull of the sling.

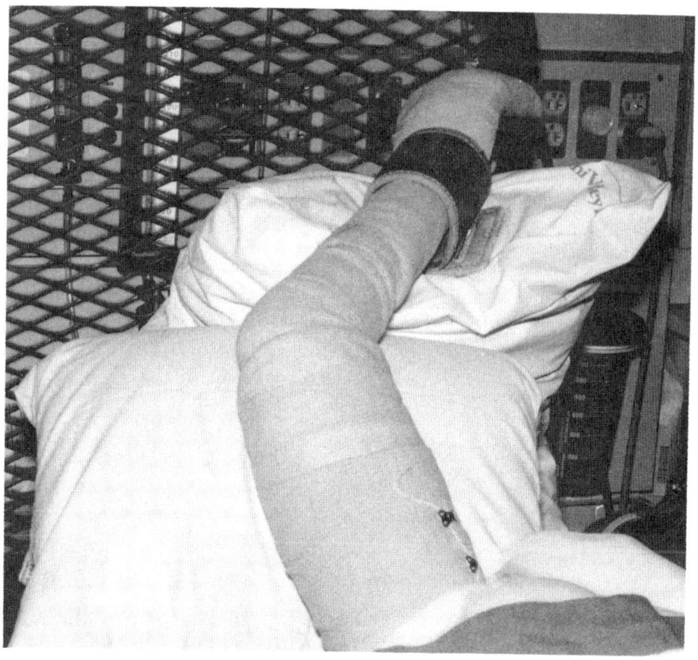

FIGURE 10–5. Multivariant positioning screen to assist with desired elbow and shoulder positioning.

tioning in bed, sitting, or during ambulation.[2] Foam wedges can be obtained commercially or fabricated by the therapist from a 6-inch block of firm density foam (Appendix E).

Several commercial shoulder abduction troughs are available as bed attachments (Appendix E). These troughs fasten onto the sides of the bed and are utilized not only for shoulder positioning but also may be used to elevate the upper extremity to decrease hand edema (Fig. 10–6). Therapists also can fabricate individual arm troughs, as described by Cooper and Paul[8] for use when the patient is in bed or sitting upright.

A creative approach for supporting the upper extremity uses surgical netting and plastic pipe to make a hammock[9] (Fig. 10–7). Hoffman[10] uses surgical netting over a sling support unit that is held in place by the mattress on a regular bed.

Occasionally skin grafts of the arm or axilla require special positioning to prevent shearing of tissue from contact with the bed. A nonskeletal system has been developed that uses an arm cuff and traction bars to protect upper extremity skin grafts (Fig. 10–8). The patient's hand and forearm are supported while the patient is placed in a side-lying position with pillows or foam wedges. The patient is not secured in this position, so co-operation is critical.[3]

Placing a patient prone with the upper extremities above the head, or side-lying on the side of the burn with the arm positioned in full flexion, are alternatives for positioning the axilla on a stretch. Patients with endotracheal tubes or central lines will be unable to lie prone.

As the patient becomes more mobile, shoulder positioning still must be maintained and emphasized. Proper shoulder positioning can be accomplished when the patient is sitting by using bedside tables or blankets to support the upper extremities (Fig. 10–9). The shoulders should be positioned at 90° in the horizontal plane and

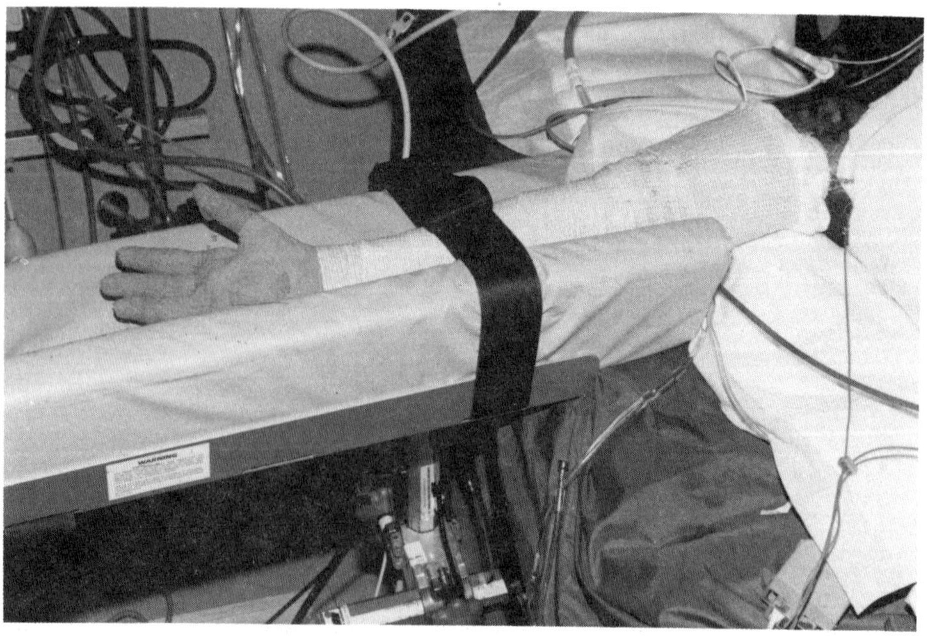

FIGURE 10–6. A commercial arm trough attached to the rail of a hospital bed provides for shoulder and elbow positioning.

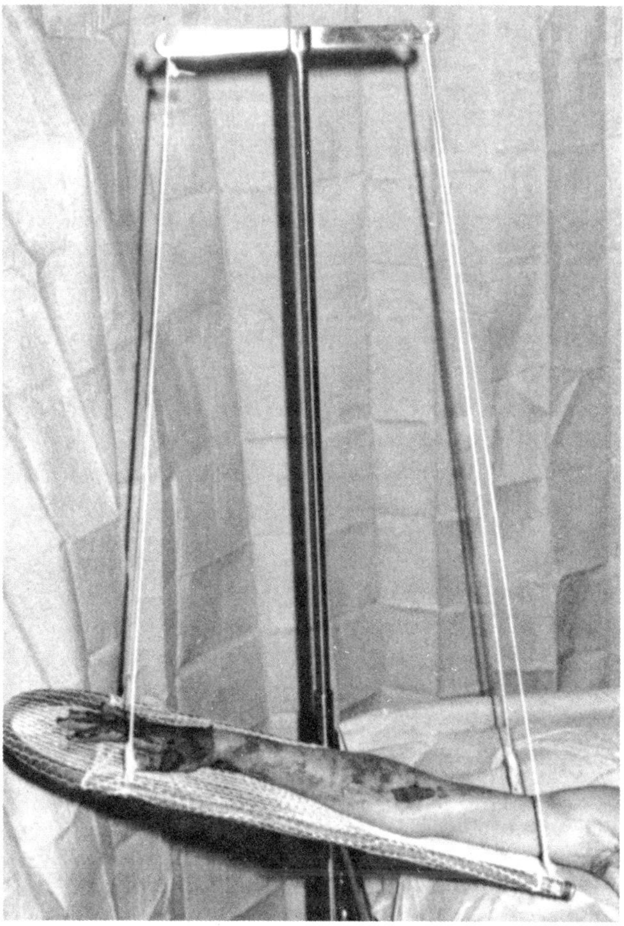

FIGURE 10–7. Shoulder positioning device using surgical netting over a metal frame and cords adjusted to proper height using an IV pole. (From Heeter et al,[9] p 145, with permission.)

between the positions of pure flexion and abduction, depending on the location of the burn. A Murphy sling or surgical netting, attached to an IV pole, can assist the patient to maintain shoulder flexion or abduction during ambulation or exercise.

Elbow

Burns to the antecubital space and circumferential burns to the upper extremity can lead to elbow flexion and forearm pronation contractures. In seeking a comfortable position, patients usually flex the elbow and predispose the joint to a flexion contracture of the antecubital area. Burns involving the posterior surface of the upper extremity may lead to extension contractures if the patient is positioned with elbows extended for prolonged periods of time. Skin grafts placed anterior to the axis of the elbow joint may cause a flexion contracture if extension is not emphasized, even when the antecubital space is spared. Because elbow extension is more difficult to regain than elbow flexion, the upper extremity is positioned with the elbow extended and the forearm either supinated or in neutral.

Many of the devices used for shoulder positioning also can be used for elbow positioning. Arm troughs allow the elbow to rest in an extended position. Overbed

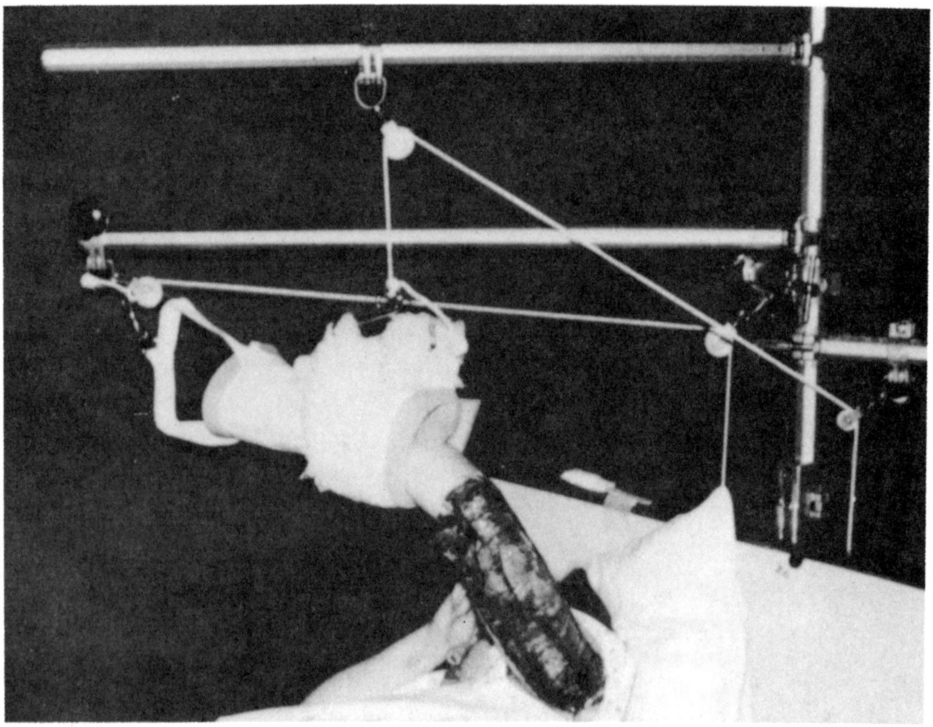

FIGURE 10–8. An arm cuff and traction bars are utilized to protect placement of a skin graft. The patient needs to cooperate in this position as the arm can be removed from the cuff. Pillows on the patient's back support the trunk to assist with positioning. (From Johnson et al,[3] p 97, with permission.)

tables can be used with patients who can voluntarily position their upper extremities. The table is placed over the patient's lap and the upper extremities are placed across the table with elbows extended. Elbow splints are an effective means of positioning, especially at night. Wrist restraints, when used in conjunction with elbow splints and attached to the head of the bed, provide a quick method for combined shoulder and elbow positioning. When elbow splints are unavailable, the use of IV boards secured with gauze or elastic wraps is an alternate method to maintain elbow extension.

The use of an air band or splint is an alternative for positioning the upper extremity during all stages of wound healing. It also can be used to provide pressure support to skin grafts or healed burn wounds (Appendix F). The air splint is easy to apply, helps control edema by applying 20 to 30 mm Hg of pressure, and is cost effective. Disadvantages to the use of air splints are excessive perspiration under the air splint and functional activity limitations. Air splints also are available for hand and lower extremity use. They are relatively inexpensive and instructions to ensure correct inflation are simple, thus making this product feasible for home use by the patient.[11]

Forearm and Wrist

Burns to the volar surface of the forearm will predispose the patient to wrist flexion and forearm pronation contractures, while burns to the dorsal surface of the

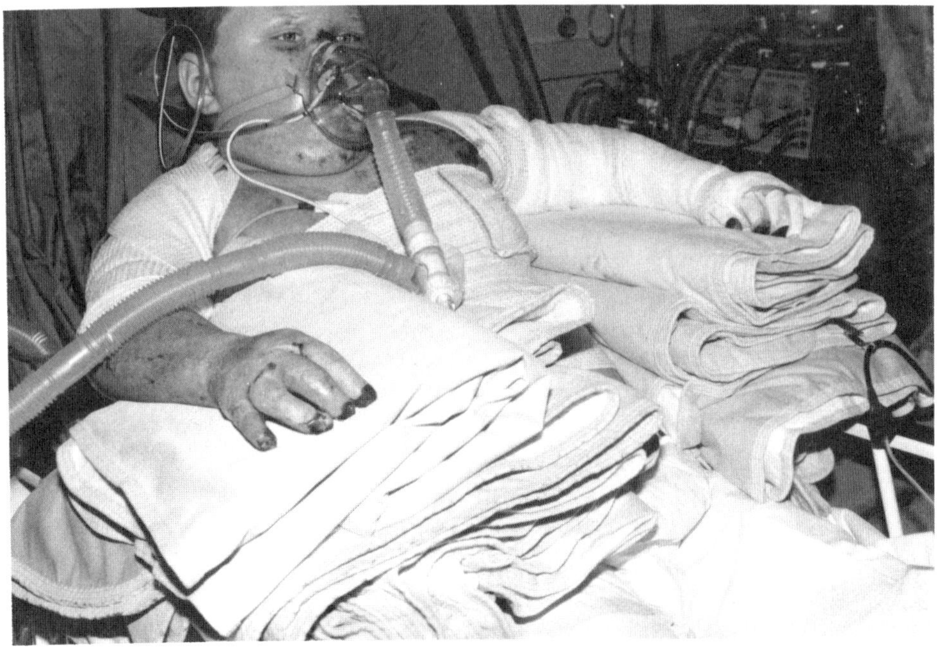

FIGURE 10–9. While the patient sits in a chair, the upper extremities are elevated using multiple layers of blankets.

forearm may cause a wrist extension contracture. The forearm frequently assumes a pronated position with the wrist in flexion when a patient elevates the forearm and hand, or rests the segment on a pillow. Therefore, the forearm is always positioned in supination and, except in the case of isolated dorsal wrist burns, the wrist should be positioned in extension. The recommended functional position of the wrist is from neutral to 30° of extension.[5] This position can be initially or temporarily accomplished by placing a small towel or gauze roll in the palm of the hand (Fig. 10–10). If wrist range of motion becomes limited in a specific direction, splinting the wrist in the opposite direction would be indicated. Usually, circumferential forearm burns require the wrist to be positioned in neutral or slight extension due to the effects of gravity and the strength of the flexor musculature.

Hand

During early hospitalization, the hand must be elevated to minimize edema formation. Elevation can be achieved using Murphy slings, surgical netting, or pillows. Elevation must be maintained while the patient is in bed, sitting, or ambulating.

The antideformity position of the hand with a dorsal burn is that of the "duckbill," "clam digger," or intrinsic plus position. Positioning of the hand may vary from one therapist to another; however, the fundamental hand positioning components are: (1) wrist extension, (2) metacarpophalangeal (MCP) joint flexion, (3) proximal interphalangeal (PIP) joint and distal interphalangeal (DIP) joint extension, and (4) thumb palmar abduction[2] (see Chapter 19). This position can be achieved by wrap-

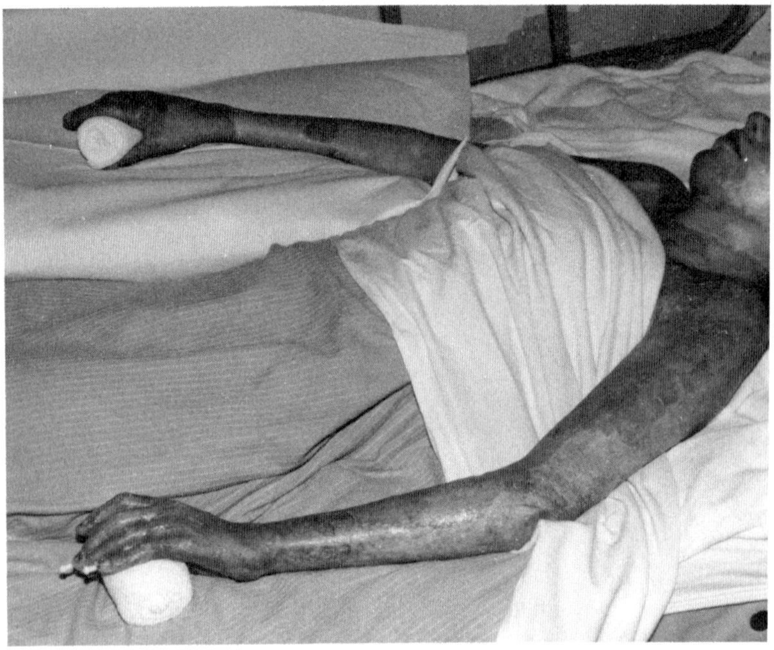

FIGURE 10–10. Gauze roll placed in patient's hand assists with positioning the wrist in extension.

ping a gauze roll or piece of foam into the palm and extending it through the thumb web space, or a hand splint can be used (see Chapter 11).

There is some controversy about whether the thumb should be positioned in radial or palmar abduction. Whichever position is used, the objective is to preserve the thumb web space. The flexor pollicis longus is a powerful muscle of the thumb and should be positioned in an elongated state.

A priority of hand positioning is to protect the dorsal expansion of the PIP joints by opposing the force of the flexor digitorum superficialis. Failure to position the extensor mechanism on a slack with deep partial- or full-thickness dorsal burns may result in rupture of this mechanism.[2]

Palmar burns may cause flexion contractures of the involved IPs, MCPs, and the thumb web space. With these burns, the hand usually is positioned with all the finger joints extended and the thumb web space on a slight stretch to preserve finger extension and thumb radial abduction. Acute palmar burns need to be positioned by a splint; when they have healed, a silicone elastomer mitt may provide both positioning and pressure support. The mitts are bivalved and applied with an elastic wrap at one-half its stretched tension. They can be used at night or intermittently during the day and can be modified by adding elastomer as edema decreases (see Chapter 11 for fabrication).

With circumferential hand burns the therapist must evaluate initially which surface is burned most deeply and is more likely to contribute to contracture formation. Hand range of motion will need to be re-evaluated often and the positioning program adjusted throughout the course of wound closure and rehabilitation.

Hip

When a burn is on the anterior or posterior hip area, the hips should be positioned in neutral rotation with slight abduction. If the patient is not positioned correctly, hip flexion, external rotation, and/or adduction contractures can result. A patient positioned with the hips in external rotation and the knees flexed for a prolonged period of time is at risk for peroneal nerve injury caused by stretch of the nerve. The results of this position can be complete paralysis with a foot drop or varying degrees of muscle weakness of the anterolateral compartments.[6]

Towel rolls or sand bags, placed lateral to the thigh, can assist to position the hip in neutral rotation. A triangular foam wedge, purchased or fabricated, or bath blankets can be placed between the lower extremities to maintain hip abduction. Lower extremity abduction splints effectively position the hips in abduction and neutral rotation, while knee extension splints can minimize hip flexion, by preventing knee flexion, when the patient lies supine. Prone is an excellent position for hip extension if the patient is able to tolerate it.

Patients should be allowed to have the head of the bed elevated or sit in a chair for only 30 minutes to 1 hour at a time, three times a day, to avoid hip flexion contractures. An alternative to elevating the head of the bed is to place the bed in a reverse Trendelenburg position. This position allows the patient to be more upright without hip flexion. To prevent the patient from sliding down in the bed, a footboard may be necessary. Anterior hip tightness may not be noticed while the patient is on bedrest, but becomes very evident when the patient begins ambulating.[3]

Knee

Burns to the posterior surface of the knee cause flexion contractures, while anterior surface burns rarely cause extension contractures. An anterior surface burn extending posterior to the axis of the knee joint has the potential to cause a knee flexion contracture.

The patient with a burn to the flexor surface of the lower extremity must be positioned with the knee in extension. The extremity may be placed in bulky dressings (especially after a skin graft) to mechanically impede knee flexion. Knee extension splints are extremely helpful to maintain extension. Pillows placed under the knees while the patient is supine are not recommended as they may cause knee flexion contractures.[3] Positioning a patient prone with the feet over the end of a mattress is a means of achieving complete knee extension. Placing a pillow under the ankle counteracts this desired effect by producing knee flexion. For edema reduction, the foot of the bed can be elevated with pillows placed lengthwise under the leg, excluding the knee, to encourage knee extension.

Ankle and Foot

Regardless of the surface area involved in a foot and ankle burn, plantar flexion contractures are the most common. Plantar flexion puts the gastrocsoleus muscle complex on slack, encouraging heel cord tightness. Therefore, placing the ankle at

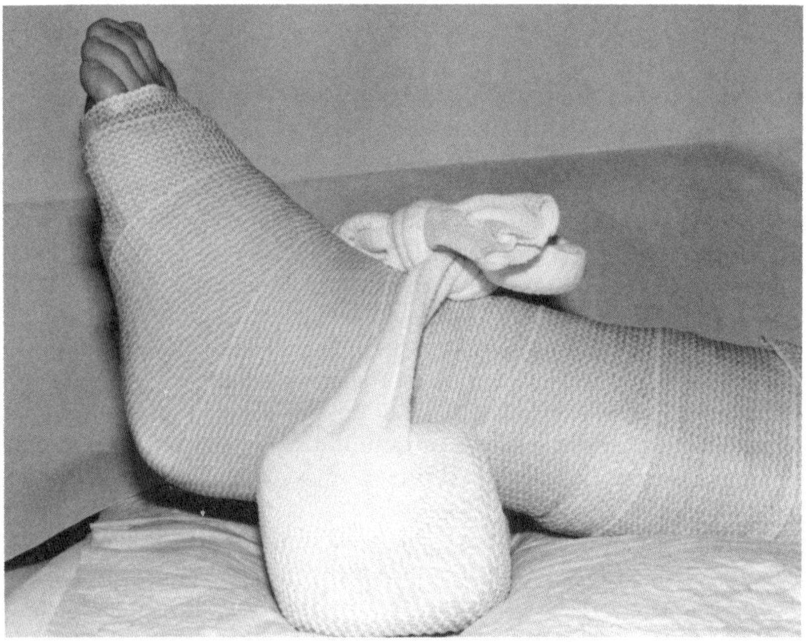

FIGURE 10–11. Foam rolls covered with surgical netting and secured around the patient's ankle maintains the heel off the bed and prevents pressure necrosis of the area.

neutral is the optimal position for posterior or circumferential burns of the ankle; however, if the burn is isolated across the anterior surface of the ankle and foot, positioning in plantar flexion is preferred while the patient is resting. If the dorsum of the foot is involved, extension contractures of the toes are likely. Subluxation at the metatarsal joints can occur.[3]

To maintain a neutral ankle position for circumferential or posterior burns of the foot and ankle, a splint is preferable to a footboard, especially with the noncompliant patient. If the patient lies prone, the feet can extend over the end of the bed, where they will rest in only slight plantar flexion. In addition, sponge booties, prefabricated splints, or custom splints with a cutout heel also may be utilized (Appendix F). When ankle position is not the main concern, but pressure on the heel is, pillows placed under the calf of the leg or thick foam covered with surgical netting, wrapped circumferentially above the ankle and tied, will help relieve pressure on the calcaneus (Fig. 10–11). Any of these devices may be necessary for a patient on prolonged bedrest who has burns over a large area, for ventilated patients who are receiving neuromuscular blocking agents (which cause total muscle paralysis), or when a 2-hour turning schedule is difficult for the patient. If the patient is ambulatory and the ankle is not burned, special positioning is not indicated.

SKELETAL TRACTION

Occasionally some facilities may use skeletal traction after skin grafting for positioning. Skeletal traction applies force through the bone by use of wires or pins placed directly into or through the osseous tissue. A fixed pulley system directs the traction force with the use of varying weight specific for each body part. All extremities can be positioned using a skeletal traction system and mandibular pins can be utilized to position the neck in extension. Hand positioning can be accomplished using a halo or banjo-type apparatus.[3] However, skeletal traction is an invasive procedure with possible pin site infection.

PEDIATRIC POSITIONING

Children are more difficult than adults to position and to maintain in a given position and therefore they present a unique challenge to burn team members. Uncooperative behavior and anxiety from pain often interfere with attempts at immobilization. Several special techniques have been developed in an effort to help position the pediatric patient. The following techniques, along with the methods described earlier, can be utilized to develop a satisfactory positioning program for the younger patient.

The upper extremity of a small child who has sustained an elbow burn can be positioned with sterile tongue depressors. This position is achieved by placing the tongue depressors 2 to 3 cm apart around the circumference of the elbow joint, wrapping with roll gauze to keep it in place, and applying adhesive tape behind the shoulders to keep the wrap from slipping distally[12] (Fig. 10–12).

A papoose has been developed to position the child with axillary burns.[13] The device is fabricated from thick foam to position the shoulders of children 6 months to 6 years of age. The papoose secures the child's shoulders in 90° to 160° of abduction with 20° of horizontal adduction to prevent brachial plexus injury. This position is maintained by foam axillary wedges and foam straps attached to the papoose and fastened around the child's arms, forearms, waist, and, if needed, legs. This technique immobilizes the child after skin grafting to prevent graft loss (Fig. 10–13).

When the child with axillary burns is able to sit, bedside tables are very useful. The table is placed across the child's lap and elevated to maintain shoulder flexion

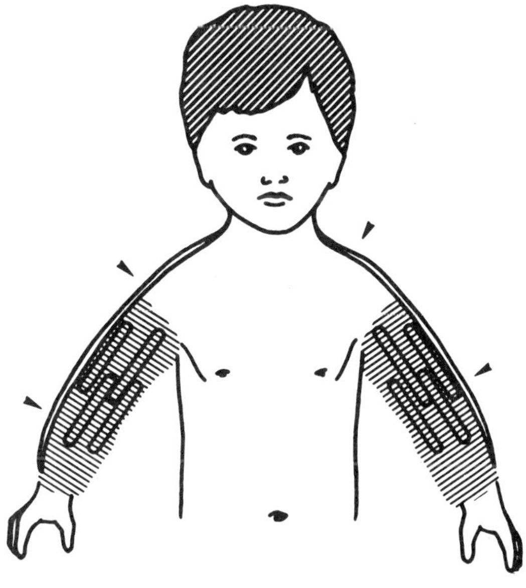

FIGURE 10–12. Schematic drawing of tongue depressors wrapped in gauze to position a child in elbow extension after skin grafting. The arrows show the adhesive tape that is placed over the wrap and behind the shoulder to keep the dressing from slipping distally. (From Kaufman et al,[12] p 462, with permission.)

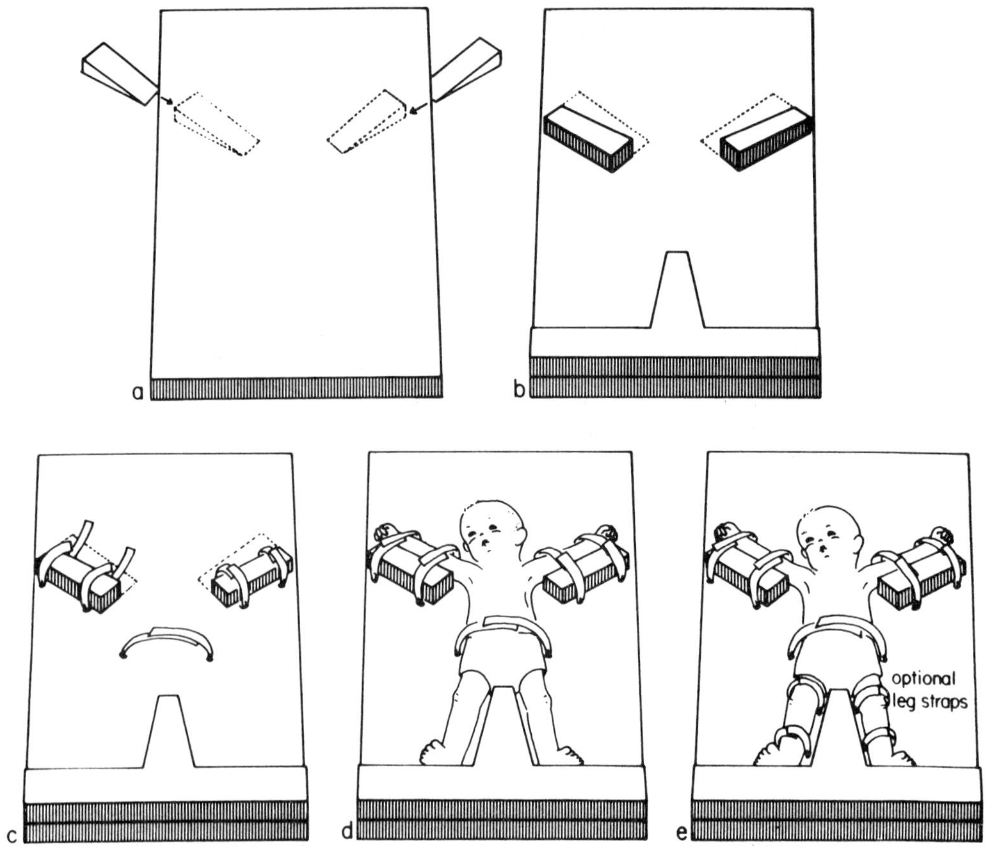

FIGURE 10–13. Stages of construction of a foam papoose positioner with (a) placement of wedges, (b) foam blocks to hold shoulders and lower edge to maintain the legs, (c) the addition to velfoam straps for waist and arms, (d) upper extremity positioning, and (e) optional leg straps added. (From MacDonald et al,[13] p 63, with permission.)

at 90°. While ambulating, an overhead walker can be used to maintain shoulder flexion.[5]

Proper hip position is especially important with children. Dislocation of the hip after burn injury has been attributed to a combination of factors including poor positioning and the contractile force of the burn scar.[5]

The papoose board shown in Figure 10–13 is an option for positioning the lower extremities. An abduction wedge and foam foot rests are fastened to this foam bed and straps secure the thighs and legs. A figure-of-8 elastic wrap should be used to maintain appropriate ankle position. The wrap is applied in the same manner as used for ambulation.[13]

POSITIONING FOLLOWING RECONSTRUCTIVE SURGERY

Although positioning is important during the acute burn phase, positioning following reconstructive surgery requires considerable attention to prevent repeated surgical procedures to the same area. For the cooperative patient who has developed a

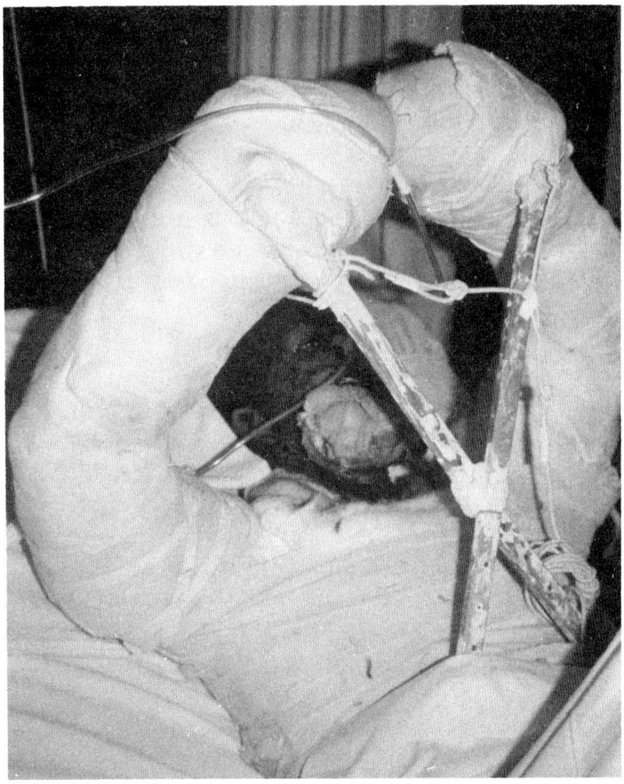

FIGURE 10–14. Surgical dressings reinforced with plaster and pieces of old crutches to hold the noncompliant patient's position after shoulder releases.

burn scar contracture or the child who has grown faster than the scar will allow, basic positioning techniques are recommended for use following reconstructive surgery.

If the patient was previously noncompliant, increased attention to detail of the positioning program will be necessary for a successful reconstructive outcome. The use of splints or other positioning aids will need to be instituted immediately following surgery. Furthermore, alternative measures may need to be instituted to ensure maintenance of proper positioning. For example, some burn centers utilize halo traction following surgical neck releases.[14] Customized neck splints can be constructed prior to surgery that allow the patient to sit or ambulate while securing the head in an immobile position[15,16] (see Chapter 11). Also, surgical dressings can be reinforced with plaster and additional supports if necessary (Fig. 10–14).

EDUCATION AND COMMUNICATION

Continual education of burn team members, patients, and their caregivers is one of the most important areas for the therapist to address in regards to positioning. In the hospital, positioning education must be conveyed to all nursing staff, because the positioning program is necessary 24 hours a day. This information is especially important for nurses who are unfamiliar with specialized burn rehabilitation techniques.

There are many effective ways of communicating the positioning program to the burn staff. They may range from simple positioning diagrams displayed at bedside to very detailed care plans. An individualized positioning program can be demonstrated by circling the specific patient positions on a comprehensive positioning chart. Staff at some burn centers may find that writing in the medical record care plan or on erasable marker boards is sufficient.

Additional methods to communicate proper positioning are photographing the correct patient position using an instant camera or using a plastic slide holder to display diagrams of individual patient positions[17] (Fig. 10–15). A positioning video could be part of an inservice library for reference or orientation of the burn unit staff.[18] Positioning could be included as part of the quality assurance (QA) nursing plan. Direct patient education, as well as staff communication during rounds, is a helpful means for achieving a good positioning program.

Instructing family members about positioning at bedside will enhance carryover following patient discharge. To assist the therapist in communicating correct positioning for the pediatric patient, developmental or baby stickers with pictures of the desired positions are available commercially through Therapy Skill Builders (Appendix G). Pictures are easily posted at the bedside for staff reference or provided to family members for home instruction. The method used to keep the positioning program current must have the flexibility to be updated frequently and communicated readily with minimal time involved.

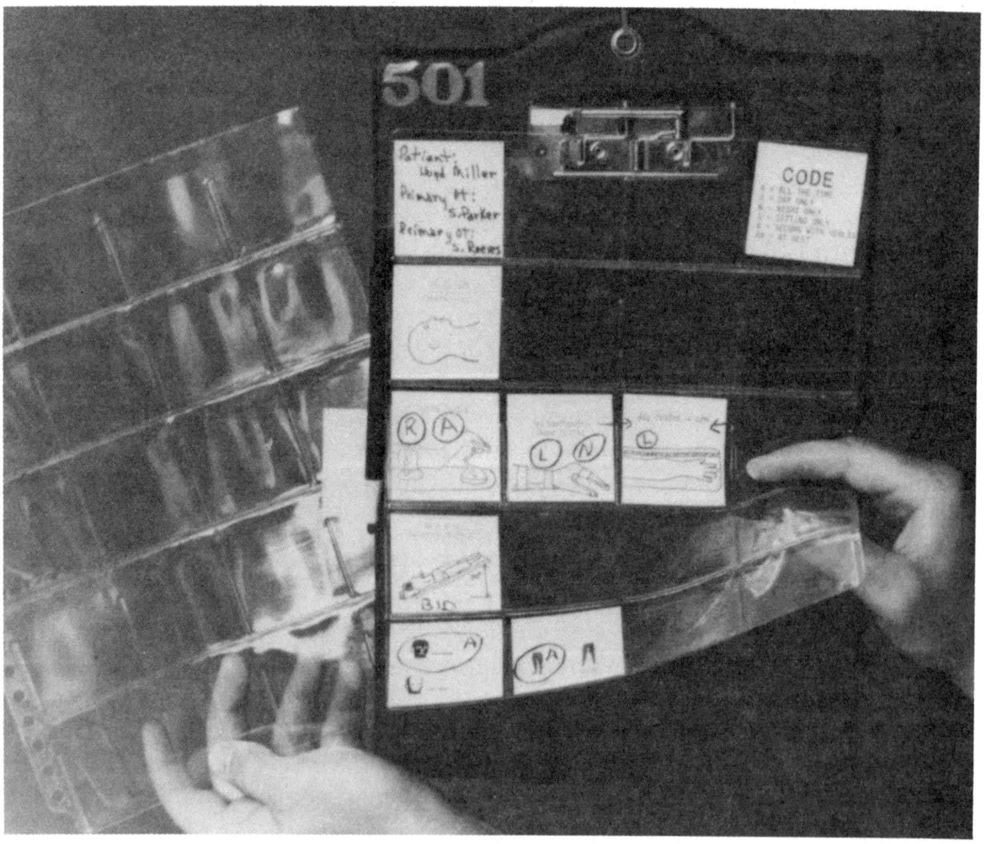

FIGURE 10–15. Pictures inserted into plastic slide sheets can be used to individualize each patients positioning program. (From Stafford,[17] p 393, with permission.)

SUMMARY

Proper patient positioning assists with edema reduction and prevention of scar contractures. Positioning consists of elevating extremities and/or placing the soft tissues in an elongated state, in opposition to a contracting burn scar. Particular consideration is paid to preventing further soft tissue damage or nerve injury. Depending on the patient's age and participation in the exercise program, the positioning program is followed while the patient is in bed, sitting in a chair, or ambulating. Multiple devices, including arm troughs, foam wedges, and sand bags, are used to assist the patient in maintaining prescribed positions. Specific positioning techniques may be necessary for the pediatric patient or following reconstructive surgery on a patient who previously was noncompliant with the rehabilitation program. Education and communication between all burn team members, patients, and their caregivers is necessary if an effective positioning program is to be successful. Consistent attention to proper positioning will aid in the prevention of scar contractures and increase the patient's potential for a functional life following burn injury.

CASE STUDY

HISTORY

TJ was a previously healthy 22-year-old male who was admitted to the hospital with a 34 percent total body burn. The burn injury occurred as a result of the patient trying to encourage the progress of a bon fire by pouring gasoline onto the fire. His mixed deep partial- and full-thickness burns included the right hand and upper extremity, the entire anterior trunk, portions of the lateral trunk and anterior cervical neck areas, and the right anterior thigh and groin area. The patient was wearing polyester shorts and a cotton short-sleeved shirt that caught fire at the time of the accident.

Upon initial evaluation by the therapist, the right hand and fingers were moderately edematous. Involved joint skin creases included both surfaces of the right wrist and elbow, anterior axillary fold, right lateral and anterior cervical neck areas, and the right inguinal fold area. The patient underwent one skin-grafting procedure 4 days after admission to the hospital.

PROBLEM LIST

Edematous right upper extremity
Multiple joint skin creases involved in burn

GOALS

Decrease right hand and finger edema within first week
Restore normal active range of motion of joint skin crease areas 7 to 10 days following healing

TREATMENT INTERVENTIONS

Right upper extremity elevation was maintained at all times until the edema resolved. The hand and fingers were kept elevated above the level of the heart by propping the hand on pillows while in bed, on a bedside table when the patient was out of bed sitting, and actively raised when upright. The elevated position was able to be maintained in combination with correct positioning of the remaining upper extremity areas of concern. The upper extremity was positioned in 90° to 100° of shoulder abduction, elbow extension, forearm supination, and wrist extension. This was accomplished by the use of sling suspension while the patient was in bed, a bedside table when sitting, and conscientious positioning by the patient when ambulating. While in bed, the patient was positioned supine with the bed horizontal. For meals, the nursing staff was instructed to have the patient sit out of bed. Sitting time was restricted to 30 minutes for meals and limited to 20 minutes at other times. The patient was instructed to lay flat in bed or ambulate the majority of the time.

RATIONALE

The prescribed positioning program was consistent throughout hospitalization, including the postoperative period. The hand was maintained in an elevated position to facilitate gravity-assisted lymphatic drainage. The remaining upper extremity positions stressed an anticontracture orientation. Burns to the anterior axillary fold tend to limit shoulder abduction, and so abduction was the position of choice. The typical pattern of restriction with circumferential burns about the elbow, forearm, and wrist is limited elbow and wrist extension with forearm pronation. Thus, the positions chosen were to offset the tendency for contracture. A position of hip extension was emphasized with the patient for two reasons. First, to deter tightness from forming across the inguinal crease and second, to maximize the stress applied to the healing tissue of the trunk and adjacent upper extremity by emphasizing a combined tissue elongation throughout all contiguous areas of involvement.

REFERENCES

1. Helm, PA, et al: Burn injury: Rehabilitation management in 1982. J Burn Care Rehabil 4:411–422, 1983.
2. Pullium, GF: Splinting and positioning. In Fisher, SV and Helm, PA (eds): Comprehensive Rehabilitation of Burns. Williams & Wilkins, Baltimore, 1984, pp 64–95.
3. Johnson, CL, O'Shaughnessy, EJ, and Ostergren, G (eds): Burn Management. Raven Press, New York, 1981, pp 48–116.
4. Eckert, PL: Physical therapy for burns of the head and neck. In Wachtel, TL and Frank, DH (eds): Burns of the Head and Neck. WB Saunders, Philadelphia, 1984, pp 122–132.
5. Fader, P: Preserving function and minimizing deformity: The role of the occupational therapist. In Carvajal, HF and Parks, DH (eds): Burns in Children: Pediatric Burn Management. Yearbook Medical Publishers, Chicago, 1988, pp 325–344.
6. Helm, PA: Neuromuscular considerations. In Fisher, SV and Helm, PA (eds): Comprehensive Rehabilitation of Burns. Williams & Wilkins, Baltimore, 1984, pp 235–241.
7. Richard, RL, Miller, SF, and Finley, RK: Positioning screen—Innovations in burn care. J Burn Care Rehabil 13:451–452, 1992.
8. Cooper, S and Paul, EO: An effective method of positioning the burn patient. J Burn Care Rehabil 9:288–289, 1988.

9. Heeter, PK and Brown, R: Arm hammock for elevation of the thermally injured upper extremity. J Burn Care Rehabil 7:144–146, 1986.
10. Hoffman, BE: Stable net slings for upper extremity elevation. J Burn Care Rehabil 6:375–378, 1985.
11. Barnett, PH and Stafford, FS: Use of plastic airbands for edema and scar control. J Burn Care Rehabil 5:469–473, 1984.
12. Kaufman, T, et al: The kerlix tongue-depressor splint for skin-grafted areas in burned children. J Burn Care Rehabil 10:462–463, 1989.
13. MacDonald, LB, Covey, MH, and Marvin, JA: The papoose: Device for positioning the burn child's axilla. J Burn Care Rehabil 6:62–63, 1985.
14. Schubert, W, et al: Halo immobilization in the treatment of burns to the head, face, and neck. J Burn Care Rehabil 9:187–189, 1988.
15. Apfel, L: Occupational therapy techniques for the patient with thermal injuries of the head and neck. In Wachtel, TL and Frank, DH (eds): Burns of the Head and Neck. WB Saunders, Philadelphia, 1984, pp 133–152.
16. Apfel, LM and Wachtel, TL: Halo neck splint. J Burn Care Rehabil 8:140–143, 1987.
17. Stafford, FS: Physical and occupational therapy: Treatment communication board. J Burn Care Rehabil 5:393–394, 1984.
18. Staley, M, Hruska, R, and Cisar, C: Consistency in burn care through the use of educational videotapes. Proc American Burn Association 18:37, 1986.

CHAPTER 11

Splinting Techniques for the Burn Patient

Mary Beth Daugherty, OTR
Judith A. Carr-Collins, OTR

Historically, splints of various materials have been used to support burned extremities, maintain joint positions following surgery, and correct or prevent deformity.[1-5] Leather, wood, and metal have been replaced with thermoplastic splinting materials, but splint design concepts remain basically unchanged. The design of splints can vary widely, but the intended results are the same. The chosen design, however, is less important than the timely application and proper fit of the splint. Splinting protocols developed by Willis[6] in 1969 continue as the basis for therapeutic intervention today.

The treatment of severe burns focuses on patient survival, functional outcome, and cosmetic appearance. Survival of an individual is dependent on the extent and depth of injury and the delivery of definitive and specialized care. The end cosmetic result is influenced by the timely closure of the wound, aggressive scar management, and the skills of the reconstructive surgeon and multidisciplinary team.[7] The degree to which function is preserved depends on early intervention and prevention of further tissue damage. A loss of joint range of motion (ROM), disruption of joint integrity, or skin graft failure may result in a temporary or permanent disability. No single therapeutic modality can preserve function. Optimal rehabilitation depends on the combined use of all treatments available to the therapist; however, this chapter will focus on splinting in the treatment of a burn patient.

INDICATIONS FOR USE OF SPLINTS IN BURN TREATMENT

Acute Phase

Prophylactic splinting usually is not required. However, if damage to tendons and joints is suspected, splinting will immobilize, provide support, and aid in positioning the affected body part. If splinting is necessary, the design of a splint should be nonconforming and methods to secure it should not be constrictive due to the dramatic fluctuation in edema during the acute phase.

Wound-Healing Phase

During the wound-healing phase of burn care, splints may prevent the development of contracture and the disruption by movement of newly applied skin grafts. Special care must be taken during this phase so that splints do not interfere with healing as a result of improper placement or fit. To ensure proper fit, a splint should be conforming, with appropriate length for leverage and edges rolled or flared away from the skin.

Rehabilitation Phase

Contractile forces within a developing scar may remain active for up to 18 months.[8] Splinting is used to reduce contracture nonsurgically, prevent deformity, maintain natural body contours, and complement pressure therapy. Ideally, only regular exercise and the consistent use of pressure are necessary to achieve normal joint mobility and scar control, but the combined treatment of splints, exercise, and pressure frequently is required. The ongoing process of scar development and contracture is, in part, managed by maintaining sustained stretch to scar tissue. Exercise may achieve normal ROM and splinting can maintain the range gained. Splints immobilize a joint at the endpoint of joint range and routinely are adjusted as increases in range are made. If the tensile strength of a scar covering a joint is poor, the site should be monitored closely for wound breakdown secondary to pressure or excessive stretch of the soft tissue by the splint.

Reconstructive Phase

Splints may be required following reconstructive procedures for restoring function or cosmesis. Contractile forces in a wound bed will distort and shorten newly healed skin grafts, cause a progressive loss of motion, and disturb body contours created by a cosmetic procedure if they are unopposed.[9] Splints applied following the release of contractures or reconstructive procedures usually are molded directly to the site and should be monitored closely for evidence of wound maceration or breakdown.

SPLINTING INDICATIONS

Protection of Anatomic Structures

A burn injury may extend beyond the level of the skin and include damage to underlying structures. The common structures at risk are tendons and joints. As with skin, the extent of permanent disability will be influenced greatly by early intervention and protection of these structures. The goal of early splinting is to securely stabilize a joint so that all external stress applied to the joint and tendon is eliminated or significantly reduced. Ideally, a position of function should be maintained; however, the position in which a joint is splinted should be determined by the extent of tendon involvement. Tendons should be splinted in a slack position to prevent rupture; joints in which the structural integrity has been destroyed should be immobilized in a position of function to facilitate fusion. Special attention also should be given to the type of dressing material applied to areas at risk. A dressing for exposed tendons should act as a moisture barrier to prevent drying of a tendon and function as splint padding to prevent further damage from the application of a rigid splint.

Prevention of Deformity

The contractile nature of the healing burn wound and subsequent scar tissue creates an ongoing battle in the maintenance of joint ROM from the acute phase of treatment through the reconstructive phase. Burn patients typically will seek a position of comfort that frequently equates to a position of deformity.[10] Splints maintain a position that is opposite of the anticipated deformity. Since pain is frequently a factor limiting patient cooperation, splints are utilized to prevent prolonged posturing in undesirable positions.

Splints to prevent deformity are applied to maintain gains in ROM achieved through exercise or as a means to apply a sustained stretch to the healing wound. The therapist should monitor closely the burn wound or the scar underlying a splint for evidence of disruption of healing or breakdown of the scar that may be due to stretch applied by the splint. Frequent re-evaluation of the maturity of a scar also is indicated to determine when a splint can be discontinued without further contracture development.

Preservation of Skin Graft Integrity

Survival of a skin graft is dependent on the establishment of circulation between the underlying wound bed and the transplanted skin. To prevent any disruption of this process, the recipient site must be immobilized completely to avoid shearing or displacement of the graft until it adheres. Immobilization can be accomplished by skeletal traction, application of a bulky dressing, or by means of a splint to prohibit motion. Consideration should be given to those joints that are located directly under a graft, and also to adjacent joints whose freedom of movement may cause shearing. Splints usually are discontinued once graft adherence is assured.

Restoration of Function

Even with intensive rehabilitation, scar contractures can occur. If treated early and aggressively, scar contractures can be reduced through splinting, thus avoiding surgical release or revision. The key to nonoperative resolution of contractures is sustained stretch and pressure. Serial splinting is used to maintain gains following active and passive exercise. Splints should be revised to accommodate any change in ROM and the wearing schedule adjusted to prevent recurrence of contracture. Plaster casting is an easy and cost-effective method of reducing contracture in a short period of time, but certain precautions may be required (see Casting).

REQUIREMENTS OF BURN SPLINTS

Many different thermoplastic and cast materials can be used to splint a thermally injured patient. The selection of material that best serves the treatment plan depends on several variables. The therapist should be familiar with more than one splinting material to best meet the needs of the patient. One material rarely will be adequate from the acute through rehabilitative phases of treatment[11,12] (Appendix H).

Compatibility with Topical Agents and Wound Dressing Materials

Selection of an appropriate material for splint construction depends greatly on the wound surface to be covered and the duration of time the splint is expected to be used. Splints constructed of solid thermoplastic materials are occlusive and can cause maceration of the wound unless an adequate absorbent dressing covers the wound or adequate skin hygiene is performed. Perforated or open-weave thermoplastics allow passage of fluids to wounds treated by wet dressings or irrigation. Wound drainage must be cleaned from the perforations because it can be a source of contamination. Plaster serves best as a one-time use item because it absorbs wound drainage and cannot be cleaned. Also, plaster is not suited for use over wet dressings.

Minimal Interference with Wound Closure or Skin Grafting

Splints should be monitored closely for evidence of pressure necrosis due to splint placement. Inconsistent dressings or a change in the level of edema present can alter the fit of a splint and subsequently disrupt healing. Any splint used repeatedly and coming into direct contact with open wounds should be constructed of a thermoplastic material for ease in cleaning the material. With each removal, a splint should be thoroughly cleansed.

Timely Application

Early splinting protocols, as outlined by Willis,[6,13] stressed the importance of "when" a splint was applied. Willis attributed the failure of early splinting techniques to either the inadequacy of the device or the delay in applying the device after damage had occurred. Early treatment for reduction or prevention of contracture yields the optimal result.

Simple Application

In the acute phase of treatment, splints are removed often and applied by a variety of personnel. In the rehabilitative phase, splints are cared for and monitored by patients and family members who often are unfamiliar with "medical appliances." A splint of simple design and application will reduce possible complications associated with improper application of the splint. A splint that is simple to apply probably will be worn more consistently.

Inexpensive or Remoldable Material

Splints should be easily adaptable to accommodate changes in a wound, edema, or in joint position. Thermoplastics are ideal for splints in which extended use is predicted because they are remoldable. Because of low cost, plaster is the material of choice for disposable splints (serial splints, postoperative splints).

Avoidance of Pressure Necrosis and Neuropathies

To prevent excessive pressure by any one portion of the splint, pressure should be distributed over a broad surface area. All proximal and distal splint edges where pressure is increased should be smooth and flared slightly. Splint placement over bony prominences should be avoided. If splinting over bony prominences cannot be avoided, as in the case of a posterior foot drop splint, the splint should be expanded to create a dome over the potential pressure area (heel). The combination of sustained stretch and pressure from splints or dressings is a common cause of neuropathies in burn patients. Most stretch- and pressure-related peripheral neuropathies are preventable by closely monitoring the splint's position and avoidance of tight dressings over superficial nerves (peroneal, ulnar, radial) and overly vigorous stretching programs.[14]

GENERAL SPLINT CONSIDERATIONS

Splinting applies an external force to a body segment and should be considered whenever full passive ROM is not obtainable. The focus of a splinting program should be on those motions that are most difficult to regain: neck extension and rotation, shoulder flexion and abduction, interphalangeal (IP) joint extension, metacarpophalangeal (MCP) joint flexion, wrist extension, elbow and knee extension, and ankle dorsiflexion. Basic splinting principles, as described by Fess and Philips,[15] are recommended when splinting a burn injured patient. These principles are as follows:

1. Mechanical principles
   a. Increasing the surface area of splint contact reduces pressure.
   b. Optimal leverage—longer lever arms decrease the amount of force or pressure needed to achieve the desired position.

c. Consideration should be given to the effect the splint has on motion of adjacent joints.
d. The effects of reciprocal forces (e.g., three-point splints) should be considered.
e. Contour shaping produces a curved surface that is stronger than a flat surface.
f. Elimination of friction—indicates poor fit, improper alignment, or ineffective fastening.
g. Avoidance of high shear stress—a splint or padding should conform closely, have round edges, be padded appropriately, and the therapist should beware of cumulative damage by repetitive stresses to tissue.

2. Principles of dynamic mobilization
   a. A 90° angle of force is optimal.
   b. Amount of force—for joints that lack normal passive motion, a splint should provide enough force to produce stretch to the tissue and allow for tissue re-alignment, but not so much as to damage tissue.
3. Design principles
   a. Determination of splint purpose(s)—immobilization; increase of passive motion; substitution for active motion; pressure; change in tightness of skin, scar, or underlying structures.
   b. Individual patient factors—location and type of problem; ability of the patient to understand the need for and use of the splint; age; life-style; and whether frequent splint revisions would cause a hardship.
   c. Duration of use—short-term splints usually have a simple design and construction and use lower-cost materials.
   d. Simplicity of design, construction, and fit.
   e. Optimum function—splint only those joints that are absolutely necessary; little interference with daily function.
   f. Ease of application and removal.
   g. The therapist must determine the surface for splint application—influenced by anatomic and mechanical factors as well as the method of wound treatment (open versus closed); pressure generally is better tolerated on the flexor surface of an extremity because of muscle and soft tissue padding over bones.
   h. Adaptation for variables—intravenous sites; a hole cut out of the antecubital area of an elbow extension splint to allow for checking blood pressure.
   i. Static versus dynamic forces. According to Colditz,[16] the use of static or dynamic splinting depends upon the stage of tissue healing. She stated that during the early inflammatory stage, static splints are useful, while both dynamic and serial static splints may be indicated during the proliferative stage of tissue healing. Although static and dynamic splints can be beneficial during the stage of scar maturation, serial static splints often prove superior. Pure skin tightness is altered best by a static splint that holds the skin at maximum length as it simultaneously provides direct positive pressure to a scar. Serial static splinting is believed to produce better results than dynamic splinting for the first web space of the hand and for proximal interphalangeal (PIP) joints which lack 30° or less of extension.[15]

      Static Splint: A static splint supports one or more joints in a specific position for the purpose of immobilization. Serial static splinting can enhance ROM of a joint through the principle of prolonged stretch,[17] which is similar to the force provided by the elastic traction of dynamic splints.

A conforming static splint is formed directly on the patient in complete contact with the contours of the body and distributes pressure along the length of the splint. A nonconforming splint also can immobilize an extremity very well but may create more problems, such as pressure points or slippage, than would a conforming splint.

Due to the ease of application and molding characteristics of thermoplastic materials, the drape and trim method of freeform splint fabrication is appropriate in all phases of burn treatment. The drape and trim method requires a minimum of measurements. Usually, only the estimated length and width of the splint are needed. The material is heated and draped directly on the patient. If the warm splint material is placed in direct contact with the patient's skin, the therapist must ensure that the material is a safe and comfortable temperature for the patient. Excess material is trimmed away and finishing, such as folding back edges and flaring proximal and distal ends, is done while the material is warm. Since fabrication time is short, the drape and trim method is ideal for fabricating splints in the operating room over a patient's operative dressings.

Dynamic splint: A dynamic splint applies a specific force in a specific plane of motion through elastic traction while allowing the patient some motion of the joint (Fig. 11–1). Dynamic splinting should be considered for those joints that demonstrate the most resistance to passive stretch and do not respond to positioning or intermittent stretching. Close supervision and monitoring of tissue is required due to the force a dynamic splint applies. A dynamic splint, particularly for the hand, can exert pressure that a patient's damaged skin may be unable to tolerate.

Prefabricated dynamic splints are used widely in burn rehabilitation. The benefits of commercially available dynamic splints, which provide low load and prolonged stretch, have been documented in case studies by Richard[18] and Richard and co-workers.[19] These splints are available for the knee, ankle, elbow, wrist, and IP joints (Appendix F) (Fig. 11–2). They can provide either a flexion or extension force, have been worn in the presence of open areas and exposed tendons, and several types are available for pediatric patients. The splint can be worn continuously with gradual increases in tension made to the level a patient can tolerate. For best results, the splint is removed only for short

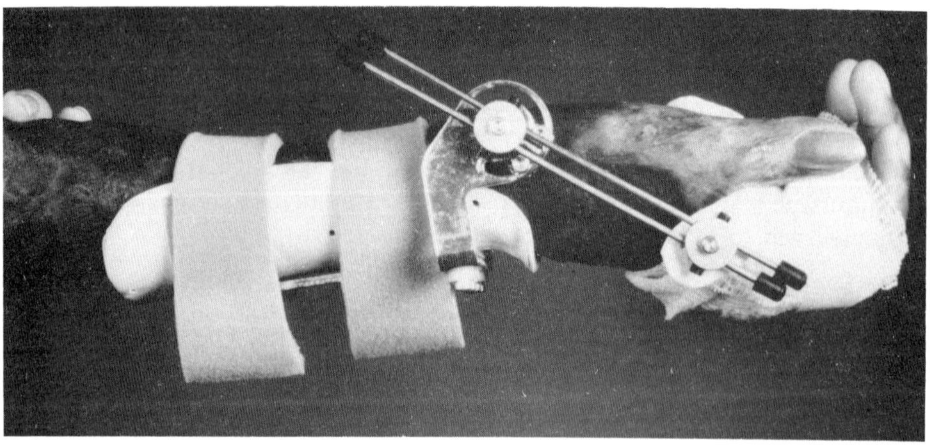

FIGURE 11–1. Custom-made dynamic splint for wrist extension.

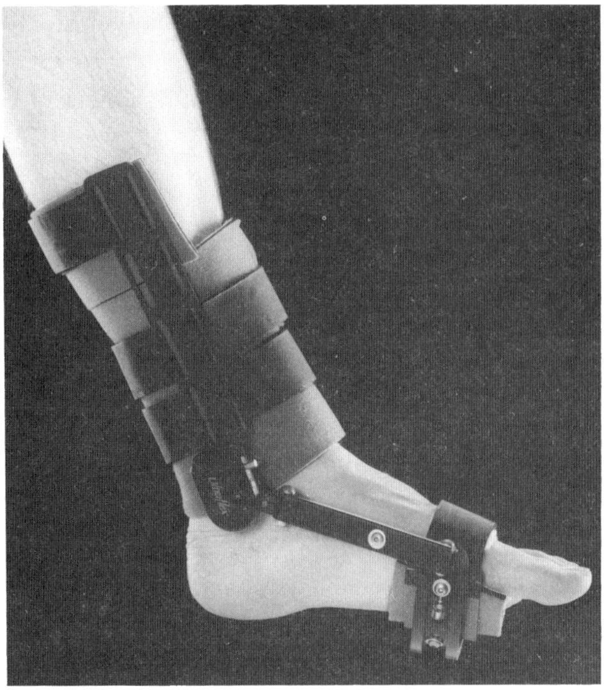

FIGURE 11–2. Commercially available ankle dorsiflexion splint with foot correction cradle.

periods of time for wound care, exercise, or therapeutic activity and gradually is discontinued once the patient can maintain increases in ROM independently or with a traditional splint.

4. Construction principles
   a. Good cosmetic effect. Most thermoplastic materials can be cleaned with soap and lukewarm water. Stains can be removed with dilute bleach or toothpaste.
   b. Most thermoplastic materials at room temperature can be cut with shears or scored with a utility knife. Warm material or $\frac{1}{16}$-inch material can be cut with scissors. Corners should be rounded and edges smoothed or rolled.
   c. Finished hardware—Rivets should be flush with the surface of the splint and covered with tape or moleskin to prevent potential skin irritation; exposed metal should be smooth.
   d. Ventilation as necessary.
   e. Padding and straps are secure.
   f. Safety precautions—The therapist must maintain a safe environment (heat guns can fall into hot water baths); a patient's sensitive skin frequently requires a buffer of dressing or stockinette to provide a barrier to the heat of the thermoplastic materials.
5. Fit considerations
   a. Relief over bony prominences.
   b. Maintenance of arches of the hands and feet.
   c. Alignment of the splint axis with anatomic axis-hinged splints.
   d. Stress on ligaments—The safe-position hand splint maintains the MCP joints in flexion to preserve the length of the collateral ligaments.
   e. Skin creases as boundaries.
   f. Adjustments for comfort.

TYPES OF SPLINTS

Various types of splints for the treatment of burn injured patients are described in this section.

Anterior Neck

Anticipated deformity: Flexion with possible lateral flexion
Secondary problems: Disturbance in mastication; distortion of facial units; difficult or hazardous intubation in subsequent reconstructive procedures

Soft Cervical Collar[20] (Fig. 11–3)

Description. Circumferential foam neck orthosis covered with stockinette; generally used when the tissue is fragile but neck requires positioning.

Advantages
- Commercially available (Appendix F).
- Used in any phase of treatment (more often post healing).
- Simple to apply and adjust.
- Comfortable for patient.
- Maintains neutral extension; prevents lateral flexion.

Disadvantages
- Absorbent—will require use of a replaceable cover.
- Tendency to rotate around neck.
- Minimally effective for scar management.

Molded Neck Splint or Collar[20–22] (Fig. 11–4)

Description. Total contact, rigid neck support.

Advantages
- Used in any phase of treatment.
- Applies definitive pressure—exact contour of surface.
- Low-temperature materials—molded directly on patient or over simple dressings. Used in serial splinting.
- High-temperature materials—formed over a positive mold of the patient's neck.
- Maintains exact position—prevents rotation and lateral flexion.

Disadvantages
- Occlusive—Frequent monitoring needed for signs of maceration or wound deterioration.
- Potential for skin breakdown exists if splint is extended over the bony areas of the chin or clavicles.

Halo Neck Splint[20,23] (Fig. 11–5)

Description. Thermoplastic orthosis that positions the neck in extension using the head and upper torso for stabilization.

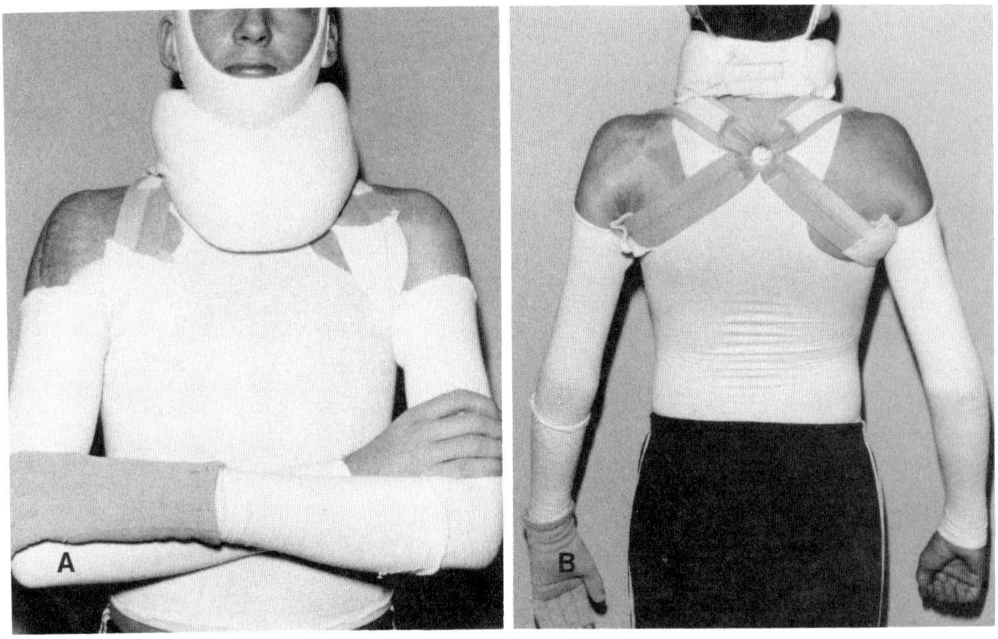

FIGURE 11–3. (*A*) Anterior view. (*B*) Posterior view. Patient wearing soft cervical collar and clavicle brace. (Courtesy of S. Reeves, 1992.)

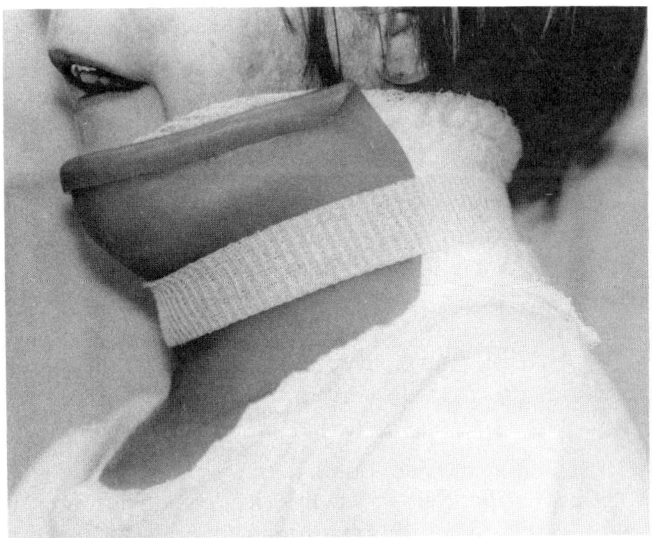

FIGURE 11–4. Neck splint custom-made from thermoplastic material.

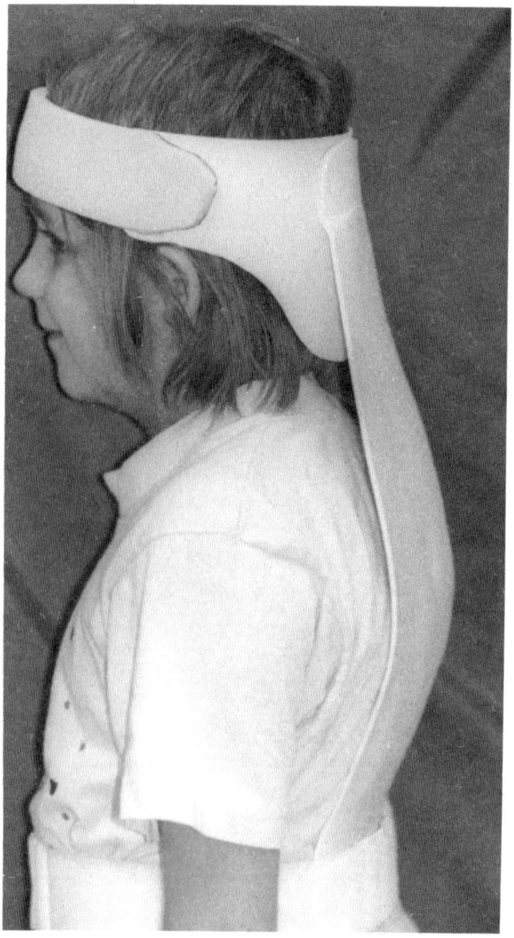

FIGURE 11–5. Custom-designed halo neck splint.

Advantages

- Used in any phase of treatment (more commonly for wounds or grafts treated with the open method).
- Permits visualization of wound.
- Allows frequent care of new skin grafts.

Disadvantages

- Contraindicated if deep burns present over forehead—strapping wound have potential to cause wound breakdown.
- Does not prevent shortening of the anterior neck secondary to opening of the mouth.
- Can be uncomfortable when patient is supine and cause skin breakdown over spinous processes in very thin patients.

Watusi Collar[20,21] (Fig. 11–6)

Description. Series of cylindrical plastic or foam tubes fastened circumferentially around the neck. Additional tubes are added as neck extension improves.

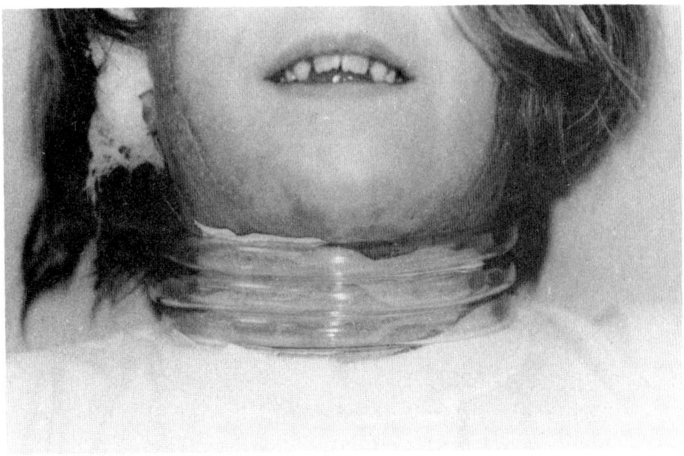

FIGURE 11–6. Watusi collar made from plastic tubes.

Advantages

- More commonly used in scar control but can be applied over a simple dressing.
- Applies good contact pressure.
- Easily adjusted.
- Maintains extension; prevents lateral flexion.

Disadvantages

- Occlusive—frequent monitoring needed for signs of maceration or wound deterioration.
- Can produce a ridged effect in scar tissue between the rings of the collar.
- Allergies to certain materials, such as latex, should be considered.

Philadelphia Collar (Fig. 11–7)

Description. Prefabricated, circumferential, foam positioning orthosis.

Advantages

- Commercially available (Appendix F).
- Easily applied.

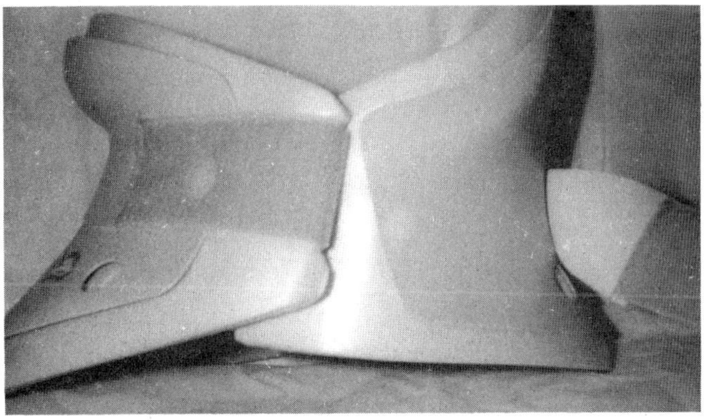

FIGURE 11–7. Philadelphia collar used for positioning neck.

Disadvantages
- For temporary use only—fit is rarely adequate.
- Occlusive.
- Only minimal dressing can be worn under collar.

Ears

Anticipated deformity: Folding of helix
Secondary problems: Auricular chondritis; excessive pressure to damaged ear

Semirigid Oxygen Mask (Fig. 11–8)
Description. Plastic oxygen mask placed over the ear and secured in position with elastic strap around head. (For pediatric use—half of bulb from bulb syringe can be substituted.)

Advantages
- Easily available and applied.
- Protects by acting as a dome over entire ear.
- Dressings applied not restricted by use.
- Used in acute care to avoid pressure.
- Used after skin grafting to prevent shear or pressure to graft.

Disadvantage
- Can be held in place with tracheostomy tape or surgical mask but position is difficult to maintain.

Mouth

Anticipated deformities: Microstomia; ectropion of upper and/or lower lips
Secondary problems: Decreased mandibular excursion both horizontally and vertically; difficulty in mastication; altered speech; drooling, may affect adjacent facial units; hazardous or impossible oral intubation

MPA—Microstomia Prevention Appliance (Fig. 11–9)
Description. Prefabricated oral orthosis used to preserve horizontal mouth opening. Acrylic endpieces fit in commissures of mouth and distance between the ends is shortened or lengthened by adjusting the sliding metal portion.

Advantages
- Commercially available (Appendix F).
- Easily applied and fitted.
- Adjustable by patient for progressive stretch.
- Variation fabricated by therapist.[24] (Fig. 11–10)

Disadvantages
- Must be removed for eating.
- Drooling is a problem.

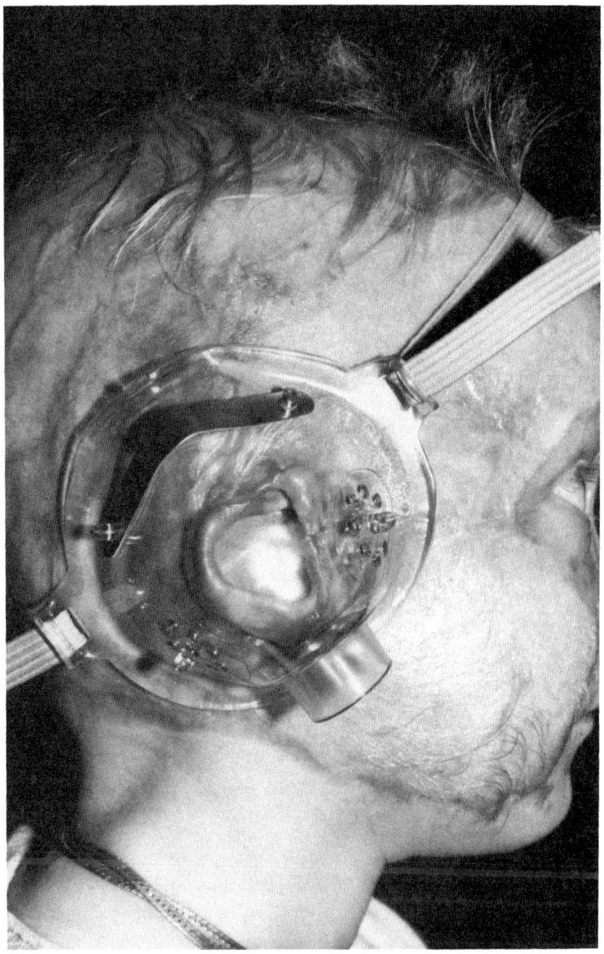

FIGURE 11–8. Semi-rigid oxygen mask used to protect tissue of burned ear from pressure.

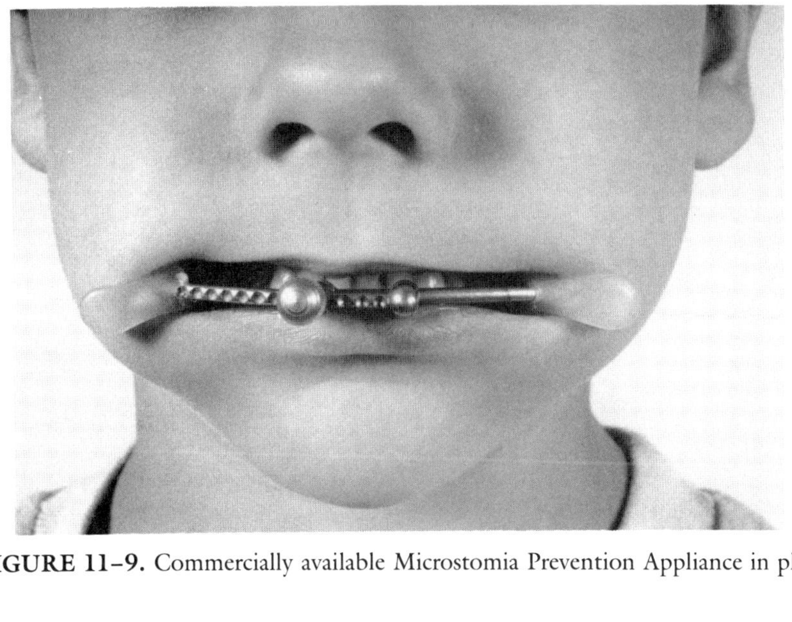

FIGURE 11–9. Commercially available Microstomia Prevention Appliance in place.

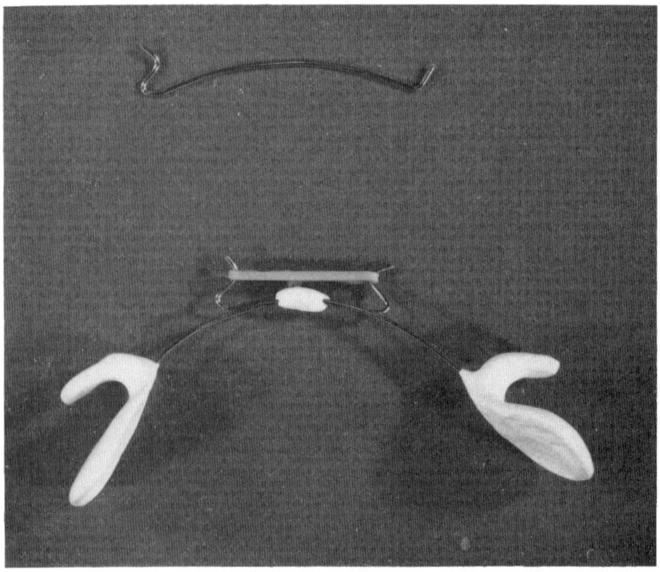

FIGURE 11–10. Microstomia prevention splint fabricated from stainless steel wire, thermoplastic material, and rubber band. Bends and curve of wire illustrated. Low cost. Not recommended for children.

- Expensive—but can be gas-sterilized for multiple patient use.
- Should not be used in small children—risk of choking if displaced.

External Traction Hooks (Fig. 11–11)

Description. Acrylic hooks that conform to a patient's commissures are attached to a molded neck collar with surgical tubing to apply horizontal pressure.

Advantages

- Fabrication using low- or high-temperature thermoplastics.
- Easily applied.
- Tension can be adjusted by patient for progressive stretch.
- Permits speech.

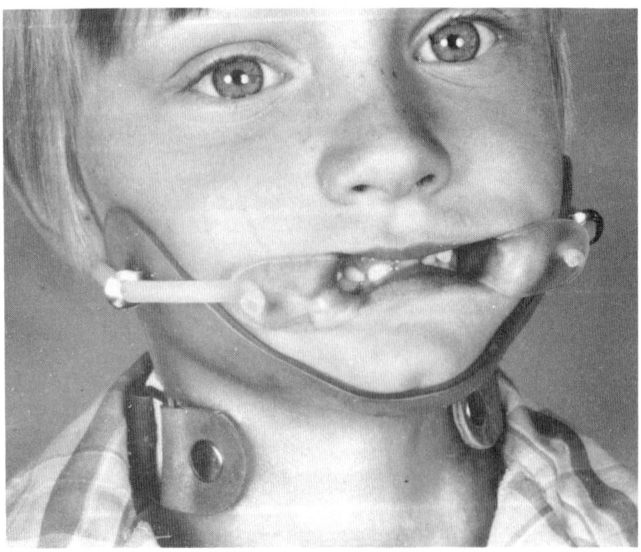

FIGURE 11–11. Acrylic hooks used to apply horizontal traction to the mouth via surgical tubing attached to a neck brace.

Disadvantages

- Drooling is frequently a problem.
- Can cause excessive pressure at commissures.
- Easily removed by young children.

Orthodontic Commissure Appliance (Fig. 11–12)

Description. Custom-fabricated commissure orthosis similar to a denture plate; "wings" on appliance statically retain the commissures of mouth.

Advantages

- Fixed style attached to the teeth or removable like an upper denture plate.
- More cosmetically acceptable than some other types of mouth appliances.
- Best for ages 6 years and younger.[25]

Disadvantages

- Requires custom dental fabrication.
- Must be applied before microstomia is developed or immediately following reconstruction.

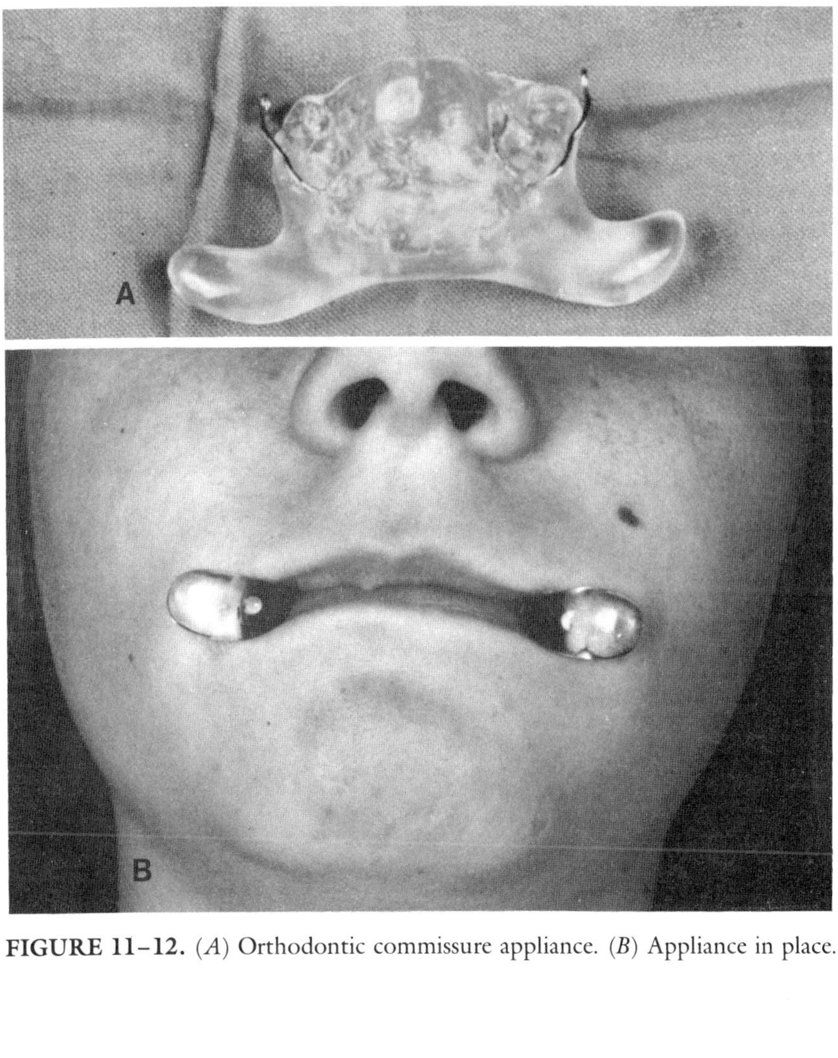

FIGURE 11–12. (*A*) Orthodontic commissure appliance. (*B*) Appliance in place.

Axillae and Anterior Chest

Anticipated deformities: Shoulder adduction, extension, and internal rotation
Secondary problem: Development of kyphosis

Axillary or Airplane Splint or Conformer[20,21] (Fig. 11–13)

Description. Thermoplastic splint for immobilization or serial splinting of the shoulder. The splint is placed on the lateral trunk and extends from above the anterior superior iliac spine to at least the elbow.

Advantages

- Used in any phase of burn treatment to maintain shoulder abduction with slight horizontal adduction.
- Can be fabricated as a conforming splint or open frame, supporting the extremity distally and at the hip, joined by a connecting bar.
- Formed on patient.
- Distributes pressure along length of splint.
- Can include elbow and wrist.

Disadvantages

- Reinforcement may be required to support arm.
- Must strap or wrap securely to avoid pressure points on distal ends of splint or rotation of splint.

Shoulder Abduction Brace[20] (Fig. 11–14)

Description. Prefabricated metal orthosis for positioning of the shoulder; attaches to the waist and supports the arm.

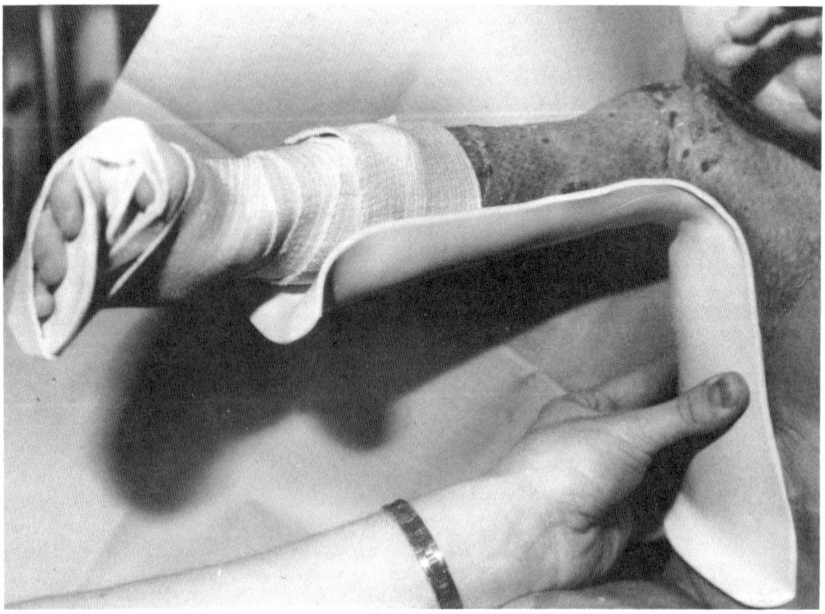

FIGURE 11–13. Axillary or airplane splint used to position right shoulder in 90° abduction.

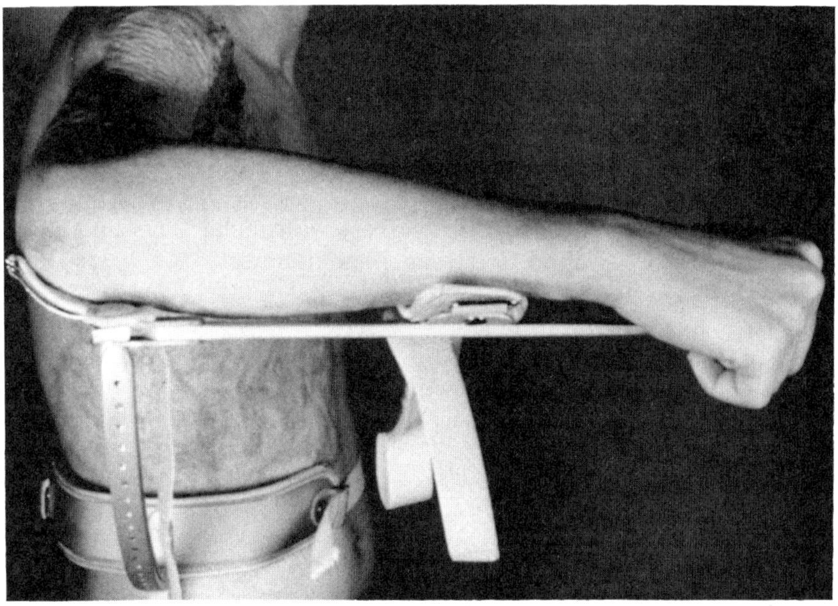

FIGURE 11–14. Shoulder abduction brace with forearm platform positions shoulder while leaving axilla exposed.

Advantages

- Commercially available (Appendix F).
- Adjustable.
- Usually metal; can be cleaned and reused on different patients.
- Includes elbow and wrist support.

Disadvantages

- Expensive.
- Must be strapped or wrapped securely around torso to avoid pressure points or rotation of brace. A small pad placed under the elbow when the patient is supine prevents anterior displacement of shoulder.
- Some limitation in size.

Clavicle Strap or Brace[20,21] (see Fig. 11–3)

Description. Prefabricated or custom-fabricated foam support that maintains the shoulders in retraction through a figure-of-8 design and applies pressure to the anterior and posterior axillary folds.

Advantages

- Commercially available (Appendix F).
- Adjustable.
- Used to apply gentle pressure to healed axilla.
- Can be used to hold pressure insert in place.
- Minimizes protraction of shoulders.

Disadvantages

- Can constrict circulation to the upper extremities in select individuals.
- Can cause chaffing or irritation of the anterior axilla.
- Can be bulky under clothing.

Back Brace or Spinal Support[26] (Fig. 11–15)

Description. Corset-type design; fabric vest with metal stays intended to limit the amount of postural deviation from scar tissue tightness.

Advantages

- Commercially available (Appendix F).
- Minimizes kyphotic posture.

Disadvantages

- Some models are difficult to apply.
- Bulky.

Elbow and Knee

Anticipated deformities: Flexion; pronation
Secondary problems: Possible ulnar nerve compression; possible peroneal nerve compression; lack of forearm supination

Gutter or Trough Splint (Fig. 11–16)

Description. A trough- or gutter-shaped splint applied to the flexor surface of the joint to maintain extension.

Advantages

- Nonconforming.
- Freeform fabrication—basic splint shape is formed without applying material to the patient.
- Can be applied in operating room over bulky dressings.

Disadvantages

- Edges must be flared to prevent pressure points.
- May rotate on extremity.

Elbow or Knee Conformer[20,21]

Description. A conforming splint applied to the flexor or extensor surface of a joint for immobilization, serial splinting, or application of pressure.

Advantages

- Formed on patient.
- Used in serial splinting; remolded to accommodate gains in ROM.
- Distributes pressure along length of splint.

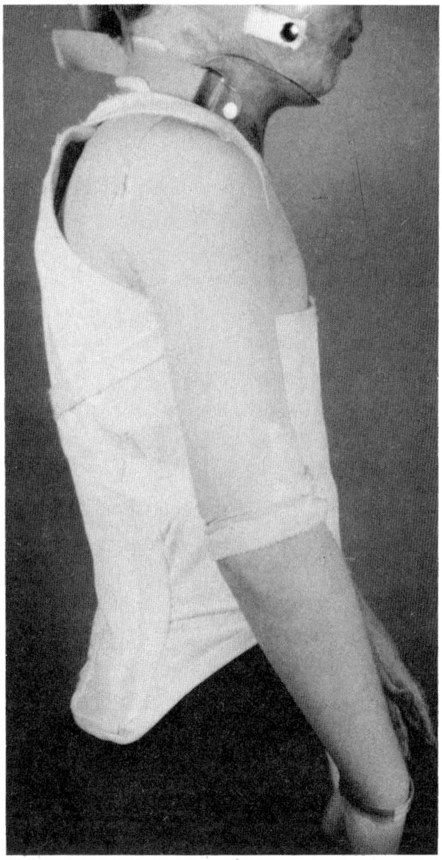

FIGURE 11–15. One type of spinal support brace used to correct trunk postural deviation.

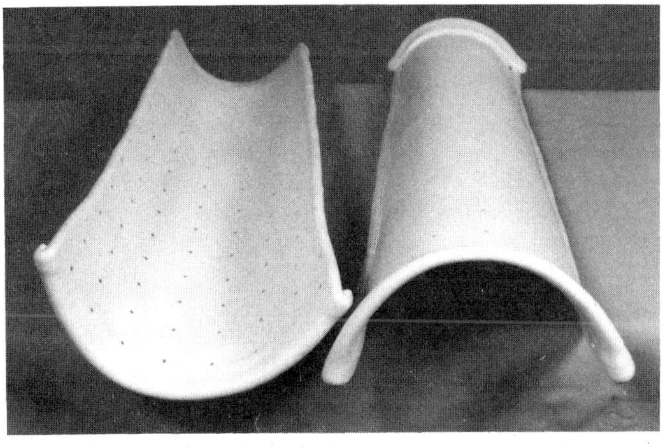

FIGURE 11–16. Gutter or trough splint to maintain joint extension.

Disadvantage
- Potential for peroneal nerve compression. Relieving or generously flaring splint over fibular head decreases risk.

Three-Point Splint[20] (Fig. 11–17)

Description. An adjustable splint that uses three points of pressure. Cuffs above and below the joint and a pad on the extensor surface of the joint increases extension.

Advantages
- Commercially available (Appendix F).
- Limits contact with flexor surface.
- Adjusts to accommodate increased extension.
- Used for elbows, knees, and IP joints of fingers.

Disadvantages
- Three points of direct pressure; can cause pressure areas.[27]
- Not effective for contractures greater than 45°.

Spiral Extension Splint (Fig. 11–18)

Description. A strip of thermoplastic material spirals around the limb so the top and bottom portions secure the flexor surface of the limb. The center of the splint applies pressure to the extensor surface of the joint. Splint can be used to increase extension of the elbow, knee, or digits of hand.

Advantages
- Simple design which easily can immobilize the elbow, knee, or IP joints of fingers.
- Common pressure points can be avoided.
- Requires minimal outer wrap to secure.

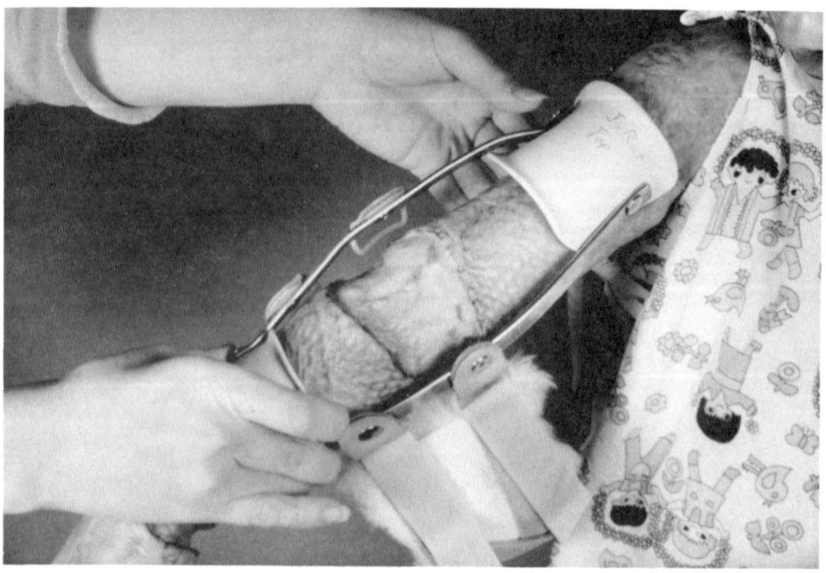

FIGURE 11–17. Three-point splint for right elbow extension. Graft over antecubital space is left exposed.

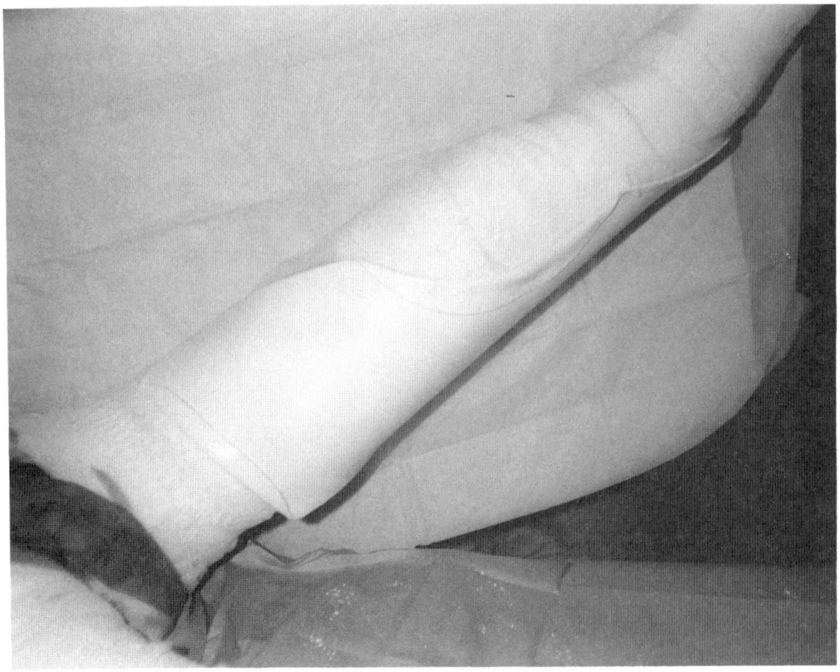

FIGURE 11–18. A type of spiral splint looped around the left upper extremity to promote elbow extension.

Disadvantage

- Can rotate out of place.

Air Splint[28] (Fig. 11–19)

Description. Transparent appliance constructed of two layers of plastic that provides immobilization and compression when inflated.

Advantages

- Commercially available for pediatric and adult (Appendix F).
- Available for upper and lower extremities.
- Provides total contact and circumferential pressure.
- Transparent and reusable.
- May assist with edema control in the acute and rehabilitation phases of treatment.

Disadvantage

- Occlusive; tissue must be monitored for maceration.

Hip and Perineal Area

Anticipated deformities: Flexion; adduction
Secondary problems: Altered gait pattern; difficulty with straddle position

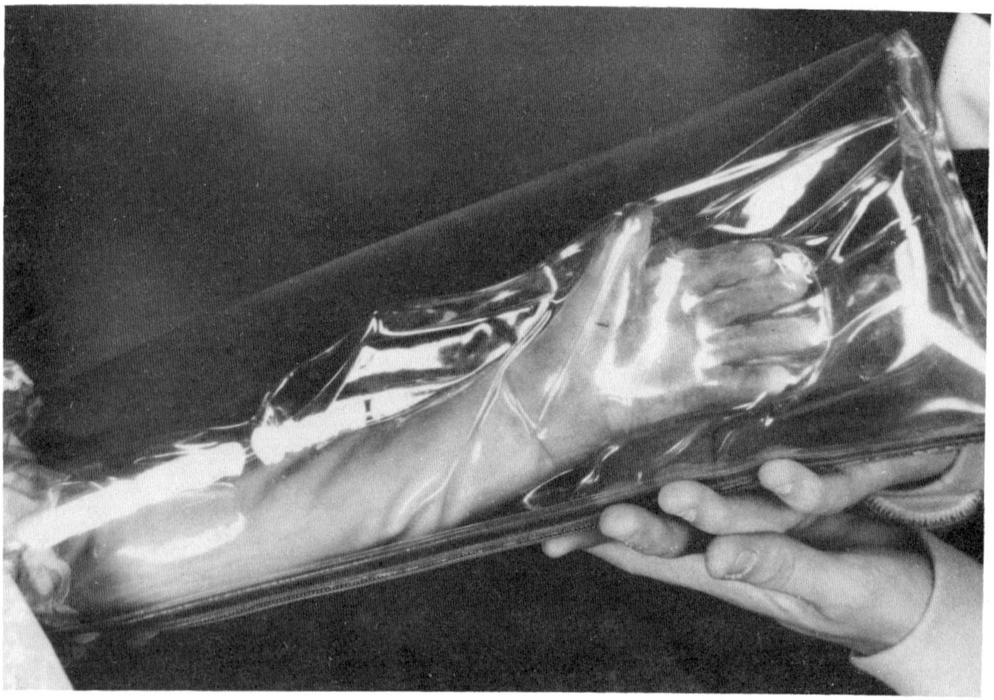

FIGURE 11–19. Air splint inflated to apply pressure to left hand and forearm.

Anterior Hip Spica (Fig. 11–20)

Description. Appliance intended to promote hip extension by blocking hip flexion. Thermoplastic material is molded on the patient from the midabdomen and extending over the anterior thighs to the knees. Straps or elastic bandages, which secure the splint, cross the buttocks to further limit flexion.

Advantages

- Used to maintain extension of one or both hips.
- Applies stretch to hip flexion contractures.
- Used postgrafting to immobilize hip in presence of anterior skin grafts.

Disadvantages

- Can be difficult to secure; requires a figure-of-8 or hip spica wrap around upper thigh and waist.
- Used only when patient is recumbent.
- Potential for pressure area over anterior superior iliac spine may require padding.

Abduction Splint (Fig. 11–21)

Description. Hip abduction is achieved through the use of thermoplastic cuffs applied to the medial and posterior aspects of the thighs and separated with a thermoplastic bar posteriorly.

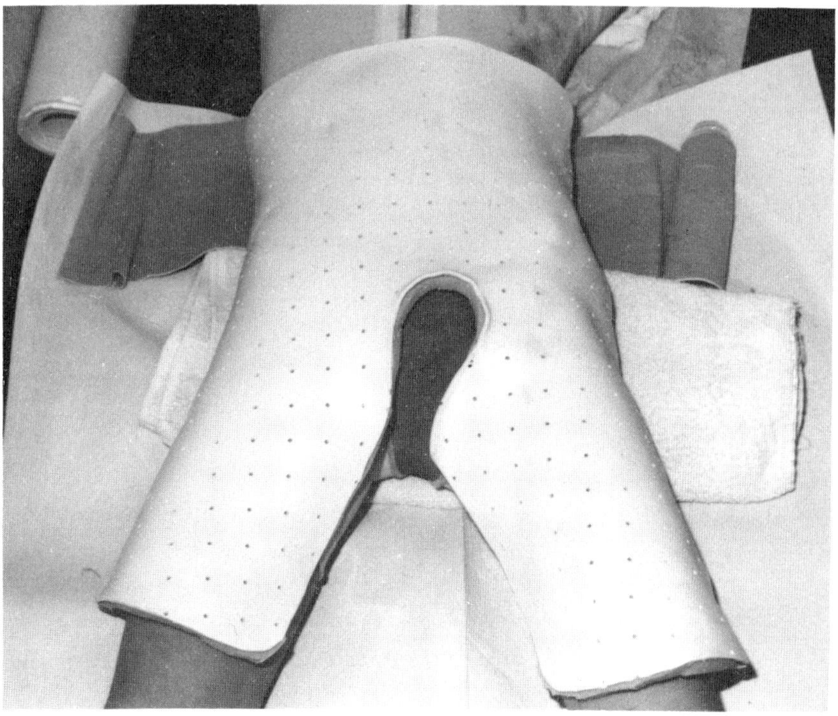

FIGURE 11–20. Anterior hip spica splint made from thermoplastic material to maintain hip extension and abduction while preventing hip flexion and adduction.

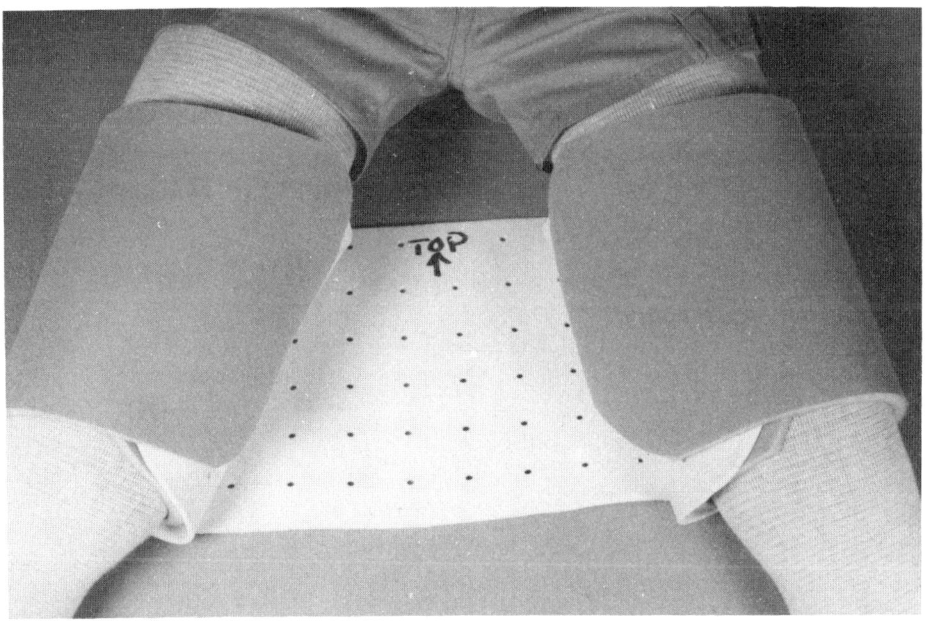

FIGURE 11–21. Hip abduction splint made from thermoplastic material and secured in place with foam straps.

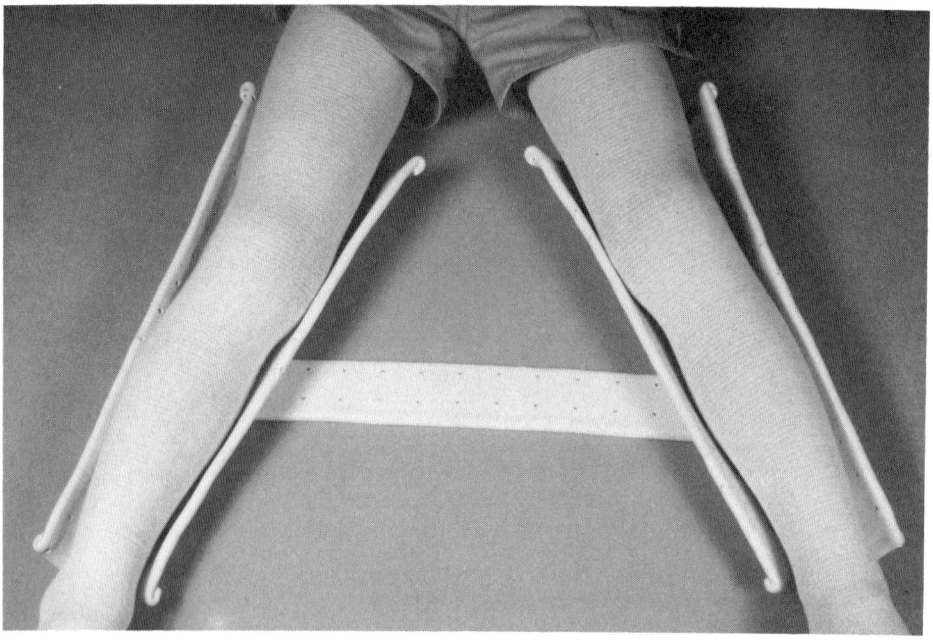

FIGURE 11–22. Spreader bar attached to knee extension gutter splints to maintain abduction of the lower extremities.

Advantages
- Freeform or molded on patient.
- Placement above knee prevents adduction of hips should the patient's knees become flexed.

Disadvantages
- Must be padded for comfort.
- A very active patient can rotate out of splint.

Spreader Bar (Fig. 11–22)

Description. A bar fastened posteriorly to two knee extension splints maintains hip abduction and limits hip flexion.

Advantages
- Metal or thermoplastic bar.
- Bar can be attached to thermoplastic cuffs above knee or to knee extension splints.

Disadvantage
- A very active patient can rotate out of splint.

Ankle

Anticipated deformities: Dorsiflexion; plantar flexion
Secondary problems: Shortening of Achilles tendon; equinus deformity; altered gait pattern

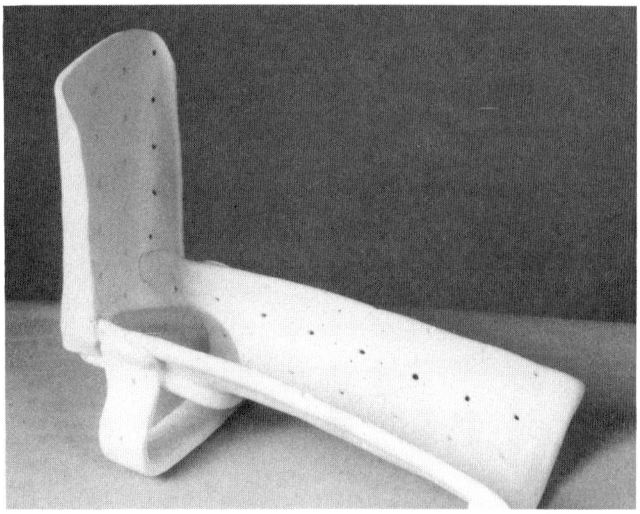

FIGURE 11–23. Posterior foot drop splint—nonconforming. Heel section cut away to relieve pressure and stand applied to splint to elevate heel off bed.

Posterior Foot Drop Splint (Fig. 11–23)

Description. Trough splint with attached footplate positions and immobilizes the ankle at neutral.

Advantages

- Freeformed from patient measurements. (See section in Basic Burn Splints)
- Calf trough may be lengthened to include knee.
- Maintains functional position of ankle.

Disadvantages

- Requires careful and generous flaring of the heel area to minimize potential for tissue breakdown.
- Potential for tissue breakdown exists over the metatarsal head of the fifth toe if the patient resists the splint and pushes against the footplate.

Posterior Ankle Conformer[20,21] (Fig. 11–24)

Description. Molded to the posterior aspect of the patient's leg and foot; conforming construction makes this splint useful in serial splinting.

Advantages

- Form fitted to follow line of posterior calf, heel, and foot.
- Maintains functional position of ankle.
- Prevents shortening of Achilles tendon.

Disadvantages

- *Precaution:* Heel must be monitored for signs of excessive pressure. Pressure is reduced by expanding the portion of the splint directly over the heel or by cutting an opening and flaring the material away from heel.
- Not used in ambulation.

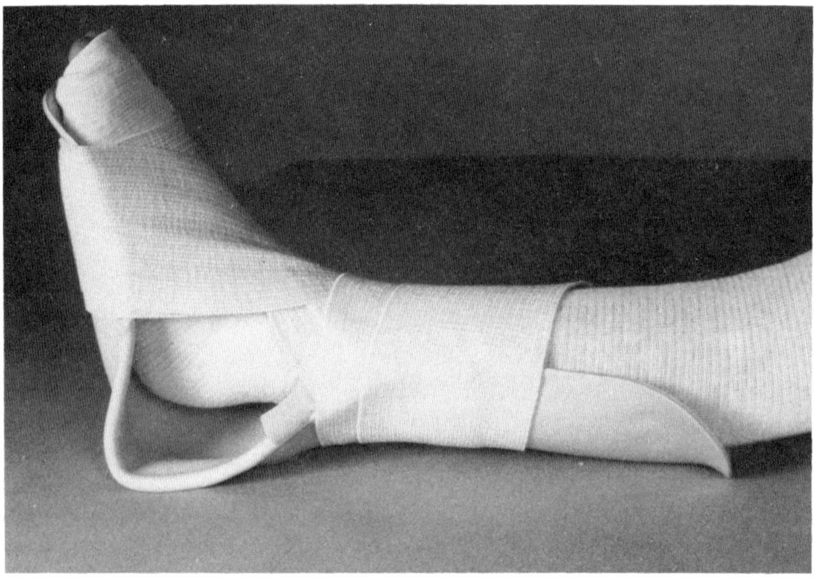

FIGURE 11–24. Posterior ankle conformer with heel section flared away for pressure relief. The splint is secured with an elastic bandage.

Anterior Ankle Conformer (Fig. 11–25)

Description. Splint is molded to the anterior aspect of the patient's leg and foot. A long lever arm along the leg is required to support the foot.

Advantages

- Form fitted to follow line of anterior leg, ankle, and foot.
- Maintains functional position of ankle without exerting rigid pressure to heel.

Disadvantages

- Pressure point can develop over anterior ankle.
- Can be difficult to secure.

High-Top Gym Shoe[20] (Fig. 11–26)

Description: Commercial high-top gym shoe in which the sole has been adapted to minimize toe-off.

Advantages

- Commercially available.
- May require additional padding or liner (slightly larger size should be purchased to accommodate padding or dressings).
- Gives gentle support to ankle during ambulation.
- Can be used to hold simple pressure inserts in place to prevent hyperextension of toes.
- Can be filled or lined with silicone elastomer or prosthetic foam (helpful to patients who have amputations of the distal foot).
- Can add metatarsal rolloff to sole to reduce toe movement during ambulation.

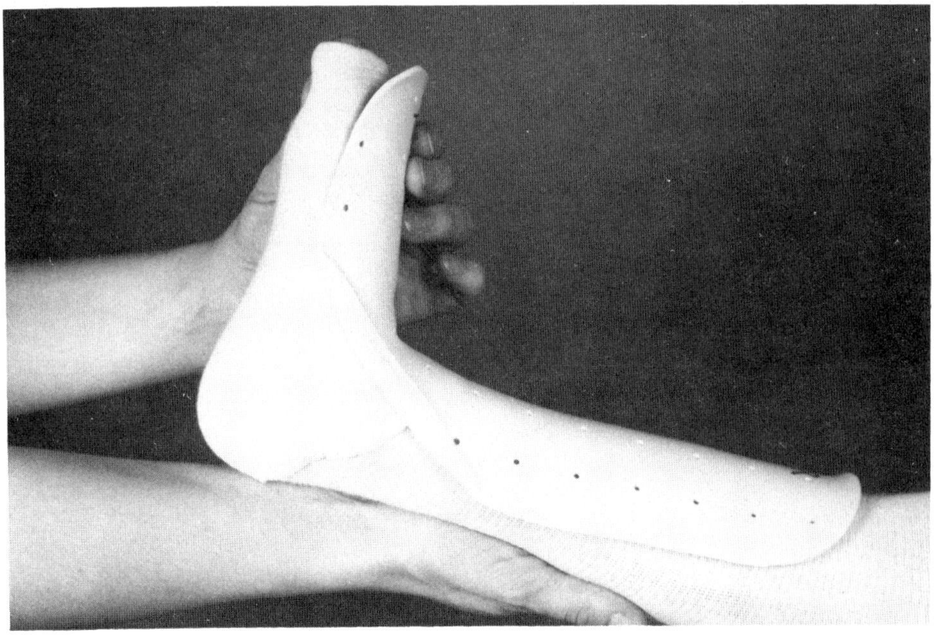

FIGURE 11–25. Anterior ankle conformer applied to patient's right lower extremity.

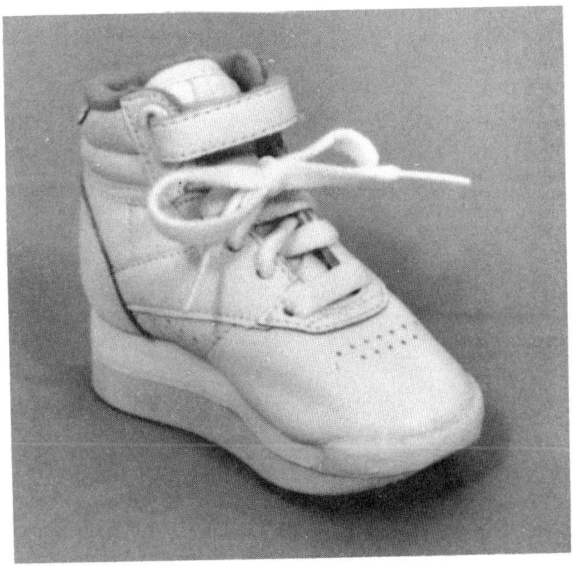

FIGURE 11–26. High-top gym shoe with metatarsal roll-off added to sole of shoe.

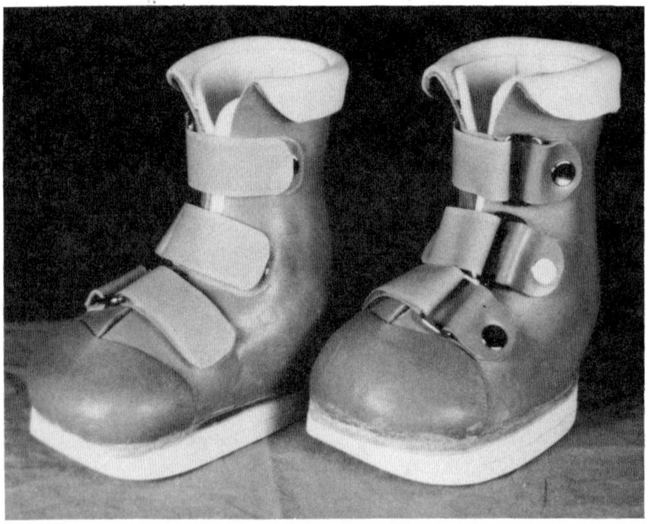

FIGURE 11–27. Custom-made molded leather shoes with foam lining, Velcro closure, and metatarsal roll-off on soles.

Disadvantage

- Does not maintain optimal ankle position.

Molded Leather Shoe[29] (Fig. 11–27)

Description. A total contact custom-fabricated leather shoe that limits foot motion and is adapted to minimize toe-off.

Advantages

- Light weight.
- Continuous ankle positioning.
- Applies circumferential pressure to the ankle and foot since it is custom fabricated from a positive mold of the leg and foot.
- Metatarsal rolloff and slight "give" of the leather allow an acceptable gait.

Disadvantage

- Can be expensive.

Foot

Anticipated deformities: Flexion or hyperextension of the metatarsophalangeal joints; flexion of the IP joints of the toes; metatarsal adduction or inversion in small children

Secondary problems: Altered gait pattern; distortion of foot arch; inability to wear regular shoes

Toe Conformer (Fig. 11–28)

Description. Conforming orthosis molded to the dorsal surface of foot to minimize extension of toes. Design does not limit standing or motion of ankle.

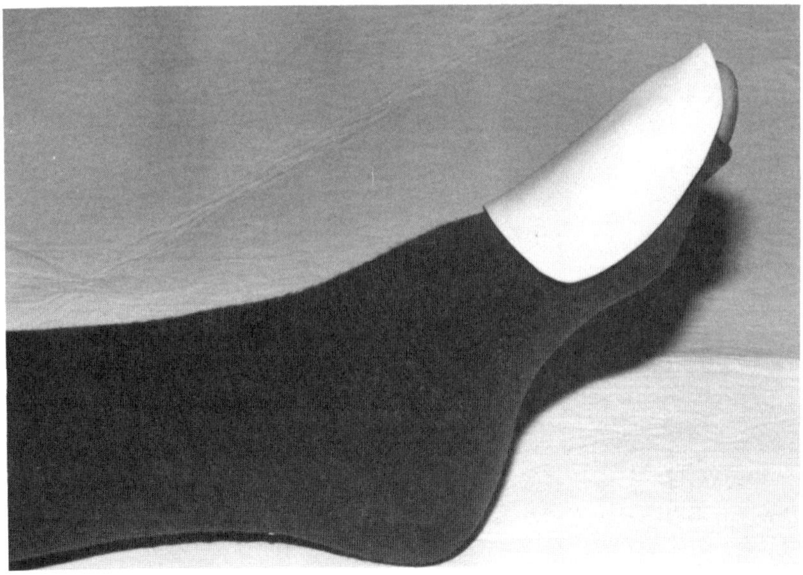

FIGURE 11–28. Toe conformer splint shaped to cover the dorsal surface of toes to prevent hyperextension. Can be secured with cohesive wrap or elastic bandage.

Advantages

- Applies consistent pressure to anterior surface.
- Can be used for night wear or under soft shoes to apply definitive pressure to contracting scar.
- Amount of pressure applied can be varied by changing outer wrap or straps.

Disadvantage

- Shearing can be a problem during ambulation unless the shoe includes a metatarsal rolloff to reduce toe movement.

Hand and Wrist

Anticipated deformities: Extension or hyperextension of the MCP joints; flexion of the IP joints; boutonniere deformity; adduction and flexion of the thumb; flexion or extension of the wrist

Secondary problems: Radial/ulnar deviation; abduction of the little finger; flattening of the palmar arches; finger adduction with syndactyle; extension of the IP joint of the thumb

Safe Position, Antideformity or Palmar Pan Splint[20,21] (Fig. 11–29)

Description. Palmar-based thermoplastic splint that positions the joints opposite of the anticipated deformity or contracture.

Advantages

- Maintains tendon balance and functional position.
- Prevents rupture of extensor mechanism.
- "All-purpose" splint for hand burns requiring protective splinting.

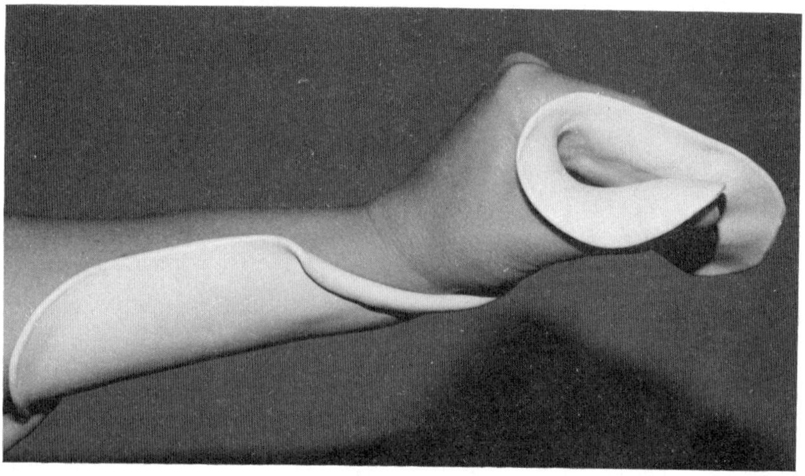

FIGURE 11–29. Antideformity hand splint positions MCP's in maximal flexion, IP's in extension, and thumb in palmar abduction.

- Should be used with a minimum of dressing bulk to maintain joint alignment.
- Maintains transverse arch of hand.

Disadvantage

- Has tendency to slip distally and must be securely applied.

Wrist Splint[20,21] (Fig. 11–30)

Description. Wrist orthosis for immobilization and positioning. Ends at or proximal to the proximal metacarpal crease of the hand.

Advantages

- Dorsal or palmar base.
- Can be used to immobilize wrist in flexion or extension.

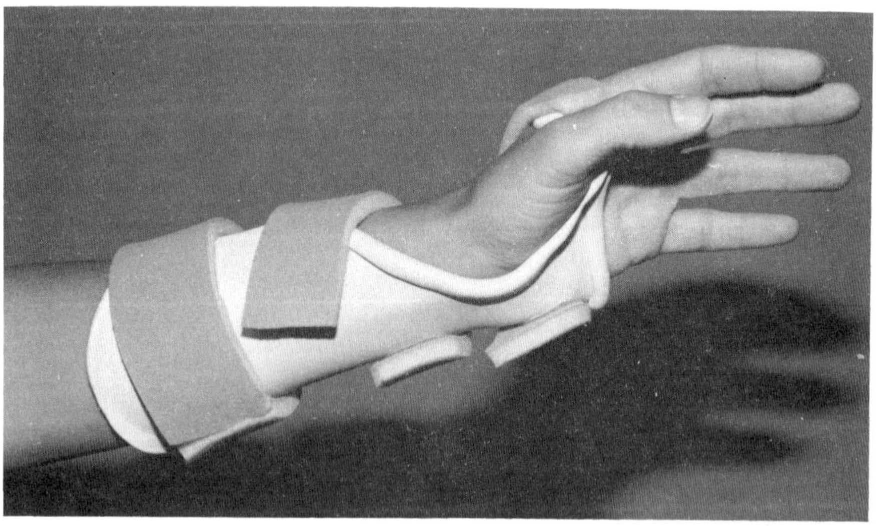

FIGURE 11–30. Wrist splint maintains wrist in extension while fingers are free to move.

- Stabilizes wrist but permits full use of fingers.
- Can be utilized in any phase of treatment when immobilization or sustained stretch is required.

Disadvantage

- Tendency to slip distally.

Thumb Spica[20] (Fig. 11–31)

Description. Orthosis for immobilization and positioning the thumb and wrist.

Advantages

- Positions wrist and thumb.
- If thumb is placed in a functional position, hand can be used in ADLs without removing splint.
- If palmar contracture is developing, splint is utilized to apply sustained stretch to thumb in radial abduction.

Disadvantage

- Tendency to slip distally.

Thumb Web Spacer[15,21] (Fig. 11–32)

Description. Thermoplastic splint that conforms to the index finger, thumb web space, and thumb to provide positioning and/or pressure.

Advantages

- Conforming.
- Used in serial splinting; remolded to accommodate gains in ROM of the carpometacarpal joint of thumb.
- The index finger may be incorporated to provide an adequate stretch to the thumb web.

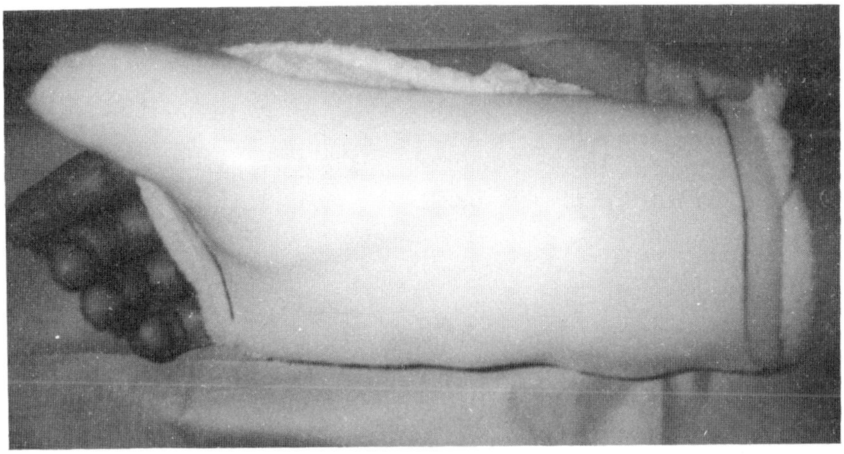

FIGURE 11–31. Thumb positioned between palmar and radial abduction with a thumb spica splint.

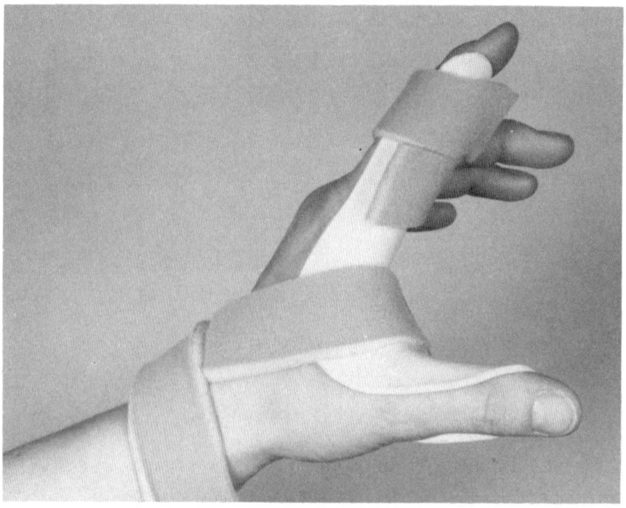

FIGURE 11–32. Thermoplastic splint conformed along index finger and thumb to preserve thumb web space. Splint is held in place with foam straps.

Disadvantage

- Care is required to avoid stretching the ulnar collateral ligament[15] by applying force to the web space rather than to the phalanx.

Palmar or Dorsal Extension Splint[20,30] (Fig. 11–33)

Description. Thermoplastic splint for extension of all digits and to provide stretch to the palmar surface of hand.

Advantages

- Best used with burns restricted to the palmar surface.
- Applies sustained stretch to healing wound or developing scar.
- Immobilizes hand in extension at all joints; children tolerate hyperextension of the MCP joints very well.
- Maintains web spaces.

Disadvantage

- Tendency to slip distally unless wrapped securely.

Traction Splint[20] (Fig. 11–34)

Description. Palmarly based splint with an extended finger section to accommodate finger traction. MCP joints may be flexed or extended.

Advantages

- Designed to immobilize hand following skin grafting of dorsal surface.
- With fingernail traction in place, grafts of the dorsal surface can be treated by open technique.
- Splint is secured distally by traction to fingertips and proximally by circular gauze wrap at the wrist.
- Traction to the fingernails can be accomplished by sutures through the nail or fingerpulp or by dressmaker's hooks glued to the nails.

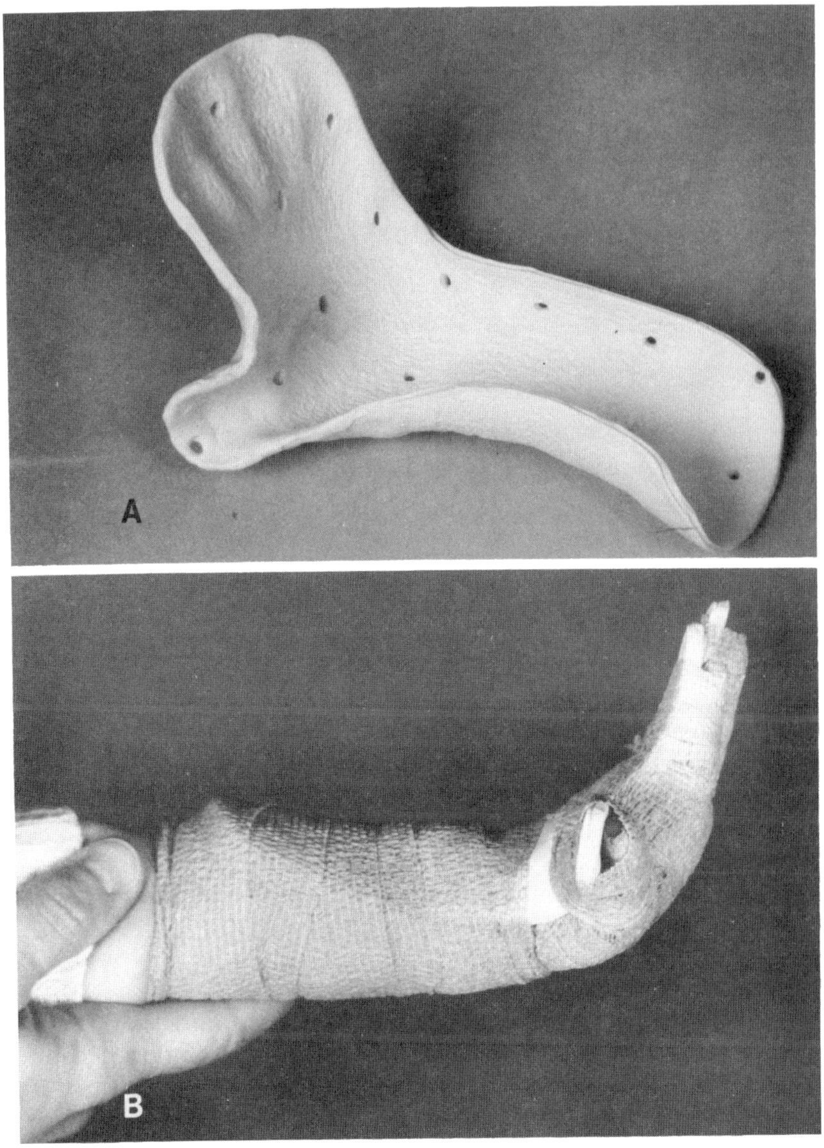

FIGURE 11–33. (*A*) Palmar extension splint for right hand. (*B*) Dorsal extension splint with padding and secured with cohesive wrap.

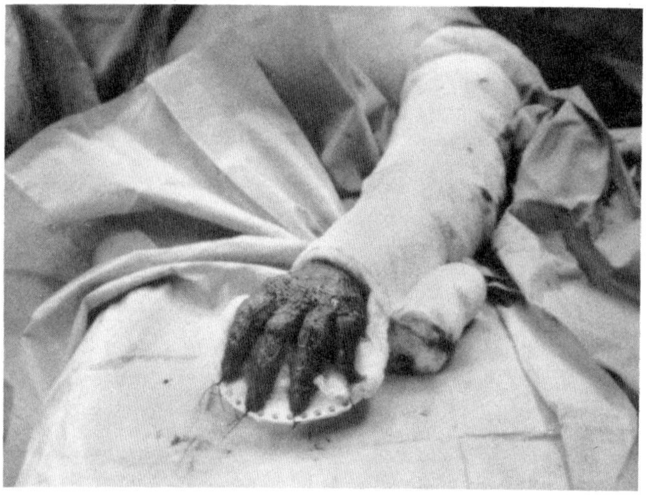

FIGURE 11–34. Traction splint—post mesh skin grafting. Finger traction is applied by rubber bands attached to dress hooks on fingernails and secured to end of splint.

Disadvantage

- Frequent monitoring is required when using dress hooks to avoid avulsion of the fingernail, particularly if the splint shifts distally.

Halo Hand Splint[20] (Fig. 11–35)

Description. Intraoperative or postoperative splint includes a forearm base with a circular outrigger to which the digits are attached by sutures through the fingernails or pulp of each fingertip.

Advantages

- Permits access to both surfaces following skin grafting when circumferential grafting is performed.
- Traction to fingers can be by suture loop or Kirschner wires.

Disadvantage

- May require use of an elbow splint (flexion) to stabilize and prevent shifting of the splint distally.

Flexion Glove (Fig. 11–36)

Description. Glove in which the digits are maintained in flexion through elastic or hook attachment of the finger sleeves to the wrist portion of glove. Requires cooperation of the patient to be effective.

Advantages

- Commercially available.
- Useful in applying sustained stretch to dorsal scar.
- Easily applied by patient for intermittent use.
- Tension applied is adjusted easily.

Disadvantages

- May require stabilization of wrist.
- Potential for pressure points over the MCP and PIP joints.

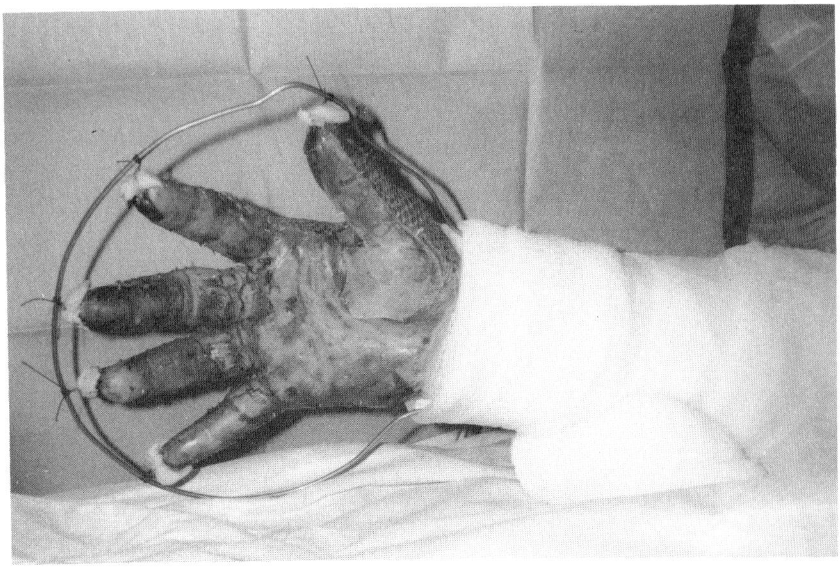

FIGURE 11–35. Halo hand splint made from wire outrigger attached to thermoplastic forearm base. Fingers attached to wire by sutures. Splint is secured with roll gauze and hand is left open to air.

Sandwich Splint[21,31] (Fig. 11–37)

Description. The hand is sandwiched between two layers of thermoplastic material, lined with foam, to maintain position of the digits.

Advantages

- Flat or bivalve construction.
- Distributes pressure over entire area, not only where straps are anchored.
- Design reduces chance of splint displacement with young children.

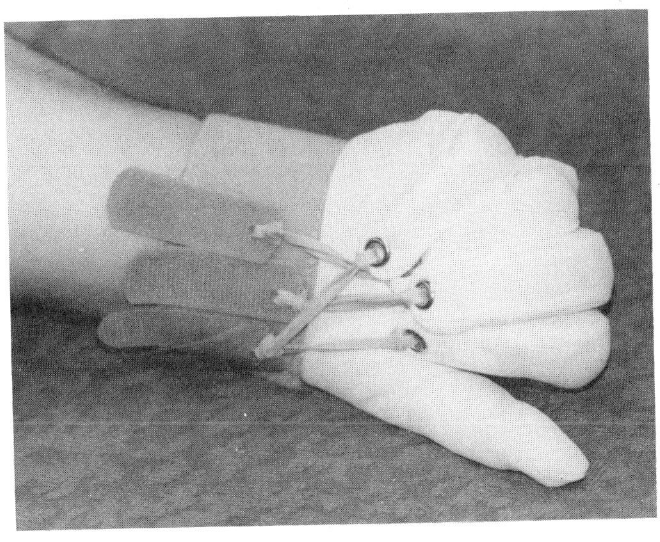

FIGURE 11–36. Commercially available flexion glove assists with finger flexion through elastic traction.

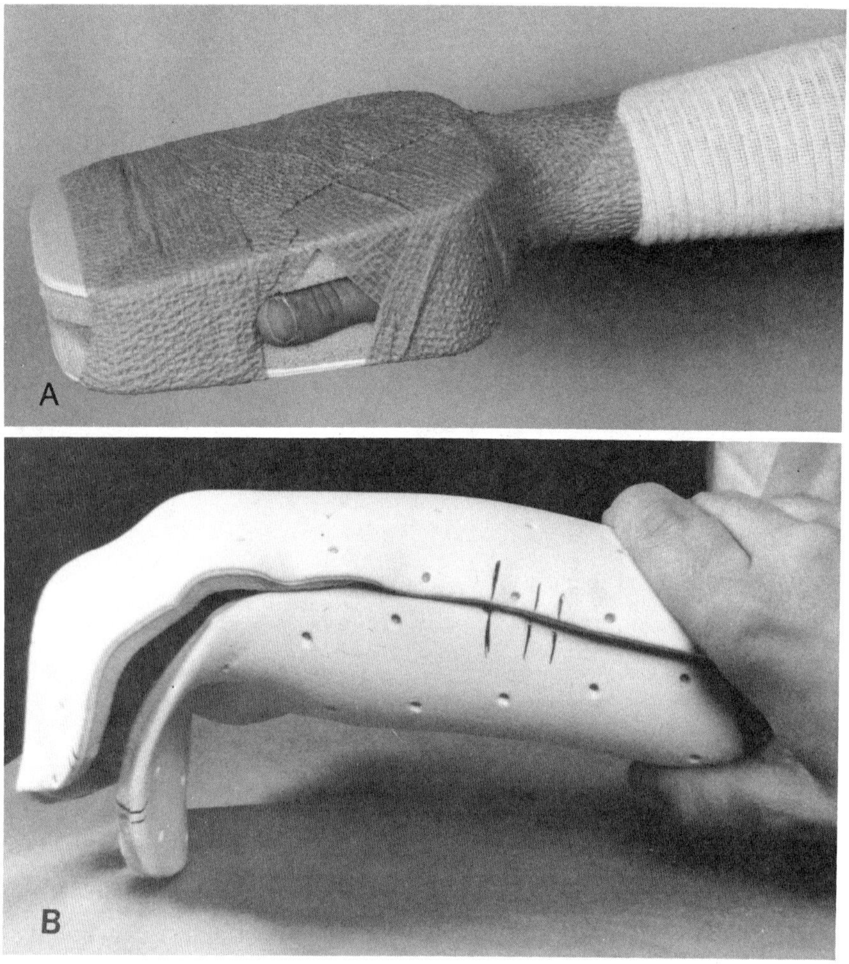

FIGURE 11–37. (*A*) Sandwich splint secured with cohesive wrap to maintain extension of digits. (*B*) Bivalved sandwich splint to maintain fingers in flexed position. Marks on both halves of splint are aligned for proper application of splint.

Disadvantage

- Potential for pressure points over dorsum of hand—foam padding required.

WEARING SCHEDULE—GUIDELINES FOR DURATION OF USE

Continuous Use

PROTECTION OF JOINTS OR TENDONS AT RISK

Splints can prevent further trauma to joints and tendons or preserve anatomical structure and function. Stabilizing joints reduces external stresses, such as shearing or pressure, which can cause tissue damage.

EXPOSED JOINTS

The joint is placed in a functional position or in a position that reduces stress to periarticular structures. A splint is used at all times, except for dressing changes and therapist-assisted exercises, until permanent tissue coverage of the joint is achieved and stability restored. Internal fixation of the joint by surgeon should be discussed if the patient is uncooperative with the splinting program or if fixation would simplify patient care. Exposed joints may take longer than 6 weeks to become stable.

EXPOSED TENDONS

Tendons are splinted in a relaxed position so tension is avoided to prevent rupture; however, the Achilles tendon is splinted with the ankle in neutral to prevent shortening. A splint is used until permanent coverage of the tendon is achieved and may be removed for wound care and supervised exercise, including ambulation.

FULL-THICKNESS DORSAL HAND BURNS

The hand is splinted with the MCP joints in flexion and the IP joints fully extended to preserve the integrity of the finger's extensor hood mechanism and maintain good tendon balance. Splinting continues until adequate coverage of the extensor mechanism is achieved. To prevent a potential rupture, the splint is removed for wound care and supervised exercise only.

THE UNCOOPERATIVE OR UNCONSCIOUS PATIENT

Splints are used to maintain a functional joint position or prevent contracture development when a patient is unable or unwilling to participate in therapy programs. Adults may develop joint stiffness following immobilization and ROM should be assessed each time the splint is removed. Children rarely develop joint stiffness as a result of prolonged immobilization.[32] Continuous use of a splint assures proper positioning until a patient is able to actively participate in the rehabilitation program or the risk of contracture is reduced.

FOLLOWING SKIN GRAFTING

Splints are applied intraoperatively to immobilize a skin graft recipient site and prevent accidental shearing of the graft. When grafts are restricted to the upper body, splints enable the patient to be ambulatory without risk of graft disruption. Splints are used continuously until graft adherence is assured, at which time they may be used at night only to prevent contracture development.

EDEMA REDUCTION

Supportive splints are used to maintain maximal limb elevation for resolution of edema. Splints used for this purpose are generally of a trough design. Exact contour of the extremity is not always necessary. The pressure support of air splints may assist edema reduction.

REDUCTION OF CONTRACTURES

In the rehabilitation phase of treatment, the development of scar contracture can occur in spite of frequent exercise and the use of gradient pressure garments. Once established, a contracture will restrict joint ROM progressively until met with an opposing force. Serial splinting facilitates the reduction of scar contracture through contact pressure and sustained stretch of the active scar. The scar can be remolded gradually with little or no trauma to the involved tissues in usually less than 2 weeks. Low-temperature splinting materials are used for their ability to be reformed multiple times to accommodate gains in range of an affected joint. Following a period of sustained stretch and exercise, the splint is molded directly over the contracture site to maintain maximal stretch. For optimal results, the splint should extend along the entire length of the contracture, which may span multiple joints. The splint is secured with straps or a compression wrap, if additional pressure is required, such as an elastic bandage or cohesive wrap. A thin layer of elastomer can be applied over the scar to provide definitive contact and pressure under the splint. The use of elastomer should be discontinued if evidence of scar maceration or wound breakdown is noted. The splint is left in place for 24 to 48 hours. The same splint is re-formed and the process is repeated until full joint ROM is achieved. Since the splint remains in place for a prescribed period of time, this method of treatment should not be used over large open wounds. Wounds underlying the splint should be free from infection and able to be managed with a simple petroleum jelly gauze dressing. Once full joint mobility is achieved, a static splint that maintains the end position of the range is fabricated. Initially, the splint should be removed only to allow bathing and self-care. Wearing time is reduced gradually as scar maturation occurs and normal joint function returns. Splints are revised frequently as a scar remodels and contracture decreases.

Intermittent Use

TO MAINTAIN GAINS IN RANGE OF MOTION

Splints are applied to patients who are active participants in their therapy program but require assistance to maintain gains in ROM achieved through exercise or sustained stretch. The involved joint is splinted at the end position of range. Splints are worn during rest periods and at night. They are removed to permit participation in functional activities and exercise.

PATIENT LACKING IN BOTH FLEXION AND EXTENSION OF JOINT

When circumferential involvement of a joint exists, resulting in a patient's inability to fully flex or extend through complete ROM, flexion and extension splints are used alternately to facilitate gains in both directions of motion. Frequent re-evaluation of ROM is necessary to adjust the wearing schedule for each splint.

Use at Night Only

MAINTENANCE OF NORMAL JOINT RANGE

When a patient is cooperative and active during the day, but experiences a loss of ROM at night, splints fabricated to maintain the end position of range will facilitate increased mobility and function in the morning. A splint is applied to maintain stretch during sleep.

OPERATIVE AND POSTOPERATIVE SPLINTING CONSIDERATIONS

Full-thickness burns require excision and skin grafting for wound closure. The success of a grafting procedure is dependent not only on the skills of the surgeon and the quality of the wound bed but also upon adequate postoperative immobilization. Immobilization of the recipient site, especially during the first 48 hours following graft placement, is essential for adherence and vascularization of a graft.

Complete immobilization can be accomplished through the use of bulky restrictive dressings or by splinting of involved joints. Using the drape and trim technique, any body surface or joint(s) can be immobilized quickly and efficiently during an operative procedure without significantly extending anesthesia time. Preoperative planning should give consideration to any potential problems so that time is not wasted should the surgical plan change during surgery.

Area Skin Grafted and Location of Donor Sites

Preplanning the number of splints needed for single or multiple joints will assist the therapist in efficient and timely application of the splints. When heating splint material in a hydrocollator unit, a length of 4- or 6-inch roll gauze can act as a sling to support the material within the unit during the heating process. Because the material does not need to be attended during the heating process, the therapist can complete one splint as the next is being heated. When donor sites are located adjacent to graft sites, splint design should permit access to the donor site.

Type of Dressing Over Skin Graft

If skin grafts are treated in a closed method, covered by dressing material, a splint can be molded directly over the graft site. When a wet dressing will be covering the graft site, a perforated or open-weave splinting material is preferred to permit continuous drainage of excess solutions and prevent graft maceration from solutions pooling under the splint. If grafts are to be treated in an open method, special consideration should be given to how the splint will be secured to prevent the splint from shifting and possibly displacing the graft. By extending the proximal and distal borders, the splint can be secured without covering the recipient site.

Immobilization of Joints

At times, movement of adjacent joints will affect splint position and diminish its effectiveness. If motion of an adjacent joint has the potential to shift the placement of a splint and disrupt a graft, this joint is incorporated into the splinting plan and immobilized in a functional position. Splints applied after skin grafting are for temporary use; therefore, the immobilization of adjacent structures will not effect long-term function. Although a skin graft may not directly cross a joint crease, movement of the joint may cause shearing or displacement of an unstable graft, particularly in the first 48 hours after grafting. For example, a skin graft to the forearm just distal to the antecubital fossa may require splinting of the wrist as well as the elbow to assure complete immobilization. Free movement of the elbow and forearm (flexion, extension and pronation, supination) may create a shearing force between the graft and the dressing over the graft.

Securing the Splint

Dressings or elastic bandages that secure intraoperative splints should be snug but not constrictive. Care must be taken to avoid excessive pressure and possible nerve compression. Extremities should be assessed periodically during the postoperative recovery period for any evidence of neurovascular compromise, such as swelling of tissues distal to surgical dressings, dusky or dark tissue coloration distal to surgical dressings, or patient report of localized pain over a bony prominence. Whenever possible, fingertips and toes should be visible to permit frequent monitoring for evidence of vascular compromise in the immediate postopertaive recovery period.

The securing dressing should adequately stabilize the splint and maintain the desired position until the first postoperative dressing change. Daily monitoring of splint position is required, and the outer dressing may need to be reinforced to prevent shifting of the splint prior to the initial dressing change.

Initial Dressing Change

During the initial dressing change, if a splint still is required, attention must be given to the amount of dressing material reapplied. The splint should not be forced into position or slide easily once in place. Excessive dressing bulk or inadequate amounts of gauze can result in pressure necrosis of the new graft or adjacent skin or neurovascular compromise. If the postoperative dressing is not duplicated, then the splint should be re-formed to assure optimal fit.

Patient Compliance

The degree to which a patient cooperates will affect the extent of "enforced" immobilization that is required. Obviously, a child or an adult who is unwilling or unable to follow a prescribed treatment plan will require a more structured splinting program than an adult who is informed and cooperative.

Splints that immobilize joints usually are discontinued once graft adherence is assured. However, in some cases, night splints, to maintain joint range or protect fragile grafts, are indicated. The duration of splint use is determined by patient participation and the degree of healing of the grafted surface.

ACUTE HAND BURNS

There is some controversy among clinicians about when splinting should be initiated for the hand. Some suggest splinting the patient's hand upon admission;[20] some prefer to wait until the acute edema subsides;[33] and some prefer not to splint during the first 72 hours post injury, and then only if the patient is unable to successfully perform active ROM exercises.[34-36]

Acute management of the burned hand must be based not only on the damage created by the thermal insult, but with consideration given to protection of undamaged structures. The ultimate goals in treatment of the burned hand, regardless of the depth of injury, are to preserve function, protect underlying anatomic structures, and to prevent contracture development as the wound heals. Splinting must be an integral part of the treatment plan and many splint designs have been documented to accomplish these goals.[37]

When the dorsal surface of the hand has sustained a full-thickness burn, the prevention of deformity should be the primary focus. Larson[38] has described the PIP joint as the most vulnerable joint in the hand due to the potential risk for rupture of the extensor mechanism. Failure to immobilize and support the hand inevitably will result in damage to the extensor mechanism. With injuries in which the extensor mechanism is suspected to be at risk, the hand should be positioned with the MCP joints in 45° to 70° of flexion and the IP joints in full extension to reduce stress applied to the extensor mechanism and to elongate the collateral ligaments. The wrist is positioned in neutral or slight extension with the thumb halfway between radial and palmar abduction to maintain normal excursion of the web space.[6]

Unsupervised flexion of the PIP joints can cause disruption of the central tendon slip and produce a boutonniere deformity.[39,40] If a boutonniere deformity occurs, the PIP joint should be splinted in a functional position of approximately 40° of flexion and permitted to arthrodese with scar. Immobilization can be accomplished with individual finger gutter splints or aluminum and foam splints.

If splints are applied in the immediate postburn period, the fit of a splint should be closely monitored and adjustments made to accommodate any increase in edema that develops. In most cases, the standard safe position or palmar pan splint will provide the correct position necessary to maintain the integrity of the extensor mechanism and a functional tendon balance when the burn occurs exclusively over the dorsum or when the entire hand is involved. The position of deformity is flexion of the wrist, extension of the MCP joints, flexion of the IP joints, and adduction and flexion of the thumb.

When a burn is restricted to the palmar surface, the hand should be splinted in extension at all joints to provide maximal stretch to the healing wound. All fingers also should be abducted to prevent contracture of the web spaces. For circumferential or palmar hand burns for the pediatric patient, Salisbury, et al.,[35] recommend immediate splinting as a preventative measure. The recommended position is the one mentioned previously for burns restricted to the palmar surface of the hand. At the

Shriners Burns Institute in Cincinnati, Ohio, circumferential burns of the small pediatric hand are splinted only if limitations in ROM are noted and in a position that opposes the contracting force.

SUGGESTIONS WHEN SPLINTING CHILDREN[30,41]

Patterns

- The therapist should assume a nonthreatening approach. A smile and harmless tools such as a marker, paper or paper towel, and tape measure can help the therapist engage the child in a painfree session of pattern making. Having extra supplies available for the child to use can be helpful.
- One technique involves asking the child to help make a picture of the tracing of their hand: "Let's make a turkey. Did you ever do this at home with mommy or daddy?," or similar conversation.
- Another method involves tracing an unaffected hand or measuring an unaffected extremity if there is resistance to touching the affected one.
- Tracing mom or dad before approaching the child may relieve some of the child's anxiety about the pattern-making procedure.
- The use of water-soluble markers allows for easy cleaning of both child and splint.
- The drape and trim method of fabrication should be considered if a pattern would be complicated.

Molding

- All materials should be placed within reach.
- Stockinette, in one or two layers, may provide some security to the child so the "boo-boos" will not be hurt and also reduces the amount of heat the child will feel from the splint material.
- The use of comfort words such as "soft" and "warm" are preferable to the word "hot."
- Securing the splint with a gauze wrap will free a therapist's hands to position the extremity. Cold spray can penetrate a light gauze wrap and speed cooling.
- Thin $\frac{1}{16}$-in splint material has a short working time since it is lightweight and cools quickly.

Finishing and Fastening

- The edges must be childproofed so that no sharp points can be used for scratching.
- Straps are convenient for splints that must be removed and reapplied frequently during the day. The option to choose the color of the straps may be appealing to the child. A strapped splint may be covered with an elastic bandage or cohesive wrap to hinder removal during the night. Color-coded straps may assist the child, parent, or staff members with splint application.
- Elastic bandages and cohesive wraps to secure the splint reduce the problem of patient removal and splint slippage. On a tiny hand, a cohesive wrap on the

hand will adhere to the cohesive wrap securing the splint, making displacement less likely.
- Encouraging the child to decorate the splint with stickers or markers may make it more appealing.
- Thin surgical tubing can replace rubber bands on dynamic splints.

General

- A therapist should limit the number of times a child is contacted or touched to decrease fear or agitation.
- Instruments should be kept out of view. A child may focus on the scissors or other objects and become fearful.
- Colored splint material and colored cohesive wrap may enhance compliance in some children.
- The therapist may enlist support of a parent or co-worker to comfort, distract, or help position the child.
- Materials should be chosen that are easy to care for and durable.
- The therapist should provide parents with extra supplies (e.g., foam, straps, or even an extra splint).
- Covering a hand or foot splint with a large sock decorated by the child may encourage compliance.
- The therapist should choose the most simple splint design and consider ease of application.
- Labeling all splints may avoid confusion. Even a simple trough splint should have top or bottom, right or left indicated.

Distal Slippage or Splint Rotation

- One technique involves sewing Velcro hook to the underside of splint straps or attaching it to the inside of the splint and sewing Velcro loop to the pressure garment the child wears under the splint (Fig. 11–38).
- Double-sided tape attached to the splint and the garment worn underneath may reduce slippage.
- Masking tape can be used to secure a splint to the underlying garment. The ends of the tape must not be joined to avoid a tourniquet effect.
- Another technique involves interlocking splints by overlapping them during fabrication (Fig. 11–39).

Precautions

- Small parts, such as rubber bands, safety pins, and the hooks sometimes found on elastic bandages, which can be removed by children age 3 years and younger, must be avoided.
- Ingestion of small pieces of splint material usually occurs when a child nibbles the end of a hand splint or silicone elastomer mitt. Because the materials essentially are

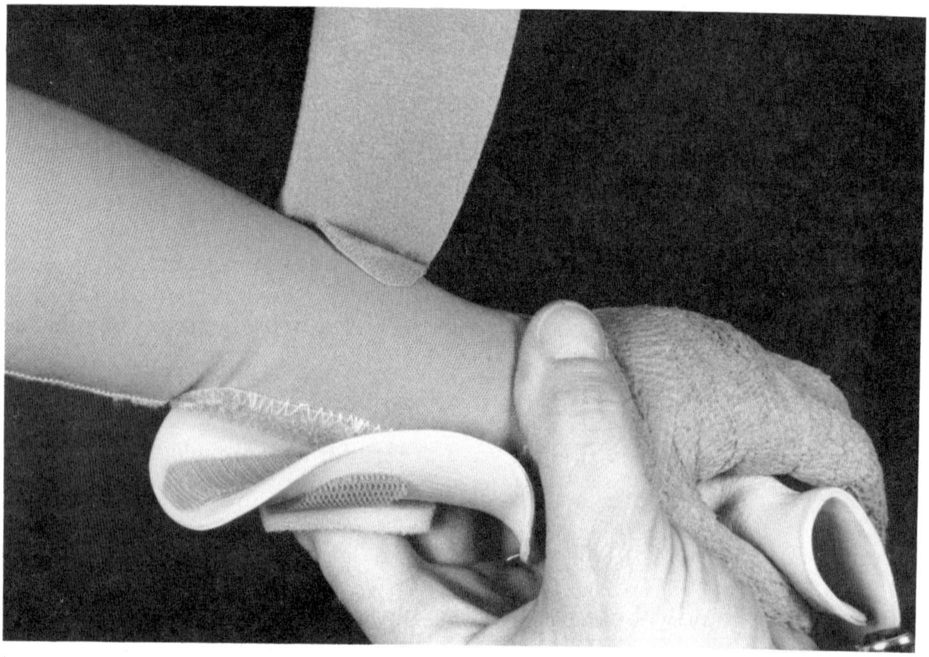

FIGURE 11–38. Velcro attached to pressure garment and splint reduces splint slippage and rotation.

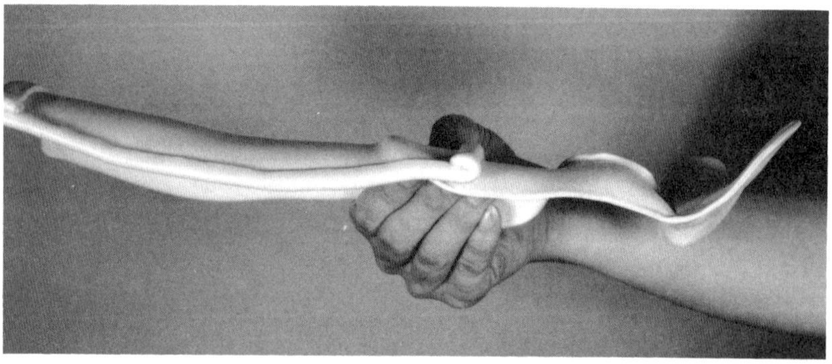

FIGURE 11–39. Flared proximal edge of hand splint will make a groove in the elbow splint formed over it.

inert, no known problems have occurred; however, the manufacturer should be contacted for material safety data sheet information.

FABRICATION OF BASIC BURN SPLINTS

Hand Splint

1. The therapist obtains a tracing of the patient's pronated hand, marking the location of the first web space, tip of middle finger, radial styloid, and distal length of splint along the radial forearm. A vertical line is drawn from the middle finger mark to intersect at a right angle with a line drawn horizontally from the mark of the first web space. From the intersecting point, a mark is placed on the horizontal line at one third the distance toward the first web space mark. To create the thumb portion of the splint, two parallel lines are drawn proximally from the two web space points equal to the length of the thumb and connected to form a rectangle. The corners of the rectangle then should be "rounded" to form the tip of the thumb. Next, the innermost rounded thumb line should extend to connect to the mark of the radial styloid by drawing a "lazy S." To complete the pattern, the width of the proximal end of the splint should be one half the circumference of the patient's forearm girth (Fig. 11–40). The finished pattern is then transferred to a thermoplastic material. Because ballpoint pen ink cannot be removed from all thermoplastic materials, use of a water-soluble marker or yellow grease pencil designed for splints provides easy cleanup.
2. The splint is cut from the material, heated, and trimmed to produce a smooth edge (Fig. 11–41).
3. The material is reheated and then flared or folded away from the thenar eminence (Fig. 11–42). The therapist places the warm material on the patient, which is held gently in place with a gauze wrap. While molding the splint into the desired shape, the therapist maintains the arches of the hand and slight flexion of the IP joint of the thumb (Fig. 11–43).
4. The therapist can remove the splint from the patient once the shape has set, but the material still should be slightly warm to make minor modifications, such as increasing the angle of MCP flexion (Fig. 11–44).
5. After examining the edges, smoothing and trimming them as necessary, the therapist heats and flares the proximal edge away from the skin. The therapist can check the arches by sighting down the forearm section of the splint. The transverse arch should slope downward on the ulnar side (Fig. 11–45).
6. The splint is applied and secured with gauze dressings, elastic bandages, cohesive wraps, or straps (Fig. 11–46). Adults may prefer straps that allow them to apply and remove the splint independently. Malick[42] illustrates several strapping designs.

Elbow or Knee Extension Splint

1. Three measurements are required to fabricate an elbow splint: the length, which is two thirds to three fourths of the arm length from wrist to the axilla (Fig. 11–47)

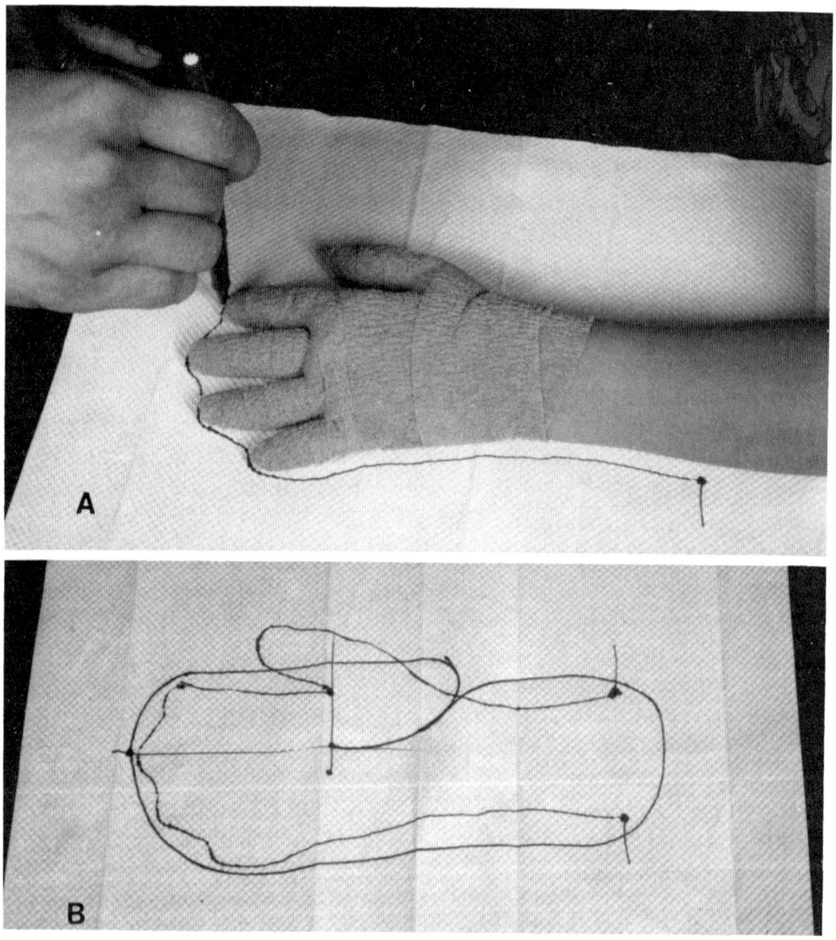

FIGURE 11–40. (*A*) Tracing the hand with wrist in neutral. Length of splint is ½ to ¾ of the forearm. (*B*) Completed pattern of hand splint superimposed on hand tracing.

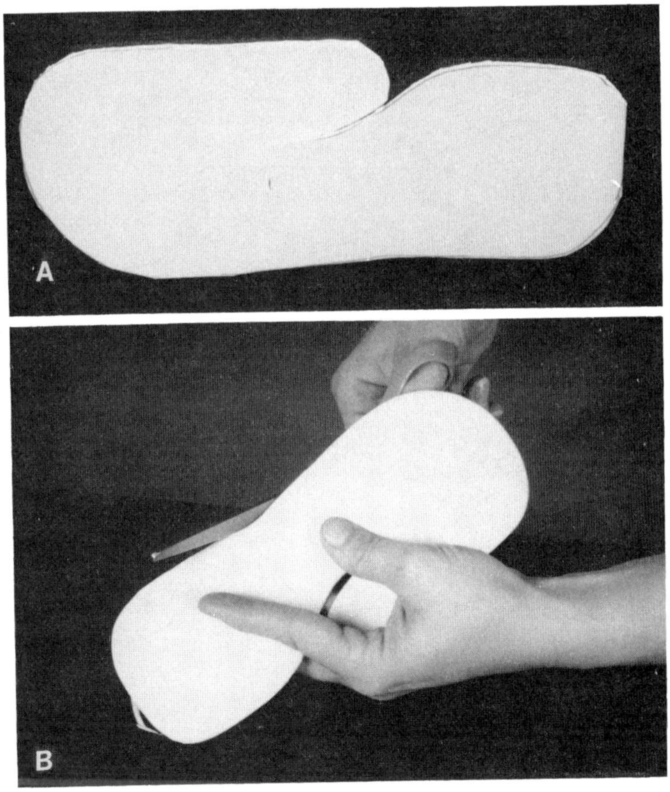

FIGURE 11–41. (*A*) Hand splint pattern cut from thermoplastic material. (*B*) Trimming the edges of heated material with scissors.

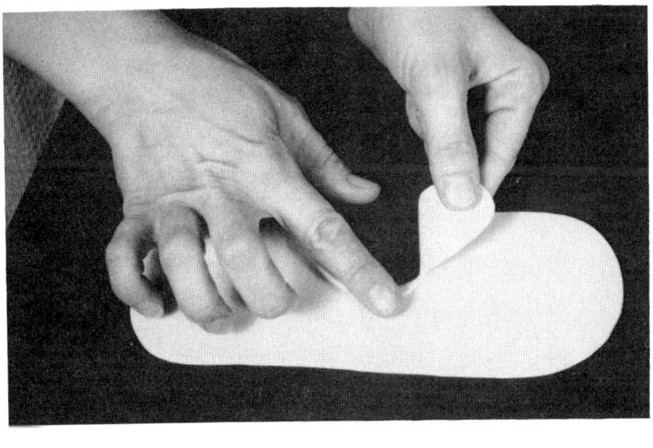

FIGURE 11–42. Thumb post is elevated and material is flared away from the thenar eminence.

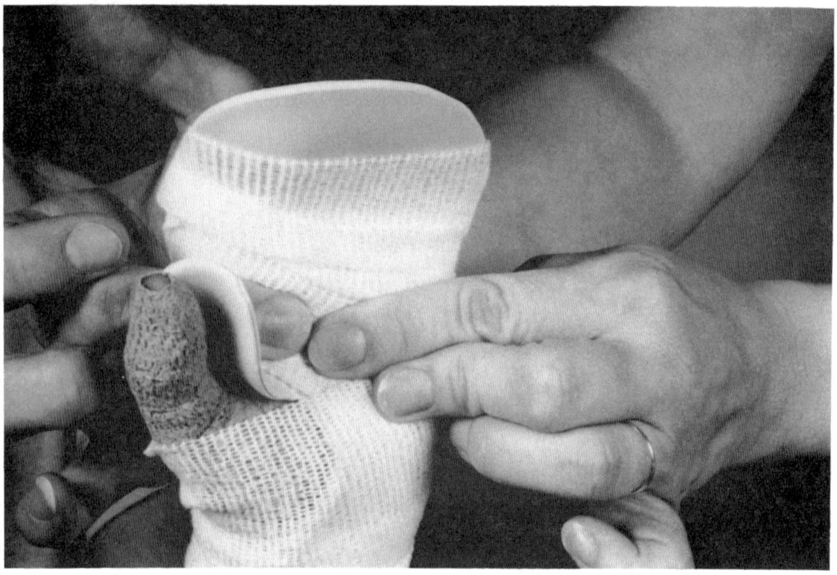

FIGURE 11–43. Molding a hand splint on the patient.

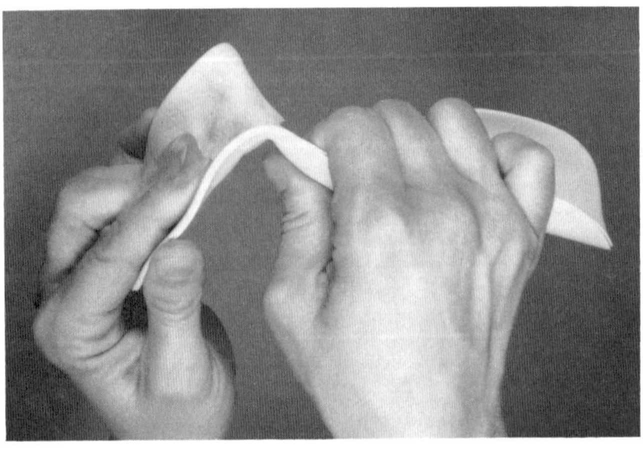

FIGURE 11–44. Increasing angle of MCP flexion.

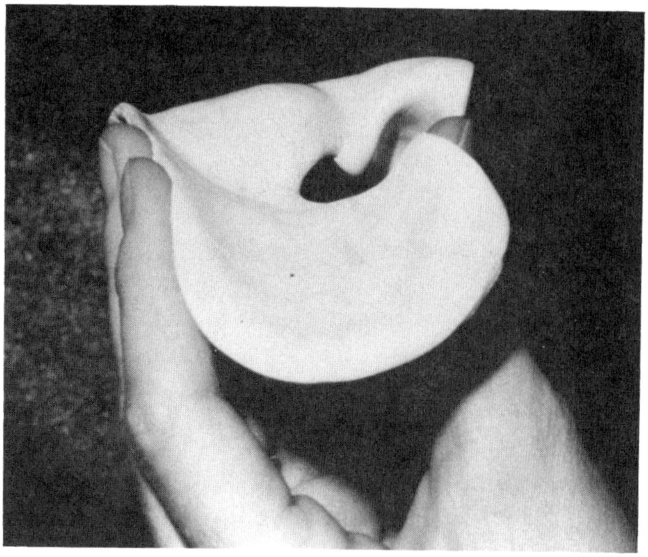

FIGURE 11–45. Examining the splint for inclusion of hand arches.

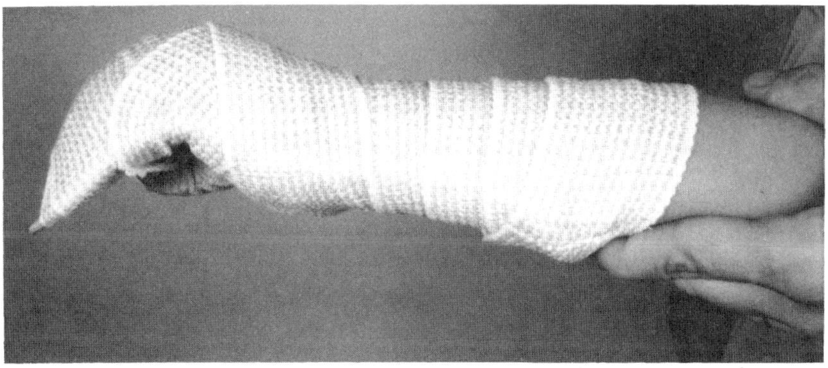

FIGURE 11–46. Hand splint secured with an elastic bandage.

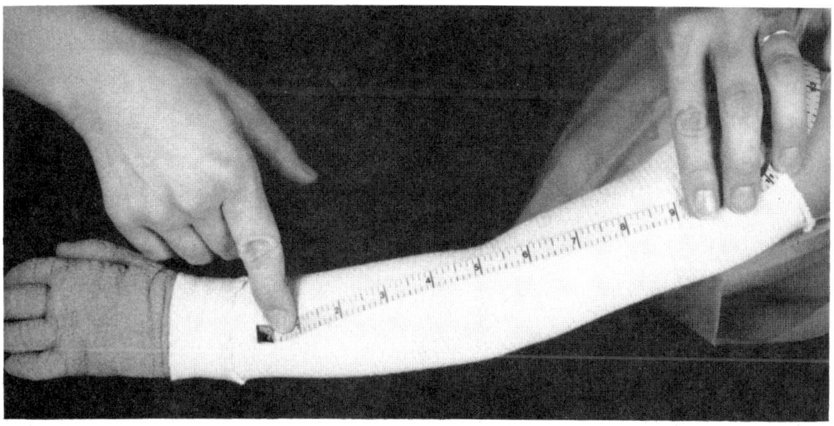

FIGURE 11–47. Elbow splint length should be $\frac{2}{3}$ to $\frac{3}{4}$ of the extremity.

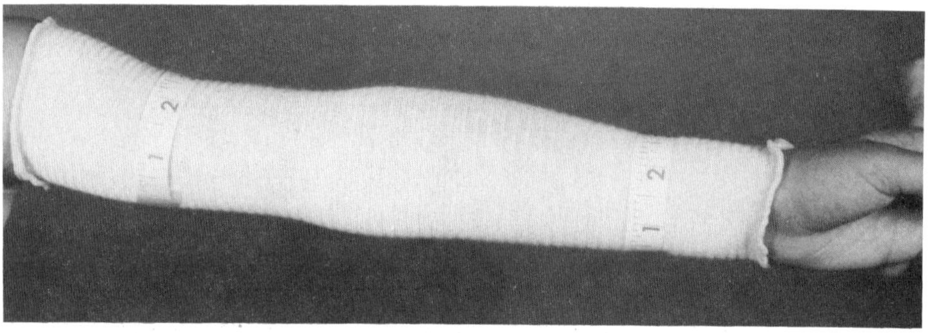

FIGURE 11–48. Proximal and distal width measurements.

and the proximal (widest) and distal (narrowest) widths which are half the circumference of the arm and forearm, respectively (Fig. 11–48).

2. The pattern is drawn directly onto the splint material by forming a rectangle with the length and proximal width measurements (Fig. 11–49). To determine the placement of the distal width and "center" the splint, the therapist locates the midpoint of the proximal width at the distal end of the rectangle and places the midpoint of the distal measurement on it (Fig. 11–50). The distal width is marked at each end and the endpoints of the proximal and distal widths are connected to complete the splint pattern (Fig. 11–51).
3. The therapist heats the material, rounds the corners, and trims the edges. If additional strength is required, the therapist can add 1 inch to each measurement, which will result in a $\frac{1}{2}$-inch foldover on each side and a rolled edge (Fig. 11–52).
4. To make a nonconforming gutter or trough splint, the therapist should allow the splint to cool enough to be manageable. A gutter shape is formed by hand and the therapist should strive for a rounded shape since flat areas can pose pressure

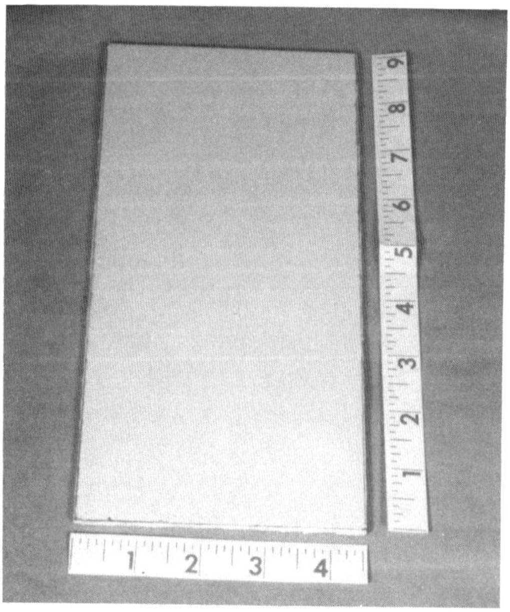

FIGURE 11–49. Rectangle formed length and proximal (widest) width.

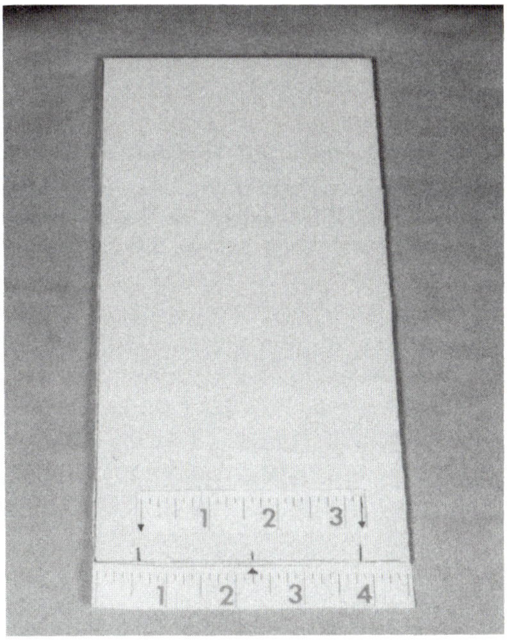

FIGURE 11–50. Distal (narrowest) width measurement centered on midpoint of splint.

problems for the patient (Fig. 11–53). Proximal and distal ends can be reheated and flared after the shape is established.

5. To make a conforming splint the therapist lays the warm material over the flexor surface of the extremity and can flare the proximal and distal edges while the splint cools on the patient (Fig. 11–54).

Note: The same process is followed to make a knee extension splint using measurements obtained from the lower extremity. However, for a conforming knee splint, the material around the fibular head should be flared generously or relieved to avoid pressure on the peroneal nerve (Fig. 11–55).

Axillary Splint or Conformer

1. Five measurements are necessary to fabricate a conforming axillary splint. The elbow and wrist should be incorporated into the splint design unless the splint is intended for very short term use (e.g., immediately after skin grafting), in which case they can be supported in another manner such as sling suspension. The overall length of the splint extends from the waist to the proximal palmar crease and is measured with the patient positioned in the desired degree of shoulder abduction. The locations of the axilla and elbow are noted along the length. Widths are recorded at the waist, midaxilla, elbow, and proximal palmar crease. Widths are half the circumference of the body part (Fig. 11–56).
2. The pattern is drawn directly onto the splinting material by plotting the widths of the four points along the overall length of the splint. The splint outline is formed by connecting all points, gradually decreasing the width from the level of the waist to the axilla, elbow, and finally the palm (Fig. 11–57).

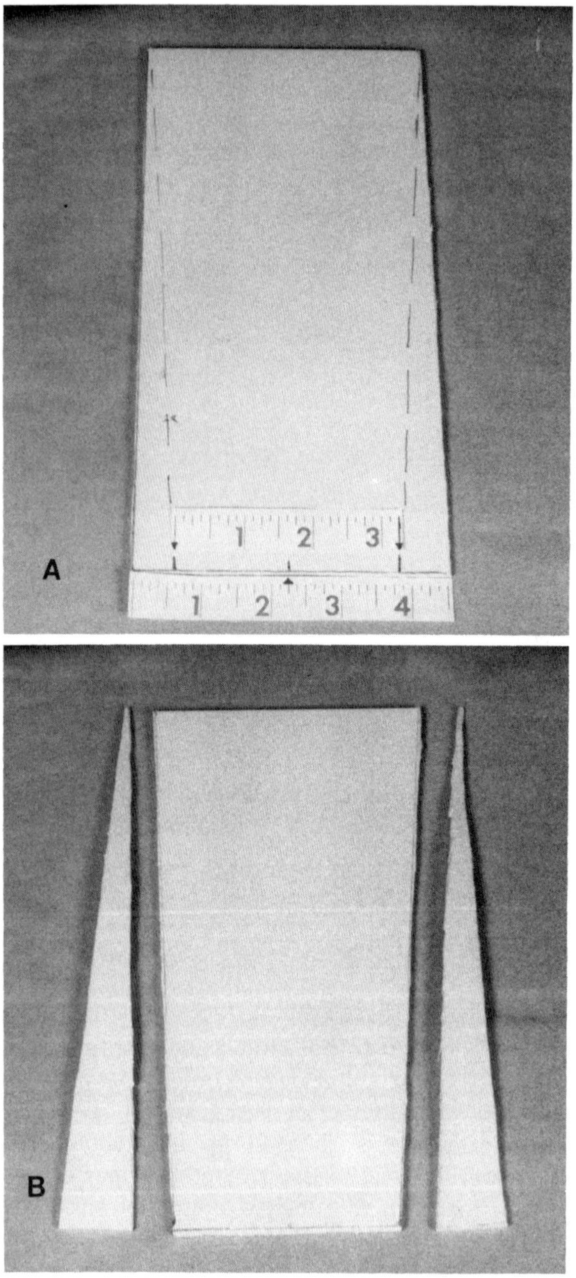

FIGURE 11–51. Completing the elbow splint pattern. (*A*) Dotted lines and widths. (*B*) Material has been cut.

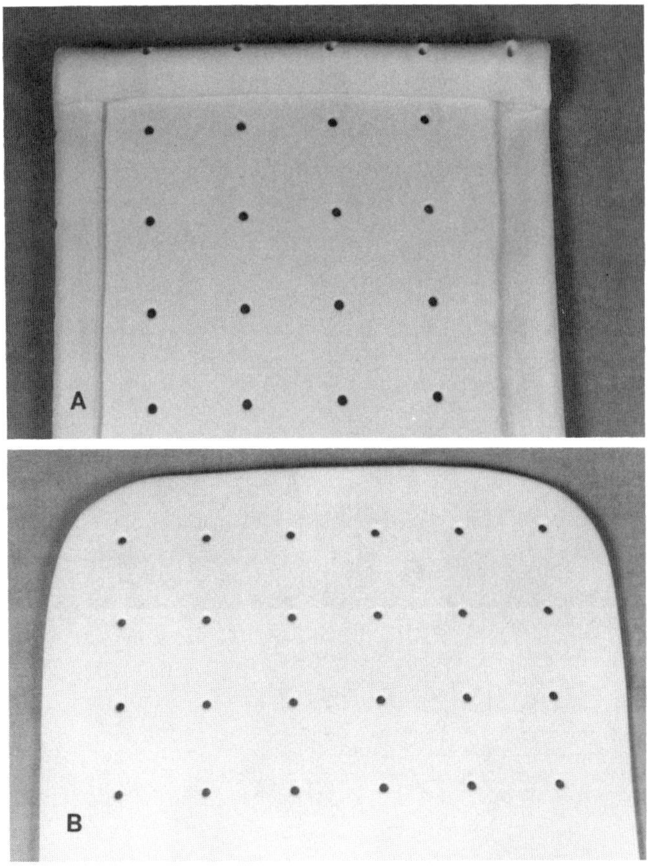

FIGURE 11–52. (*A*) Splint with folded edges. (*B*) Rounded corners with trimmed edges.

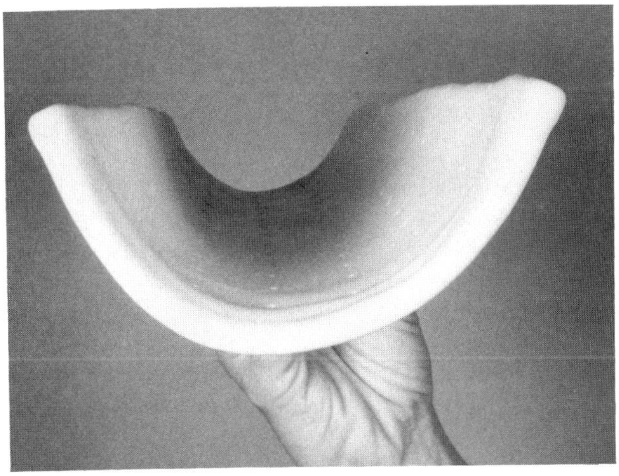

FIGURE 11–53. Rounded shape and symmetry is checked by looking down the midline of the splint. Sides should be an equal distance from the midline.

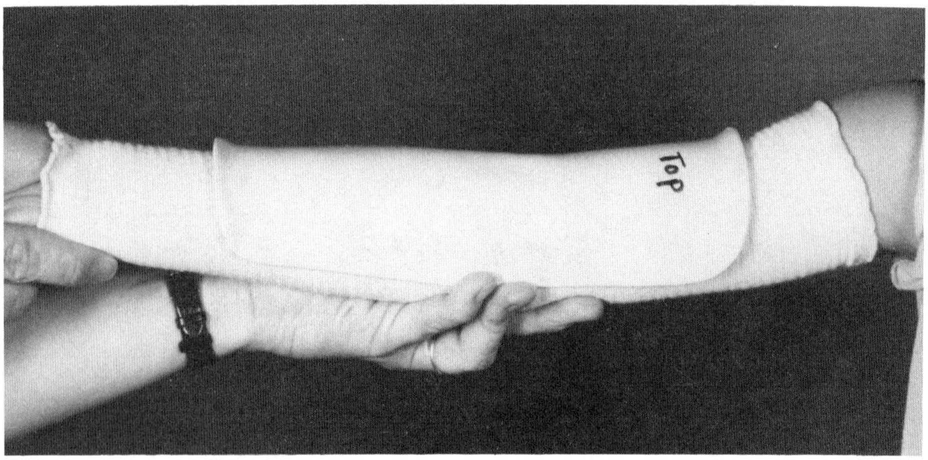

FIGURE 11–54. Conforming elbow extension splint.

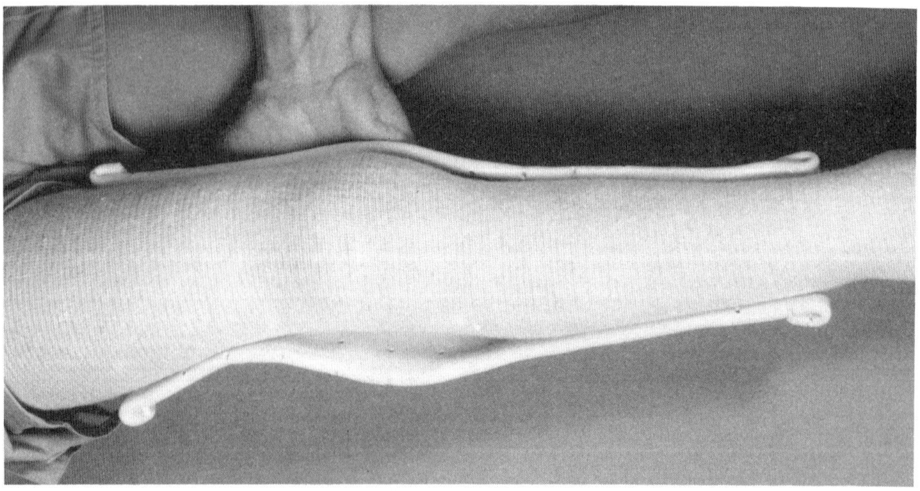

FIGURE 11–55. Conforming knee extension splint with relief over the fibular head.

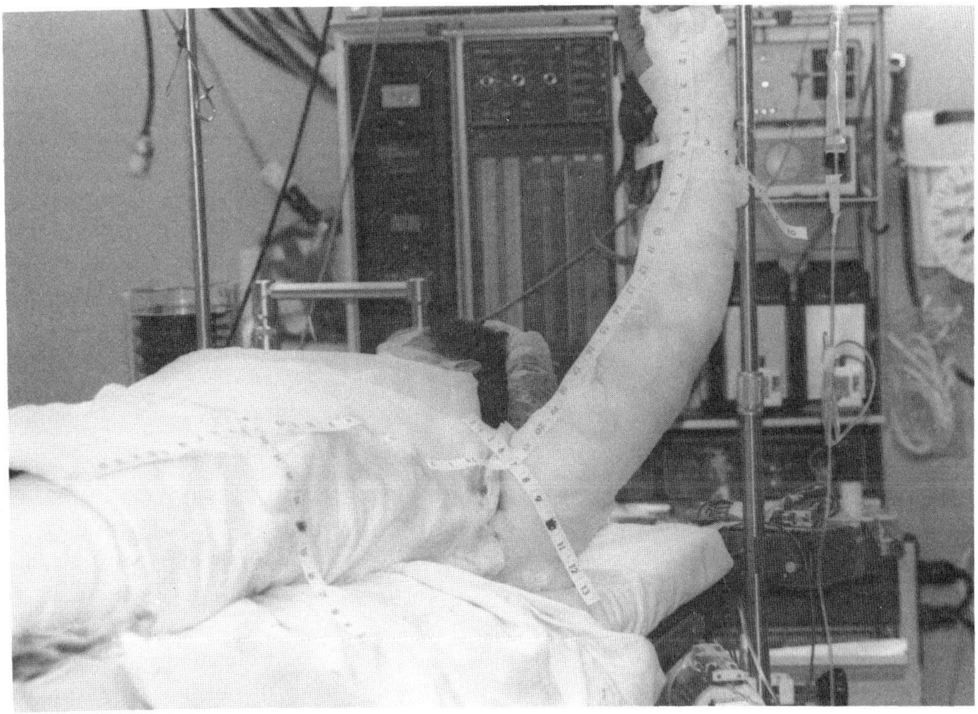

FIGURE 11–56. Length and width measurements of axillary splint taken with patient in proper position. (Elbow measurement not indicated.)

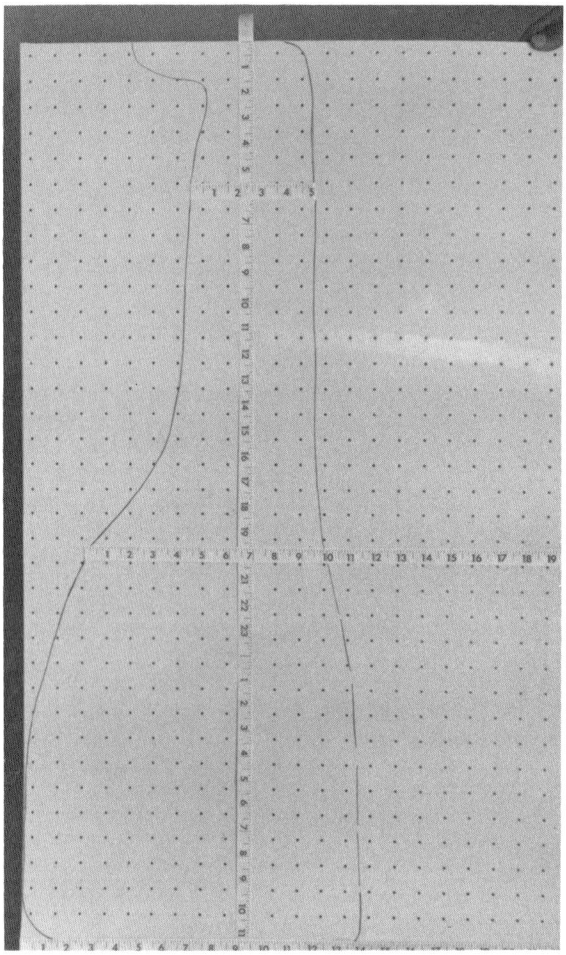

FIGURE 11–57. Axillary splint pattern drawn on thermoplastic material.

3. The patient is positioned in bed with the head of the bed elevated to aid in support of the extremity while the splint is being molded. In addition to abduction (90° to 140°), the shoulder also should be positioned in slight horizontal adduction to avoid stretch to the brachial plexus.
4. Heating the splint in its entirety can pose a problem due to its overall length. By heating the splint in sections and folding it into thirds, using a cotton material or wide length of gauze as an interface, the entire splint can be heated without adhering to itself (Fig. 11–58).
5. The therapist heats the material, rounds the corners, and trims the edges. Prior to molding the splint, the therapist can fold the edges of the material in the axillary area back on itself. Folding the material in this fashion strengthens the splint at its weakest point and allows easier molding on the patient by decreasing bulk in the axillary area (Fig. 11–59).
6. The therapist aligns the splint on the patient and begins forming it at the level of the hand. A circular wrap of gauze or elastic bandage will hold the shape of the splint along the extremity so that the therapist, working distal to proximal, can form the splint with only one heating. Once the arm portion of the splint is

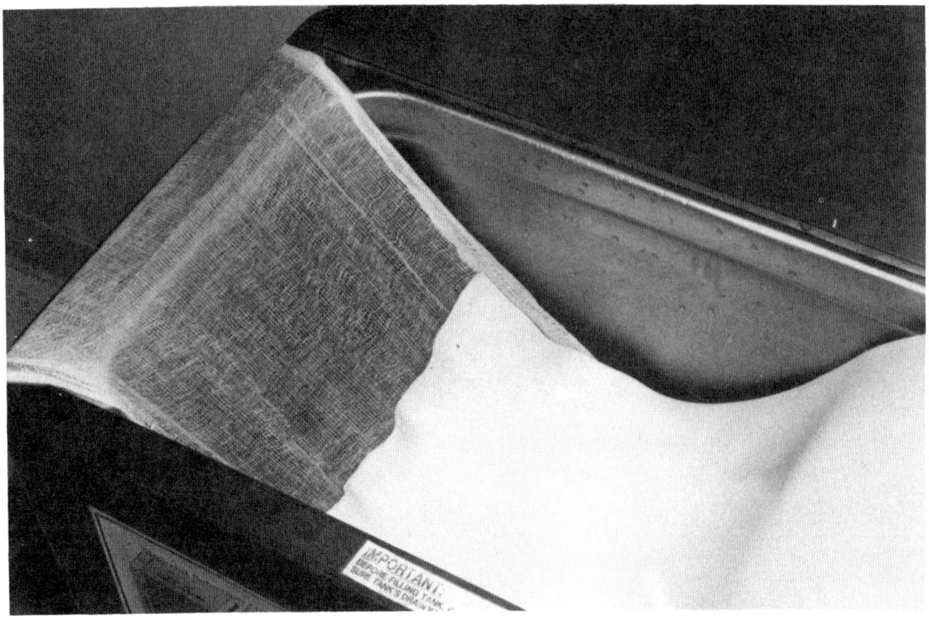

FIGURE 11-58. Heating a large length of splint material in a water bath.

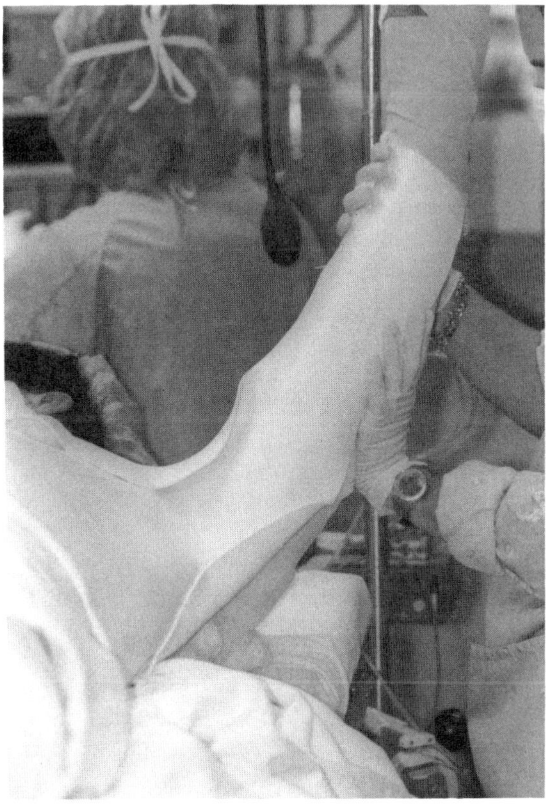

FIGURE 11-59. The axillary portion of the splint is strengthened by folding the edges of the material.

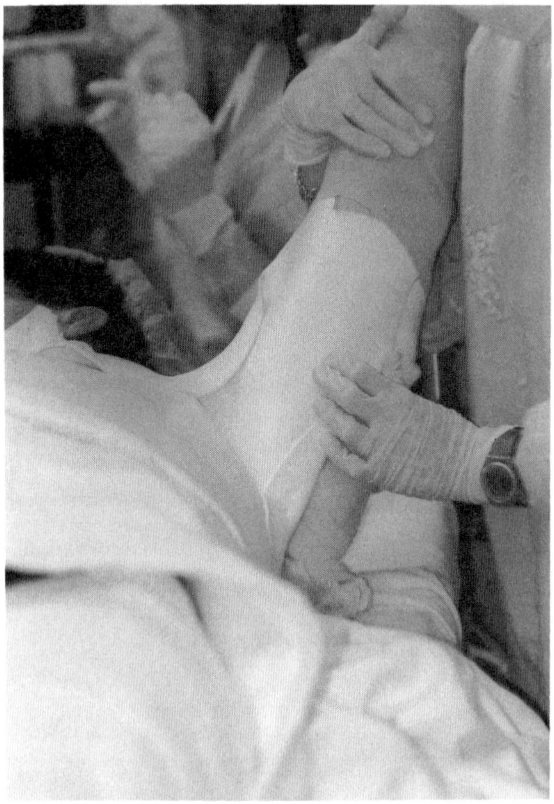

FIGURE 11-60. Molding the splint to the patient.

formed, the trunk portion can be held in place by hand as the material cools (Fig. 11-60).

7. Once completed, the edges should be examined and the proximal and distal edges flared (if not done during the initial fitting) to avoid pressure points.

Posterior Foot Drop Splint

1. Four measurements are required to fabricate a posterior foot drop splint. The overall length of the splint extends from just distal to the popliteal fossa to the toes. The therapist notes the location of the heel along the length measurement (Fig. 11-61). Width measurements are taken at the calf, heel, and metatarsophalangeal (MTP) joints of the foot (Fig. 11-62). Widths are half the circumference of the body part.
2. The pattern is drawn directly onto the splint material by plotting the widths and the location of the heel on the overall length. The splint outline is formed by connecting all points, gradually decreasing the width from the calf to the heel and extending the line to match the width of MTP joints (Fig. 11-63).
3. The therapist heats the material, rounds the corners, and trims the edges.
4. *Nonconforming splint:* The therapist should allow the splint material to cool enough to be manageable. The basic shape of the splint is formed by hand, avoiding all sharp angles that may create pressure points. The therapist checks the fit of

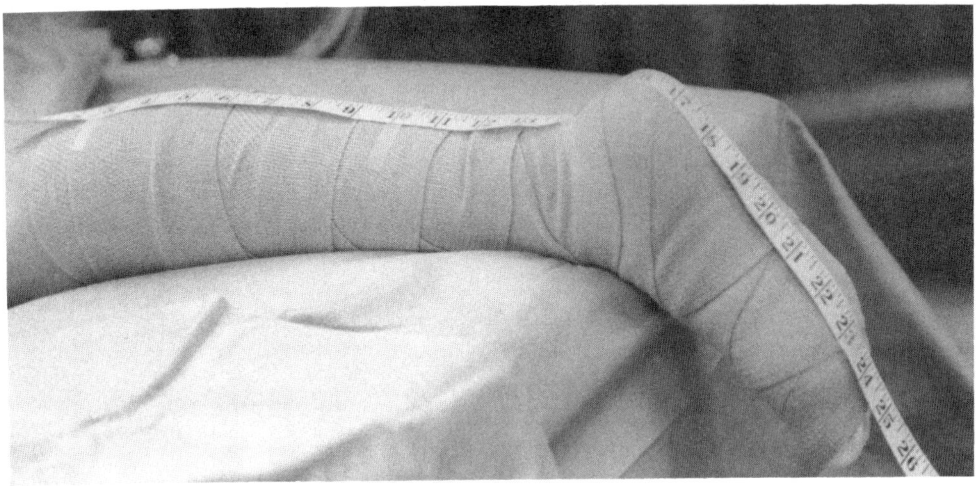

FIGURE 11–61. Length measurements of posterior foot drop splint.

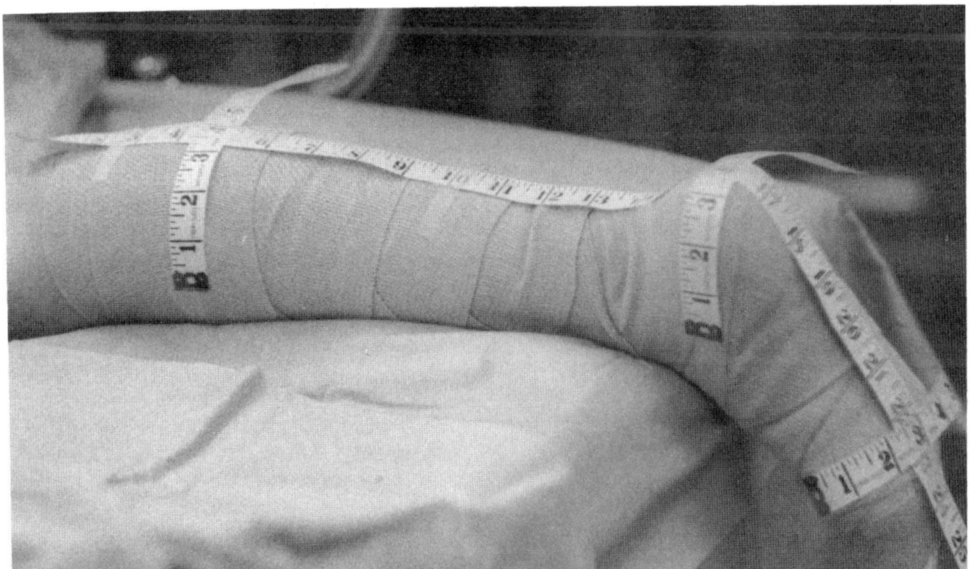

FIGURE 11–62. Width measurements of foot splint.

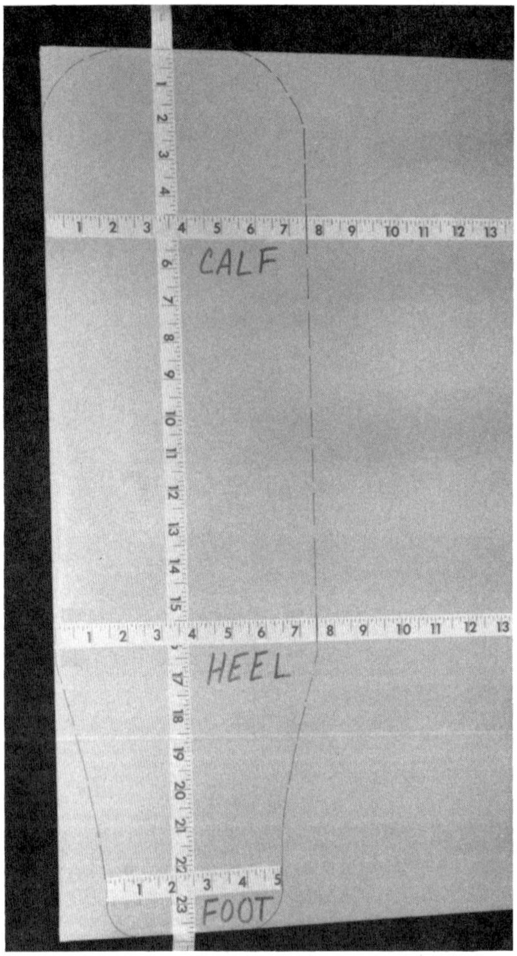

FIGURE 11–63. Foot pattern is plotted on splint material.

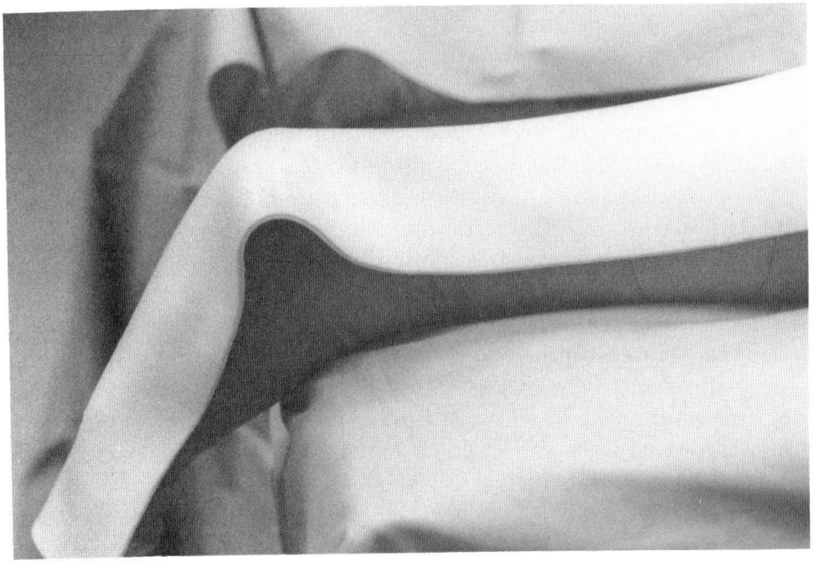

FIGURE 11–64. Splint material is molded on patient in position.

the splint on the patient, makes any necessary adjustments by spot heating, and flares the proximal edge.

5. *Conforming splint:* The therapist lays the warm material over the posterior aspect of the extremity, which is most easily accomplished with the patient in the prone position (Fig. 11–64). The position of the ankle must be maintained as the material cools. The ankle angle is reinforced by external pleating of the material or by folding the material back on itself (Fig. 11–65). Care must be taken to avoid pressure to the malleoli. The proximal edge of the splint is flared to create a rounded edge. The therapist should check that knee flexion is not restricted by the splint.
6. Once the basic shape of the splint is completed and any necessary adjustments made, the therapist should spot heat and expand the heel portion to prevent excessive pressure over the heel.

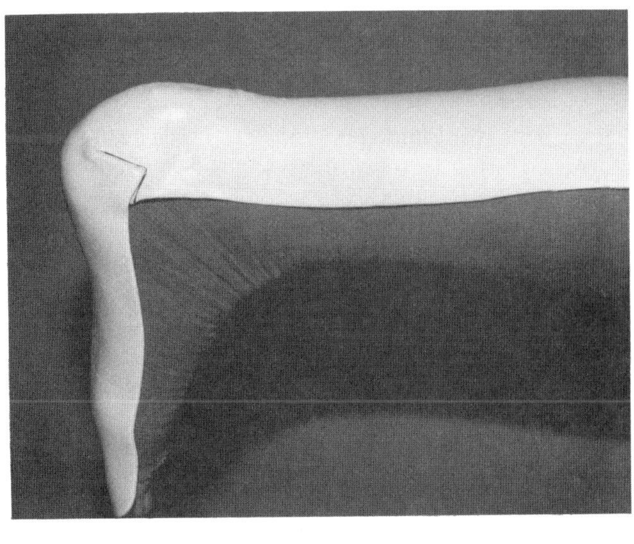

FIGURE 11–65. Finished splint with pleated and folded material at the ankle. Note the expanded heel area for pressure relief.

CASTING

Casting has been used successfully with both children and adults when traditional methods of treatment have failed.[43,44] Indications for use include persistent limitation in ROM or progressive loss of motion due to patient noncompliance; multiple joint involvement; or when a traditional program is overwhelming or beyond the ability of the patient or family. Casts maintain a static position while providing protection, a constant stretch, and pressure, depending upon the materials and manner in which they are applied. They are effective in the management of children and unreliable adult patients because they generally are accepted well but are difficult for the patient to remove. A cast applied to a child can provide some relief to the parents who can leave the direct care of the casted extremity to the therapist. Parents can spend more time on the less-involved or difficult-to-maintain areas of the child's burn injury, which allows parents and child to experience some success with the lesser-involved areas. Cast materials include plaster bandages, synthetic casting tapes, and silicone elastomer.

Plaster Bandage

Plaster, a gypsum-impregnated cloth bandage, is the most common casting material. Excellent ease of molding, low incidence of allergic reactions, and low cost are advantages. Common disadvantages are its weight, drying and curing time, poor water resistance, and the fact that application can be messy. The use of gloves during casting will facilitate cleanup. Bandage widths range from 2 to 6 inches. Types include fast-setting, extra-fast-setting, and elastic plaster rolls that are manufactured with the addition of elastic fibers. The setting time is 2 to 4 minutes for extra-fast-setting plaster and 5 to 8 minutes for fast-setting and elastic plaster. Setting time is measured from the point at which the plaster is saturated with water until the cast has become firm.[45] Casts are affected by:

1. Temperature
   a. Warm dipping water hastens setting; cool water delays it.
   b. Room temperature dipping water that feels cool to the touch, about 70° to 75°F, is recommended.
2. Moisture
   a. Very wet bandages delay setting; those wrung out excessively hasten setting.
3. Accelerating or retarding additives
   a. *Accelerating additives:* potassium sulfate, common salt.
   b. *Retarding additives:* sodium citrate, borax.
   c. Additives are not recommended because they can reduce the strength of the plaster and increase the exothermic reaction.
   d. Use clean dipping water as plaster residue acts as an accelerator.

A cast may seem dry on the surface but contain considerable moisture in its deeper layers. A cast will become stronger with drying, which is affected by:

1. Thickness
   a. The average cast is less than $\frac{1}{4}$-inch thick; four to six layers of evenly applied plaster are required.

b. Thin casts may dry in several hours; thick casts of $\frac{1}{4}$-inch can take up to 72 hours.
c. Depending upon the size of a patient, weight-bearing casts may require additional plaster (five plies of the plaster bandage cut to the length of the cast) incorporated on the weight-bearing surface. Weight bearing usually is not recommended until the cast has dried for a minimum of 24 hours.

2. Ventilation
   a. Lack of free circulation of air around a cast retards drying.
   b. *Poor ventilation is caused by the following:* wrapping the cast with an elastic bandage, placing the cast on a pillow or mattress, covering the cast with a sheet or blanket.
3. Moisture
   a. Very wet bandages will delay drying.

The activation of plaster by water produces an exothermic or heat-releasing reaction. The cast will reach its maximum temperature in approximately 5 to 15 minutes following application. The temperature increases:

1. With the thickness of the cast (eight or more plies).
2. When bandages with faster setting times are used.
3. If room temperature and humidity are high.
4. With warmer temperatures of dipping water.
5. With restricted ventilation.

Synthetic Casting Tape

Synthetic casting tapes consist of polyester or fiberglass fabric, woven or knitted, impregnated with polyurethane resin (Appendix I). Short drying and curing time, light weight, strength, and water resistance are advantages of synthetics. Their ease of molding is average and not appropriate where exact impressions are required. Disadvantages include a relatively high cost, potential for allergic reaction, and an abrasive surface with fiberglass. Tape widths range from 2 to 5 inches. Manufacturers are competitive and continue to improve this product. As a result there is no standard labeling for products with similar setting times. Setting times range from 2 to 8 minutes and are affected by:

1. Temperature of the dipping water, similar to plaster
2. Moisture
   a. Manipulating the roll in the dipping water will accelerate setting.
   b. Exposure to moisture in room air will activate the tape and result in a setting time of approximately 8 minutes.

Three to four layers provide a strong cast. Two to three extra layers around the foot and ankle are adequate for a weight-bearing cast and the addition of casting tape reinforcement is not required. The patient can bear weight after 20 minutes as opposed to a minimum of 24 hours for plaster. Activation produces an exothermic reaction similar to plaster and is affected by the same variables: thickness, fast setting time, room temperature and humidity, temperature of the dipping water, and ventilation.

Precautions should be taken to avoid potential burns to a patient's sensitive skin by controlling the variables. The most important variables to control are the cast thickness, setting time, temperature of the dipping water, and ventilation.[46,47] A combination of the variables poses the greatest hazard to the patient. Under experimental conditions, temperatures of up to 68.5°C (155.3°F) were recorded for up to 24 minutes when variables were combined.[46] Stockinette or padding is required under synthetics to prevent resins from adhering to the patient's skin. The therapist must use gloves. Sharp edges or points of a fiberglass cast can be removed with sandpaper or a fingernail file. A length of stockinette can cover the cast at night to protect bed sheets.

Synthetics are available in a rainbow of colors that may enhance a patient's acceptance of the cast. To reduce expense, a colored roll is applied as the last layer. Flash Cast is a polyester-based tape intended for use as the top layer of a fiberglass cast to eliminate its abrasive surface and is available in pediatric and adult patterns as well as colors (Appendix I). Due to plaster's absorbent quality, it can be used as the first layers of a cast and a synthetic tape as the last layer. This notion is helpful particularly when early weight bearing is desired.

Padding

Because plaster conforms precisely and adheres slightly to the skin, thus eliminating shear forces, plaster casting was used for years without padding. Due to burn patient's fragile, sensitive skin and possible presence of open areas, padding is recommended. However, padding can increase the possibility of shear forces and cast slippage and should be kept to a minimum. Standard rolls of cotton cast padding and stockinette are appropriate under both plaster and synthetic casts. Thicknesses of $\frac{1}{8}$ to $\frac{1}{2}$ inch of felt also can be used to pad as appropriate, including all bony prominences. The therapist should be aware of areas that may become bony prominences due to loss of tissue or atrophy following a burn injury (e.g., the anterior tibia). Appropriate skin care, padding, and proper application of a cast will decrease the potential for skin irritations or pressure areas. Standard wound care treatment (e.g., topical antimicrobial, petroleum jelly, gauze, dome paste), edema control, and scar management (e.g., elastic bandages, cohesive wrap, silicone elastomer) can be used under a cast for burn patients.

Serial Casting

When used correctly, serial casting is a nontraumatic method of increasing joint motion. The contracted tissue is positioned near the end of its elastic limit (e.g., when the tissue blanches) with a gentle force without causing pain. For children and very sensitive or frightened patients, the initial cast simply may encase the deformity. In this instance, further contracture is prevented while the patient accommodates to wearing the cast. Therapists must be cautious if casts are applied while a patient is anesthetized. Force applied beyond a tissue's elastic limit can result in ischemic areas and tears.

Serial casting to increase ROM is accomplished by periodically removing and replacing the cast at the subsequent end of the patient's increased joint range, or by wedging the cast between cast changes and patching the opening that results from

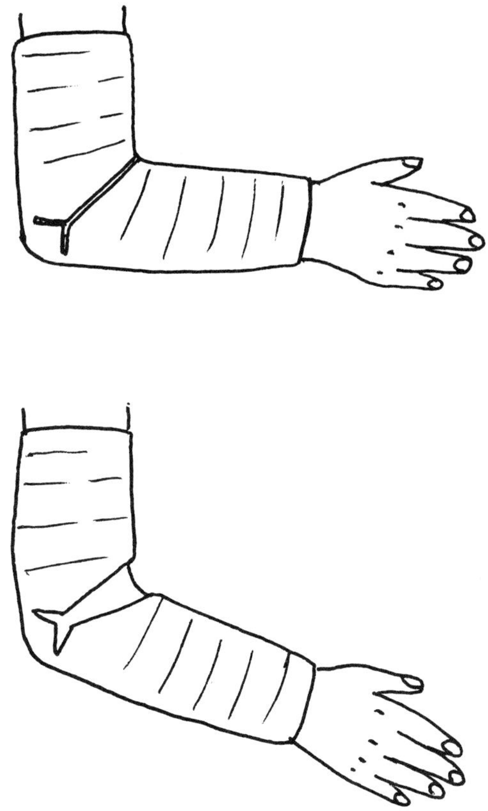

A

B

FIGURE 11–66. Wedging a cast with a Y-shaped cut on either side of the cast. (*A*) Closed cut. (*B*) Opened cut.

the improved range. There are several methods of wedging a cast.[43,48,49] Wu[48] recommends a double Y-shaped cut through approximately 75 percent of the circumference of the cast (Fig. 11–66) to minimize pressure problems on the convex side of the joint (Fig. 11–67). Wedging usually is used to correct flexion contractures of larger joints. The frequency of cast changes can vary from daily to monthly. Daily changes may be required by conditions such as presence of large or multiple open areas, anticipation of rapid resolution of contracture, or questionable patient tolerance of the cast. Less

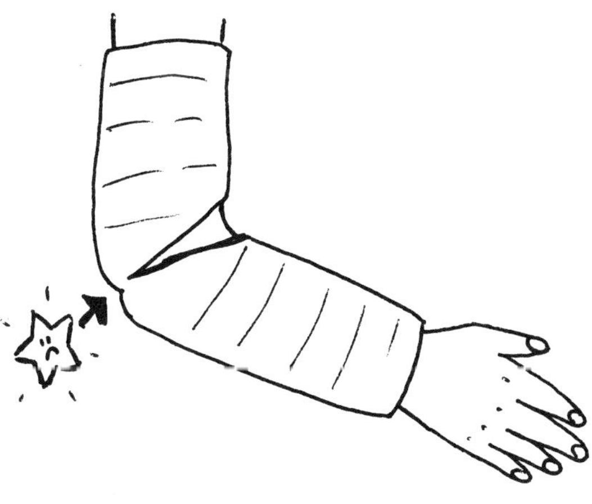

FIGURE 11–67. Using a straight cut to wedge a cast can produce a pressure point when the cut is opened.

frequent changes are possible when there are no problems with the patient's skin condition and the patient tolerates the cast well but is unavailable for wedging of an existing cast.

Assessment of a patient's needs and attention to basic splinting principles will help to determine the style of the cast. Several styles are illustrated in Figure 11–68.

Considerations for Casting a Burn Patient

1. Ideally, a cast is applied immediately following standard treatment to improve ROM. The extremity is cleaned, dry skin areas are moisturized, and any wounds are dressed lightly. A topical agent and petroleum jelly gauze usually are sufficient. Dome paste can be used under a cast for fragile skin with multiple open areas.
2. If an extremity becomes ecchymotic or edematous, and pressure wraps or garments will be worn proximal to the cast, the extremity, including fingers and toes, should be wrapped with a cohesive wrap and elastic bandages. The wrap is extended 1 to 2 inches beyond the proximal end of the cast. Fragile skin over bony areas can break down under pressure wraps and must be padded appropriately before wrapping (e.g., a strip of felt on each side parallel to a prominent anterior tibia).
3. A thin layer of silicone elastomer can be incorporated under the cast if the skin can tolerate it and additional scar remodeling is desired.
4. The patient often can continue to wear pressure garments distal to the cast, such as gloves or anklets.
5. Generally, stockinette is the first material used against a patient's skin when a cast is applied. However, it is not necessary if other materials such as an elastic wrap or silicone elastomer are used.

Fabrication of a Basic Cast

Supplies are listed in Table 11–1.

1. Stockinette must be cut sufficiently longer than the cast so there is approximately 1 to 2 inches extra on each end and applied to the extremity without wrinkles. The therapist can cut any wrinkles at the dorsum of the ankle or popliteal or antecubital spaces so that the fabric is overlapped rather than folded (Fig. 11–69). A slit must be cut for the thumb if the hand is included in an arm cast (Fig. 11–70).
2. Two people frequently are required to position an extremity. The extremity is wrapped with cast padding in a smooth spiral fashion overlapping about half its width and with care taken to avoid wrinkles. Two to three layers are sufficient. Felt pieces are applied to all bony areas and secured with one wrap of cast padding (Fig. 11–71).
   a. *Hand:* The padding is torn partially or cut through its width and smoothly wrapped through the thumb web space (Fig. 11–72). The padding can be cut to a 1 inch width to wrap the thumb (Fig. 11–73).
   b. *Ankle, flexed knee, or elbow:* The therapist can wrap the padding in a figure-of-8 fashion and fill any gaps with additional padding.

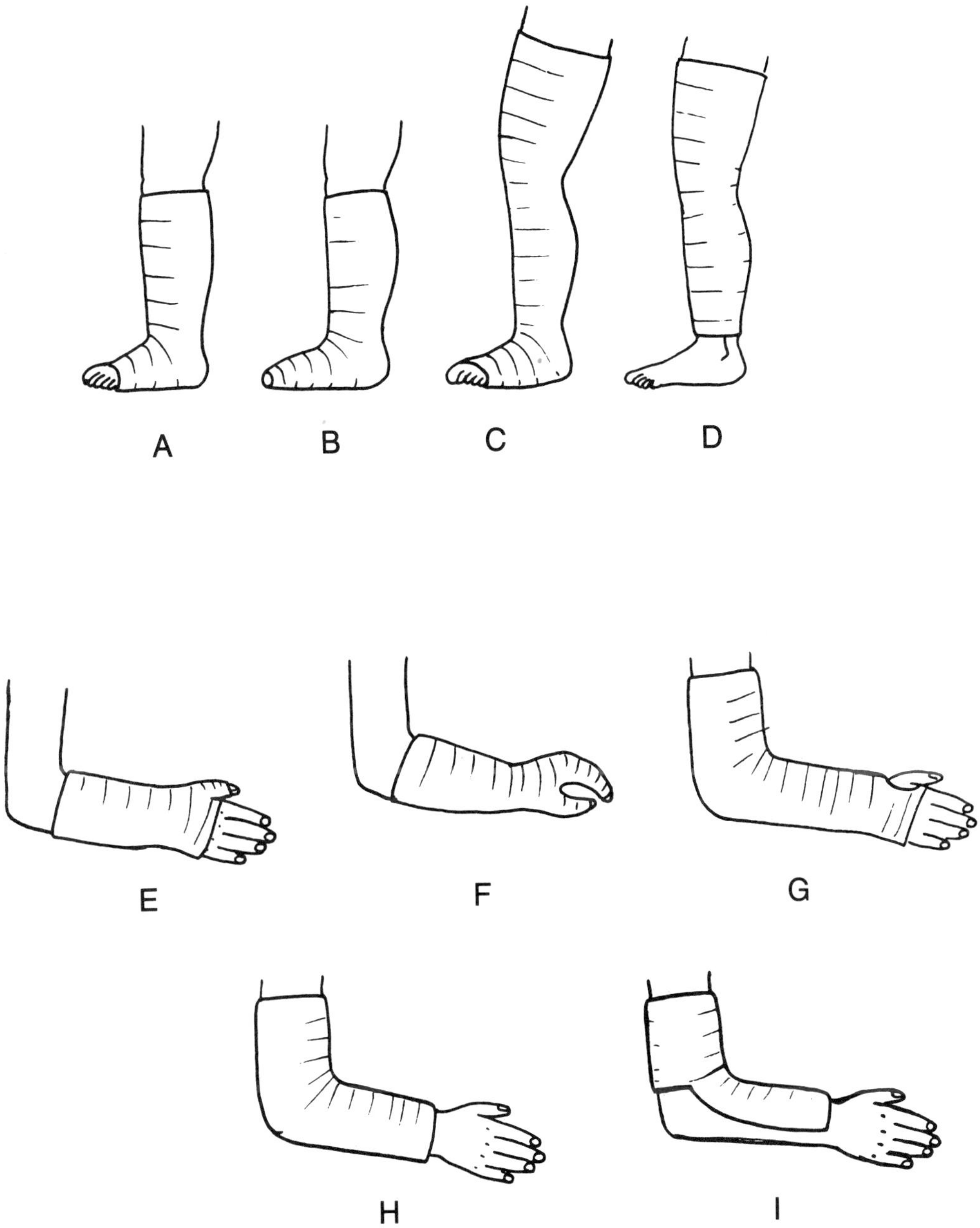

FIGURE 11–68. (*A*) Short leg cast. (*B*) Short leg cast including toes. (*C*) Long leg cast. (*D*) Long leg cylinder cast. (*E*) Short arm cast with thumb spica. (*F*) Short arm cast with thumb spica and MCP flexion. (*G*) Long arm cast. (*H*) Long arm cylinder cast. (*I*) Fall-out or drop-out cast.

TABLE 11–1. Casting Supplies and Materials—Adult Sizes (Widths)

	Arm (inches)	Leg (inches)
Stockinette	3	4
Cast padding	3	4
Cast material		
Plaster	3–4	4–6
Synthetic	3–4	4–5
Felt pieces	Gloves	
Bucket/bowl	Scissors	
Water	Cast saw	
Plastic/cloth sheet	Cast spreader	

3. A roll of plaster or synthetic cast material is immersed in water until saturated, then removed and gently squeezed to eliminate extra water. The therapist rolls the plaster or synthetic cast material snugly but not firmly around the extremity overlapping about half of its width (Fig. 11–74).
   a. *Hand:* The roll is cut partially through its width and smoothly wrapped through the thumb web space.
   b. *Arm:* A short arm cast ends approximately 1 inch distal to the antecubital crease and a long arm cast at approximately two thirds the length of the arm. A cylinder cast is started proximal to the radial and ulnar styloid processes.
   c. *Leg:* A short leg cast ends below the fibular head and a long leg cast at approximately two thirds the length of the thigh. A cylinder cast is started proximal to the malleoli.
4. After the first one or two layers of cast material are applied, the stockinette and padding are folded snugly back over the cast and secured with additional layers of cast material (Fig. 11–75). The plaster is rubbed with the palms to smooth and strengthen the cast. The therapist molds, shapes, and trims the cast as necessary. During the casting process, the therapist must avoid pressing a hand or fingers into the material as pressure areas can result. The patient's position must be maintained until the material has set.

A cast saw and cast spreader will remove both synthetic and plaster casts. The padding and stockinette are cut with scissors. Some therapists place a strip of felt along the length of the extremity under the cast. This strip serves as a guide and buffer for the cast saw during cast removal (Fig. 11–76). The poor water resistance of plaster can be an advantage when working with children since the cast can be soaked off in warm water, eliminating the noise and fear of the cast saw. Serial casting is discontinued once a contracture has been corrected or no further gains are achieved. A splint frequently is used in a patient's maintenance program following casting.

Bell-Krotoski[50,51] provided detailed instruction on the fabrication of plaster casts to correct flexion contractures of the IP joints and boutonniere deformities. Tribuzi[52] illustrated a circumferential cast to increase or maintain MCP flexion.[52]

Applying a cast to a child requires special considerations. Two individuals usually are required whether the other person is a cooperative parent or another staff member who assists with positioning, calming, or distracting the child. Due to a

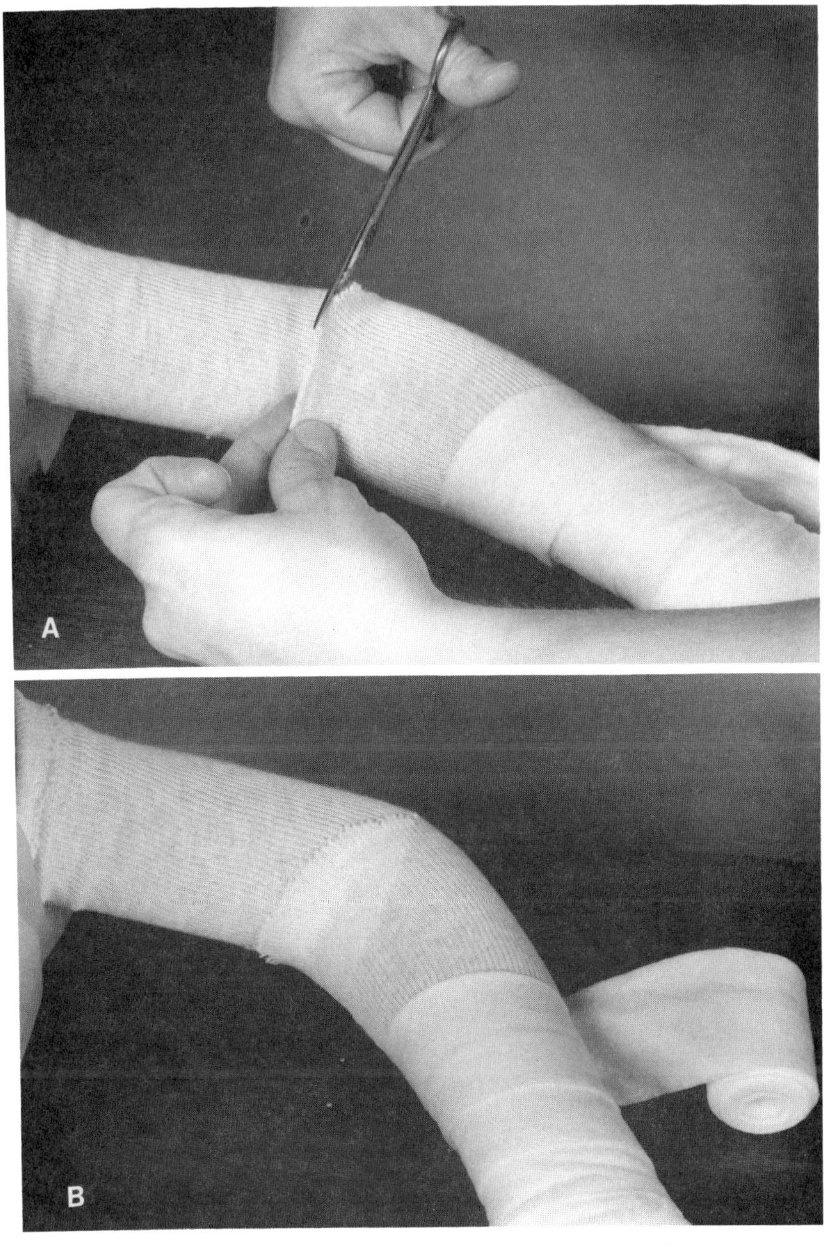

FIGURE 11–69. (*A*) Wrinkle in stockinette is cut. (*B*) Edges overlap.

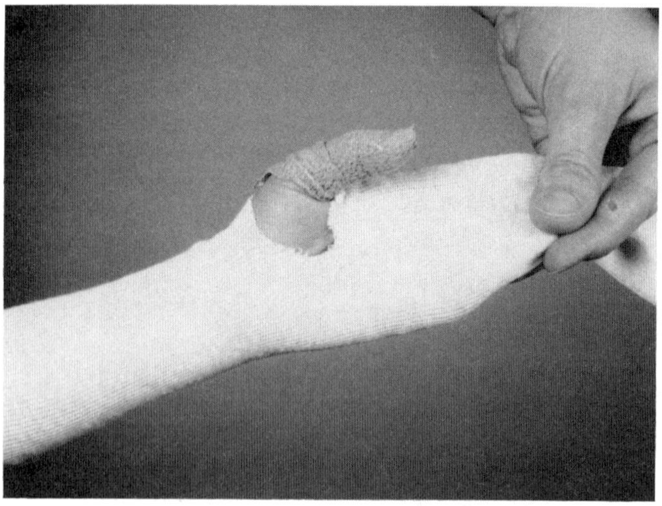

FIGURE 11–70. Slit cut in stockinette for thumb.

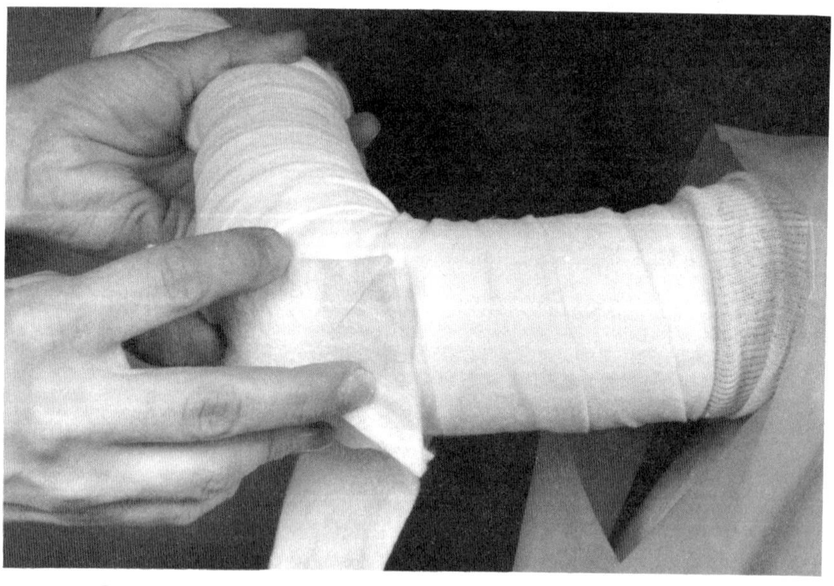

FIGURE 11–71. Felt pieces applied to bony area of the olecranon.

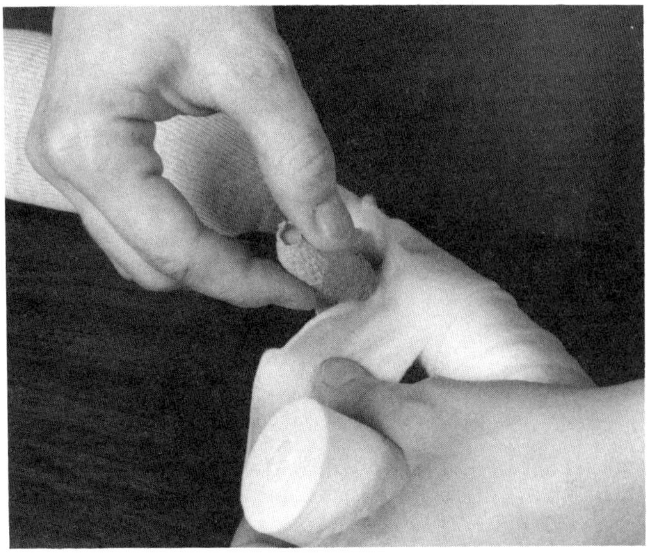

FIGURE 11–72. Cast padding torn through $\frac{1}{2}$ the width to smoothly wrap the thumb web space.

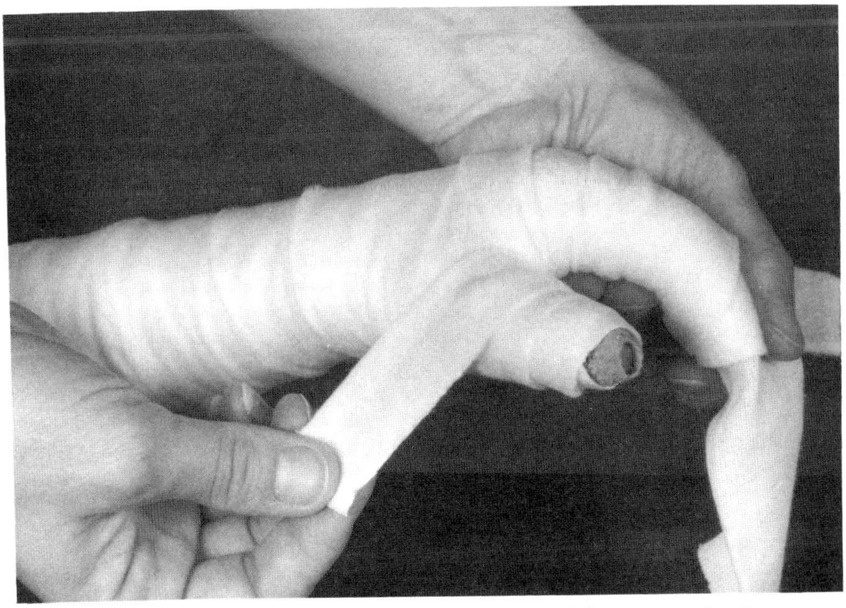

FIGURE 11–73. Cast padding cut to a narrow width to wrap the thumb.

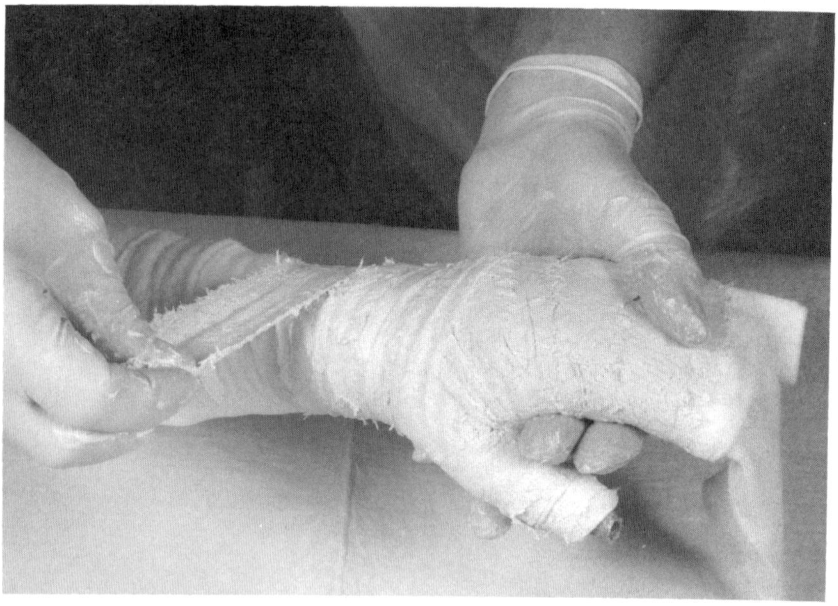

FIGURE 11–74. Cast material is overlapped by $\frac{1}{2}$ its width for an even thickness.

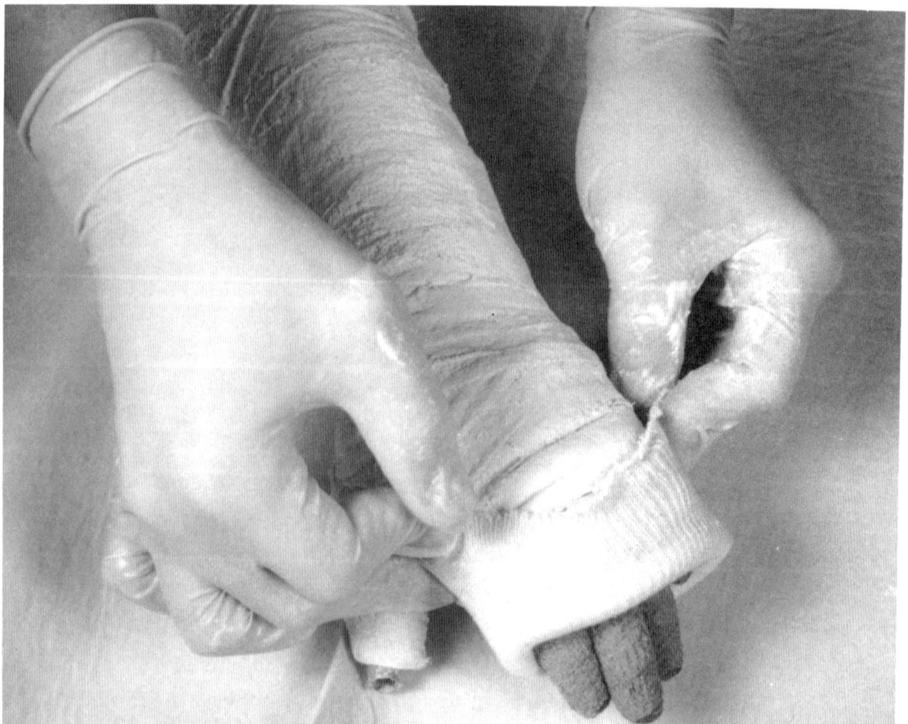

FIGURE 11–75. Stockinette pulled back to provide a smooth edge.

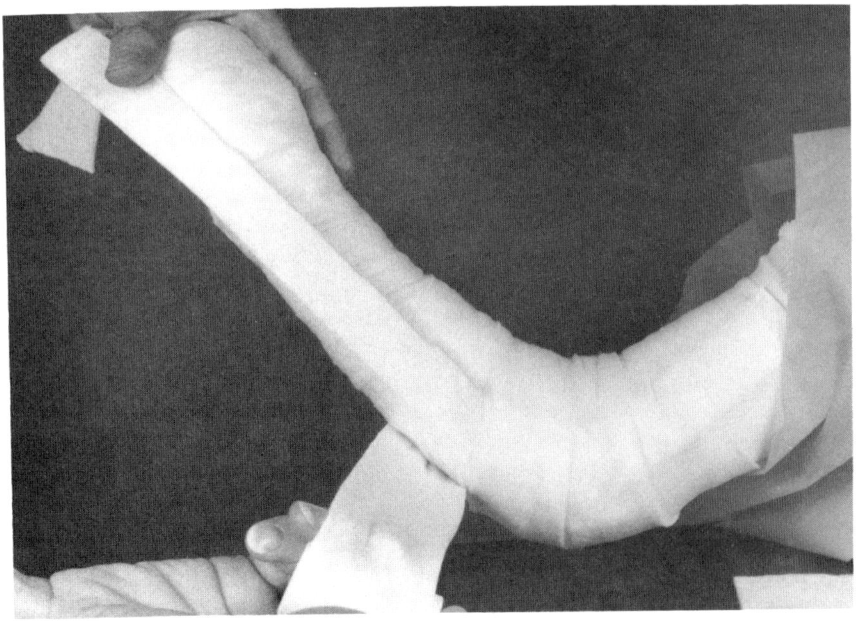

FIGURE 11–76. A strip of felt incorporated into the cast acts as a buffer for a cast saw during removal.

child's small body size, the conforming quality of plaster makes it preferable over the synthetic materials, although Flesch[53] has reported success with synthetics. Smaller rolls of cast material must be used. Two-inch rolls may be too wide for the hands and feet of children less than 3 years of age. Plaster rolls can be cut in half while still in their wrappers with a hacksaw. This technique is possible with the synthetics but they will become activated as soon as the wrapper is opened reducing the time available to apply the material. Fiberglass also tends to shred when cut in this manner. A common error is to apply too much padding beneath a cast causing it to shift distally as a child moves. Occasionally, a short arm cast may need to include a triceps strap (Fig. 11–77) or be changed to a long arm cast with the elbow in approximately 90° of flexion to prevent slipping (Fig. 11–78). A sling should be used to support the upper extremity when the elbow is included in a cast. A photograph of the cast with a line drawn on a finger or toe showing how much is exposed, or a line drawn on the skin at the proximal end of the cast can indicate if the cast has slipped. Any cast that has slipped out of position must be removed. Parents are instructed to look for any change in their child's skin color, swelling, or behavior as if in pain, such as inconsolable crying. Children may not be able to verbalize their discomfort other than by crying and must be monitored following the application of a cast. The cast should be removed if any of these events occur. The initial cast should be changed within 24 hours to evaluate skin condition.

Silicone Elastomer

The use of silicone elastomer in the rehabilitation and reconstructive phases of care for the management of hypertrophic scar was described by Malick and Carr[20,54] and by Feldman[55] as early as 1972. In addition, elastomer is effective in the immobili-

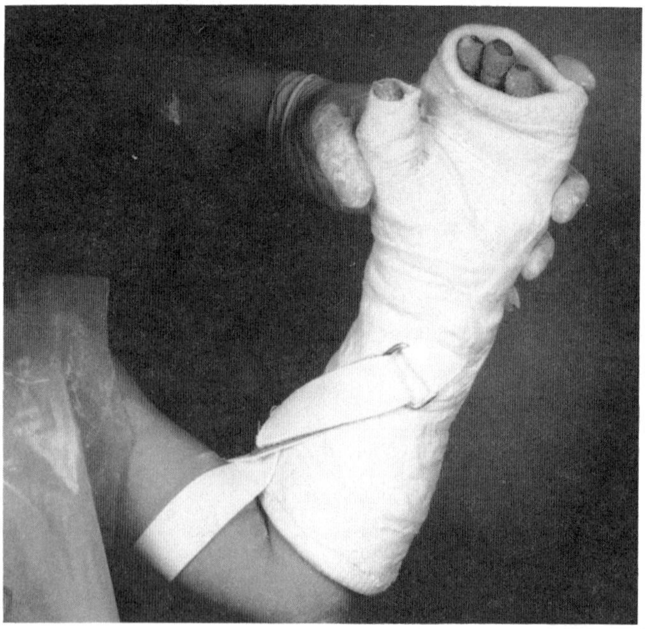

FIGURE 11–77. Triceps strap added to a short arm cast.

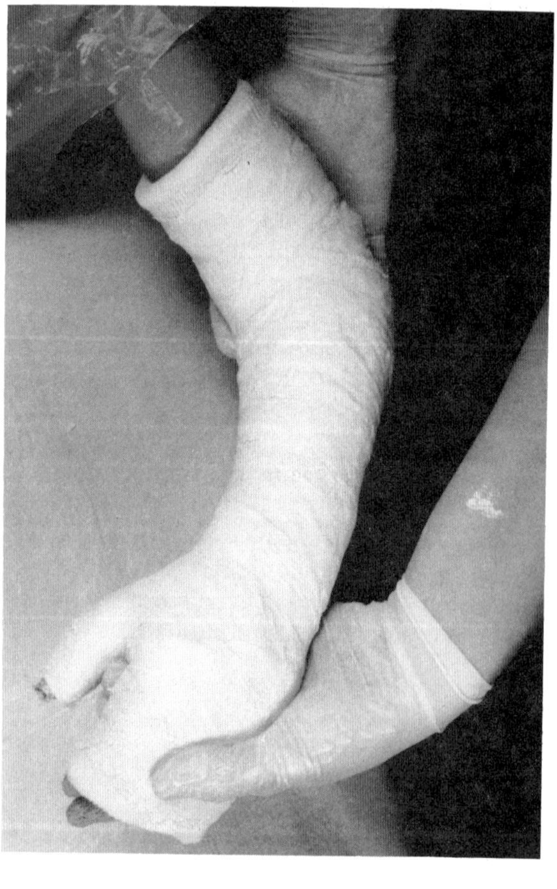

FIGURE 11–78. Long arm cast with flexed elbow.

zation of skin grafts for areas in which the application of a dressing or splint is difficult.[56] This material is excellent for casting when an exact impression of a tissue is required or when forming a negative mold for positive casts.[15]

Silicone elastomer is a two-component product consisting of a liquid elastomer base and a liquid catalyst (stannous octate). When combined, a rubberlike solid is produced without heat production that is flexible, nontoxic, and nonirritating. The time the product needs to cure is affected by the amount of catalyst used (more catalyst for a shorter cure time) and the temperature of the base. A base at room temperature will cure faster than a base that has been refrigerated if the same amount of catalyst is used. Curing is unaffected by moisture. Elastomers have a shelf life of approximately 6 months. Silicone elastomer should be used with caution over open areas or fragile tissue, as it is occlusive and maceration can occur.

Casts of silicone elastomer are ideal for use with tiny hands when alternative forms of therapy are ineffective (Fig. 11–79). The cast adheres slightly to the skin but can be made removable if slit and the suction developed is released. Unfortunately the finished cast or silicone mitt is often heavy and very immobilizing for a child, but it is effective for night splinting.

Another use is for serial casting of the hand or digits when an ideal position is difficult to maintain or the hand is severely contracted. The elastomer is poured over the hands of both the patient and person holding the patient's position. When cured, the individual's hand holding the position is released from the cast. The resultant holes are patched with additional elastomer. An elastic bandage or cohesive wrap secures the elastomer cast.

CASE STUDY

HISTORY

NP, a 41-year-old male, was admitted to the burn unit following a house fire. He sustained a 40 percent total body surface area burn of which 25 percent was full-thickness. His injury involved areas of all extremities distal to the mid-arm and thigh regions and small areas on his face.

The patient was evaluated by a therapist within 24 hours of admission. The patient could actively flex and extend all involved joints upon command, although flexion of the fingers was limited due to edema, and elbow, knee, and ankle ROM was limited due to pain. The therapist made assessments daily of the patient's ROM and function during regularly scheduled therapy sessions. As the first week progressed, the patient began loosing terminal extension of both the elbows and knees with more limitation on the left.

During the second week of hospitalization, the patient had excision and skin grafting of all full-thickness wounds. The left Achilles tendon area necessitated debridement down to tendon and the left dorsal hand required excision to fascia. Dressing changes took place on the second and fifth postoperative days and twice daily thereafter.

All skin grafts were successful except over the exposed Achilles tendon area, which progressed to more limited ankle dorsiflexion. This area slowly

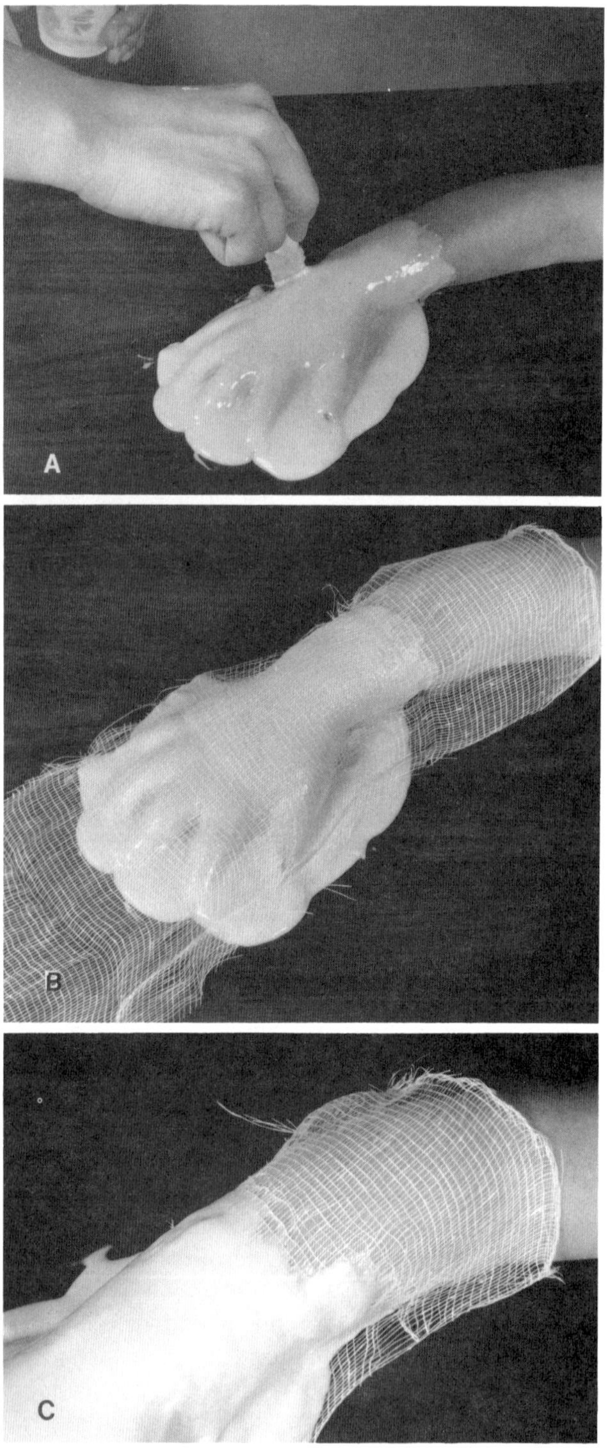

FIGURE 11–79. (*A*) The hand is positioned. Elastomer is spread over the entire hand and proximal to the wrist. The elastomer is tapered to as thin a thickness as possible at the wrist. (*B*) A gauze interface is set into the elastomer to minimize ripping of the final product. (*C*) A second thin layer of elastomer is applied and tapered at the wrist.

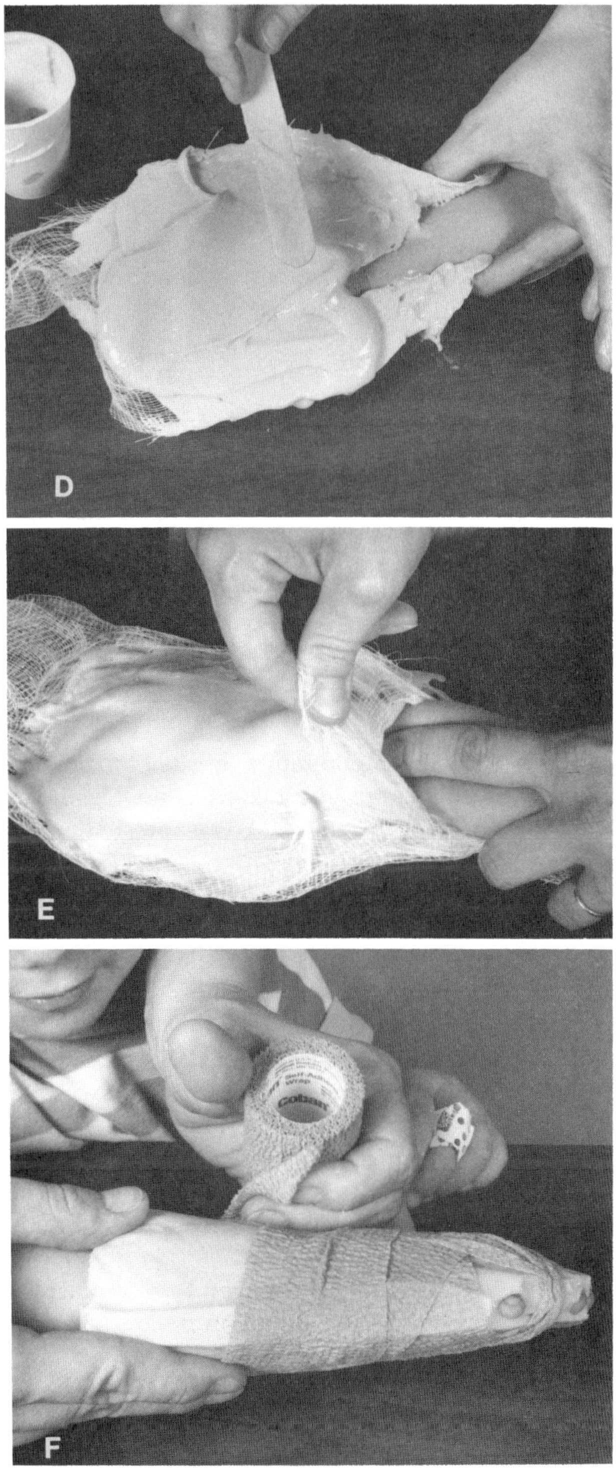

FIGURE 11–79. (*D*) The process is repeated on the palmar surface. (*E*) The therapist loosens the elastomer from the patient's skin by pushing the patient's skin away from the firm elastomer. The elastomer is cut with blunt tipped bandage scissors at least to the level of the MCP joints so that the hand can slip out. (*F*) The mitt is trimmed to expose fingertips which will act as landmarks for re-application. The therapist must carefully reapply the mitt to avoid pinching the skin where the mitt is cut. It is secured with a cohesive wrap.

granulated to fill the defect and the area was successfully spot-grafted a second time.

PROBLEM LIST

Extremity edema especially of the hands
Pain limiting ROM
Operative exposure of left Achilles tendon
Left-hand excision to fascia

GOALS

Minimal edema
Prevent scar tissue contracture development
Prevent deformity of left hand and fingers
Restore functional use of left ankle

TREATMENT INTERVENTION

Initially, the therapist chose not to splint the wrists, fingers, and hands due to the edema present. Likewise, neither the elbows nor the knees were splinted because full active ROM was present. However, bilateral ankle dorsiflexion splints were fabricated prophylactically for use while the patient was in bed.

As both knees and elbows became limited in extension, posterior knee and anterior elbow conforming splints were fabricated to prevent a further loss of motion. The wearing schedule was established as full-time use of the knee splints, while the elbow splints were alternated each hour during the day to allow the patient to perform functional tasks and were left on full time at night. All splints were removed for dressing changes and therapy.

Following surgery, the right hand was placed in a functional position splint and the left hand in an antideformity splint. The elbow and knee splints were changed from a semiporous to an open basketweave thermoplastic material. At the time of the first and second dressing changes, all splints were remolded. The splint schedule was changed to continuous wear in skin-grafted areas until the fifth postoperative day.

The patient was changed to a commercial dynamic ankle splint for his left ankle as limitations in motion progressively worsened. This splint was resumed following the patient's second surgery to skin-graft this area and used during outpatient care for an additional 3 weeks.

The other splints were changed to the preoperative wearing schedule after 1 week following surgery and discontinued as each area healed and the patient was able to demonstrate preservation of motion through exercise and ambulation.

RATIONALE

The patient's hands and wrists were not splinted initially because of fluctuations in edema during the first several days after burn injury. The therapist refrained from splinting the other areas of involvement, except for the ankles, until the patient began displaying a loss of motion so that mobility could be encouraged. The ankles were splinted immediately in dorsiflexion due to the depth of the burns and the natural plantarflexed position the ankles assume when a patient is lying in bed.

Full-time use of the knee splints kept the lower extremities extended at all times as this is the desired position. Knee extension splints also can be used during ambulation. The elbow splints were alternated to allow functional use of one of the upper extremities.

Contractures tend to develop more as burn wounds deepen. Excision to fascia of the left hand placed this hand in a more vulnerable state for limitations in motion than the right hand, so a more extreme antideformity position was chosen to splint the left hand compared to a more functional type of splint for the right.

The splint material for the elbows and knees was changed following surgery to an open weave to allow wetting of the postsurgical dressings. Modifications of all splints were needed at the time of the early postoperative dressing changes to accommodate the change in dressing bulk and to ensure proper fit of the definitive splints.

The patient continued to loose left ankle dorsiflexion while wearing standard static splints. Therefore, a splint that provided a constant force or tension was needed to counteract the changes occurring in the area of the exposed Achilles tendon. A dynamic ankle splint was utilized to achieve this goal. Additionally, the dynamic splint was worn for a longer period of time to counteract the deforming forces associated with a deeper wound and a prolonged healing time.

SUMMARY

Splinting is only one component of a comprehensive rehabilitation program and can be used in all phases of burn treatment for the purposes of protection, prevention of deformity, and preservation and restoration of function. Burn splints must meet specific requirements, including compatibility with wound dressings, ease of application, and reasonable cost. General mechanical, design, and construction principles must be followed along with specific considerations for the fit of the splint. Multiple splints for each body part are outlined with a description as well as specific advantages and disadvantages of each. Splint-wearing schedules are dependent upon patient participation and burn wound status and guidelines for continuous or intermittent use are included. Considerations for splinting during the operative and postoperative period, as well as splinting patients with hand burns and children are addressed. Fabrication guidelines for a basic hand, elbow, or knee extension; axillary and foot drop burn splints, and a basic cast are provided. By appropriately identifying the purpose(s) of a splint, wisely selecting the material, using the basic principles of splint construction, and fabricating a splint that is patient-specific rather than injury- or therapist-specific, the use of splinting can have a positive impact upon the rehabilitation of the burn-injured patient.

REFERENCES

1. Robotti, EB: The treatment of burns: An historical perspective with emphasis on the hand. In Grossman, JA (ed): Burns of the Upper Extremity. Hand Clinics 6:163–190, 1990.
2. Von Deines, Grapow, and Westendorff (ed and trans): Ubersetzung der medizinischen texte, vol. 4. Berlin, Akademie-Verlag, 1958, pp 214–221.
3. Paré, A: Opera chirurgica, a docto viro plerisque locis recognita et latinitate donata. Iacibi Guillemeau. . . . Labore et Diligentia. Frankfurt am Mein, Ioannem Feyrabend, 1594.
4. Warden, GD: The burned upper extremity—Historical perspective. In Salisbury, R and Pruitt, B (eds): Burns of the Upper Extremity. WB Saunders, Philadelphia, 1976, pp 16–23.
5. Cockshott, WP: The history of the treatment of burns. Surg Gynecol Obstet 102:116–124, 1956.
6. Willis, B: The use of orthoplast isoprene splints in the treatment of the acutely burned child: Preliminary report. Am J Occup Ther 23:57–61, 1969.
7. Evans, EB, Larson, DL, and Yates, S: Preservation and restoration of joint function in patients with severe burns. JAMA 204:843–848, 1968.
8. Larson, DL, et al: Contracture and scar formation in the burn patient. Clin Plast Surg 1:653–666, 1974.
9. Bryant, WM: Clinical symposia—wound healing. Ciba Pharmaceutical Company, 29, 1977.
10. Larson, DL, et al: The prevention and correction of burn scar contraction and hypertrophy. Shriners Burns Institute, University of Texas Medical Branch, Galveston, 1973.
11. Roberts, L, et al: Analysis of materials used for splinting the thermally injured patient. Proc Am Burn Assoc 22:143, 1990.
12. Staley, M, et al: A comprehensive evaluation of available splinting materials. Proc Am Burn Assoc 23:173, 1991.
13. Willis, B: Follow-up: The use of orthoplast isoprene splints in the treatment of the acutely burned child. Am J Occup Ther 24:187–191, 1970.
14. Helm, PA, et al: Burn injury: Rehabilitation management in 1982. J Burn Care Rehabil 4:411–422, 1983.
15. Fess, EE and Philips, CA: Hand splinting, principles and methods, ed 2. CV Mosby, St. Louis, 1987.
16. Colditz, JC: Dynamic splinting of the stiff hand. In Hunter, JM, et al (eds): Rehabilitation of the Hand, Surgery and Therapy. ed 3. CV Mosby, St. Louis, 1990, pp 342–352.
17. Kottke, FJ, Pauley, DL, and Ptak, RA: The rationale for prolonged stretching for correction of shortening of connective tissue. Arch Phys Med Rehabil 47:345–352, 1966.
18. Richard, RL: Use of the Dynasplint to correct elbow flexion burn contracture: A case report. J Burn Care Rehabil 7:151–152, 1986.
19. Richard, RL, et al: Treatment of exposed bilateral achilles tendons with use of the Dynasplint, a case report. Phys Ther 68:989–991, 1988.
20. Malick, MH and Carr, JA: Manual on Management of the Burn Patient, Including Splinting, Mold and Pressure Techniques. Harmarville Rehabilitation Center, Pittsburgh, 1982.
21. Walters, CJ: Splinting the Burn Patient. RAMSCO Publishing Company, Laurel, Maryland, 1987.
22. Fader, P: A self-instructional package: Neck conformer. J Burn Care Rehabil 6:124–127, 1985.
23. Apfel, LM and Wachtel, TL: Halo neck splint. J Burn Care Rehabil 8:140–143, 1987.
24. Fowler, D: Personal communication with Mary Beth Daugherty, 1984.
25. Silverglade, D and Ruberg, RL: Nonsurgical management of burns to the lips and commissures. Clin Plast Surg 13:87–94, 1986.
26. Smith, MN: Post-operative bivalved spinal fusion jacket. In Schreiber, S: Splinting with Aquaplast: The Basics and Beyond. WFR Aquaplast Corporation, Wyckoff, New Jersey, 1988.
27. Gore, D, et al: Comparison of complications during rehabilitation between conservative and early surgical management in thermal burns involving the feet of children and adolescents. J Burn Care Rehabil 9:92–95, 1988.
28. Barnett, PH and Stafford, FS: Use of plastic air bands for edema and scar contracture. J Burn Care Rehabil 5:469–473, 1984.
29. Keehnen, J, Daugherty, MB, and Warden, GD: Special shoes for the problem foot and ankle. Proc Am Burn Assoc 22:135, 1990.
30. Schwanholt, C, et al: Splinting the pediatric palmar burn. J Burn Care Rehabil 13:460–464, 1992.
31. Ward, RS, et al: Have you tried the sandwich splint? A method of preventing hand deformities in children. J Burn Care Rehabil 10:83–85, 1989.
32. Herndon, JH: Hand injuries—special considerations in children. Emerg Medi Clin North Am 3:405, 1985.
33. Puddicombe, BE and Nardone, MA: Rehabilitation of the burned hand. In Grossman, JA (ed): Burns of the Upper Extremity. Hand Clin 6:281–292, 1990.

34. Schnebly, WA, et al: A nonsplinting approach to the care of the thermally injured patient. J Burn Care Rehabil 10:263–266, 1989.
35. Salisbury, RE, Reeves, SU, and Wright, P: Acute care and rehabilitation of the burned hand. In Hunter, JM, et al (eds): Rehabilitation of the Hand, Surgery and Therapy, ed 3. CV Mosby, St. Louis, 1990, pp 831–840.
36. Miles, WK and Grigsby, L: Remodeling scar tissue in the burned hand. In Hunter, JM, et al (eds): Rehabilitation of the Hand, Surgery and Therapy, ed 3. CV Mosby, St. Louis, 1990, pp 841–857.
37. Richard, R, et al: The wide variety of designs for dorsal hand burn splints. Proc Am Burn Assoc 24:162, 1992.
38. Larson, DL, Abston, S, and Evans, EB: Splints and traction. In Polk, HC and Stone, HH (eds): Contemporary Burn Management. Little, Brown, Boston, 1971, pp 419–431.
39. Malick, MH: Management of the severely burned patient. Br J Occup Ther 38:76–80, 1975.
40. Tanigawa, MC, O'Donnell, OK, and Graham, PL: The burned hand—A physical therapy protocol. Phys Ther 54:953–958, 1974.
41. Byron, PM: Splinting the hand of a child. In Hunter, JM, et al (eds): Rehabilitation of the Hand, Surgery and Therapy, ed 3. CV Mosby, St. Louis, 1990, pp 1147–1152.
42. Malick, MH: Manual on Static Hand Splinting: New Materials and Techniques, ed 5. AREN Publications, Pittsburgh, 1985.
43. Bennett, GB, et al: Serial casting: A method for treating burn contractures. J Burn Care Rehabil 10:543–545, 1989.
44. Ridgway, CL, Daugherty, MB, and Warden, GD: Serial casting as a technique to correct burn scar contractures: a case report. J Burn Care Rehabil 12:67–72, 1991.
45. Indications and directions for use, plaster of Paris. Johnson & Johnson Products Inc, package insert.
46. Lavalette, R, Pope, MH, and Dickstein, H: Setting temperatures of plaster casts: The influence of technical variables. J Bone Joint Surg 64A:907–911, 1982.
47. Gannaway, JK and Hunter, JR: Thermal effects of casting materials. Clin Orthop Rel Res 181:191–195, 1983.
48. Wu, KK: Techniques in Surgical Casting and Splinting. Lea & Febiger, Philadelphia, 1987.
49. Jordon, MH, et al: Dynamic plaster casting for burn scar contracture—an alternative to surgery. Proc Am Burn Assoc 16:17, 1984.
50. Bell-Krotoski, JA: Plaster cylinder casting for contractures of the interphalangeal joints. In Hunter, JM, et al (eds): Rehabilitation of the Hand, Surgery and Therapy, ed 3. CV Mosby, St. Louis, 1990, pp 1128–1133.
51. Bell, JA: Plaster casting for the remodeling of soft tissue. In Fess, EE, Philips, CA: Hand Splinting, Principles and Methods, ed 2. CV Mosby, St. Louis, 1987, pp 449–466.
52. Tribuzi, SM: Serial plaster splinting. In Hunter, JM, et al (eds): Rehabilitation of the Hand, Surgery and Therapy, ed 3. CV Mosby, St. Louis, 1990, pp 1120–1127.
53. Flesch, P: Casting the young and the restless. Proc Am Burn Assoc 17:120, 1985.
54. Malick, MH and Carr, JA: Flexible elastomer molds in burn scar control. Am J Occup Ther 34:603–608, 1980.
55. Feldman, AE, Thompson, JT, and MacMillan, BG: The moulded silicone shoe in the prevention of contractures involving the burn-injured foot. Burns 1:83–95, 1974.
56. Engrav, LH, et al: Do splinting and pressure devices damage new grafts? (appliances and new grafts). J Burn Care Rehabil 4:107–108, 1983.

CHAPTER 12

Soft Tissue Management and Exercise

Cathy Humphrey, PT
Reginald L. Richard, MS, PT
Marlys J. Staley, MS, PT

Exercise, in conjunction with positioning and splinting, is an essential part of a burn patient's rehabilitation program. Static splinting and positioning usually are used to maintain a patient's range of motion or to prevent further loss of motion, while exercise imparts a stress to the patient's healing tissues to preserve or restore movement and improve the patient's physiologic and functional status. Exercises for a burn patient should be based on sound biomechanic and physiologic principles. Without exercise, results such as scar contracture, muscle atrophy, cardiopulmonary difficulties, and self-care limitations will occur.

Many therapists feel uneasy exercising burn patients due to the presence of extensive wounds, the extreme pain experienced by patients, and the fear of causing additional tissue damage.[1] In the literature, much of the information to support the use of exercise with burn patients was gained empirically through clinical experience.[2,3] The purpose of this chapter is to present current information about burn patient exercises and to describe the methods and interventions that can be used to initiate and progress a burn patient's exercise program.

An initial evaluation of the patient should be performed as soon as possible after a patient's hospital admission and an exercise program should be designed specifically for the patient. Initially, burn patients and their families may not understand why such painful treatments are necessary. Repeated explanations and reassurances may be required until the patient and family realize that exercise is an essential part of burn rehabilitation and long-term functional recovery. At first, the discomfort and protests voiced by a patient may be difficult for a therapist to manage psychologically. However, the realization that the physical alternative to exercise for a burn patient may be scar tissue contractures and deformity can assist the therapist to persevere

TABLE 12–1. Timelines for Development of Various Tissue Tightness

Tissue Type	Days
Burn scar contracture	1–4
Intramuscular adhesion from bleeding	3–5
Tendons and sheaths	5–21
Muscle adaptive shortening without trauma	14–21
Ligaments and joint capsule	30–90

with an exercise program. In addition, the therapist must develop a creative exercise program based on the unique characteristics of each patient and the burn wound.

Burn patient exercises are designed primarily to prevent the development of burn scar contractures and to avoid the deleterious effects of in-patient hospitalization. Additionally, burn patients may be susceptible to other types of soft tissue tightness with varying times of onset (Table 12–1).[4] However, if there is an absence of direct trauma or bleeding to these other tissues, limitations in motion usually take a longer period of time to develop. Close monitoring of a patient's range of motion will enable the therapist to determine which tissues are causing restrictions in motion.

An exercise program should begin immediately following a patient's admission to the hospital to counteract the contracting force of the wound and subsequent scar tissue.[2,5,6,7] Clinically, one cause of scar tissue contracture may result simply from a lack of tissue to accommodate movement. Exercises are used to keep the wound from contracting so that additional scar tissue can be produced to fill the wound. With more tissue available, movement should be easier to achieve.

EXERCISE PRESCRIPTION FACTORS

The ultimate goal of a burn rehabilitation program is to assist patients to return to society at the most optimal functional level as possible compared to their preinjury status. This all encompassing goal can be subdivided into more specific goals depending on the patient's stage of recovery as listed in Table 12–2.[2,3,8]

In addition to setting treatment goals, an exercise plan takes various factors into consideration (Table 12–3). Each of these factors impacts the others.

Phase of Recovery, Intent of Exercise, Patient Medical Status

The severity of a burn injury determines how quickly a patient passes through the emergent and resuscitative phases. The primary intent of the initial exercise program will be to treat any resulting edema. If a patient is alert and able to assist mentally and physically with an edema reduction program, active exercises may be used. Conversely, if a patient has experienced an extensive burn or is unresponsive, other methods for edema reduction are used and the initial exercises will need to be performed passively.

During the acute or pregrafting phase of recovery, the focus of an exercise program is to preserve a patient's range of motion and functional strength. As before, if the patient is able to participate in the exercise program without undue physio-

TABLE 12–2. Goals of Burn Patient Exercise Program

Reduce edema and promote circulation.
Prevent scar tissue contractures and deformity.
Preserve muscle strength and joint mobility.
Promote maximum functional independence.

TABLE 12–3. Factors Affecting the Establishment of a Burn Patient Exercise Program

Goals to achieve
Phase of recovery
Intent of exercise
Patient's medical status
Age of patient
Social support
Frequency of treatment
Location of burn
Extent of burn
Depth of burn
Precautions and contraindications
Type of exercise

logic stress, exercises can be performed actively. If, however, a patient continues to experience a decreased level of consciousness, passive exercise intervention is appropriate.

A patient's level of pain should be considered to determine the intensity of the exercises. As the patient progresses into the postacute or recovery phase, the program emphasis should include more functional types of activities, with the patient performing the majority of exercises independently.

Age, Social Support, and Frequency of Treatment

The age of a patient, particularly the extremes of the young and aged, impacts the extent of an exercise program. Infants, toddlers, and children are unable or too unreliable to actively participate in an independent exercise program. Although they are physiologically capable of tolerating high levels of activity under normal conditions,[9] children will be limited in the daily total amount of exercise time unless their therapy program is supplemented with outside assistance from persons other than the therapist.

After age 25 to 30, the physical capacity of adults to exercise declines approximately 8 to 10 percent each decade.[9] Adults may be more reliable to perform an individually prescribed exercise program, but their absolute strength and aerobic capacity decreases with age.

During the painful recovery process from a burn, patients of all ages should be advised to exercise more frequently for shorter periods of time rather than less frequently for longer treatment periods. Once a patient's range of motion (ROM) and flexibility have been increased, scar tissue immediately will tend to return to its pref-

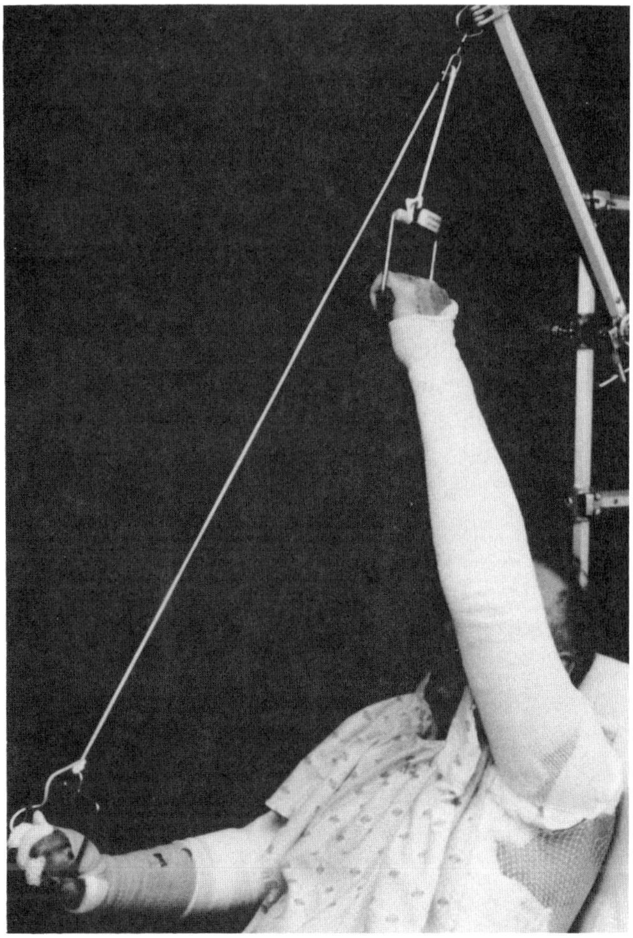

FIGURE 12–1. Patient uses reciprocal pulleys independently at bedside to supplement formal exercise program.

erential shortened state.[5] Unless a patient's scar tissue is maintained in an elongated state through splinting, positioning, or additional exercise, the patient's ROM again will become limited in a relatively short period of time. With proper instruction, informal therapy can be administered by a competent adult or parent for a youngster, or by compliant patients with the use of assistive devices such as reciprocal pulleys or cuff weights (Fig. 12–1).

Location, Extent, and Depth of Burn

Due to the relentless contractile nature of scar tissue, it would be difficult for patients to overexercise,[5] especially when a burn injury is deep. The deeper the burn injury, the greater the chance of scar tissue contractures developing.[10] Dobbs and Curreri[11] have documented the incidence of scar contracture for both deep partial-thickness and full-thickness burns and showed a progressive increase in contracture formation in the more severe burn injury. As the depth of the burn injury increases, so should the emphasis on exercise.

The need for burn patients to exercise also exists due to a direct relationship between the total body surface area burned and the number of burn contractures that can develop.[12] As the percent of body burn increases, the emphasis placed on exercise should increase. Burn scar is approximately one third as pliable as normal skin. Therefore, as more of the body's normal skin is replaced by scar tissue, a greater emphasis needs to be placed on maintaining immature scar tissue in an elongated state.

Exercise for a burn patient should focus on those areas that are most likely to develop scar tissue contractures (see Chapter 9, Table 9–2). Equally important is the need to elongate scar tissue that forms over multiple and adjacent joint skin creases.[1,13] Contiguous areas of scar tissue that cross neighboring joint surfaces should be elongated in combination with each other. For example, if a burn lies on the lateral trunk surface and extends to the anterior axillary fold and includes the entire arm and forearm, the exercise session should conclude with the patient in a supine position of shoulder abduction with the wrist and elbow in extension (Fig. 12–2).

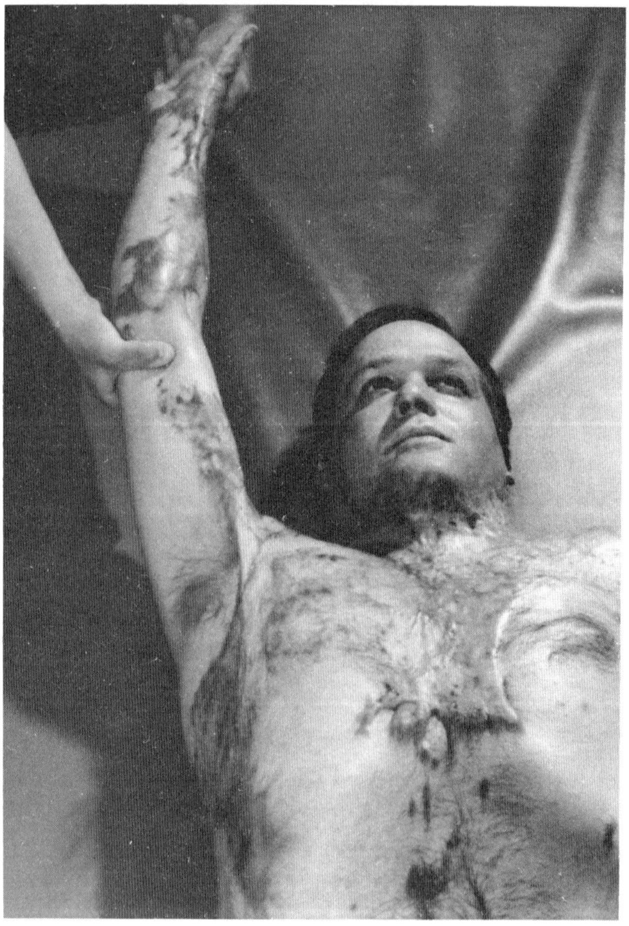

FIGURE 12–2. Tissue elongation over multiple involved areas of patient's torso and right upper extremity. This stretching exercise emphasizes shoulder flexion/abduction, elbow extension, and wrist extension. Note the extent of scar tissue blanching through the entire length of involvement.

Precautions and Contraindications

Normally, when a person becomes wounded, the body part or segment is placed at rest for a specific period of time so wound healing may occur. This time may be 7 to 10 days for sutured wounds and 6 weeks or longer for fractured bones to heal. However, for burn patients, except in cases where a burn wound is either skin-grafted or primarily closed, exercise of burn areas is allowed to progress with little regard for the healing process. This treatment approach is a major difference between treating burn patients and patients with other soft tissue injuries.

Modifications of an exercise program may be indicated in some circumstances[7] (Table 12–4). Patients with a significant past medical history for cardiac or orthopedic conditions, such as surgical repair of joints, should be screened carefully.[14] Immediately following a major burn injury, there is a great demand placed on the cardiovascular system as a result of fluid shifts and hemodynamic changes. Caution should be taken to avoid strenuous exercise of patients with pre-existing cardiac or pulmonary problems. Similarly, particularly in the elderly, patients should be screened for arthritis and other dysfunctional limitations. Burn rehabilitation emphasizes regaining full ROM and one needs to note where previous limitations existed.

Because the hands are so vital to function, one of the greatest concerns with exercises involves the extensor tendons of the fingers. When there is any question concerning the depth of a burn to the dorsum of the fingers, repeated flexion and extension of the joints, particularly the proximal interphalangeal joints, should be avoided.[1] Forced composite fisting of a hand and digits should be avoided to prevent rupture of the extensor mechanism. However, if a burn wound is determined to be superficial, or previously exposed extensor tendons are covered with viable tissue, then gentle ROM to increase flexion may begin.[1]

Caution when performing ROM exercises in areas involving exposed tendons is justified but needs to be qualified. There is a significant difference between a "button-hole" type of tendon exposure and one in which the entire length of the tendon is exposed. Also, the thickness, or surface area of the tendon should be considered when contemplating performing exercises with exposed tendons.

A button-hole type of tendon exposure means a tendon is visible through a small opening in the surrounding tissue or becomes visible as the wound separates with motion. A common place to observe a button-hole type of exposure is on the dorsum of the hand with flexion of the metacarpalphalangeal joint or at the distal end of the Achilles tendon. Some therapists agree that ROM exercises are continued despite exposed tendons in the lower extremity.[15] Justification included the fact that the cross-sectional area of the tendon, and hence the tensile strength, was sufficient that tendon rupture was of minor concern; or, the location of tendons, such as the toe exten-

TABLE 12–4. Burn Patient Exercise Precautions

Significant past medical history
Joint disease
Exposed tendons
Dystrophic calcification
IV lines or ventilatory support

TABLE 12–5. Burn Patient Exercise Contraindications

Exposed joints
Tendon exposure over the proximal interphalangeal joint of the finger
Thrombophlebitis
Deep venous thrombosis
Compartment syndrome
Fresh skin graft

sors, minimized risk during exercise or gait. However, exposed tendons are difficult areas to treat, and caution is advised to err on the side of conservatism if a therapist is inexperienced or in doubt of a clinical situation.

Another precautionary condition involves the formation of excessive bone (see Chapter 20). When dystrophic calcification is suspected as a problem, any form of forced exercise is contraindicated although active ROM is permitted.[16,17]

When treating burn patients, there are few instances forbidding exercise. Strict contraindications to burn patient exercises are listed in Table 12–5. In the instance of exposed joints, any form of exercise should be halted and strict immobilization of the joint is indicated.[7,8,18] The joint should be immobilized in a neutral position or in the position that will be most functional for the patient without risking further joint damage.

To avoid the possibility of an embolus developing, any patient suspected of thrombophlebitis or diagnosed with a deep venous thrombosis should not exercise the involved extremity until the patient has received appropriate medical treatment and has been permitted by the physician to resume exercise.[3,19,20]

A compartment syndrome is another circulatory problem that necessitates the cessation of exercise. Excessive edema may cause severe circulatory compromise. If a therapist suspects that a muscle compartment syndrome is developing, exercise should be halted immediately and the physician notified. Signs of a compartment syndrome include paresthesia or numbness, poor capillary refill of nail beds, decreased peripheral pulses, pain, or a change to a cooler temperature or paler color of the skin.

Depending on the postoperative policy of each burn facility, exercise to areas following skin grafting may not be permitted immediately. This delay in reinstituting exercise is true particularly where skin grafts cover joint creases or multiple adjacent joints.[1,3] Burn wounds that have been primarily closed by sutures, either in the acute phase of healing or following a reconstructive procedure, usually remain immobilized at least until the sutures are removed. However, areas not skin-grafted can continue to be exercised particularly if they are distant from a skin grafted site.[3]

The time frame for initiation of exercise following the application of cultured skin depends on the type of skin used and guidelines established by the provider of the skin. In many cases, when cultured skin is used for grafting (see Chapter 8), strict adherence to a policy of no exercise therapy for up to 10 days is advised by the manufacturer to allow undisturbed time for the skin cells to adhere. Cultured skin displays little resistance to mechanical forces for a minimum of 3 weeks, so progression of an exercise program must be very gradual.[21–23]

TYPES OF EXERCISE

Most of the exercises used to treat burn patients can be grouped into three basic categories: ROM, conditioning, and functional exercises. Although there can be an overlap as to when each type of exercise is implemented, some of the various exercises have specific indications for use.

ROM Exercises

PASSIVE ROM EXERCISES

Passive exercise is used to maintain ROM, assess joint motion, elongate tissue and requires little energy expenditure by a patient.[3,8,24] Although passive range of motion (PROM) may be the least desirable form of exercise, this exercise has a definite place in burn care (Table 12–6). Some clinicians believe that PROM may cause tissue damage from microtears, leading to increased scarring, but this theory has not been substantiated.[3,5,7] PROM frequently is used with a patient who is comatose or in an intensive care unit (ICU) to maintain joint mobility and lubrication.[3] Burn patients who are obtunded need to have their limbs moved, which can be accomplished by an external source. Likewise, patients who are heavily medicated or critically ill may be unable to actively participate in an exercise program. PROM should be performed gently, slowly, and cautiously by the therapist. Precautions should be taken to avoid overstretching joint structures.

PROM is a useful method to obtain full joint ROM, particularly if soft tissue is restricting movement. Scar tissue responds well to passive force when applied in a steady, controlled manner over a prolonged period of time. Anytime there is paralysis of a limb segment, the segment and surrounding tissue only can be moved passively.[3] This situation is the case when PROM is performed while a patient is under anesthesia as discussed later.

There are a few special instances where PROM is indicated. One situation is when an escharotomy has been performed.[3] Frequently, therapists are hesitant to perform ROM to limbs where an escharotomy has been made due to the amount of tissue damage. However, once hemostasis has occurred, range of motion is permis-

TABLE 12–6.
Considerations for Use of PROM Exercise

Patient level of consciousness
Medication level
Severity of condition
Decreased ROM
Scar contractures
Peripheral nerve injury
Preservation of joint mobility
Anesthetized patient
Area of escharotomy
Preservation of tendon glide

sible. Also, limited PROM can be performed to preserve tendon glide and prevent the formation of tendon adhesions. However, caution is advised when using this approach with exposed tendons. The degree of joint ROM should be restricted to the amount required for an observable tendon excursion to occur. After full ROM is obtained, and if the patient is responsive, PROM should be replaced with active or active-assistive exercises.

ACTIVE-ASSISTIVE ROM EXERCISES

Clinical indications to perform active-assistive range of motion (AAROM) with burn patients are listed in Table 12–7. AAROM exercises are performed when a patient has difficulty completing full ROM.[2,8,24] This lack of motion may be due to weakness, fear, pain, or tight tissue and usually occurs near the end of joint range. The therapist should encourage as much active movement as possible and provide as little assistance as necessary.

AAROM also is permitted in areas where escharotomies have been performed.[3] Some clinicians believe that AAROM following skin grafting should be reserved until there is good graft adherence to avoid loosening the graft from its wound bed.[2]

To decrease the physiologic energy demands on patients during times of high metabolic stress, performing AAROM has been recommended.[3,7] Wilmore[25] has reported a direct increased relationship between metabolic rate in burn patients and the extent of body surface area burned when compared to normal persons. Black and colleagues[26] reported an approximate 55 percent increase in resting oxygen consumption of burn patients with a mean burn size of 38.3 percent. However, when performing a set of short-arc quadricep knee extension and straight leg raise exercises, burn patients demonstrated a relatively equal increase in oxygen consumption required to perform these exercises when compared to a control group of nonburned subjects. Leman and colleagues[27] also reported at the 1992 American Burn Association Meeting that no statistically significant difference was found when comparing resting and exercise oxygen consumption values of 10 burn patients with a mean 26 percent total body surface area burn.[27]

Both passive and active-assistive exercises encompass the elongation of tissue or "stretching." The preferred method of tissue elongation to avoid tissue damage is a sustained stretch delivered in a slow, prolonged manner to an area of decreased motion or contracture.[2,3,7,8,24] Healed tissue is stretched to the point of frank blanching, within a patient's pain tolerance, and maintained until the tissue becomes more

TABLE 12–7. Considerations for Use of AAROM Exercises

Limited ROM
Scar contractures
Area of escharotomy
Skin graft adherence
Increased physiologic demands
Decreased cardiac reserve
Poor ventilation and respiratory status
Decreased strength secondary to prolonged hospitalization

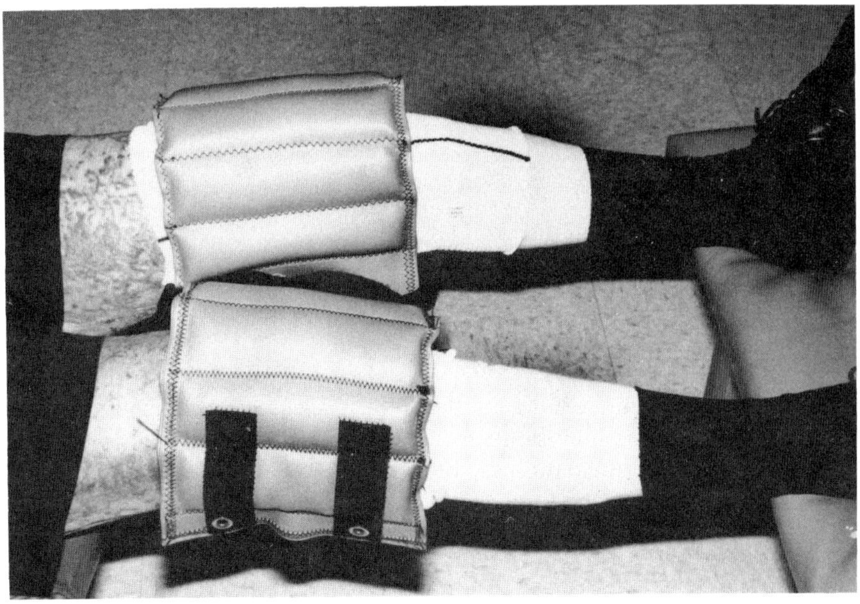

FIGURE 12–3. While patient sits on a chair with feet supported on a stool, cuff weights are applied to the anterior knees to assist with passive elongation of bilateral knee flexion contractures.

pliable or tissue color returns.[8,24] Approximately 1 to 2 pounds of force is required to cause blanching, but this force must be maintained for long durations, as discussed in Chapter 4. Additionally, 6 to 10 preliminary repetitions of tissue elongation should be performed to ensure that a tissue is at its optimal length before a sustained force is applied.

It has been suggested that stretching is more effective when preceded by or used in conjunction with heat modalities such as paraffin or ultrasound.[1,3,7,24,28]

The therapist can apply a gentle sustained stretch at the end range using a contract-relax technique, or pulleys and weights. Contract-relax is a technique requiring as isometric contraction of a muscle followed by relaxation of the same muscle while the therapist gently stretches the overlying involved tissue.[1,3,8] The procedure should be performed near the end of a patient's available range and repeated until full ROM is achieved or no further increase in ROM is noted.

Active-assistive exercises using pulleys or the patient's body weight can be very effective to stretch axillae, elbows, wrists, knees, or Achilles tendon areas and allows the patient some control over the treatment.[3,10,24] Static weights can be used to elongate scars of elbows, knees, and wrists. For example, with a knee flexion contracture, the patient can sit in a chair with the foot of the affected leg supported on another chair. The knee is unsupported between the two chairs. Weights, to patient tolerance, are applied gradually to the knee to obtain knee extension (Fig. 12–3). Alternatively, a weight around the ankle of a patient while lying prone could be used.

Some patients will want to stop stretching before blanching of a scar occurs or before the therapist perceives the maximum range has been attained. Encouragement and relaxation reminders, such as deep breathing and visualization, are helpful to the patient in these circumstances.[7] With experience, a therapist usually develops a perception of how extensively to stretch scar tissue.[8]

TABLE 12–8. Considerations for Use of AROM Exercises

Edema reduction from muscle pumping
Increasing circulation
Initiation of exercise first week after skin grafting
Conditioning of uninvolved areas
Exposed tendons (except the proximal interphalangeal joint)
Prevention of soft tissue shortening
Prevention of muscle atrophy

ACTIVE ROM EXERCISES

Active range of motion (AROM) is the preferred type of exercise in several situations[7] (Table 12–8). AROM may be less painful for a patient than active-assistive or passive range and is used for patients who can achieve full ROM of a particular joint within a reasonable amount of time. AROM can assist in edema reduction through activation of the muscle pump that enhances venous and lymphatic return.[2] Also, active motion can promote circulation in an area to prevent circulatory problems, such as deep venous thrombosis.

AROM by a patient should be encouraged for any body area or segment that is not burned to preserve joint ROM, to prevent muscle atrophy, or to strengthen weakened muscles that result from the burn.[2] Usually, a patient's volitional muscle contraction is insufficient to rupture a tendon, so AROM is preferred when tendons are exposed.[7] ROM of the proximal interphalangeal joints is exempted because of possible rupture of the extensor tendons overlying these joints (see Chapter 19). However, any tendon that is suspected of having extensive damage should be treated conservatively by immobilizing the tendon in a slack position.[3]

In some burn facilities, only AROM during the first week following skin grafting is permitted.[2,7,8] The rationale for this approach is to avoid applying forces to the skin graft that might disrupt the graft from its bed and to allow the skin graft more time to adhere. Patients usually will not move beyond their own pain tolerance, which limits the stress applied to a skin graft.

Conditioning Exercises

Several types of exercise can be grouped under the category of conditioning exercises and subdivided into strengthening and endurance exercises[3] (Table 12–9). These exercises usually are implemented during the rehabilitative phase of a burn patient's exercise program to preserve or increase muscle strength or to improve a patient's endurance.[2] These exercises should be instituted after complete ROM has been achieved consistently.[7] If ROM is lacking, the therapist's priority should be to

TABLE 12–9. Considerations for Use of Conditioning Exercises

Improvement in cardiovascular capacity
Strengthening muscles opposite contractures
Maintain strength in uninvolved extremities

treat the limitation in motion rather than strengthening the patient as a normal healthy muscle is unable to generate the force required to elongate burn scar tissue.

Isometrics are a form of conditioning exercise that can be used early in a patient's exercise program.[2,3] They are comfortable to perform and require a minimal amount of energy expenditure. Isometrics are beneficial to maintain muscle strength in patients on bed rest. In addition, isometric exercises can be performed by muscle groups with newly applied skin grafts without fear of disrupting the graft since no stretching, buckling, or shearing force is applied. Isometric exercises also are a means to promote circulation in an area.

When burn patients have achieved an anabolic state of metabolism and can perform AROM exercises successfully, they can progress to resistive exercises and begin an independent exercise program. The physical capacity of a patient, which includes strength, aerobic power, and flexibility, should be evaluated prior to beginning a resistive exercise program, with the patient's age being taken into consideration. Standardized tests for work capacity can be used to establish satisfactory baselines for future comparison.[29] Cronan and associates[30] found significant deficits in the isokinetic strength of burn patients following discharge from the hospital. Resistive exercise is of tremendous benefit to a patient to increase muscle strength, but should be used only when the patient can tolerate the increased metabolic stress.[3,7] In addition, prior to the initiation of resistive exercises with a patient, the area to be exercised should have full AROM, which can be achieved consistently.[7] In general, the therapist should wait until a majority of the burn wound is healed prior to initiating a resistive exercise program.[3,7] Previously healthy adult patients with less than 15 percent total body surface area burns and no concomitant medical problems should tolerate resistive exercise.[7] The use of resistance can be initiated sooner to extremities or individual joints not involved in the burn injury. For example, patients with lower extremity burns can perform progressive resistive exercises with the upper extremities.

When implementing a strengthening program, the muscles opposing scar tissue contractures should be strengthened.[1,3,7] For instance, if the antecubital space of an elbow is burned, then exercises designed to strengthen the triceps for elbow extension should be emphasized. Throughout a patient's hospital course, strengthening muscles of uninvolved extremities should be encouraged.[2,3] These exercises should be performed as part of a patient's independent exercise routine to make better use of the time established for formal therapy sessions.

Similarly, endurance-type exercises should be reserved for that period in the patient's course of recovery when other primary needs have been satisfied. Satisfactory endurance and strength both can be regained once normal activities are resumed.[31,32]

Functional Exercises

Functional exercises can begin early in a patient's hospital course to reinforce the ultimate goal of physical independence for the burn patient (Table 12–10). The initial intent of functional exercises should be directed at promoting a carryover effect of the ROM program.[7] Activities designed to mirror the direction of movement necessary to avert scar contracture formation should be stressed. Likewise, when sequencing a patient's treatment program, functional activities are more beneficial if they follow

TABLE 12–10. Functional Exercise Considerations

Reinforce carryover of exercise program.
Perform following achievement of maximal ROM.
Increase patient self-satisfaction.
Increase patient endurance.

tissue elongation exercises so that a greater ROM may be used while performing the functional demands of tasks.

Functional exercises also serve to increase the self-esteem and satisfaction of burn patients when they are able to accomplish activities of daily living once inhibited by weakness or scar contracture tightness.[33] Because hospitalization has a deleterious effect on a patient's cardiovascular and aerobic capacity, functional activities should stress endurance.[8,30–32] In preparation for discharge from the hospital, functional activities, such as personal hygiene, dressing, cooking, and light housekeeping, may become the primary focus of a patient's daily treatment. This emphasis ensures that the patient is able to manage physically at home and to ease the transition from the hospital to home environment.

Beyond basic activities of daily living, burn patients should progress to more strenuous forms of functional activities when mutually agreed upon by the therapist, patient, and physician. Programs such as work-hardening or vocational rehabilitation for adults provide a gradual transition back into the workforce (see Chapter 16). Children can be challenged gradually in the level of their play activity to the point of age-appropriate recreation.

Joint Mobilization

Joint mobilization and distraction techniques can be used effectively with a burn patient when special precautions are taken.[8] Because of the extensive damage to the skin with resulting scar formation, decreased ROM of a particular joint may be mistaken for capsular involvement. In general, capsular involvement will not be seen in the acute stage of a burn injury, unless there was trauma to the joint from a fall or other type of impact at the time of the burn injury (see Table 12–1). Usually the capsule becomes affected during the scar maturation phase after an extended period of decreased ROM. Joint mobilization is contraindicated for an open joint or a joint with exposed tendons. Due to the amount of physical contact required for mobilization techniques, a burn patient's tissue might not be able to tolerate the forces involved with a therapist's hand placement. Therefore, caution should be used when applying a mobilization force.

ADDITIONAL EXERCISE CONSIDERATIONS

Pool Therapy

If a hospital is equipped with a swimming pool, or a public pool is available, swimming can supplement a burn patient's exercise program following wound closure. Swimming can be an enjoyable means for a patient to achieve total body exercise and increase cardiovascular endurance. Crawford[34] cited the benefit of a burn rehabilitation swimming program as having low risk of damaging newly healed skin, weak muscles, or weak joints and attributed positive aspects of swimming to the buoyancy of the water. Community swimming programs also promote a gradual and controlled exposure of the burn patient to the public. In addition, various hydrofitness devices for upper and lower extremity strengthening are available for use in the pool.[35,36] However, due to the amount of chlorine required for use in public pools by departments of public health, caution is advised if a patient has particularly sensitive skin or develops a rash.

Circuit Training

Recently, a growing interest in group activities and circuit training for burn patients has developed.[37,38] Parrot and associates[37] described a program that included 10 work stations each requiring a different activity such as pulleys, chin-up bar, macrame or belt work, and stair climbing. According to their research, the use of a circuit program resulted in: (1) increased functional independence of patients in a shorter time period, (2) increased level of patient self-confidence, (3) improved exercise habit patterns, (4) increased time efficiency for patient treatment, (5) identification of otherwise unnoticed problem areas, and (6) more specific goal setting for the patients.

Education

Part of a therapist's treatment goal should be to assist the patient to become as independent as possible with an exercise program and activities of daily living (ADL) skills.[8,24] The patient's family or primary caregiver can be a great aid in achieving this goal. Instructing the family as caregivers teaches them the importance of exercise and prepares them to assist the patient when the therapist is absent. Unfortunately, family members may become part of the problem of decreased patient compliance because of their concern for their loved one and their fear of causing the patient pain. When this is the case, the therapist needs to spend extra time teaching and encouraging family members.

SPECIAL EXERCISE CONSIDERATIONS

Exercise Under Anesthesia

Therapists agree that a patient's poor tolerance of pain makes the goal of maintaining full ROM difficult. Patients often become extremely fearful of any activity that increases their pain. They may refuse to move and may resist a therapist's attempt to assist with exercises. Children also can become so fearful of pain that achieving full ROM may be impossible. In these cases, joint ROM under anesthesia is recommended.[1,3,39-42] This intervention is performed in conjunction with a patient's scheduled surgery. Following the administration of anesthesia and while the operating room staff prepares the patient for surgery, the therapist performs slow, sustained

PROM with the affected extremity. Precautions should be taken to avoid tears, joint dislocation, damage to the joint capsule, or fractures. The amount of time the therapist spends on one area will depend on the extent of contracture or tissue resistance and the time allotted for the surgical procedure. Performing PROM while the patient is anesthetized provides the therapist with the following advantages: (1) to determine the source of the restricted ROM, (2) to assess the actual amount of joint ROM available, (3) to identify the soft tissue cause of any limitation in motion, and (4) to provide the patient with a thorough ROM treatment without pain. These determinations will help a therapist to guide a patient's daily exercise program.

Auto-Release

Auto-release is a term used to describe a scar, usually situated near a joint, which separates during exercise or some type of forceful stress. When this tissue separation occurs, an open wound results (Fig. 12–4). Usually, there is little pain involved when an auto-release occurs and the patient's ROM improves instantly. Some physicians may elect to allow the auto-release area to heal spontaneously, while others will skin graft the area. Allowing small open wounds to heal while maintaining the newly achieved ROM often is the best alternative. If an open wound is large and continues to increase in size with movement, a skin graft will be needed.

Exercise Following Skin Grafting

The patient should resume a daily exercise program to areas that were skin-grafted as soon as the graft will tolerate movement. Adherent skin grafts will have a pinkish hue to them, indicating vascular inosculation of the graft, which is necessary for healing. Skin graft adherence can be judged by placing one's finger on various parts of the skin graft and attempting to gently move the graft from side-to-side. Protocols from various burn units differ on the time frame for initiating exercise

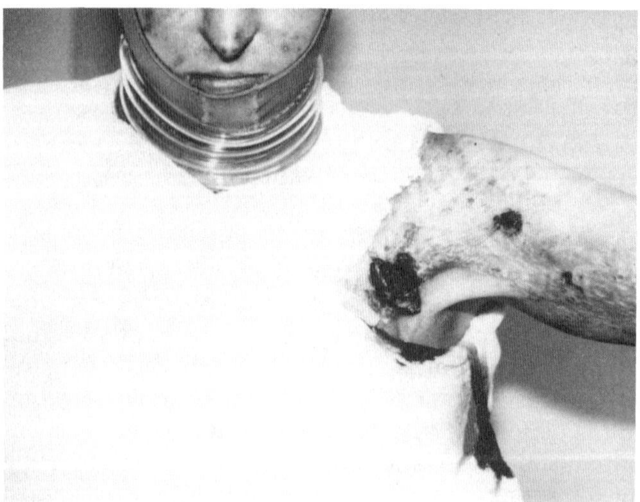

FIGURE 12–4. Site of auto-release of scar tissue of left anterior axillary fold.

following skin grafting.[3,8,41,43,44] The reported length of immobilization usually varies from 4 to 10 days.[1,2,8,44,45] However, the accepted length of time for immobilization currently has been decreasing.[46,47]

The therapist should view the skin grafts prior to reinitiating exercise to determine: (1) the integrity of the graft (e.g., does the graft appear thin and fragile or hematomas in several areas?), (2) the presence of exposed tendons, (3) any joint creases that are involved, and (4) the extent of graft adherence. When exercise is resumed, AROM is preferred to limit the amount of stress applied to the new skin.[2,8] If a patient had good AROM prior to surgery, the therapist can expect to regain this motion within 7 to 10 days following the resumption of exercise.[3] Frequently, the patient's AROM is limited after surgery by pain if surgical staples were used to secure the skin grafts. The aggressiveness of ROM provided should be tempered if staples are present to avoid causing patients undue pain. After 2 to 3 days of active motion, AAROM can be added to the program for those patients having difficulty regaining motion. Exercise should continue to those areas not directly involved in the skin graft procedure unless the exercise causes movement of the grafted areas.[3,14]

Donor Sites

Exercise intended to improve the ROM of areas that are exercise-limited because they were donor sites needs to be clarified. Typically, donor sites are taken from areas of skin that do not cross joint skin creases. However, due to the thickness of a skin graft harvested from a donor site, these resulting wounds can be very tender and painful depending on the type of donor site dressing. Frequently pain associated with a donor site interferes with a patient's movement. If a painful donor site is the cause of a limitation in motion, the limitation generally will resolve once the donor site heals. Unless the donor site is in direct line with a band of scar tissue limiting motion at a particular joint, the area of a donor site may not require exercise. If there are skin grafts located next to a donor site, exercise may have to be delayed until the graft shows evidence of adherence.

The Patient in an Intensive Care Unit

The goals for a burn patient in an intensive care unit (ICU) are the same as other burn patients, but achieving these goals can be more challenging. Due to the severity of the burn injury, a patient can have multiple intravenous (IV) lines in the arms, feet, or neck. In addition, the patient may have a feeding tube, urinary catheter, pulse oximeter, and heart monitor in place. Also, if there is an inhalation injury, the patient could be on a ventilator with a tracheostomy or endotracheal tube. Some patients may be medicated with a drug that temporarily paralyzes the skeletal muscles to prevent resistance to mechanical ventilation. In this case, the patient will not be able to offer assistance or resistance to movement or indicate pain with movement.

Initially, PROM is the recommended type of exercise performed. Any joint area not compromised by medical devices should be exercised. Fortunately, IV sites are changed frequently to prevent infection; therefore, any particular joint area where ROM is compromised by an IV site usually will be available for exercise in a few days. With a tracheostomy, endotracheal tube, or subclavian arterial line, gentle neck ROM usually can be performed. If there is doubt concerning the stability of these devices, consulting with the appropriate medical personnel is recommended. However, movement to the extreme ends of the range should be avoided.[3]

Even with multiple lines and tubes, some burn patients are alert and able to follow commands. In these cases, the patient can be instructed in AROM and AAROM.

As a patient's medical status improves and increased activity is tolerated, the patient can be progressed to sitting on the side of the bed, standing, and walking in place. Even when space is limited, walking in place can help to increase the patient's endurance. A restorator or light hand weights can be useful for these patients.

While working with ICU patients, the therapist must use caution to avoid overstressing the patient.[3] The use of a continuous passive motion machine for the upper or lower extremity can be of assistance in maintaining mobility of the joints with minimal stress to the patient.[48] Heart rate and blood pressure should be monitored prior to, during, and following exercise. If systolic blood pressure increases over 20 mm Hg, exercise should be halted.[3] Changes in heart rate can vary from patient to patient but should not exceed the predicted maximum for any given patient. If the heart rate does not return to pre-exercise levels within 30 minutes, the exercise program should be modified to patient tolerance.

The Pediatric Patient

For the child who has sustained a burn injury, pain and fear complicate the rehabilitation process because of the child's difficulty with understanding the necessity for therapeutic interventions.[49] The exercise goals for children are similar to adults, but the methods for achieving these goals may need to be modified according to the age and developmental level of the child.[50] Knowledge of the physical development of a child can assist in establishing an exercise program that will achieve full ROM and maintain a child at an appropriate level of development. Frequently an exercise approach needs to be in the form of play activities to stimulate the child's participation in the exercise program (see Chapter 18).[3,51]

Pressure Garments

Often, patients will report that their pressure garments are restrictive and interfere with their ability to perform their exercise program. Ward and colleagues[52] investigated this complaint by measuring AROM activities both before and following pressure garment application. No measurable or clinically reliable difference was found in the patients' overall movement.

Sometimes, however, the weave of the pressure garment fabric can cause irritation to patient's skin. The texture of pressure garment material and devices should be progressed according to the patient's skin tolerance, as discussed in Chapter 14. Skin irritation or breakdown should be monitored closely by the therapist so that it does not interfere with a patient's exercise program.

MASSAGE

Scar tissue essentially is nonelastic and, without treatment, scar can limit movement. The simultaneous use of massage and exercise can help to elongate and soften immature scars and increase their pliability.[2,53-55] However, newly healed scars are fragile and can blister easily. Massage can be started early, but should be gentle to avoid shearing forces, blistering, or tearing of the skin. The use of a lubricant is helpful to decrease friction (see Appendix C). After a scar has matured, deep massage can begin. Massage can improve pliability and aids in decreasing the sensitivity of healing skin and scar tissue.

INDIVIDUAL AND GROUP TREATMENT TIME

There are many instances when a therapist works one on one with a patient. This time is essential to establish the trust needed between a therapist and a burn patient. Individual therapy sessions give the therapist an opportunity to learn about the patient as a person. Similarly, the patient has an opportunity to get to know the therapist and to realize this caregiver sincerely is interested in helping.

Patients may have difficulty relaxing during a stretching session, especially if there are other people in the area or distracting noises. Using an isolated room or treatment booth, where the environment is quiet, gives a patient the opportunity to relax. Burn patients often lack fluid movements during functional activities. This rigid movement results from their continual pain experienced with movement, exercises that emphasize movement in the extremes of range, and static interventions of positioning and splinting. Practice on combining movements in a rhythmic fashion should be included as part of an overall exercise program and may be best accomplished in a quiet environment.

There are several advantages to developing group exercise programs for burn patients. Group exercise enables a therapist to see more patients in a shorter period of time, facilitates patient independence, provides an opportunity for socialization, and allows peer pressure to encourage patients to work harder. The use of various types of music can add enjoyment to a group. Also, specialty classes can be effective, such as using one session to emphasize the upper body and one to emphasize the lower body. Allowing patients to lead an exercise class can further challenge them.

SPECIFIC EXERCISES FOR SPECIFIC AREAS

Some areas of the body are more prone than others to develop burn scar contractures, as indicated in Table 12–11. When these body areas are involved as part of the burn injury, stretching exercises should be performed in a direction opposite to the surface of the burn. Initial strengthening exercises should focus on muscles that oppose the shortening scar tissue. In cases where a burn crosses adjacent joint skin creases, the exercises ultimately should be in a combined manner to elongate the scar tissue over all successive joints. Examples and explanations of exercises to prevent scar tissue tightness for various areas of the body follow to assist therapists treating patients with burns.

TABLE 12–11. Direction of Exercise Emphasis

Body Area	Specific Site	Contracted Position	Direction of Exercise to Avert Contracture
Face	Eyes	Eversion of lower eyelid (ectropion)	Close eyes
		Temporal corners of eyes	Open eyes wide with an elongated face
	Mouth	Corners of mouth (commissures)	Vertical and lateral opening of mouth
Neck	Anterior/lateral surface	Anterior neck Lateral neck	Cervical extension, lateral flexion, and cervical rotation away from burn site
Shoulder	Anterior axillary fold	Frontal and horizontal adduction plane	Shoulder abduction
	Posterior axillary fold	Shoulder extension	Shoulder flexion
Elbow	Antecubital space	Elbow flexion	Elbow extension
Forearm	Volar surface	Pronation	Supination
Wrist	Volar surface	Wrist flexion	Wrist extension
Hand	Dorsal surface	MCP extension	MCP flexion
	Palmar surface	MCP flexion, palmar cupping	MCP extension Preserve arches
	Dorsal finger	IP extension	IP flexion
	Palmar finger	IP flexion	IP extension
	Small finger	Abduction	Adduction
	Thumb	Adduction	Radial and palmar abduction
	Web spaces	Finger adduction	Finger abduction
Trunk	Chest	Shoulder protraction	Shoulder retraction
		Dorsal kyphosis	Spinal extension
	Flank	Lateral flexion/scoliosis toward burn	Lateral flexion away from burn
Hip	Anterior surface	Hip flexion	Hip extension
	Inguinal area	Hip adduction	Hip abduction
Knee	Popliteal space	Knee flexion	Knee extension
Ankle	Achilles tendon area	Plantarflexion	Dorsiflexion
	Anterior radius	Dorsiflexion	Plantarflexion
Toes	Dorsal surface	Extension	Flexion
	Plantar surface	Flexion	Extension
	Web spaces	Adduction	Abduction

Face

Facial burns can lead to contractures and scar deformities of the eyelids and mouth. Facial contractures are difficult to prevent because tissue of the face is fairly mobile and lacks any points of fixation against which a stretching force may be opposed. The most common contracture of the eyelid is eversion of the lower lid, known as *ectropion*. If a burn involved the cornea of the eye, the physician may perform a tarsorraphy to prevent desiccation of the cornea. This procedure involves suturing the upper and lower lids together, leaving only a small opening for the patient to see. While the sutures are in place, all exercises that might pull on the sutures are avoided. Following the release of a tarsorraphy, exercise for the eyelids should be initiated. Exercise may not prevent ectropion, but may lessen the extent of contracture.

Exercises for the mouth are designed to prevent the occurrence of *microstomia,* which is a narrowing of the oral orifice. Microstomia is common with full-thickness facial burns, but can occur with partial-thickness burns when the patient refuses to exercise the perioral area. This condition can result in difficulty with eating, vocalizing, salivating, and oral hygiene.

Problem Area	Patient Exercise Suggestions
Eyes	Tightly close eyes (Fig. 12–5) Open eyes as wide as possible Wink
Mouth	Open mouth as wide as possible Smile Say "EEE" Open mouth while eyes are closed (see Fig. 12–5) Horizontally stretch mouth using fingers in commissures (Fig. 12–6) Draw lower lip over bottom teeth Progressively place an increased number of tongue blades between the upper and lower teeth (Fig. 12–7)

Neck

Burn patients in an ICU or in critical condition for an extended time are susceptible to neck contractures due to prolonged immobility. The anterior neck is the surface most prone to contracture development. Neck flexion contractures can interfere with breathing, salivation, vocalization, and sight. When exercising the neck region, the position of the shoulders and chin must be monitored. Patients tend to elevate their shoulders or open the mouth to relieve tension on the neck. Massaging the neck with an upward stroke toward the chin or mouth may help minimize the distortion of the mouth with neck-stretching exercises. Placing the patient supine on a mat table or plinth with the head off the edge, supported by the therapists hands, is an effective and energy-saving position to elongate the tissue of the anterior neck. If a mobilization table is available, the patient can lie supine and the headpiece can be lowered gradually.

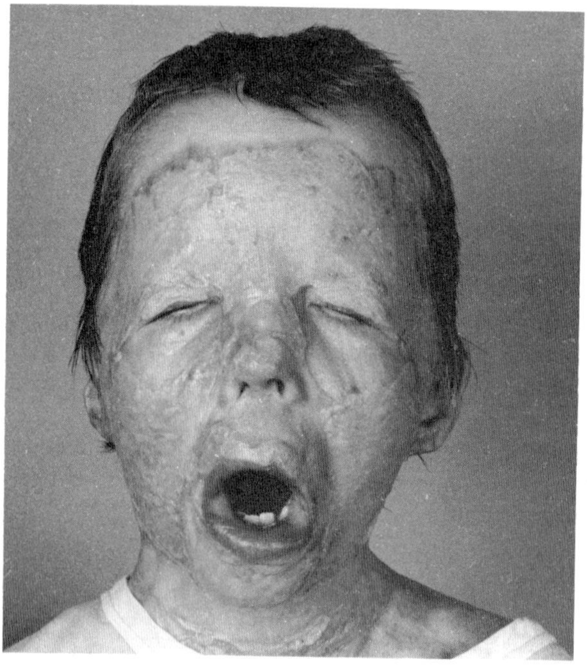

FIGURE 12–5. Patient closes eyes tightly while opening mouth to stretch perioral area.

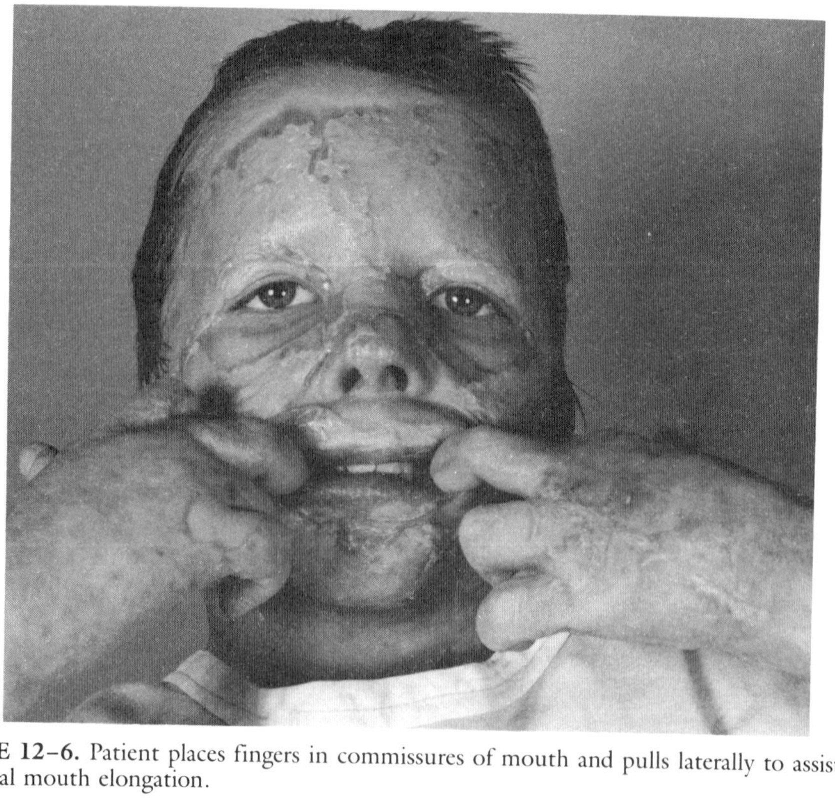

FIGURE 12–6. Patient places fingers in commissures of mouth and pulls laterally to assist with horizontal mouth elongation.

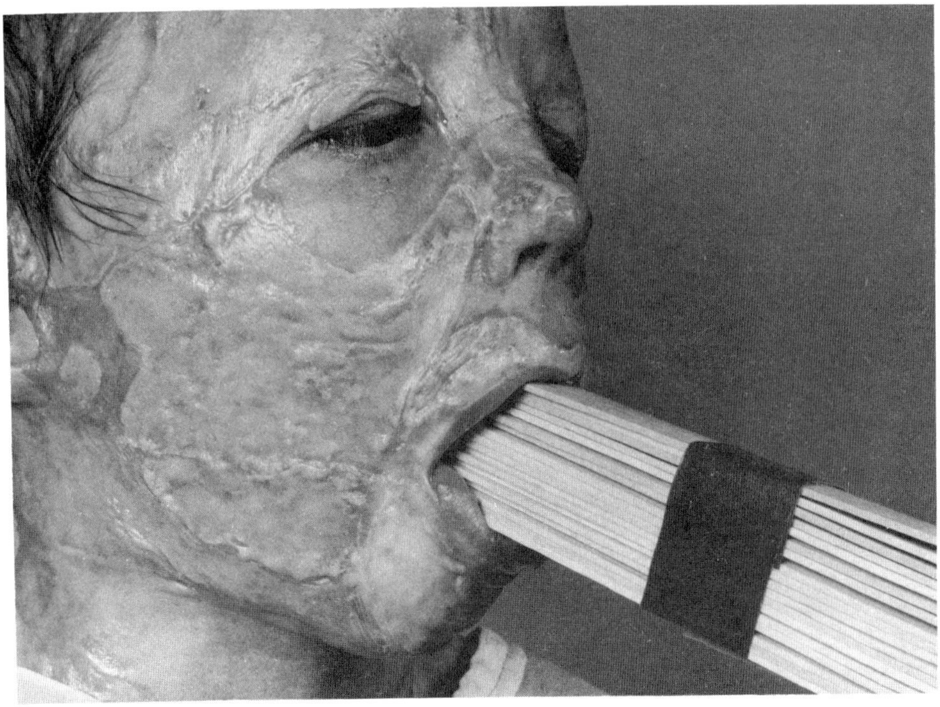

FIGURE 12–7. A stack of tongue blades is placed in the patient's mouth to maintain vertical opening of mouth. As tissue tightness decreases, additional tongue blades can be added.

Problem Area	Patient Exercise Suggestions
Anterior and lateral neck	While sitting in a straight back chair, have the patient look up to the ceiling with jaw and lips closed. Lie supine, hang head over the edge of a bed, wedge, or mat table (Fig. 12–8). With mouth closed, turn chin toward each shoulder while sitting or supine. Laterally flex neck so that ear moves toward the shoulder while sitting or supine. Shoulder should not rise to meet ear. Proprioceptive Neuromuscular Facilitation (PNF) neck pattern.

Upper Extremity

Therapists may need to stabilize various upper extremity segments to prevent substitution movements while performing upper extremity exercises. For example, a patient may plantarflex at the ankles to reach overhead. Because of the many joints involved in the upper extremity, exercises that involve multiple joints should be emphasized after isolated joints have been exercised.

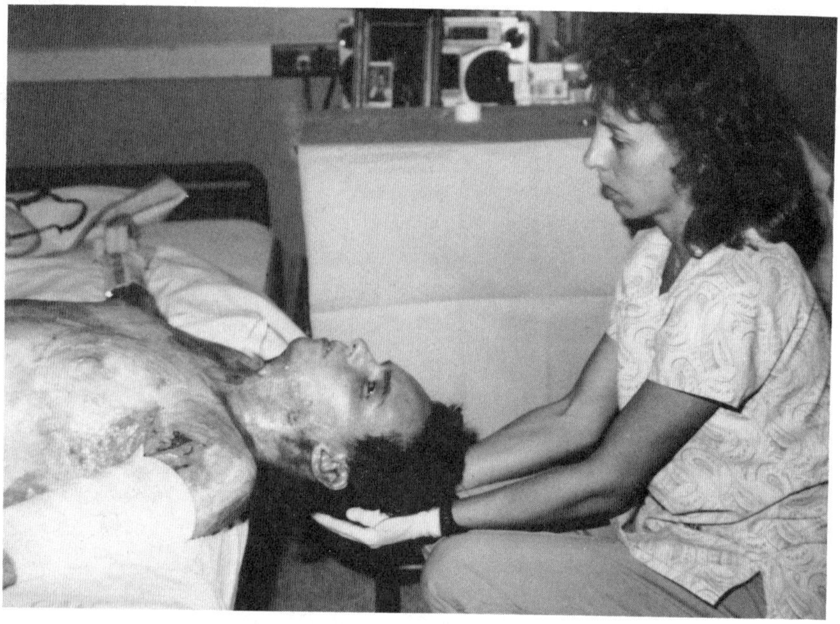

FIGURE 12–8. Patient with head over edge of bed supported by therapist during neck range of motion exercise. The head is lowered slowly to stretch the anterior neck.

Problem Area	Patient Exercise Suggestions
Axillary folds	Grasp overhead bar and bend knees (Fig. 12–9). While sitting with trunk supported, raise arms toward ceiling keeping elbows extended. With back supported, hold cane with both hands and lift above head with elbows extended. Move cane to left and to right. With arms by the side, abduct shoulders until hands touch overhead. PNF patterns. Jumping jacks (good with children). Pulleys, shoulder wheel, finger ladder, Valpar equipment or Baltimore Therapeutic Equipment (BTE), catching and throwing balls from overhead.
Elbow	Weighted wrist cuff (Fig. 12–10). Carrying weighted buckets. Wall pushups.
Forearm	Single-sided dumbbell (Fig. 12–11). Turn or rotate trapeze bar on the bed. Open doorknob. ADLs such as eating, brushing teeth, combing hair, dressing.
Wrist	Rest forearm either pronated or supinated on table with hand off edge. Flex or extend wrist. With hands together at chest height, raise elbows while keeping palms together (Fig. 12–12). Stretch to achieve palm of hand against wall or table top with supinated forearm. Wall or mat pushups, crawling on hands and knees, mimicking painting strokes, or conducting an orchestra with children.

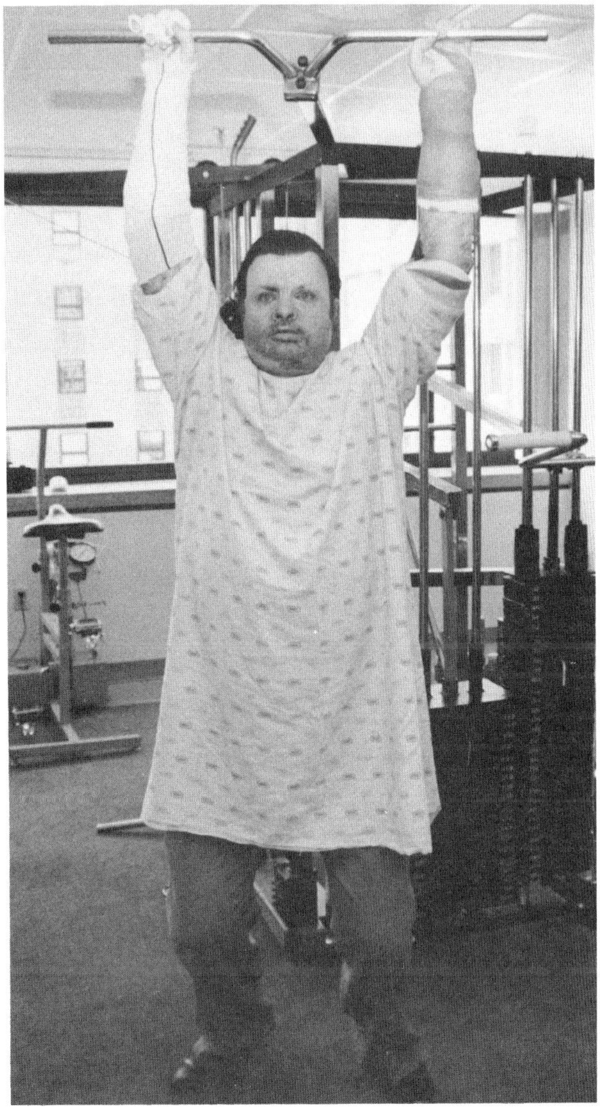

FIGURE 12–9. Grasping an overhead bar, the patient bends his knees to increase stress placed on axillary fold scar tissue. This method of stretching also provides a combined stretch to the upper extremities and torso while giving the patient control over the exercise intensity.

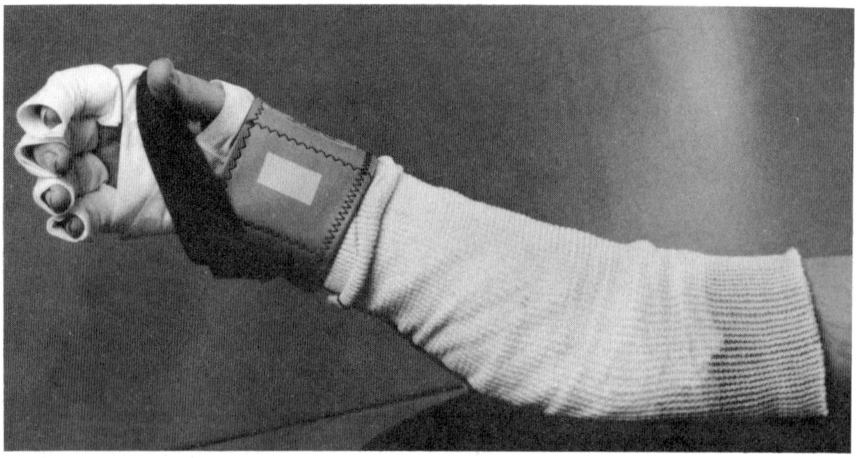

FIGURE 12–10. Weighted cuff at the wrist used to stretch tight scar tissue across the anticubital space. The arm is supported and the forearm is left unsupported to allow for maximal elbow extension.

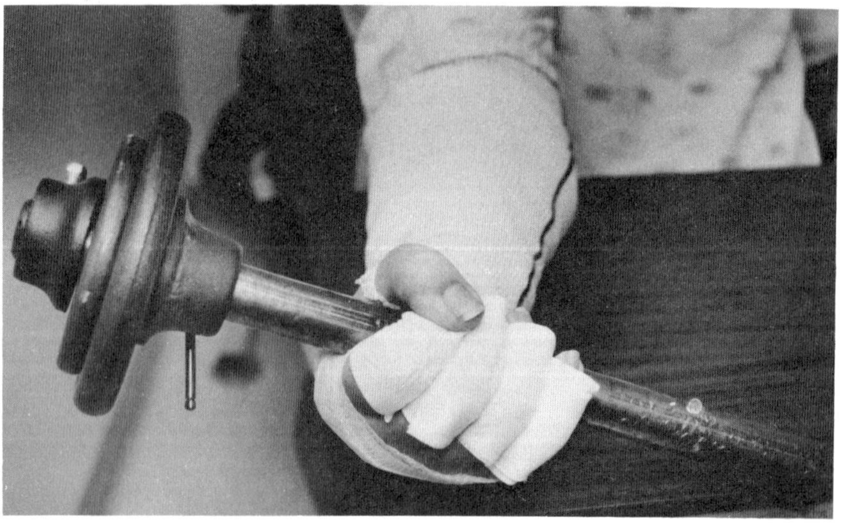

FIGURE 12–11. Patient holds a dumbbell in hand, weighted only on the radial side, to assist with forearm supination.

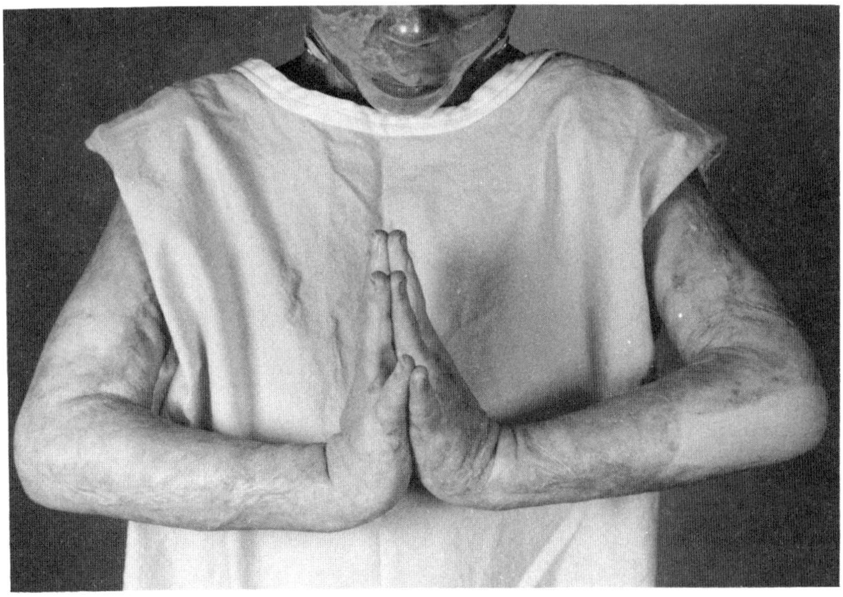

FIGURE 12–12. "Prayer position" for self-assisted bilateral wrist extension. Palms remain in contact with each other while forearms move from a vertical to horizontal position.

Hand

The hand possesses multiple joints and it is necessary to exercise each joint area individually as well as collectively. Individual joint ROM measurements may be within normal limits, however, total combined movements may reveal functional limitations.

Problem Area	Patient Exercise Suggestions
Fingers and thumb	While extended, abduct fingers. Touch each finger tip to thumb. Isolate MCP joint flexion and extension. Place dorsal surface of the proximal phalanges on soft surface and flex MP joint (Fig. 12–13). Isolate IP joint flexion and extension (Fig. 12–14). Oppose thumb and flex fingers over (for children, "hide thumb" under fingers). Hold a soda can, insert various-width bottlenecks between fingers. Practice writing, use pegboard, mold putty, hang clothes with clothespins.

Lower Extremity

For lower extremity exercise, ambulation, bicycles, isokinetic units, or other types of exercise equipment can be used. However, specific stretching exercises may be necessary to achieve full ROM.

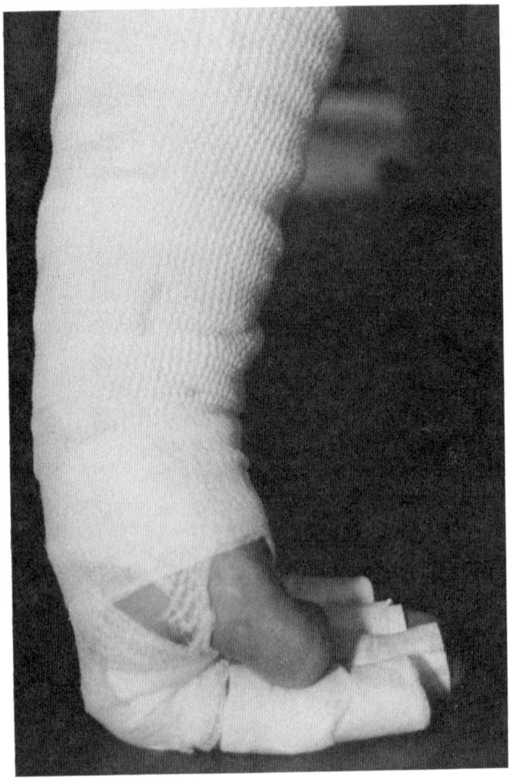

FIGURE 12–13. With fingers extended at the interphalangeal joints, the dorsal surface of the fingers are kept in contact with a flat, smooth surface. The patient delivers a downward force to stretch the scar tissue across the MP joints to increase flexion.

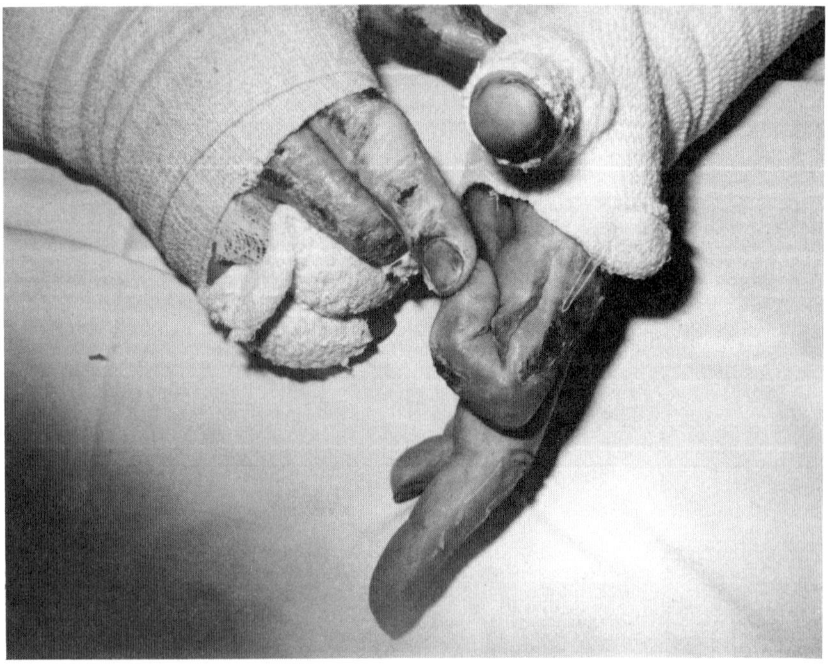

FIGURE 12–14. Patient performs independent self-ROM of isolated IP joint flexion.

Problem Area	Patient Exercise Suggestions
Anterior hip	Lie prone on firm surface (floor, table). Do not lie on soft mattress. While prone, lift one leg off the mat at a time with knee extended or flexed. While prone, keep legs extended and push trunk up with arms (if patient is too weak, place small bolster under upper trunk). Lie supine on mat table with leg off side of mat. Lie supine, place pillow, towel roll, or bolster under buttocks. Bridging.
Posterior hip	While supine, bring one knee at a time toward chest. While supine, perform straight leg raises. Marching, squatting. Long sit and reach for toes.
Perineum	While supine, abduct legs with knees extended. While sitting or supine, cross legs "man" (ankle on opposite knee), Indian, and frog style (Fig. 12–15). Squatting using stall bars for assistance.
Knee	Straight leg raises with ankle dorsiflexed. Long sit. Short arc quad sets: bolster under knee, then extend knee. While prone, extend knees. While prone, extend lower part of leg off end of table and place cuff weight at ankle (Fig. 12–16). Stairs, bicycle, rowing machine, ramp.
Anterior ankle	While on mat table, sit on heels with dorsum of foot on mat surface (Fig. 12–17). Point toes like a ballerina, press down as on a gas pedal (for child).
Posterior ankle	Long sit. Place a towel, belt, theraband, or strap around the ball of the foot and while holding both ends, pull foot into dorsiflexion (Fig. 12–18). While standing, slowly bend at the knees without lifting heels (patient may need to hold on to a stable object for support). While facing a wall with feet parallel, lean on wall with hands keeping heels on floor. With one foot slightly in front of the other, lean into wall bending knee of hind foot. Keep feet flat on the floor. Walk up and down ramp forward, backward, and sideways. Dip heel off edge of stair step.
Toes	While sitting, point toes or pull toes up off the floor. Spread toes apart manually. If area is healed, squeeze sand with toes or try to pick up small objects.

Trunk

An inflexible trunk will alter a patient's gait, ability to perform ADLs, posture, and general mobility. The typical posture of a patient with anterior trunk burns is a flexed trunk, protracted shoulders, and a forward and flexed head. This posture can cause difficulty with breathing as well as mobility problems. Strong scar bands can develop at the base of the neck, extend across the anterior chest and abdomen, and pass over the anterior hip. The patient with a posterior trunk burn usually walks erect but has difficulty with sitting, forward flexion, and reaching forward or using

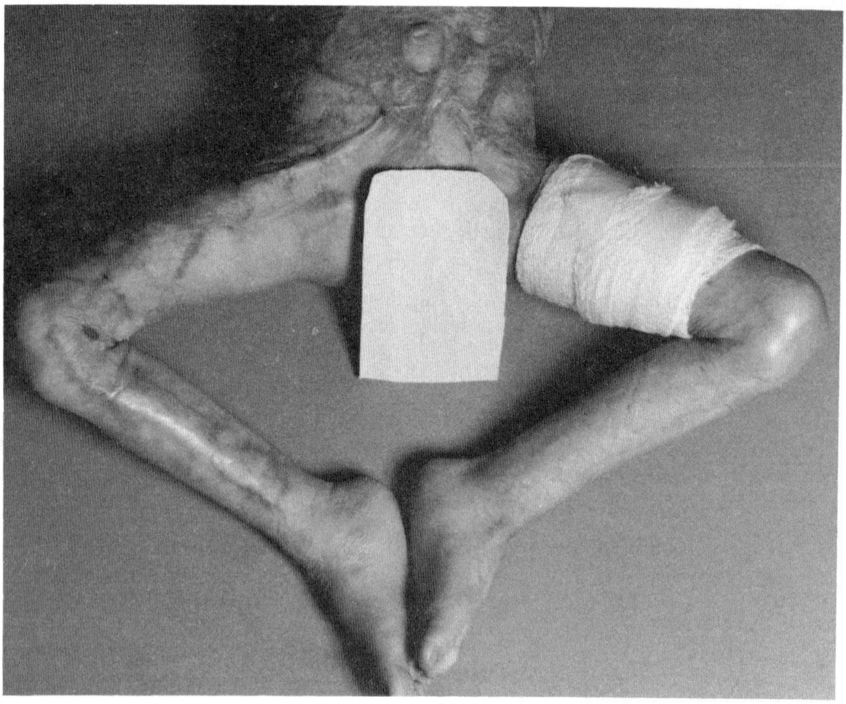

FIGURE 12–15. Frog-leg position to stretch perineum. While patient lies supine, hips and knees are flexed and plantar surface of feet are brought together, the perineum is stretched by externally rotating the hips and lowering the knees to the floor.

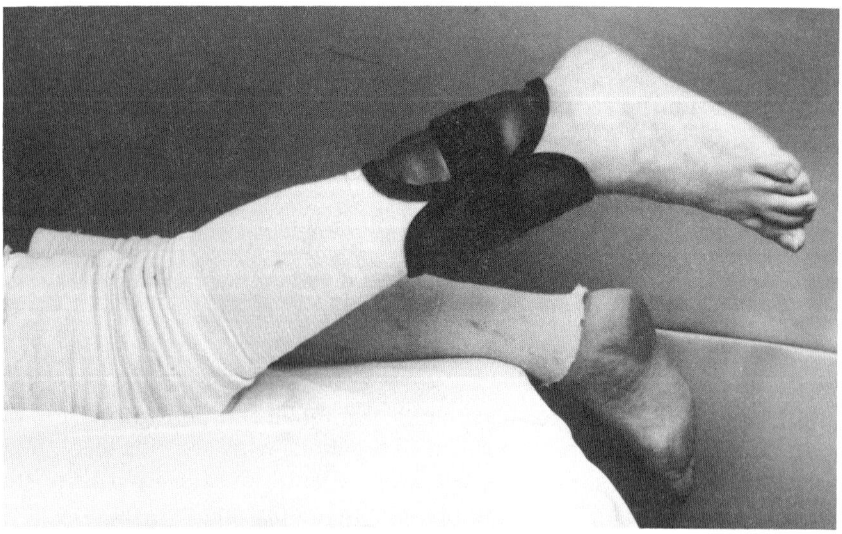

FIGURE 12–16. With the patient lying prone and the foot positioned off the edge of a mat table, a cuff weight is placed on the ankle. The weight provides an elongation stress to the flexor surface of the knee to promote knee extension.

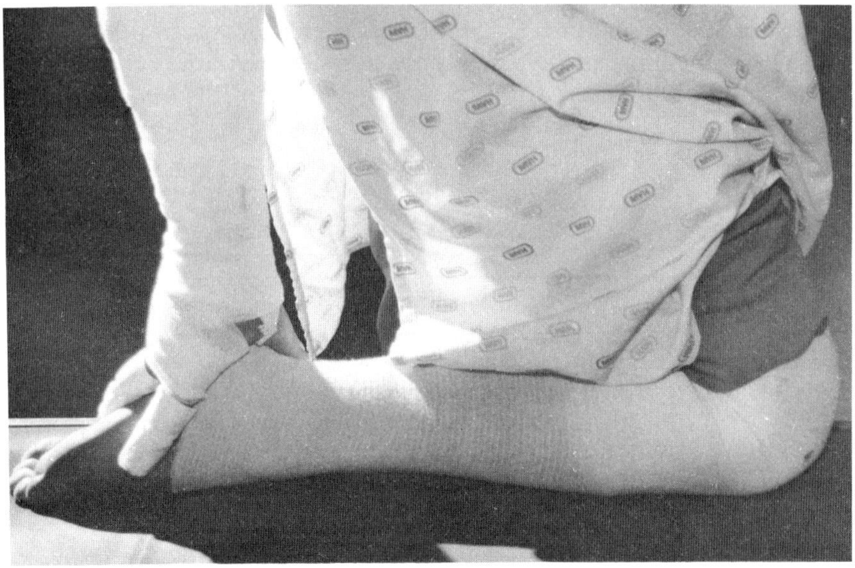

FIGURE 12-17. While patient kneels on the right leg with foot plantar flexed, a force is applied to the heel using the body weight to stretch the anterior surface of the ankle.

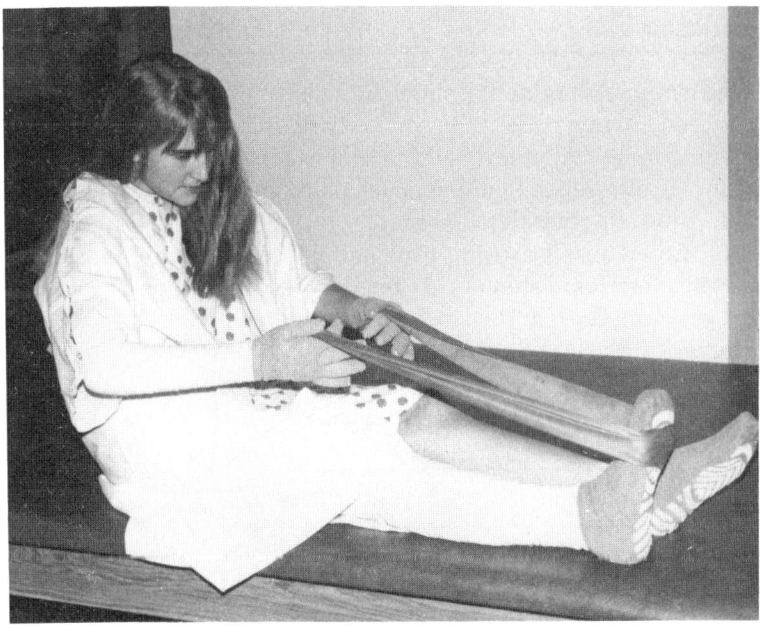

FIGURE 12-18. Patient performs active-assistive right ankle dorsiflexion exercise.

the upper extremities at midline. Lateral trunk burns can cause a lateral deviation toward the side of the burn as the patient tries to relieve tension of the scar at the site of the burn or skin graft. This trunk shift may result in postural deformities that could affect a patient's balance in gait and possibly lead to long-term musculoskeletal problems due to structural imbalances.

Problem Area	Patient Exercise Suggestions
Anterior trunk	Hands behind head or back—wing elbows back. Prone pushups while extending neck. Place pillows under hips while supine or under chest while prone. With patient supine, place bolster lengthwise under spine or perpendicular to spine at waist level for stretching.
Posterior trunk	Cross arms in front of body (bear hug) (Fig. 12–19). Sitting or standing, forward-flex trunk and touch toes. "Windmill" pattern of stretching.
Lateral trunk	While standing, slide arm down the side of leg opposite burn. (Use teapot analogy for children). Practice golf swing. Sidelie over bolster (Fig. 12–20). Reach one arm up toward the ceiling and then the other.

Relaxation Exercises

Due to the extreme amount of pain burn patients experience and for the length of time it is endured, many patients become tense and find relaxation difficult. This feeling of needing to be "on guard" all the time stems from the fact that almost every aspect of burn care and rehabilitation causes pain. Typically, patients walk in a semi-rigid manner with their shoulders elevated.

As part of the exercise program, time should be set aside to instruct patients in gentle relaxation exercises. Patients first need to recognize this "protective or defensive posture" in themselves and then be instructed in exercises they can perform to relieve muscle tension.

Problem Area	Patient Exercise Suggestions
Relaxation	Gentle shoulder shrugs. Shoulder rolls—forward and backward. Head circumduction. Ankle rotation.

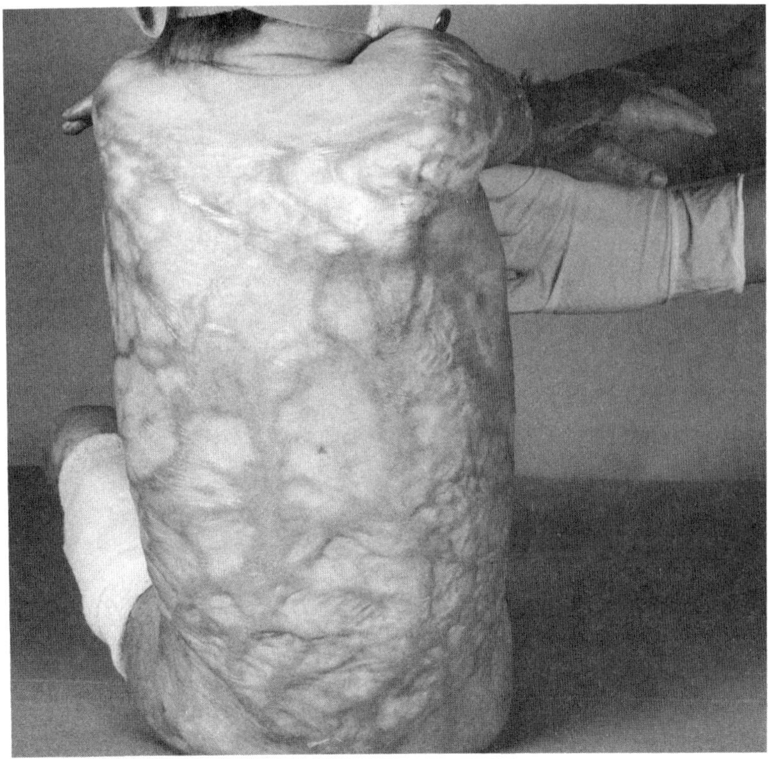

FIGURE 12–19. Patient crosses arms anteriorly (bear-hug) to elongate posterior trunk scar.

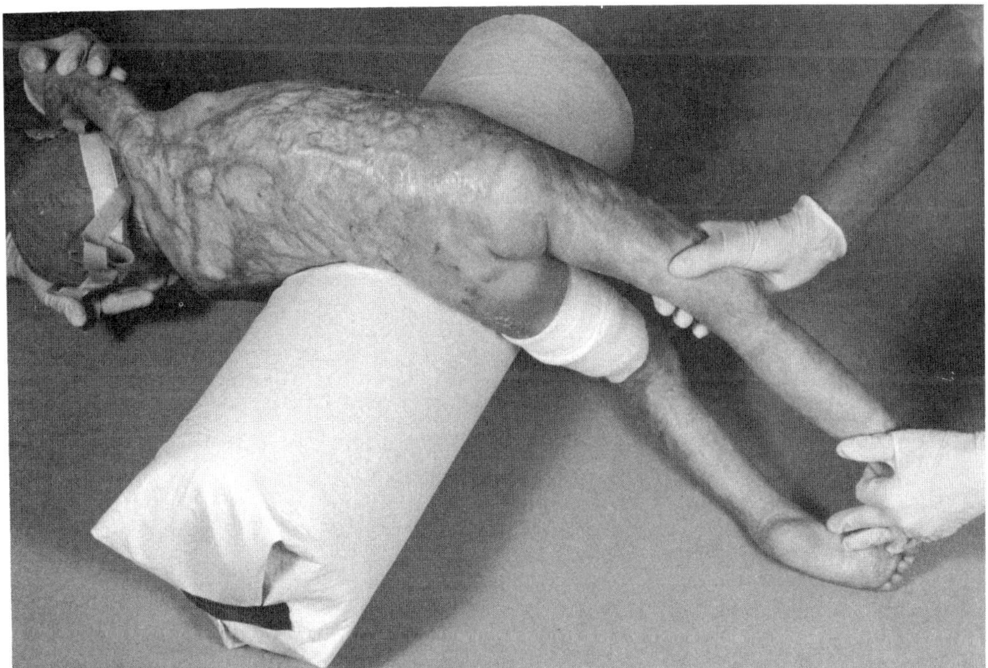

FIGURE 12–20. Patient sidelies over bolster to elongate lateral trunk tissue. The right shoulder is abducted to place maximal tension on tight scar tissue.

CASE STUDY

HISTORY

LR is a 40-year-old male who sustained a 38 percent full-thickness scald burn to his anterior neck and trunk and circumferential bilateral arms and forearms. The patient underwent excision and split-thickness skin grafting to these areas on postburn days 7 and 17 and had spot grafting to some remaining open areas on postburn day 27.

Prior to his first surgery, active range of motion (AROM) was as follows:

Neck extension—24 cm (chin to manubrium)
Neck rotation bilaterally—60°
Shoulder abduction bilaterally—145°
Right elbow—minus 5° extension to 110° flexion
Left elbow—minus 10° extension to 100° flexion
Forearm supination bilaterally—45°
Bilateral wrist ROM was within normal limits (WNL)

Under anesthesia, following excision of his burn wound, bilateral shoulder abduction was 170°, elbow ROM was zero to 135° and forearm supination was 70°.

LR was discharged from the hospital 38 days following the burn injury. At the time of discharge, AROM was as follows:

Neck extension—22 cm
Neck rotation bilaterally—60°
Right shoulder abduction—170°
Left shoulder abduction—165°
Right elbow—zero to 125° flexion
Left elbow—zero to 120° flexion
Forearm supination bilaterally—WNL
Bilateral wrist ROM—WNL

LR's overall strength was good and endurance was fair. He and his wife were able to demonstrate his home exercise program independently. He was scheduled for outpatient therapy three times a week.

PROBLEM LIST

Anterior neck burn with a predisposition for a neck flexion contracture
Bilateral anterior axillary fold scar with a predisposition for a shoulder adduction contracture
Circumferential upper extremity scars with a predisposition for overall decrease in elbow ROM and forearm supination

GOALS

Increase neck extension to 24 cm
Maintain bilateral neck rotation at 60°
Increase active bilateral shoulder abduction to 170°
Increase active bilateral elbow ROM to zero extension and 135° flexion
Maintain active wrist ROM at WNL
Increase active forearm supination to 70° bilaterally
Strength rating of good to normal at discharge
Endurance rating of fair to good at discharge
Patient and family independent in home exercise program

INTERVENTIONS

Following his admission to the burn unit, LR was on bed rest. He was seen bedside and instructed in an active exercise program. Exercises included neck extension and rotation while sitting in bed and shoulder abduction, elbow flexion and extension, forearm supination, and wrist flexion and extension while supine. In addition, he was instructed in ankle pumps and heel slides. The therapist assisted with shoulder abduction and forearm supination as LR was unable to achieve acceptable active ROM of these areas.

PROM was performed in the operating room prior to placement of skin grafts. On the fifth day following each skin-grafting procedure, LR began AROM once again within the tolerance of the graft. The following day active-assistive ROM (AAROM) was initiated. The therapist now assisted with all upper extremity ROM and incorporated massage into the stretching program. The patient continued with AROM exercises to the lower extremities; however, bridging and straight leg raises were added to the program. LR's wife began to learn how to assist him with stretching and perform massage to the upper extremities. When LR was allowed off bed rest, pulleys while sitting and wand exercises while supine on a mat table and standing were initiated. LR also began walking the hallways and using a restorator with his wife supervising. LR was discharged with a written home exercise program, a set of pulleys, and some Theraband to begin minimal resistive exercise.

RATIONALE

Prior to surgery, the patient was encouraged to perform AROM exercise to maintain ROM and strength and decrease edema. If a patient has limited ROM or is unable to complete full AROM because of increased physiologic demands from a burn injury, then AAROM is indicated. When a patient does have limited ROM prior to surgery, the therapist should evaluate the patient's true ROM under anesthesia. This approach also allows for a pain-free exercise session for the patient.

AROM usually is initiated after skin grafting to minimize the potential for graft disruption. AAROM can be included as part of the exercise program as the graft becomes adherent and can tolerate more movement. Massage and stretching are incorporated into the exercise program after the graft is well adhered and finally resistive exercises are initiated when the patient has acceptable AROM. Resistive strengthening exercises can be instituted earlier for those extremities not involved in the burn injury as long as the patient is physiologically able to tolerate the stress. Involving a family member early in the exercise program may increase the total amount of therapy a patient receives throughout the day and helps to maintain the strength of uninvolved extremities.

SUMMARY

Exercise is one of the necessary interventions of burn rehabilitation. Without exercise, debilitating deformities can occur that are detrimental to the patient's physical and functional recovery and can be cosmetically unappealing. Although painful, exercise must be initiated as soon after admission to the burn unit as possible, or at the initial visit for an outpatient. Families and patients will have difficulty understanding why exercises are so important, but with education and encouragement from the therapist, the exercises will become routine.

The therapist chooses passive, active-assistive, active, or resistive exercises depending on the status of the patient. Various equipment and exercise techniques are used to provide a prolonged, gentle force to elongate scar tissue and then to condition the patient once full ROM is achieved. Exercise, in conjunction with other aspects of burn care, can help minimize the permanent effects of a burn injury and maximize the person's physical and functional potential.

REFERENCES

1. Johnson, CL, O'Shaughnessy, EJ, and Ostergren, G: Burn Management. Raven Press, New York, 1981, p 47.
2. Braddom, RL, et al: The physical treatment and rehabilitation of burn patients. In Hummel, RP (ed): Clinical Burn Therapy. John Wright-PSG, Boston, 1982, pp 279–299.
3. Nothdurft, D, Smith, PS, and LeMaster, JE: Exercise and treatment modalities. In Fisher, SV and Helm, PA (eds): Comprehensive Rehabilitation of Burns. Williams & Wilkins, Baltimore, 1984, pp 96–147.
4. Cummings, GS, Crutchfield, CA, and Barnes, MR: Orthopedic Physical Therapy Series, Volume 1. Stokesville Publishing, Atlanta, 1983.
5. Matson, K: Physical Therapy Management of the Burned Patient. In Wagner, MM (ed): Care of the Burn-Injured Patient. PSG Publishing, Littleton, Mass., 1981, pp 141–162.
6. Wright, PC: Fundamentals of acute burn care and physical therapy management. Phys Ther 64:1217–1231, 1984.
7. Kozerefski, PM: Exercise and ambulation in the burn patient. In DiGregorio, VR (ed): Rehabilitation of the Burn Patient. Churchill Livingstone, New York, 1984, p 58.
8. Wright, PC: Physical therapy in burn injury. In Salisbury, RE, Newman, NM, and Dingeldein, GP (eds): Manual of Burn Therapeutics. Little, Brown, Boston, 1983, pp 165–178.
9. Astrand, P and Rodahl, K: Textbook of Work Physiology. McGraw-Hill, New York, 1977, pp 291–329.
10. Dobbs, ER: Physical therapy. In Artz, CP, Moncrief, JA, and Pruitt, BA: Burns—A Team Approach. WB Saunders, Philadelphia, 1979, pp 492–499.
11. Dobbs, ER and Curreri, PW: Burns: Analysis of results of physical therapy in 681 patients. J Trauma 12:242–248, 1972.
12. Kraemer, MD, Jones, T, and Deitch, EA: Burn contractures: Incidence, predisposing factors, and results of surgical therapy. J Burn Care Rehabil 9:261–265, 1988.
13. Helm, P, et al: Burn injury: Rehabilitation management in 1982. Arch Phys Med Rehabil 69:9–16, 1982.
14. Adams, RB, et al: Cardiovascular rehabilitation of patients with burns. J Burn Care Rehabil 11:246–255, 1990.

15. OT/PT Special Interest Group, American Burn Association Annual Meeting, Baltimore, April 3, 1991.
16. Hartford, CE: Surgical management. In Fisher, SV and Helm, PA (eds): Comprehensive Rehabilitation of Burns. Williams & Wilkins, Baltimore, 1984, pp 28-63.
17. Evans, EB: Heterotopic bone formation in thermal burns. Clin Orthop 263:94-101, 1991.
18. Jackson, DM: Burns into joints. Burns 2:90-108, 1976.
19. Pruitt, BA: Other complications of burn injury. In Artz, CP, Moncrief, JA, and Pruitt, BA (eds): Burns—A Team Approach. WB Saunders, Philadelphia, 1979, pp 523-552.
20. Hammond, MC, Merli, G, and Zierler, RE: Rehabilitation of the patient with peripheral vascular disease of the lower extremity. In DeLisa, JA (ed): Rehabilitation Medicine. JB Lippincott, Philadelphia, 1988, pp 795-820.
21. Munster, AM, Weiner, SH, and Spence, RJ: Cultured epidermis for the coverage of massive burn wounds. Ann Surg 211:676-680, 1990.
22. Weekley, R and Klein, R: Clinical nursing experience with cultured epidermal autografts. J Burn Care Rehabil 13:138-141, 1992.
23. Herndon, DN and Rutan, R: Comparison of cultured epidermal autograft and massive excision with serial autografting plus homograft overlay. J Burn Care Rehabil 13:154-157, 1992.
24. Johnson, CL: The role of physical therapy. In Boswick, JA, Jr (ed): The Art and Science of Burn Care. Aspen Publishers, Rockville, 1987, pp 299-306.
25. Wilmore, DW: The Metabolic Management of the Critically Ill. Plenum, New York, 1977, p 34.
26. Black, S, et al: Oxygen consumption for lower extremity exercises in normal subjects and burned patients. Phys Ther 60:1255-1258, 1980.
27. Leman, CJ, et al: Exercise physiology in the acute burn patient: Do we really know what we're doing? Proc American Burn Association 24:91, 1992.
28. Head, MD and Helm, PA: Paraffin and sustained stretching in the treatment of burn contractures. Burns 4:136-139, 1978.
29. Sharkey, BJ: Physiology of Fitness. Human Kinetics Publishers, Champaign, Illinois, 1979.
30. Cronan, T, Hammond, J, and Ward, CG: The value of isokinetic exercise and testing in burn rehabilitation and determination of back-to-work status. J Burn Care Rehabil 11:224-227, 1990.
31. Saltin, B, et al: Response to exercise after bed rest and after training. Circulation (Suppl)1:1-78, 1968.
32. Cisar, C, Staley, M, and Gillespie, R: Physical fitness adaptations of the severe burn patient following discharge. Proc American Burn Association 18:23, 1986.
33. Covey, MH: Occupational therapy. In Boswick, JA, Jr (ed): The Art and Science of Burn Care. Aspen Publishers, Rockville, Maryland, 1987, pp 285-298.
34. Crawford, C: The burn rehabilitation swimming program. J Burn Care Rehabil 9:290-291, 1988.
35. Abidin, MR, et al: Hydrofitness devices for strengthening upper extremity muscles. J Burn Care Rehabil 9:199-202, 1988.
36. Goitz, RJ, et al: A new hydrofitness device for leg musculoskeletal conditioning. J Burn Care Rehabil 9:203-206, 1988.
37. Parrott, M, et al: Structured exercise circuit program for burn patients. J Burn Care Rehabil 9:666-668, 1988.
38. Greenspan, B, et al: The design and implementation of a burn exercise and activity group in the acute care setting. Proc American Burn Association Meeting, Salt Lake City, 24:163, 1992.
39. Nicosia, J, Stein, ED, and Stein, JM: The advantage of physiotherapy for burn patients under anesthesia. Burns 6:202-204, 1980.
40. Petro, JA, et al: Hospitalization of burned patients. In Nicosia, JE and Petro, JA (eds): Manual of Burn Care. Raven Press, New York, 1983, pp 15-88.
41. Wright, PC: Fundamentals of acute burn and physical therapy management. Phys Ther 64:1217-1231, 1984.
42. Blassingame, WM, et al: Range of motion of the shoulder performed while patient is anesthetized. J Burn Care Rehabil 10:539-542, 1989.
43. Jaeger, DL: Maintenance of function of the burn patient. Phys Ther 52:627-633, 1972.
44. Giuliani, CA and Perry, GA: Factors to consider in the rehabilitation aspect of burn care. Phys Ther 65:619-623, 1985.
45. Howell, JW: Management of the acutely burned hand for the nonspecialized clinician. Phys Ther 12:1077-1089, 1989.
46. Richard, RL, et al: Early range of motion following skin grafting. Proc American Burn Association 21:136, 1989.
47. Burnsworth, B, Krob, MJ, and Langer-Schnepp, M: Immediate ambulation of patients with lower-extremity grafts. J Burn Care Rehabil 13:89-92, 1992.
48. Richard, RL, Miller, SF, and Staley, MJ: The physiologic response of a patient with critical burns to continuous passive motion. J Burn Care Rehabil 11:554-556, 1990.
49. Hanson, NN: Burns in Children. In DiGregorio, VR (ed): Rehabilitation of the Burn Patient. Churchill Livingstone, New York, 1984, pp 131-150.

50. McDonald, K, Johnson, B, and Prasad, JK: Collaborative physical therapy for a 4-month-old infant with 80% full-thickness burns. J Burn Care Rehabil 9:193–195, 1988.
51. Mahaney, NB: Restoration of play in a severely burned three-year-old child. J Burn Care Rehabil 11:57–63, 1990.
52. Ward, S, et al: Influence of pressure supports on joint range of motion. Proc American Burn Association 23:182, 1991.
53. Head, MD: Wound and Skin Care. In Fisher, SV and Helm, PA (eds): Comprehensive Rehabilitation of Burns. Williams & Wilkins, Baltimore, 1984, pp 148–176.
54. Howell, JW: Posthospitalization Care. In DiGregorio, VR (ed): Rehabilitation of the Burn Patient. Churchill Livingstone, New York, 1984, pp 151–171.
55. Reeves, SU: Occupational Therapy in Burn Treatment. In Salisbury, RE, Newman, NM, and Dingeldein, GP (eds): Manual of Burn Therapeutics. Little, Brown, Boston, 1983, pp 179–195.

CHAPTER 13

Lower Extremity Burns and Ambulation

Margaret Schmitt, PT
Reginald L. Richard, MS, PT
Marlys J. Staley, MS, PT

The ability to stand and ambulate efficiently is an integral part of human activity. Present-day life-styles often require long periods of being "on our feet" at home, work, or school, and in the community. Likewise, many recreational activities depend on how quickly a person can change directions. The lower extremities must provide a strong yet flexible base for ambulation activities. When a person sustains a burn injury to the lower extremities, this mobile base can be compromised severely.

A careful and comprehensive burn rehabilitation program must be developed to restore a patient's foundation for efficient ambulation. The therapist plays a key role in the burn rehabilitation process and must plan an individualized treatment program that balances proper splinting and positioning with early mobility depending upon the patient's phase of wound healing. The rehabilitation of a patient with lower extremity burns can be a complex challenge for a therapist, but meeting this challenge can mean an active and productive life-style for the burn patient. This chapter attempts to consolidate the current treatment philosophies of rehabilitation for the patient with a lower extremity burn into a basic treatment format that can be adapted into any burn treatment setting.

The literature related to burn care contains many references about the general management of lower extremity burns, but focuses mainly on wound care and skin grafting.[1-3] The rehabilitation literature emphasizes positioning, exercise and scar control with less attention paid to mobility and ambulation.[4,5] Currently, there is a lack of objective, measurable documentation on the success or failure of therapy treatment and ambulation protocols for the patient with a lower extremity burn.

EVALUATION AND TREATMENT GOALS

Every rehabilitation program begins with a patient evaluation. When evaluating a patient with a lower extremity burn, the history should include details of the patient's preburn mobility level, including home and work or school activities. Pre-existing lower extremity problems such as peripheral vascular disease, joint injuries, neuropathies, or strength deficits should be determined. Objective measurements of passive and active range of motion (ROM) and strength should be completed. If possible, bed mobility and gait should be assessed. Goals of a therapy program for the patient with a lower extremity burn usually include edema control, maintenance or restoration of ROM and strength, early mobility to prevent bedrest complications, and ambulation without gait deviations.

INITIAL TREATMENT PROGRAM

Following an evaluation of the patient, a comprehensive treatment program is developed. This program includes positioning, exercise, and ambulation. As with all burns, positioning is dependent on the surface area affected. Usually, with a lower extremity burn, the antideformity position includes hip extension with neutral rotation and approximately 20° to 30° of abduction. The knee most frequently is placed in extension and the ankle in neutral. Possible interventions to attain these positions include the use of splints, wedges, footboards, and prone lying.

To enhance lower extremity circulation, ankle pumps are indicated while the patient is on bed rest. Quadricep and gluteal muscle isometrics can help maintain strength when the patient is prohibited to move due to recent skin grafting. When movement is allowed, lower extremity exercises may include hip extension, straight leg raises, heel slides, and squatting.

A therapist may need to consider multiple factors when planning an ambulation program. These factors can include the total body surface area burned, depth of burn and location, the patient's respiratory and circulatory status, location of any intravenous lines or monitoring devices, extent of edema and the presence and location of escharotomies or fasciotomies. Early mobility is advocated in the literature and specifically is cited as a means to reduce blood clot formation, maintain lower extremity strength and ROM, and to increase a patient's functional independence.[1,2,5–7] However, there can be problems associated with early ambulation, including pain, bleeding, increased edema, venous stasis, and delayed or poor wound healing.[8–10]

In the literature, there are various early ambulation protocols. The information that follows is a partial listing of current practice.

1. Patients can be ambulated after 48 hours when the cardiovascular system stabilizes and there are no medical complications.[10]
2. Independent transfers and ambulation should be initiated as soon as medically permissible.[11]
3. Ambulation should begin on the day of admission and performed two to three times a shift.[6]
4. Ambulation should commence as soon as possible after hospital admission.[9]

TABLE 13–1. Considerations for Safe Patient Ambulation Following a Burn Injury

Consideration	Requirement
Mental status	Alert, able to follow directions
Vital signs	Blood pressure, heart rate within range of criteria set for patient
Edema	Mild to moderate
Inhalation injury	Good measurable oxygenation
Intravenous catheters	Patent peripheral and central lines; however, patients with lines in their groin or foot may not be permitted to ambulate
Pain	Patient tolerance
Range of motion	Adequate to allow gait cycle
Strength	Able to bear weight on lower extremities

5. Ambulation should begin as soon as the patient's physical condition warrants, usually by 48 to 72 hours after injury, when vital signs are stable and fluid resuscitation complete.[7]
6. As soon as the patient's vital signs are stable, ambulation should be initiated. Most patients are medically stable after the first 3 days, which is the period of initial fluid resuscitation.[12]
7. Ambulation is begun as soon as possible after admission when the patient is hemodynamically stable after the resolution of the burn shock phase.[13]
8. One to three days post burn, ambulation is begun if the patient is physiologically stable and the burns permit.[1]

Although there is a variance in the timing of early ambulation reported in the literature, patients usually can ambulate if certain requirements are met (Table 13–1).

Factors Influencing Ambulation

A patient's general physical status following burn injury is the most critical factor in early ambulation. The patient should be mentally alert and able to follow simple directions. The patient's vital signs of blood pressure and pulse rate should be stable.[7] Usually, if a patient has sustained an inhalation injury and is on a ventilator or has had a tracheostomy, he or she may be confined to bed.[2,11] However, some physicians encourage a more aggressive treatment approach and permit the supervised ambulation of ventilator-dependent patients.[6,12] The presence of an intravenous line in the foot or a central arterial line in the groin may prohibit ambulation.[11] This decision usually is made by the physician.[2,4] Early massive edema also can be a contraindication to ambulation due to increased compartment pressures and potential episodes of hypotension.[6,7,11] A final factor influencing ambulation is the patient's ability to tolerate pain with activity. Pain should be assessed critically by the therapist and other members of the burn team.[11] Distinctions should be made between generalized and localized lower extremity pain and between burn wound pain and other sources of pain, such as calf pain from thrombophlebitis. The patient's individual response to pain must be recognized also. The therapist must evaluate any subjective and objective pain factors and decide what influence pain has on the initiation of ambulation.

AMBULATION FOLLOWING A PARTIAL-THICKNESS BURN

Partial-thickness burn injuries of the lower extremities may heal without skin grafting if they are treated properly. Because of the lack of dermal support for blood vessels, a patient with a partial-thickness injury is prone to edema and venous stasis when the lower extremity is in a dependent position.[7,9–12] Patients may experience pain that can be quite severe and usually is described as tingling, throbbing, or stinging.[6,7] They may be at an increased risk to develop cellulitis surrounding the burn wound.[3,14] The patient with a partial-thickness burn can ambulate successfully if a careful program of progressive lower extremity dependency, combined with the use of elastic wraps to the lower extremities, is followed.* Often, ambulation is limited in time and distance until wound epithelialization is complete.[14]

If the patient and family are able to manage wound care, pain control, and transportation to and from the burn treatment facility, the patient with a partial-thickness burn of the lower extremities can be treated as an outpatient.

AMBULATION FOLLOWING A FULL-THICKNESS BURN

Similar to patients with a partial-thickness burn injury, patients with full-thickness burns of the lower extremities may develop edema, venous stasis, and have pain when ambulation is attempted. Patients with circumferential burns may require an escharotomy or fasciotomy, which can delay ambulation. A full-thickness burn on the sole of the foot may prohibit ambulation, but some patients can walk with the use of adapted shoes or padded slippers.[3,7,9]

Ambulation may be contraindicated when exposed tendons have become frayed because the forces generated by walking may lead to tendon rupture.[7] This situation is particularly important if larger tendons such as the Achilles or tibialis anterior are involved. Smaller tendons or small exposed areas of larger tendons can be supported sufficiently with elastic wraps during ambulation. Most patients with full-thickness burns are permitted to ambulate prior to skin graft application.

Patients with partial- and full-thickness lower extremity burns will require careful elastic bandage wrapping prior to ambulation or whenever the lower extremities are in a dependent position. Elastic bandages provide support for the vascular system and help to control edema, venous stasis, and dependent pain.[17] Application of an elastic wrap should begin just proximal to the toes and extend to the groin.† A figure-of-8 wrap pattern should be used to provide maximal support and pressure distribution (see Chapter 14).‡ The width of the elastic wrap used is related proportionately to the size of the patient's lower extremity.[16] A 4-inch bandage on the leg and a 6-inch bandage on the thigh work well for adults. Infants and children may require the use of 2 or 3-inch bandages.

AMBULATION FOLLOWING SKIN GRAFTING

The initiation of ambulation following lower extremity skin grafting usually is dependent upon the establishment of competent circulation to the grafted area. Inosculation is the process of anastomosis of blood vessels between the recipient site and

*References 3–7, 9–13, 15, 16
†References 4, 6, 7, 12, 13, 16
‡References 4–7, 12, 13, 16, 18

the skin graft by vessels growing into the graft from the underlying vascular bed.[19] This blood vessel connection allows a nutritive blood flow to the graft that usually is established within 2 to 3 days following a skin grafting procedure. Initially the new blood vessel connections are very fragile. If a lower extremity is placed in a dependent position too soon following skin grafting, the arterial and venous blood in the graft will not be exchanged effectively. This occurrence can lead to venous pooling beneath the graft, which eventually can cause graft disruption.[13] Research findings have not yet determined the exact time when venous pressure ceases to be a problem, but the graft probably remains at risk for at least 10 to 12 days after skin grafting.[19] For this reason, ambulation protocols following skin grafting usually have not been initiated until the tenth to fourteenth postoperative day.* The exact timing for the initiation of ambulation varies greatly between burn centers and in the literature.[3,6,17] Recently, there has been great interest in decreasing the time from grafting to ambulation and several protocols are being used.[21-23]

Supporting the Lower Extremity Skin Graft

Regardless of when ambulation is initiated following skin grafting, most therapists begin the process by gradually placing the grafted lower extremity in a dependent position.[7] This procedure is called *dangling* (Fig. 13–1).[6] From the time a skin graft is applied until dependent positioning is allowed, the patient should have the grafted extremity elevated.[3,9] The lower extremities can be elevated while the patient lays supine in bed by gatching the lower portion of the bed or by propping the legs on pillows or wedges. Pillows and wedges are not indicated for use with an air-fluidized bed because they decrease the pressure-relieving effect of the bed. When in a chair, the patient also should sit with the lower extremities elevated. This position can be attained by using a footstool, a wheelchair with elevating footrests, or a lounge chair that has an elevating leg feature. Care must be taken so the skin graft is not in a dependent position for a prolonged period during bed-to-chair transfers. This position can be avoided by teaching the patient a parallel sit transfer from bed to chair. This procedure can be difficult if the patient is on an air-fluidized bed and the patient may need to be lifted to the chair. Another option is to transfer the patient to an adjustable stretcher, lower the stretcher to chair height, and then complete a parallel transfer.

The key factor in safely and successfully placing a skin grafted lower extremity in a dependent position is to provide support to the graft and its underlying vascular system. The three most frequently used methods of support are as follows:

1. *Elastic wrapping:* This method of skin graft support is common for the lower extremity as previously noted. Support is accomplished by using a figure-of-8 wrap with an elastic bandage. The elastic bandage can be placed over a dressing or directly on the newly grafted area. Small open areas should be covered with a nonadherent dressing before the elastic bandage is applied.[6,13] An advantage of using an elastic wrap is the wrap can be removed easily and quickly for graft inspection. A disadvantage is the wrap must be reapplied each time the extremity is placed in a dependent position.

---

*References 2, 6, 7, 13, 14, 19, 20

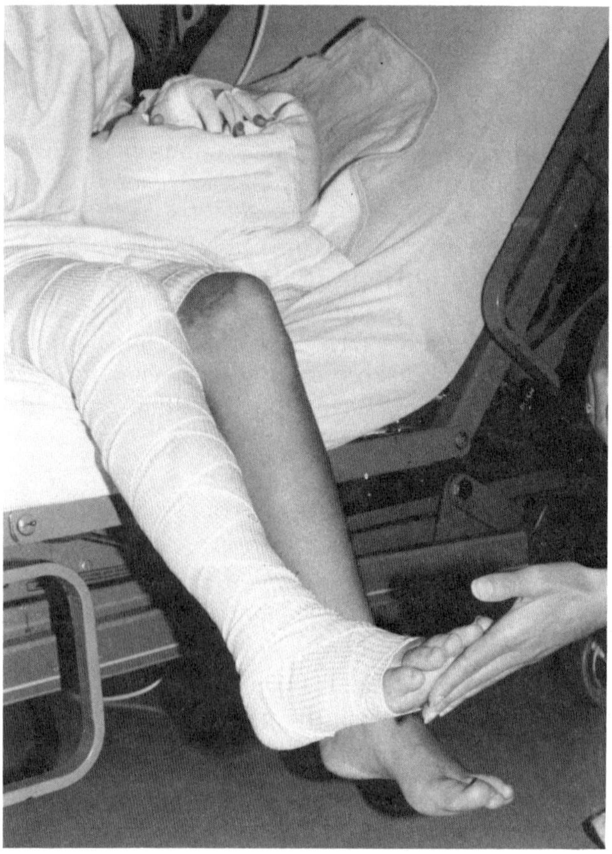

FIGURE 13–1. Patient demonstrating lower extremity "dangling" position off side of bed. Active ankle movements can assist circulation.

2. *Unna's boot (Domeboro paste):* This gauze, impregnated with calamine lotion and zinc oxide, is commercially available (Fig. 13–2) (see Appendix B).[24] Upon drying, the gauze provides a semirigid support to a skin graft. Unna's boot provides excellent venous support and can be applied immediately following a skin graft procedure or shortly thereafter, thus eliminating the need for a postoperative dressing. The successful use of Unna's boot for small grafted areas has been documented.[3,24–26] A disadvantage is that Unna's boot is not readily removed for graft inspection. The boot can be left in place for up to 7 days but usually is changed every 3 days so that the graft can be visually inspected. The boot can be discontinued 7 to 14 days after the initial application and an elastic bandage or a custom-made stocking then can be used for venous support.
3. *Plaster casts:* Casts can be applied in the operating room immediately following the skin-grafting procedure. Either a short or long leg cast can be used depending on the size and location of the graft. A layer of dressing should be placed between the graft and the cast. Advantages are that the cast provides good venous support and eliminates the need for a postoperative dressing. A disadvantage is that the cast is difficult to remove for graft inspection. The cast can be left in place for up to 14 days following the skin graft but may be removed sooner. Special care should be taken when applying the cast to avoid problems with pressure and shear forces.

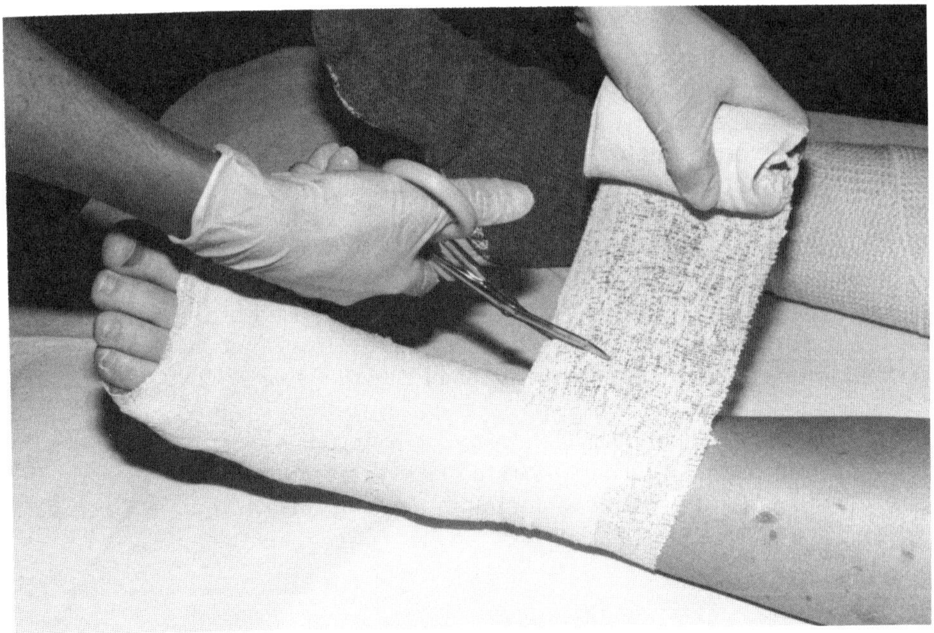

FIGURE 13–2. Application of Unna's boot to left foot and leg for pressure support of vasculature.

Ambulation Protocols and Timing

After a technique to support and protect the skin graft has been selected, the timing of ambulation can be determined. Patients treated with Unna's boot can begin ambulation as soon as the boot dries. Although some patients may need to use crutches initially, Unna's boot may allow immediate postoperative ambulation and early hospital discharge. A cast also allows for ambulation as soon as the cast dries and permits early discharge, but the patient may be required to use crutches.[27]

If an elastic wrap technique for graft support has been chosen, a progressive dangling program is initiated prior to allowing the lower extremity to be placed in a dependent position (see Fig. 13–1). Once wrapped, the patient usually sits with the extremity in a dependent position for approximately 1 minute. The extremity is then elevated, the elastic bandage removed, and the graft observed for color change, bleeding, or breakdown. If no adverse condition is noted, the extremity is rewrapped and the process repeated with the extremity incrementally dependent for longer periods of time up to 3 to 5 minutes. Patient discomfort, edema, bleeding, or tingling in the lower extremity may indicate inadequate pressure support or difficulty with the establishment of circulation to the graft.[7]

When the process of dangling has been successfully completed, ambulation can begin. The time to initiate ambulation following skin grafting varies from 1 day to 2 weeks. Munster[14] advocated ambulation at 2 weeks and Feller and Jones[2] on the tenth postoperative day. Schmitt and associates[21] ambulated patients on the seventh postoperative day. McDonald and co-workers[23] reported successful ambulation with a small group of patients on the fifth postsurgical day.

Burnsworth, Krob, and Langer-Schnepp[22] conducted a retrospective study of 58 patients who ambulated immediately postoperatively without exhibiting any significant problems associated with the graft. The average time following grafting before a patient ambulated approximately 30 feet was 1.7 days. In 98 other burn units, 7.1 days elapsed following grafting prior to a patient ambulating that distance. Patients in this study were discharged on the seventh postoperative day compared to an average 9.3 days for the other reporting units.

Whatever protocol is selected for ambulation following skin grafting to the lower extremities, the grafts should be inspected carefully following each ambulation trial. Severe discomfort or pain during or after ambulation can be an indicator of potential graft problems. If discoloration, bleeding, breakdown, or edema occur, the frequency or distance the patient ambulates may need to be decreased or the vascular support to the lower extremities may need to be increased. A five-point assessment scale can be helpful to objectively evaluate the status of a graft (Table 13–2).

Following skin grafting, some patients will be unable to safely stand due to orthostatic hypotension if immobilization and bed rest has occurred. These patients may require the use of a tilt table to gradually achieve an upright position.[6,7] The patient's blood pressure should be monitored during this procedure. Once patients

TABLE 13–2. Five Point Assessment Scale

Color	0	None
	1	Slight redness after dangle; alleviated on elevation
	2	Mild redness alleviated <1 minute
	3	Moderate redness alleviated >1 minute
	4	Dark red/purple color alleviated >1 minute
Discomfort	0	None
	1	On initial dependency; alleviated while limb still dependent
	2	Mild on dependency; alleviated with elevation
	3	Moderate on dependency; alleviated >1-minute elevation
	4	Severe; does not allow limb to be dependent
Tingling	0	None
	1	On initial dependency; alleviated while limb still dependent
	2	Mild on dependency; alleviated with elevation
	3	Moderate on dependency; alleviated >1-minute elevation
	4	Severe; does not allow limb to be dependent
Edema	0	None
	1	Minimal; alleviated quickly on elevation
	2	Mild; alleviated <1-minute elevation
	3	Moderate; alleviated >1-minute elevation
	4	Severe; not alleviated with elevation
Bleeding	0	None
	1	Minimal from graft
	2	Mild; alleviated on elevation
	3	Moderate; alleviated >1-minute elevation
	4	Severe; prohibits dependency
Breakdown	0	None
	1	Minimal; graft edges only
	2	Mild; small area < dime size
	3	Moderate; > dime-size area
	4	Severe; > quarter-size area

Adapted from Schmitt et al.,[21] p 34, with permission.

are able to tolerate standing on the tilt table, they can ambulate from the table. Patients who have been allowed to sit out of bed prior to dangling usually do not require the use of a tilt table. Some patients may need to begin ambulating in the parallel bars while others can begin from bedside or a chair.

Once ambulation has been initiated following skin grafting, the patient should be advanced to independent ambulation as rapidly as possible.[6,13,16] Walkers, canes, and crutches can be used, but they should be discontinued as soon as possible to facilitate the resumption of a normal gait pattern.[6,7,9,11,16] Upon assuming an upright position, patients should be encouraged to walk immediately rather than stand, because standing increases the likelihood of venous stasis and can lead to increased discomfort in the lower extremities.[9] The distance and frequency of ambulation should be increased gradually and patients should be able to tolerate 5 to 15 minutes of ambulation prior to discharge from the burn center. The patient should be instructed how to ascend and descend stairs with and without the use of a railing. Instruction and practice also should include how to ascend and descend ramps and to walk on surfaces of different textures (e.g., grass, concrete, carpet).

GAIT TRAINING AND DEVIATIONS

The ultimate goal of ambulation for the patient with a lower extremity burn is the ability to walk efficiently so that all daily activities can be accomplished easily. Normal gait patterning is essential for efficient ambulation and includes control of the head and trunk, arm swing, and pelvic movement. The lower extremities must function properly during swing and stance phase, including the complex ankle and foot movements during heel strike and toe-off.

The first step in a gait training program is a comprehensive evaluation. This evaluation should be performed during the first ambulation session following skin grafting and re-evaluated frequently as ambulation progresses. The patient can be taught simple gait techniques, such as proper weight shift to each lower extremity, step alternation, and stance time. Many patients benefit from gait instruction while in the parallel bars. As a patient improves, hip, knee, ankle, and foot motion during the stance and swing phases can be emphasized. Finally, the cadence and rhythm of walking can be incorporated into the program.[7] The patient also will need to be taught to move quickly. Children and the athletically inclined may benefit from instruction in running and other locomotor skills such as jumping, hopping, skipping, and leaping.[7,10] A wide variety of physical therapy equipment (e.g., treadmill, BAPS board, bicycle, ramps) can be used to enhance gait training (Fig. 13–3).[15,16,28] Most importantly, the patient should be instructed in a home program to be performed daily.

Several gait deviations occur frequently in the patient with a lower extremity burn,[6,7,13] although many may correct themselves once the patient's wounds heal and pain diminishes.[9] Table 13–3 summarizes these deviations. Some of these deviations can be minimized by proper positioning and aggressive exercise during the acute phase of burn care. Problems that remain after the initiation of ambulation often can be corrected with an appropriate exercise program. The use of mirrors as a means of feedback for the patient can help to identify deviations in gait or posture.[6,7,16]

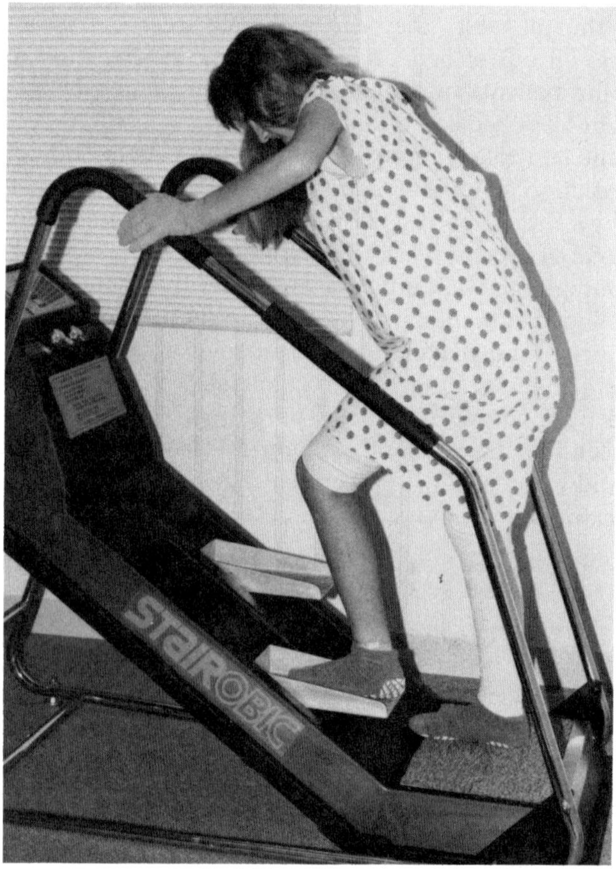

FIGURE 13–3. Patient utilizing stair climbing machine for lower extremity exercise.

TABLE 13–3. Common Gait Deviations Following Burn Injury

Forward trunk position
Decreased trunk rotation
Decreased pelvic mobility
Increased arm swing
Increased hip flexion
Inadequate hip abduction
Increased hip external rotation
Hip circumduction
Knee flexion or extension maintained throughout cycle
Ankle plantar flexion with no heel strike
Poor weight shift
Decreased stance phase on affected lower extremity
Decreased swing phase on nonaffected lower extremity
Improper step alternation
Decreased step length
Wide base of support
Decreased or no toe-off

LONG-TERM PROBLEMS AND SOLUTIONS

After being discharged from the burn center, a patient with lower extremity burns can be confronted with a wide variety of problems that may require therapeutic intervention. While some of these problems are common to most burn patients, others are specific to those patients with lower extremity burns.

Scar Control

Burn scars can become a problem for patients when they include the posterior knee, ankle, dorsal foot, or toe web spaces (Fig. 13–4). Elastic bandages used for initial graft support can be used for early hypertrophic scar control. They can be replaced later by tubular bandages and eventually by custom-made elastic pressure garments.[9] Additional pressure can be applied through the use of inserts such as elastomer molds, construction of special shoes, or adaptations of regular footwear.[3,7,9,29–32] Children who develop hypertrophic scarring of the dorsal foot are prone to develop hyperextension of the metatarsophalangeal joints.[31,33,34] Without proper intervention, this condition can lead to dislocation of the metatarsal heads and an eventual "rocker bottom" foot (Fig. 13–5). This deformity can limit ambulation and require extensive reconstructive surgery.[33] Shoes with a rocker bottom or metatarsal bar added can help to avoid this complication (see Chapter 11). Patients with a peroneal nerve palsy or plantar flexion deformity may require the long-term use of a splint or orthosis.[3,7,9,17,35]

Normal gait and safe ambulation depend upon the use of proper shoes. Initially, patients will require shoes with nonslip soles that are comfortable to wear. If patients use elastic bandages, they may require a larger-than-normal shoe size to accommodate the added bulk of the bandage. Athletic or soft-sided shoes work well at this stage. Shoes can apply contact across the dorsal foot and serve as an adjunct to

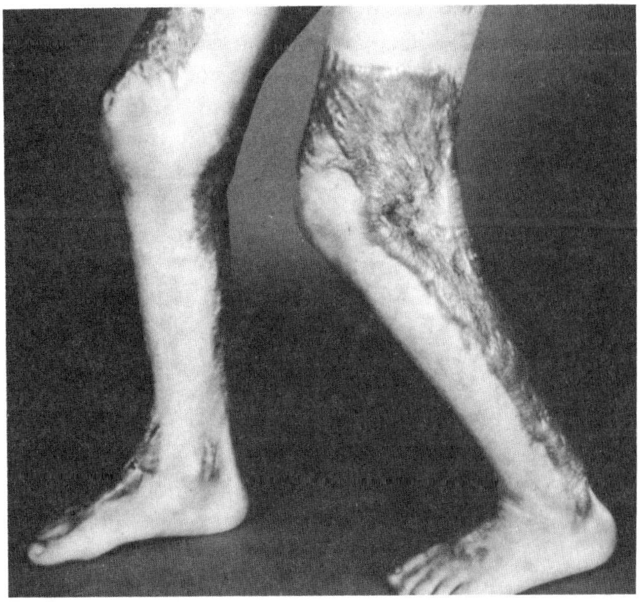

FIGURE 13–4. Thick hypertrophic burn scar of posterior leg preventing complete knee extension in an adolescent.

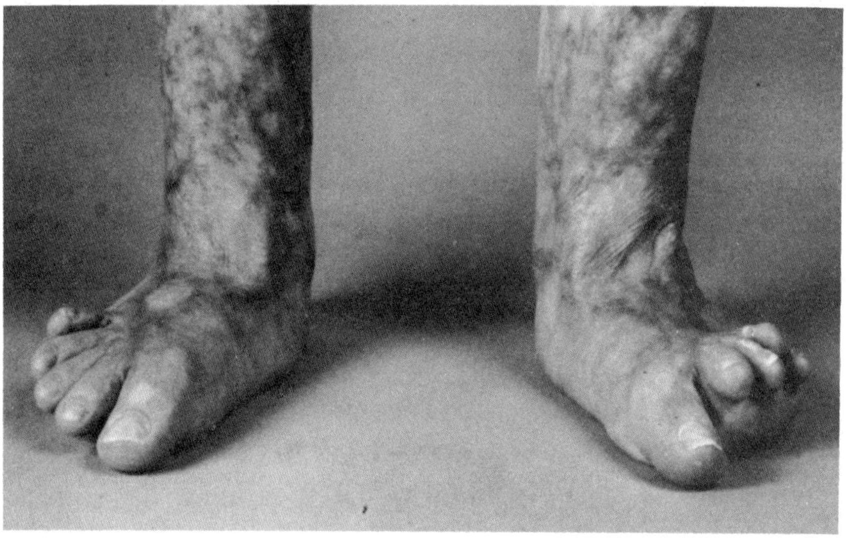

FIGURE 13–5. "Rocker-bottom" foot deformity secondary to scar tissue contracture formation on dorsal surface.

pressure therapy for this area. High-topped shoes can be beneficial for patients who require increased stability and pressure in the ankle area.[30] Later, patients will most likely return to the type of footwear worn before the burn injury.

Venous Stasis

Patients who have had lower extremity skin grafting may experience long-term problems with return of venous circulation.[2,7,9] Patients with deep burns to the lower extremities that required fascial excision will have more difficulty than patients whose burn wounds were tangentially excised.[3] Venous blood tends to pool in skin grafts due to either the lack of superficial veins or poor capillary function.[6,7,13] The area may exhibit a purple discoloration and can be prone to skin breakdown.[6,13] (Fig. 13–6) Pain, when the extremity is in a dependent position, may be the most disturbing symptom for a patient.[7] This complication is due to the progressive increase in vascular pressure in the foot compared to the hip in the lower extremity and may limit the patient's ability to stand and ambulate.[36] Pain may be intensified when the patient stands still, but improves during ambulation because the muscles act to assist the venous pump mechanism.

The patient should be instructed in a program of lower extremity exercises that can be performed to alleviate these symptoms when they occur. One method is to have a patient place his or her foot of the involved leg on the seat of a chair when needing to stretch the Achilles tendon area (Fig. 13–7). Flexing the hip and knee appears to decrease the total amount of columnar pressure exerted by blood. Performing static exercises of gluteal and quadricep setting, straight leg raises and ankle pumps immediately prior to ambulation can help greatly in reducing a patient's dependent pain when assuming an upright position.[7,15] Once standing, the patient should be instructed to begin ambulation immediately to maintain a pumping action of the lower extremity musculature so as to avoid an increase in circulatory pressure.[36]

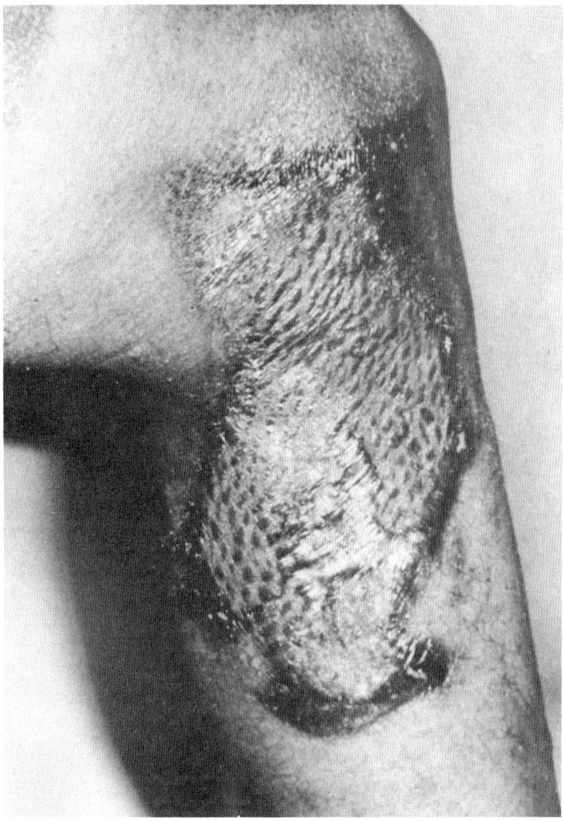

FIGURE 13–6. Venous stasis in a healed meshed skin graft of the leg when dependent. Note the amount of marked discoloration.

Gradually increasing the time of standing or walking, interspersed with lower extremity elevation, also can help.[13,16] If a patient has a job that requires prolonged standing, a job modification or change in occupation may be required to avoid symptoms the patient cannot tolerate.

Well-fitting compression garments can be very helpful in alleviating symptoms of venous stasis. Many patients will prefer to wear some type of elastic support garment even after their scars have matured.[13] For some patients, support pantyhose are adequate, while others will require custom-made pressure gradient garments.

Skin Breakdown

Lower extremity skin grafts and healed burn areas can be prone to breakdown. Open areas will require continual wound care and dressings. Additional skin grafting may be required for wounds that do not heal within an acceptable time period. Care should be taken to reduce pressure on areas with the potential for skin breakdown (e.g., malleoli, heel, or plantar surface of the foot at the metatarsal heads) (Fig. 13–8). Support garments and footwear must fit properly. Padding and inserts can be used to alleviate pressure areas provided they do not cause undesired pressure elsewhere.

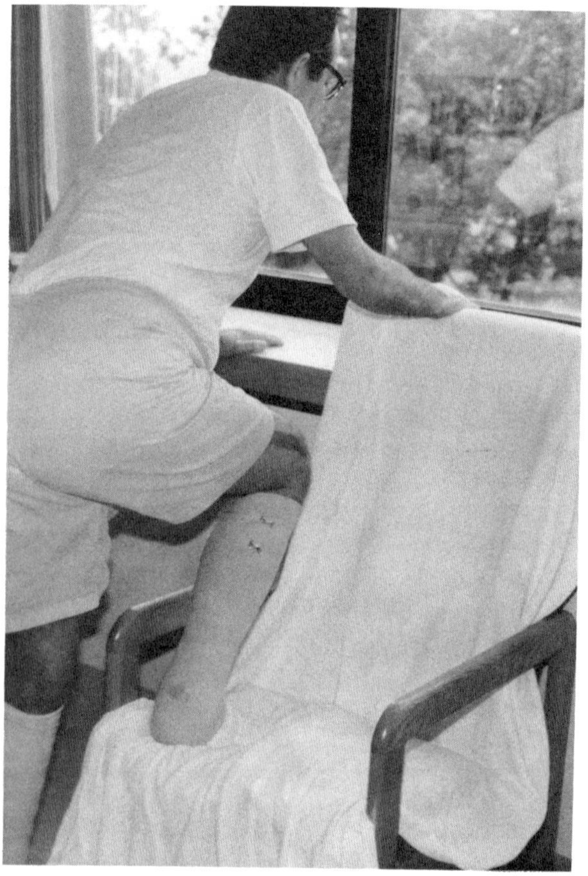

FIGURE 13–7. Patient with foot on chair and hip and knee flexed to exercise ankle area more comfortably. This position assists in decreasing the amount of dependent pain in the lower extremity experienced by patients.

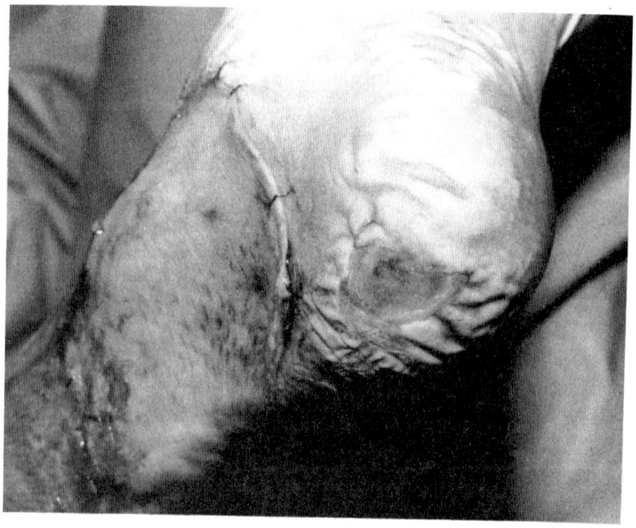

FIGURE 13–8. Pressure sore on left heel.

Altered Sensation

The patient with a lower extremity burn may experience difficulties from a lack of sensation or hypersensitivity. The patient must become aware of areas where sensation is lacking and instructed how to prevent further injury. If the sole of the foot is insensate, a patient may require special footwear and instruction on how to protect the foot. Patients with tarsal tunnel syndrome or peripheral neuropathy may require surgical or medical intervention to relieve the condition.

Patients with hypersensitivity may benefit from a desensitization program. Physical therapy modalities including paraffin, cryotherapy, and transcutaneous electrical nerve stimulation may help to alleviate symptoms. Many patients experience improvement in symptoms as scar maturation occurs.

Pain

Recurrent pain and discomfort often are complaints voiced by patients with lower extremity burns. Careful evaluation can determine the source of the pain (e.g., venous stasis, hypertrophic scar, nerve involvement) and a treatment program can be planned. Treatment with medication and physical therapy modalities often can decrease the symptoms.

CASE STUDY

HISTORY

WM is a 73-year-old man who was burned when his pants ignited from a ground fire he was tending while burning leaves. He sustained a 23 percent body burn with 9 percent being full-thickness. The patient was wearing shorts and ankle-length socks with shoes, which spared the skin distal to the malleoli bilaterally.

The patient had a significant history of cardiomyopathy and secondary hypotension that made his period of fluid resuscitation difficult. Additionally, the patient reported having "arthritis" in both knees.

After 1 week of stabilization, WM was taken to surgery for skin grafting. Grafts were placed on the wounds of the right posterior leg and extended proximally to just above the popliteal space. The left leg required placement of skin on the posteriomedial aspect.

Therapy was initiated on the day following his weekend admission. A review of the patient's medical record revealed the nursing staff had recorded a syncopal episode of the patient when they were attempting to transfer him from his bed to a wheelchair for transport to the treatment room for his dressing change.

Upon initial evaluation, WM's feet were moderately edematous. Right knee active-assistive range of motion (AAROM) measured −15° extension to 100° flexion with the left knee displaying −5° terminal extension and 95° flexion.

Bilateral active ankle dorsiflexion was −10°; however, a neutral position was achieved with assistance. All patient limitations in motion were accompanied by pain. All other ROM and strength were within functional limits for the patient's age.

PROBLEM LIST

Cardiac disease
Hypotension
Syncopy
Bilateral foot edema
Limited bilateral knee and ankle ROM
Full-thickness burns
Scarring potential

GOALS

Minimal bilateral foot edema
Maintain bilateral knee ROM
Increase bilateral ankle dorsiflexion to neutral plus position
Normal ambulation
Minimal scar formation

TREATMENT PLAN

Preoperative physical interventions for the patient included elevation and support of bilateral lower extremities on pillows, instruction in ankle pump, quadricep and gluteal muscle isometrics and straight leg raises, general upper extremity and trunk strengthening, instruction in bed mobility, and application of bilateral ankle dorsiflexion splints following each twice-daily therapy session for 2 hours and for continuous night use.

In the intraoperative period the therapist accompanied WM to surgery to determine the true extent of his ankle and knee limitations. After anesthetic induction, PROM of the ankles and knees was performed. The ankles continued to be limited to approximately a neutral position, but with a soft end feel that suggested the limitation was due to the edema still present. Knee limitations in both flexion and extension bilaterally were determined due to arthritis bony blockage. Following skin graft application to all full-thickness areas, the bilateral ankle dorsiflexion splints were reapplied and conforming posterior knee extension splints were fabricated bilaterally.

In the postoperative period WM remained on bed rest for 2 days following surgery. His first dressing change after surgery was performed at bedside. On the second and subsequent days, he was transported to the treatment room for dressing changes. The therapist assisted WM and the nursing staff with safe bed-to-gurney transfers to avoid shearing the skin grafts for 2 days. On the fourth postoperative day, the therapist assisted with bed-to-wheelchair transfers keeping the patient's legs elevated and knees extended. During the first 4 days following surgery, lower extremity and general body exercises were performed at bedside twice daily, similar to the preoperative period.

After the fifth postoperative day's dressing change, all skin grafts were determined to be stable enough to permit the lower extremities to assume a dependent position and the patient could begin stand-pivot wheelchair transfers.

The next day, by arrangement with the nursing staff, a therapy session was scheduled prior to the morning dressing change. During this time, a tilt table was brought to WM's room. He was transferred to the tilt table and vital signs were taken by the therapist. Splints were removed and the patient's legs were wrapped with compression bandages. Following the dangling program described in this chapter, he was sequentially tilted to various semivertical positions in 20° increments and vital signs were monitored at each stage. Prior to the tilt table being elevated and during each elevation, the patient was instructed to continue moving his toes and contracting his quadricep muscles.

WM successfully completed two bouts of progressive tilting, but during the third trial he became "light-headed." He was returned to a horizontal position and vital signs were taken. His blood pressure was slightly lower than usual with a rapid heart rate. After his vital signs restabilized, the patient was transported on the tilt table to the dressing room for wound care. The same sequence was performed each day, with the same blood pressure and heart rate effects but at progressively higher upright angles, until the patient was able to transfer off the standing platform of the tilt table to a wheelchair 4 days later. In addition to performing his regular exercise routine, WM also was progressed through a typical bedside dangling program a second time each day.

Once his skin grafts had adhered, the knee extension splints were discontinued and the ankle splints changed to nighttime application only. WM had tolerated the upright position and the emphasis of his therapy was shifted toward ambulation. However, prior to each ambulation attempt, he performed all his routine lower extremity exercises. Eventually he was able to progress from a walker to contact guarding for assistance.

At the time of discharge, WM's wounds were healed and his edema had subsided. His ankle ROM had improved sufficiently to allow a normal gait pattern and his limitations in knee ROM had not progressed. WM was wearing intermediate pressure support stockings while awaiting his definitive pressure gradient garments and he had progressed to independent ambulation with standby assist. WM was discharged back to his son's family with whom he was living at the time of his accident.

RATIONALE

Due to WM's initial syncopal experience and pending surgery, the patient's presurgical rehabilitation program was limited to lower extremity elevation and positioning to reduce edema and preserve his knee ROM, and dorsiflexion splints were used to prevent further loss of ankle motion. Exercises were prescribed to assist in ROM goals and, due to his cardiac and circulatory history, to promote circulation to reduce edema and prevent blood clot formation. Further attempts at stand-pivot transfers or ambulation were delayed for three reasons. First, to allow additional time for hemodynamic stabilization; second, questionable added benefit would have been derived from such an intervention because of the patient's pending surgery; and finally, to avoid any undue dependent pain for the patient since he would be on bedrest following surgery.

Knee splints, in addition to ankle dorsiflexion splints, were provided following surgery to limit potential further loss of motion after determining his knee limitations were due to his arthritic condition. His active bilateral lower extremity exercise program was permitted immediately following surgery because it was felt the ankle motions would not disturb the proximally placed skin grafts. In addition, the static quadricep and straight leg raise exercises did not cause disturbance of the skin grafts because the muscle contractions and hip joint motion did not impact the grafts. Performing these exercises also helped encourage circulation to the lower extremities and aided in limiting postsurgical edema.

The tilt table was selected for use to begin the patient's lower extremity dependent positioning program instead of bedside dangling. The reason for this alternative treatment approach was to avoid flexion of the right knee where skin grafts had been placed, to avoid a more instantaneous upright head position considering the patient's prior syncopal event, and to decrease the patient's apprehensiveness regarding ambulation.

Before any attempt at early ambulation, a series of lower extremity exercises were performed to promote circulation and to maintain a muscle pump action to aid venous return and prevent the secondary threat of hypotension. In addition, the patient wore compression dressings at all times. Pressure gradient support garments likewise were ordered for vascular support as well as to prevent excessive scarring.

The patient was allowed use of a walker to begin independent ambulation for security and safety reasons. Splints were discontinued as the patient's wounds and skin grafts healed and ROM was being maintained. The continual exercises, along with ambulation, were sufficient for maintaining ROM in the lower extremities.

SUMMARY

A burn injury to the lower extremities potentially can cause severe limitations in a patient's ability to function in the home and work environment. The restoration of efficient ambulation can be a long and arduous process. Comprehensive treatment planning, including positioning, exercise, vascular support, and appropriate progressive ambulation and gait training can speed the burn patient's return to an independent, quality life "on his (or her) feet." Specialized footwear, inserts, or splints may be necessary depending on the extent of the burn. Problems such as scarring, venous stasis, chronic edema, and altered sensation provide a challenge for the patient and therapist after discharge. However, through education and the use of therapeutic exercise and modalities, the patient's lower extremity symptoms may be minimized.

REFERENCES

1. Roberts, ML and Pruitt, BA: Nursing care and psychological considerations. In Artz, CP, Moncrief, JA, and Pruitt, BA (eds): Burns: A Team Approach. WB Saunders, Philadelphia, 1979, pp 370–389.
2. Feller, I and Jones, CA: Nursing the Burned Patient. The Institute for Burn Medicine, Ann Arbor, 1973, p 73, 151.
3. Heimbach, DM and Engrav, LH: Surgical Management of the Burn Wound. Raven Press, New York, 1984, pp 83–98.

4. Malick, M and Care, JA: Manual on Management of the Burn Patient. Harmarville Rehabilitation Center, Pittsburgh, 1982.
5. Johnson, CL, O'Shaughnessy, ET, and Ostergreen, G: Burn Management. Raven Press, New York, 1981, p 79.
6. Kozerefski, PM: Exercise and ambulation in the burn patient. In DiGregorio, VR (ed): Rehabilitation of the Burn Patient. Churchill Livingstone, New York, 1984, pp 55–73.
7. Nothdurft, D, Smith, PS, and LeMaster, J: Exercise and treatment modalities. In Fisher, SV and Helm, PA (eds): Comprehensive Rehabilitation of Burns. Williams & Wilkins, Baltimore, 1984, pp 96–147.
8. Achauer, BM: Management of the Burn Patient. Appleton and Lange, Norwalk, 1987, p 128.
9. LeMaster, J: Treatment of Burns of Specific Areas. In DiGregorio, VR (ed): Rehabilitation of the Burn Patient. Churchill Livingstone, New York, 1984, pp 99–130.
10. Petro, JA, et al: Hospitalization of burned patients. In Nicosia, JE and Petro, JA (eds): Manual of Burn Care. Raven Press, New York, 1983, pp 15–88.
11. Zane, LJ: Evaluation of the Acutely Ill Burn Patient. In DiGregorio, VR (ed): Rehabilitation of the Burn Patient. Churchill Livingstone, New York, 1984, pp 5–31.
12. Wright, PC: Fundamentals of acute burn care and physical therapy management. Phys Ther 64:1217–1231, 1984.
13. Wright, PC: Physical Therapy in Burn Injury. In Salisbury, RE, Newman, NM, and Dingeldein, GP (eds): Manual of Burn Therapeutics. Little, Brown, Boston, 1983, pp 165–178.
14. Munster, AM: Burn Care for the House Officer. Williams & Wilkins, Baltimore, 1980, pp 12–60.
15. Braddom, RL, et al: The physical treatment and rehabilitation of burn patients. In Hummel, RP (ed): Clinical Burn Therapy. John Wright PSG, Boston, 1982, pp 279–300.
16. Johnson, CL: The Role of Physical Therapy. In Boswick, JA (ed): The Art and Science of Burn Care. Aspen, Rockville, 1987, pp 299–306.
17. Helm, P, et al: Burn injury: Rehabilitation management in 1982. Arch Phys Med Rehabil 63:6, 1982.
18. Whitmore, JJ, et al: Bandaging the lower extremity to control swelling: Figure 8 versus spiral technique. Arch Phys Med Rehabil 53:487, 1972.
19. Hartford, CE: Surgical management. In Fisher, SV and Helm, PA (eds): Comprehensive Rehabilitation of Burns. Williams & Wilkins, Baltimore, 1984, pp 28–63.
20. Moncrief, JA: Grafting. In Artz, CA, Moncrief, JA, and Pruitt, BA: Burns: A Team Approach. WB Saunders, Philadelphia, 1979, pp 273–298.
21. Schmitt, MA, French, L, and Kalil, ET: How soon is safe? Ambulation of the patient with burns after lower-extremity skin grafting. J Burn Care Rehabil 12:33–37, 1991.
22. Burnsworth, B, Krob, MJ, and Langer-Schnepp, M: Immediate ambulation of patients with lower extremity grafts. J Burn Care Rehabil 13:89, 1992.
23. McDonald, K, et al: Ambulation and lower leg autografts following thermal injury. Proc Am Phys Ther Assoc 70:R170, 1990.
24. Harner, T, et al: Dr. Paul Unna's boot and early ambulation after skin grafting the leg: A survey of burn centers and a report of 20 cases. Plast Reconstr Surg 69:359–360, 1982.
25. Grube, BJ, Heimbach, DM, and Engrav, LH: Molten metal burns to the lower extremity. J Burn Care Rehabil 8:403–405, 1987.
26. Ainsworth, P, et al: The evaluation of the Unna boot in autografted burn wounds. Proc American Burn Association, Baltimore, 23:181, 1991.
27. Ricks, NR and Meagher, DP: The benefits of plaster casting for lower extremity burns after grafting in children. J Burn Care Rehabil 13:465–468, 1992.
28. Duncan, CE: Use of a ramp surface for lower extremity exercise with burn-injured patients. J Burn Care Rehabil 10:346–349, 1989.
29. Law, EJ: Minimizing burn scar and contracture. In Hummel, RP (ed): Clinical Burn Therapy. John Wright PSG, Boston, 1982, pp 301–320.
30. Dobbs, ER: Physical therapy. In Artz, CP, Moncrief, JA, and Pruitt, BA: Burns: A Team Approach. WB Saunders, Philadelphia, 1979, pp 492–499.
31. Rivers, EA: Management of Hypertrophic Scarring. In Fisher, SV and Helm, PA (eds): Comprehensive Rehabilitation of Burns. Williams & Wilkins, Baltimore, 1984, pp 177–217.
32. Yeakel, M: Occupational therapy. In Artz, CP, Moncrief, JA, and Pruitt, BA (eds): Burns: A Team Approach. WB Saunders, Philadelphia, 1979, pp 500–511.
33. Howell, JW: Posthospitalization care. In Fisher, SV and Helm, PA (eds): Comprehensive Rehabilitation of Burns. Williams & Wilkins, Baltimore, 1984, pp 151–172.
34. Larson, D, et al: Prevention and treatment of scar contracture. In Artz, CP, Moncrief, JA, and Pruitt, BA (eds): Burns: A Team Approach. WB Saunders, Philadelphia, 1979, pp 466–491.
35. Pullium, GF: Splinting and positioning. In Fisher, SV and Helm, PA (eds): Comprehensive Rehabilitation of Burns. Williams & Wilkins, Baltimore, 1984, pp 64–95.
36. Hammond, MC, Merli, G, and Zierler, RE: Rehabilitation of the patient with peripheral vascular disease of the lower extremity. In LeLisa, JA (ed): Rehabilitation Medicine: Principles and Practice. JB Lippincott, Philadelphia, 1988, pp 795–810.

CHAPTER 14

Scar Management

Marlys J. Staley, MS, PT
Reginald L. Richard, MS, PT

When I was 8 years old, my sister and I were fighting and she scratched me on the cheek near my eye. She was grounded and I was scarred. What is a scar? *Stedman's* medical dictionary defines scar as "the fibrous tissue replacing normal tissues destroyed by injury or disease."[1] *Funk and Wagnalls* defines scar as "the mark left on the skin after the healing of a wound or sore."[2] Scars have multiple etiologies. A scar may occur naturally, as with stretch marks from obesity or pregnancy, as a result of accidental trauma to the skin, or self-inflicted, as in tattooing or deliberate body decorations as seen on natives in African tribes. Infections also may cause scarring as seen with boils or severe acne.[3]

Throughout our lives numerous minor injuries occur to each of us that leave a permanent reminder of the incident. The burn patient incurs a similar reminder; however, the extent is generally much greater and the scar can be more emotionally and physically devastating. In 1988, in his American Burn Association Presidential Address, Dr. David Heimbach predicted that scar management of the burn patient will be a continued problem well into the year 2000.[4]

The purpose of this chapter is to provide therapists with information regarding burn scar formation and current treatment interventions. Scar management of the burn patient is the responsibility of the entire burn team and a major concern of the burn therapist because poor cosmesis, contractures, and itching associated with scarring often impair the patient's ability to return to a normal life of work and play. The responsibilities of a therapist in management of the scar formation process are to control scar hypertrophy and hasten scar maturation. Through various prophylactic and therapeutic methods, itching and soft tissue contracture are minimized and cosmetic outcome is optimized. Education of the patient, family, and other burn team members regarding their roles in controlling burn scar formation is another service the therapist provides.

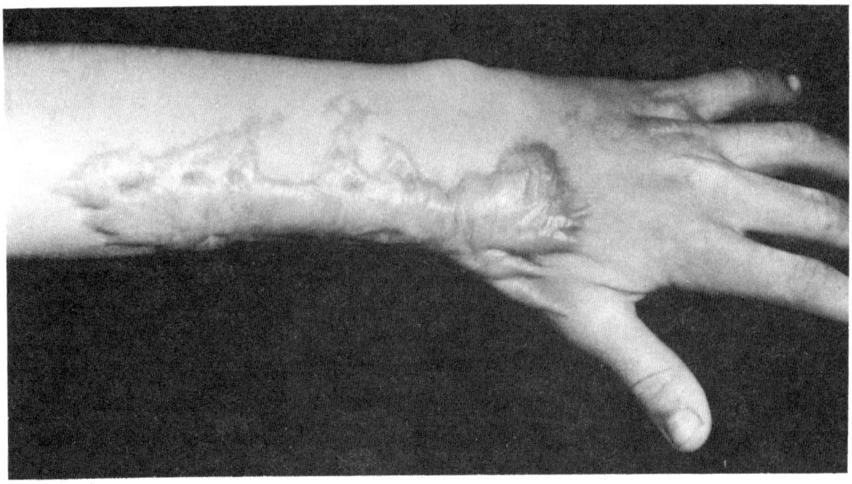

FIGURE 14–1. Typical appearance of a hypertrophic scar.

SCAR HYPERTROPHY

In normal epidermal healing, the skin is replaced with minimal discrepancies in the original texture, color, or surface height. The epidermis does not thicken and therefore does not contribute to the height of a scar.[5] However, if a burn injury extends into the dermis, the skin is repaired through scar formation. Two types of excessive scar may develop. A *hypertrophic* scar is an overgrowth of dermal constituents that remains within the boundaries of the wound. A *keloid* is a scar that extends beyond the boundaries of the original wound (Figs. 14–1 and 14–2). From 1802, when Alibert first described the keloid, until today, discussion continues as to the difference between these two scars.[6] Linares,[7] in his review of hypertrophic healing,

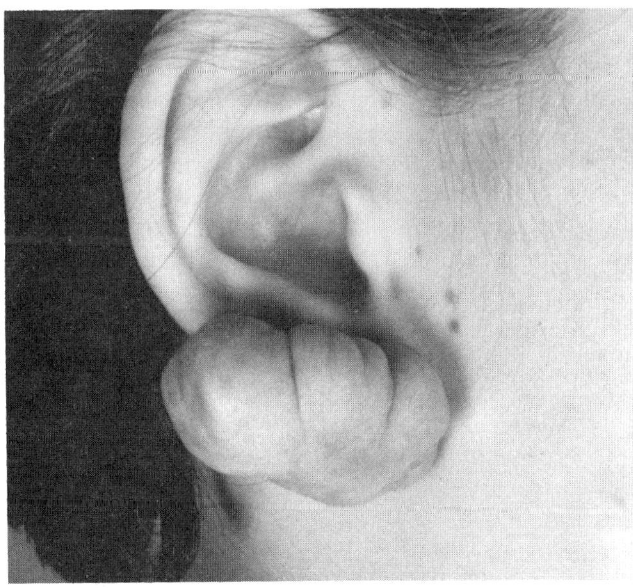

FIGURE 14–2. Right earlobe keloid with characteristic appearance of scar extending beyond wound margin.

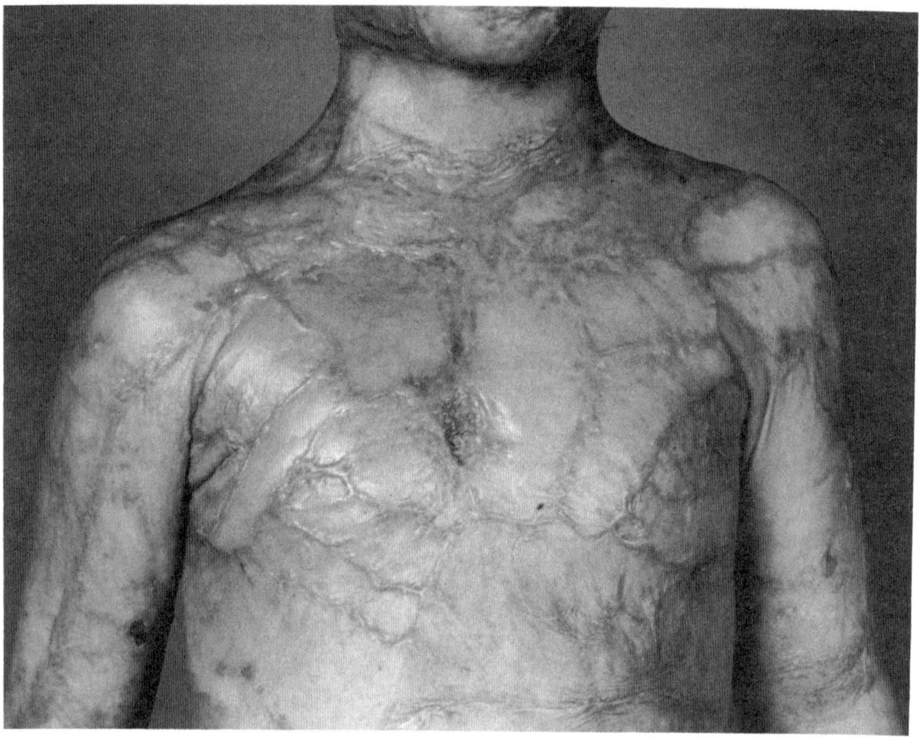

FIGURE 14–3. Scar hypertrophy development in seams between sheet grafts on chest and arms.

stated that hypertrophic scars vary from keloids only quantitatively and that keloids represent the most severe degree of hypertrophic scarring. If an injury extends into the deep (reticular) layer of the dermis, as in the case of a deep partial-thickness burn or if there is delayed wound healing of greater than 3 weeks, hypertrophic scars frequently occur.[7,8] Hypertrophic scars also tend to occur in areas where full-thickness burns have healed by re-epithelialization, granulation tissue formation and contraction or where donor sites have been harvested too deeply, reharvested several times, or are otherwise delayed in healing due to infection or trauma.

Hypertrophic scars usually do not occur in burned areas that have been repaired with split-thickness or full-thickness skin grafts. However, such scars may be located at the junction of grafted and ungrafted tissue, at the seams between skin grafts, and in the interstices of a meshed split-thickness skin graft[8,9] (Fig. 14–3). Researchers have speculated on possible reasons for hypertrophic scar formation[10-13] and why skin grafting appears to minimize scarring,[8,9,14] but no conclusive rationale to explain hypertrophic scarring exists at this time (Table 14–1).

CHARACTERISTICS OF SCARS

Immediately following wound closure, either by skin grafting or the body's own reparative process, the newly formed immature scar is generally smooth and flat. During the next 6 weeks to 3 months, hypertrophic scarring may appear as cellular and biochemical changes in the healing tissue occur.[15] The clinical signs or character-

TABLE 14–1. Possible Causes of Hypertrophic Scar Formation

Prolonged healing time
Granulation tissue
Increased blood flow
Chronic inflammatory process
Trapped foreign material
Infection
Genetics
Increased serum protein
Increased proline hydroxylase
Mast cell degranulation
Myofibroblast
Immunologic factors
Altered ground substance
Repeated harvesting of donor sites
Mechanical tissue deformity

istics that depict an immature (active) hypertrophic scar are the "three R's": red, raised, and rigid. These characteristics of immature scar are due to an increase in vascularity,[16,17] an increase in the number of fibroblasts,[7,17] reduced interstitial spaces,[18] and abundant and altered ground substance.[6,7,16,17,19] Although the clinical signs of hypertrophic scarring may not be evident until 6 weeks or more after healing, the eventual appearance of a scar is probably dependent upon the initial wound healing process.[5]

Scar hypertrophy, or "overhealing," caused by increased scar production, frequently occurs when the repair process involves the formation of granulation tissue,[5,7,9] which begins within a few days following injury.[20,21] Granulation tissue consists of a dense population of macrophages, fibroblasts, and neovasculature embedded in a loose matrix of collagen, fibronectin, and hyaluronic acid.[21] Some investigators have reported that the orientation of the collagen fibers in the resulting scar mirrors the orientation of fibers in the granulation tissue.[22-24] In granulation tissue and scar tissue of burn wounds that produce nonhypertrophic scars, collagen fibers are oriented in a parallel fashion to the surface of the skin. In granulation and scar tissue of burn wounds that produce hypertrophic scars, collagen fibers are about half to three fourths the size of those found in normal skin and they are randomly oriented in a nodular or whorl-like pattern[7,17,22,25,26] (see Chapter 4). The keloid has even less organization than a hypertrophic scar[16] (Fig. 14–4).

Although a clear histologic distinction between keloids and hypertrophic scars is difficult, several differences are noted between these two types of scars and normal skin (Table 14–2). Rockwell, Cohen, and Ehrlich[16] in their review of hypertrophic scars, stated that collagen synthesis in keloids is greater than in hypertrophic scars, and both are accelerated when compared to normal skin. At the same time, there is an increase production of collagenase (an enzyme that breaks down collagen), but to a lesser extent. Thus, there is an accumulative imbalance between collagen synthesis and degradation that leads to excessive scarring. There is an abundance of chondroitin-4-sulfate which Linares[7] speculated may be a stimulus for the production of collagen. Furthermore, collagen fibers produced in this environment may be more resistant to digestion by collagenase. The tissue level of prolyl hydroxylase, the enzyme that catalyzes the changing of proline into hydroxyproline in the formation of

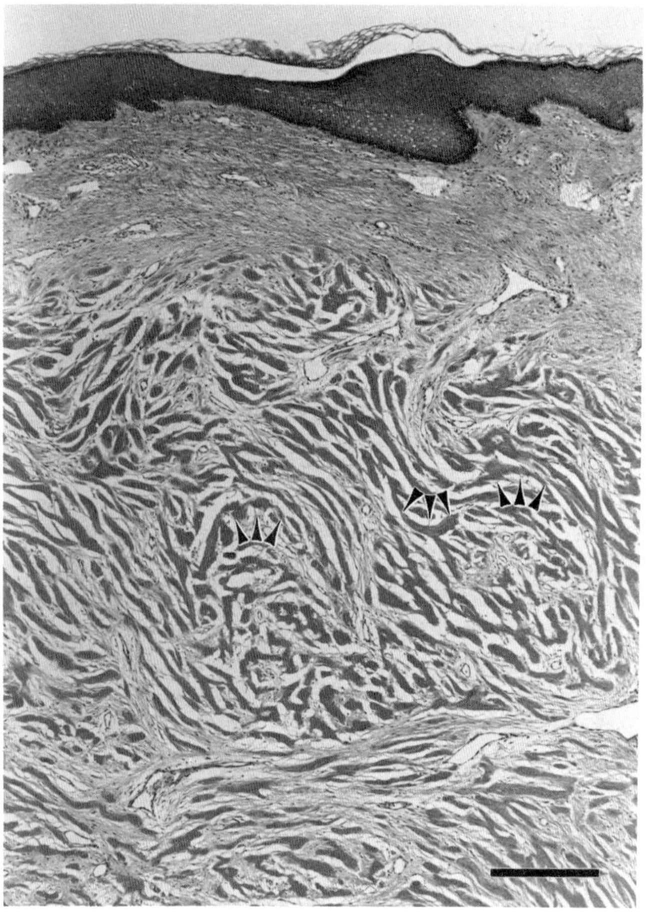

FIGURE 14–4. Collagen fibers in hypertrophic scar randomly oriented in whorl-like pattern.

TABLE 14–2. Characteristics of Hypertrophic Scar versus Normal Skin

Collagen fiber diameter decreased in papillary dermis
Large bundles of collagen fibers in reticular dermis
Collagen aligned in whorls
Increased ratio of type III to type I collagen
Higher proportion of nonsaturated, reducible cross links
Decreased tensile strength
Increased chondroitin sulfate-A
Increased propyl hydroxylase
Increased water content
Decreased transcutaneous pO_2
Increased number of myofibroblasts
Increased number of mast cells

collagen peptide chains, has been shown to correlate with the rate of collagen synthesis. Hayakawa and associates[27] found the amount of prolyl hydroxylase was 25 to 50 times greater in granulation tissue than in normal skin. After skin grafting, the tissue level of prolyl hydroxylase showed a decrease, but remained elevated at 5 to 20 times above normal for 2 years and decreased to slightly below normal levels at 4 years after injury. Therefore, the rate of collagen synthesis can remain high for a very long period of time and most likely starts with high levels of activity in granulation tissue.

Hayakawa reported that the ratio of type III (embryonic) to type I (adult) collagen is increased in granulation tissue as well as in hypertrophic scars when compared to normal skin.[28] This increase lasts approximately 2 to 3 years post burn, but if the area is skin grafted, the ratio decreases within 3 weeks. This result suggests increased wound maturation with the grafted burn wound. As the scar or skin graft matures, less type III collagen is noted and there is an accumulation of large bundles of type I collagen with a stronger resultant scar.[21,28]

High levels of soluble collagen in a wound indicate active collagen synthesis. Gibson and Kenedi[29] reported that soluble collagen reaches a maximum level from 6 weeks to 2 months following injury. The formation of covalent cross-linkages transforms soluble collagen to insoluble collagen. Hayakawa and associates[30] found the concentration of insoluble collagen was much less in hypertrophic scar when compared to normal skin 1 year post burn, but this concentration was greater than in normal skin after 2 years. Thus, collagen synthesis is very active soon after wound closure. Therefore, the best time to attempt to alter collagen is within the first few months up to the first year post burn before strong cross-linking has been established. After 2 years the ability of scar tissue to be modified is significantly reduced.

As the hypertrophic scar matures, there is a decrease in vascularity and the number of fibroblasts. Collagen begins to become oriented in a more parallel fashion and a decrease in the number of whorls occurs. By the time a scar is fully mature, or inactive, there is a diminished number of capillaries and fibroblasts in the scar and collagen fibers lie in predominately parallel bands.[5,7,15,22] Clinically, the mature scar is described by the "three Ps": pale, planar, and pliable. In a burn scar with nonhypertrophic healing, maturation may be complete in 4 to 8 weeks. However, hypertrophic healing may take up to 2 years to mature.[6,17]

FACTORS AFFECTING SCAR FORMATION

Hypertrophic healing cannot be reliably predicted; however, certain variables can be used as guidelines to help therapists identify potentially high-risk individuals. Deitch and associates[31] investigated five variables that contributed to hypertrophic scarring. The results of this study indicated that the length of time to accomplish wound closure was the single most important factor to predict which patients would develop hypertrophic scars. Overall, 78 percent of the burns that required greater than 21 days to heal developed hypertrophic scars. For this reason, surgery was advised for those patients whose wounds would not heal within 3 weeks of injury. Additional factors that may influence scar formation follow.

Race

Generally, darker-pigmented races (Asian and black) are more susceptible to hypertrophic scarring.[6,16,31,32] Leung and Ng[33] reported that the flattening and softening of hypertrophic scars in the Chinese often takes over 4 years to complete. Deitch and associates[31] noted a two times greater incidence of hypertrophic scarring in black populations when compared to Caucasians. According to Rockwell, Koonin, et al[16] this phenomenon is attributed to a possible abnormality in the production of melanocyte-stimulating hormone (MSH). Increased incidence of keloids has been noted during periods of physiologic or pituitary activity (i.e., pregnancy or puberty) at which time MSH levels are increased.[16,32] Keloids also are rare on the palms and soles where few melanocytes exist.

Age

Although Deitch and co-workers[31] noted that age was not a predictor of hypertrophic scarring, clinically, younger people scar more than older people. Ketchum, Cohen, and Masters[6] noted that approximately 88 percent of hypertrophic scars and keloids occurred in people less than 30 years old. The high incidence of scarring in this age group was thought to be due to the fact that younger people are more susceptible to trauma, have greater skin tension, and the rate of collagen synthesis is greater in this group. The elderly may have less scarring due to decreased collagen metabolism, less elasticity, and more skin redundancy.[32]

Location

Certain areas of the body appear more predisposed to the formation of hypertrophic scars. The areas most commonly involved are the sternum, upper back, and shoulder (deltoid).[6,7,31,32] The buttocks and dorsal aspect of the foot also show a greater incidence of scarring.[31] Keloids also can occur anywhere on the body but are predominantly located from the level of the ears to the waist, and from the shoulder to the elbow.[6,9] Hypertrophic scars rarely occur on the eyelids, genitals, palms, or soles, where skin is relaxed or splinted by its attachment to underlying structures.[6,31,34] Donor sites on the middle or low back appear to scar less than donor sites located on the thigh.[35]

Depth

Deeper burns, which involve the reticular dermis, scar more than superficial burns that involve only the epidermis or the papillary dermis. This increased scarring is due to the formation of granulation tissue and prolonged healing time.[9,24,31]

Tension

There is a certain amount of inherent skin tension where the skin drapes over the skeleton.[6,32] Some areas are higher in tension than others and increased scarring frequently is seen in these high-tension areas such as the shoulder and upper back.[6,16,32] Increased tension, with subsequent microtrauma, is a stimulus for inflammation that triggers the fibroblast to secrete more collagen. If tissue loss occurs, there will be increased tension if the wound is primarily closed. The larger the loss, the greater the tension. Tension is increased if the direction of the scar is perpendicular to the lines of maximal tension (see Chapter 4). Excessive motion or stretching also will increase tension in an area. Tissue tension must be minimized to reduce the amount of scarring.

Gender

Gender does not appear to be a predictor of scarring, with male/female ratios being approximately equal.[16,32]

Other Predisposing Factors

Other conditions to note when monitoring a patient for possible hypertrophic scarring are areas where skin grafts did not adhere, infection, persistent presence of necrotic tissue, or excessive motion of the skin graft edges during healing.[6,32] Lawrence[3] stated that "redheads scar less than blondes, and both scar worse than brunettes." However, Robertson and associates[36] did not find hair color to be useful in predicting the formation of raised scars. There appears to be a familial predilection for hypertrophic scar formation due to genetic inheritance of this trait.[3,7,9,37] In general, the manner in which a patient's body scarred with previous injuries may give some indication as to how he or she is apt to scar from a burn.

All of the preceding factors may play a role in determining the outcome of a scar. However, the time from injury to wound closure is probably the most significant variable for prediction of hypertrophic scarring.

SCAR ASSESSMENT

Researchers are using several methods to determine the state of scar maturation, although some techniques lend themselves better to the research environment than to the clinical setting. Esposito and associates[38] have used a modified tonometer to measure skin tone, which correlates to skin pliability and tension. Results from this work produced a firmness index (FI), which is zero in normal skin and increases with the firmness of scar. This study compared a subjective clinical rating to the FI, which may assist the investigators in design of an electronic tonometer to quickly and accurately calculate average scar tension values.

Katz and co-workers[39] appeared to have greater success when they compared scar thickness, determined by high-resolution ultrasonic scanning, with firmness and flexibility of a scar, as measured by a tonometer. Decreased skin thickness correlated with decreased tension within the scar 62 percent of the time. In both studies, the devices were useful in measuring scar change over time, but they were unable to compare one site to another or different individuals to each other. Also, Katz and associates[39] felt the ultrasonic scanning method was better suited for research, while the tonometer was more useful in the clinic.

The elastometer, a hand-held noninvasive device that quantifies the elastic properties of normal skin or hypertrophic scar, has been used by Bartell and colleagues.[40] The device detects differences in elasticity between normal skin and hypertrophic scars and yields reproducible results. As scars matured, their elasticity increased. By measuring the elasticity of scars over time, the effectiveness of a scar management program could be monitored. This study also showed that some scars improved over time even if left untreated.

While the redness or erythema of immature scars previously has been assumed due to increased blood flow, there are conflicting studies on this topic. Hosoda and associates[41] and Leung and colleagues[42] utilized laser doppler flowmetry to determine the perfusion of hypertrophic scars in relation to nonhypertrophic scars. Both studies reported a twofold increase in microcirculatory blood flow in hypertrophic scars. Areas of increased erythema demonstrated an increased blood flow that gradually decreased over time as the scar became pale. From these results the authors felt that laser doppler evaluations could be used as an indicator of hypertrophic healing. On the contrary, Berry and associates[43] used thermographic measurements in a study of hypertrophic scar maturity and found no significant difference in surface temperature between erythematous, or immature, scars and normal skin. They concluded from these results that erythematous scars have basically the same blood flow as normal skin.

Sloan and colleagues[44] measured low levels of oxygen in immature scar and related this to increased metabolic activity in the scar. The high levels of activity would lead to increased oxygen consumption and therefore less oxygen would diffuse through the skin. Berry[43] also looked at levels of transcutaneous oxygen tension ($tcpO_2$) in hypertrophic scars. He postulated that low levels of $tcpO_2$ in immature scars resulted from low oxygen diffusibility through scar tissue and not from increased metabolic consumption of oxygen by the tissue. As maturation of the scar proceeded, thickened capillary walls began to thin, densely cemented masses of collagen fibers became less cohesive, and the $tcpO_2$ rose toward normal levels.

These studies suggest that laser doppler flowmetry and monitoring of $tcpO_2$ levels may be possible means of measuring scar maturation in the future. However, at present, there is controversy regarding their use. Further studies in this area would be valuable.

A rating scale for assessing scar maturation was developed by Sullivan and associates.[45] The scale consists of rating four burn scar characteristics: pigmentation, vascularity, pliability, and height. In general, the higher the total score the more immature or active the scar. As a scar becomes more mature or inactive, the scores return to zero. The rating scale is a rather subjective means of evaluating burn scar, but can be a useful clinical tool, especially for monitoring outpatient progress toward scar maturity.

At the Shriners' Burns Institute in Cincinnati, a modification of the Vancouver form currently is being used to monitor outpatients. The scar characteristics assessed are vascularity, pliability, and height. Pigmentation was not believed to offer useful

Burn Scar Assessment

Name:	
Hair Color:	
Age:	Eye Color:
Race:	
Burn Date:	% Burn:
Graft Date:	Donor Site Date:

Type of Pressure	Date

Date	Scar #	Vascularity	Pliability	Height	Total	OT/PT Init	Compliance

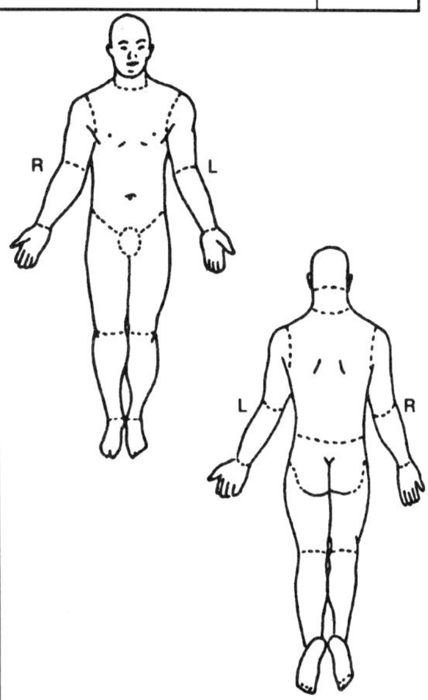

VASCULARITY (V)
0 normal - color that closely resembles the color over the rest of one's body
1 pink
2 red
3 purple

PLIABILITY (P)
0 normal
1 supple - flexible with minimal resistance
2 yielding - giving way to pressure
3 firm - inflexible, not easily moved, resistant to manual pressure
4 banding - rope-like tissue that blanches with extension of scar
5 contracture - permanent shortening of scar producing deformity or distortion

edge / graft

HEIGHT (H)
0 Normal
1 <2 mm
2 <5 mm
3 >5 mm

scale in mm

* Record actual height

COMPLIANCE
Record number of hours garments and splints worn per day

garments / splints

Based on assessment form developed by the Vancouver General Hospital

Shriners Hospitals for crippled children — Burns Institute
Burn Scar Assessment

■ Form

FIGURE 14–5. Burn scar assessment form used at Shriners Burns Institute, Cincinnati, to record a patient's progress through the scar maturation process.

information regarding maturity or immaturity of a scar. Patients are evaluated at the time of discharge and at monthly intervals. One split-thickness skin grafted area and one donor site are assessed on each patient. For visual comparison, photographic slides of each area are taken at each assessment. Compliance with the patient's pressure program is recorded as the number of hours pressure garments are worn each day. This simple method demonstrates to the caregiver and the patient the importance of the pressure program to enhance scar maturation (Fig. 14–5). Regardless of whether a formal assessment tool is used to monitor scar maturation, color slides or photographs taken at intervals provide the clinician, patient, and family member with a visual representation of scar progression.

TREATMENT OF HYPERTROPHIC SCARS

Currently, therapists have limited methods to control hypertrophic scar formation. Physical intervention is based on trying to alter the mechanical or physical properties of scar through the use of compression, silicone products, and massage. Other options, which may alter collagen metabolism or remove the scar altogether, are available to the physician. A brief review of these medical treatment approaches is provided, followed by guidelines for the mechanical or physical alteration of scar.

Drugs

Some chemicals that act similar to proline, such as colchicine, D-penicillamine, and beta-aminoproprionitrile (BAPN), have been shown to retard some phases of collagen synthesis or cross-linking and to decrease secretion of collagen from fibroblasts.[9,16,46,47] These effects would decrease the amount of scar tissue formed.

Steroids

The use of some steroids causes the dermis to become thinner and steroids have been used for many years to prevent keloid formation or encourage keloid regression.[6,9,16,32,48] The most commonly used and effective steroid is the corticosteroid triamcinolone. Intralesion injections of triamcinolone frequently are used following surgical excision of a keloid or in conjunction with pressure techniques.[9,16] Although steroids decrease the inflammatory phase of wound healing and are thought to decrease collagen production, triamcinolone appears to enhance collagenase production rather than inhibit collagen synthesis, thus increasing collagen degradation.[6,16,32] Side effects associated with steroid use, such as atrophy, depigmentation, and occasionally Cushing's syndrome, are related to high doses and usually are reversible. Local steroid treatment for small scars has minimal side effects.[9,16]

Surgery

Hypertrophic scars generally can be corrected through surgical excision with either primary closure or skin grafting, while excised keloids frequently reoccur.[9] Surgery is considered when other conservative measures (e.g., pressure, steroids) have failed. However, surgical outcome frequently fails unless pressure or steroids are used following the procedure.[6,16]

Radiation

Depending upon dosage, irradiation of a wound immediately following keloid excision either destroys local fibroblasts or causes suppression of fibroblast cell proliferation. Thus, irradiation may help to restore the balance between collagen production and degradation.[16,32] Some researchers believe that radiation may have a place in the treatment of keloids. However, since the effects and complications associated with the use of irradiation are permanent and cumulative, some believe irradiation should be used only as a last resort and only in the elderly.[6,9,32]

Lasers

The possible beneficial use of lasers for treating keloids has appeared in the literature infrequently and no large controlled studies with follow-up data have been reported.[49,50] Apfelberg and associates[49] in their study of 13 patients with keloids, observed no long-term beneficial effects from the use of argon and CO_2 lasers. Additional controlled studies are necessary to determine the efficacy of laser treatment of keloids.

Ultrasound

The literature is sparse regarding the use of ultrasound in the treatment of hypertrophic scars or keloids. One study[51] noted good results with two patients in flattening keloids using continuous ultrasound at 0.8 W/cm^2 for 4 minutes. Neither the number nor the frequency of treatments was noted.

Other Treatments

Multiple topical agents, such as retinoic acid, zinc oxide, and asiatic acid, have been investigated for their effect on hypertrophic scar, with some beneficial results reported.[16] However, subsequent comparative studies have not been performed. Also, many herbs, vitamins, and enzymes have been tried through the years to soften and flatten scars but with disappointing results.[6,16,52]

Compression Therapy

Historically, in 1835, Rayer successfully used pressure in the treatment of keloids, while Unna, in 1881, applied pressure to burns scars.[53] In 1968, Fujimori, Hiramoto, and Ofuji[54] used a technique of sponge fixation to control scarring after skin grafting procedures. In 1971, Silverstein observed that vascular support garments decreased scarring associated with a burn and Larson noted the same effect with pressure-exerting splints on scar tissue.[55] Subsequently, the practice of utilizing compression therapy for burn scar control became a widely accepted intervention.

TABLE 14–3. Hypothetical Effects of Compression Therapy on Burn Scar

Accelerates the scar maturation process
Superficial blanching
Flattening of the scar
Increased pliability
Decreased blood flow
Decreased edema
Decreased rate of collagen synthesis
Collagen bundles realign parallel to epidermal surface
Absent or less prominent nodules
Decreased cohesiveness of intercollagen fibers
Increased collagenase-mediated collagen breakdown
Gradual decrease in myofibroblasts
Stabilization and gradual decrease in mast cells
Decreased deposition and change in ground substance
Thinning of dermis

Despite the fact that no study confirms the mechanism by which pressure alters the structure of scar, pressure has been noted to have a thinning effect on the dermis.[16] Mechanical compression of a scar causes a visible blanching that indicates decreased blood flow through the scar.[5,32,56–59] This decreased flow leads to tissue hypoxia with a resultant reduction in cell proliferation.[60,61] Decreased blood flow reduces the number of collagenase inhibitors and the rate of collagen lysis is enhanced. The overall effect of applying pressure is an improved balance between collagen synthesis and lysis of a scar.

In addition, compression of scar tissue produces the following: reduction in tissue edema with less ground substance production,[5,33,58,59,62] scar nodules disappear, collagen bundles are reoriented parallel to the epidermal surface,[5,32,57] and large bundles of collagen fibers convert to smaller groups of fibers arranged in a less compact fashion.[56] Compression therapy appears to accelerate the scar maturation process by inducing changes in the physical properties of scar tissue in a period of months rather than years (Table 14–3 and Fig. 14–6).

The geometry of the body surface influences the amount of compression applied by pressure garments and is governed by Laplace's law. Laplace's law is defined as

$$\text{Pressure} = \text{Tension/Radius of curvature}$$

Concave surfaces, such as the presternal or interscapular area, possess negative radii and no pressure is exerted in these areas unless an insert is included to change the radius of curvature[63] (Fig. 14–7). Convex body surfaces and those with smaller radii, such as the chin, receive greater pressure than an area with a larger radius, such as the top of the head.

GUIDELINES FOR PRESSURE APPLICATION

The formation of hypertrophic scars begins shortly after injury, so the earlier pressure is applied, the better the results. Engrav and associates[64] found that splints and pressure devices did not damage new skin grafts when applied directly over a graft in the operating room. Although this practice is not widespread, pressure appli-

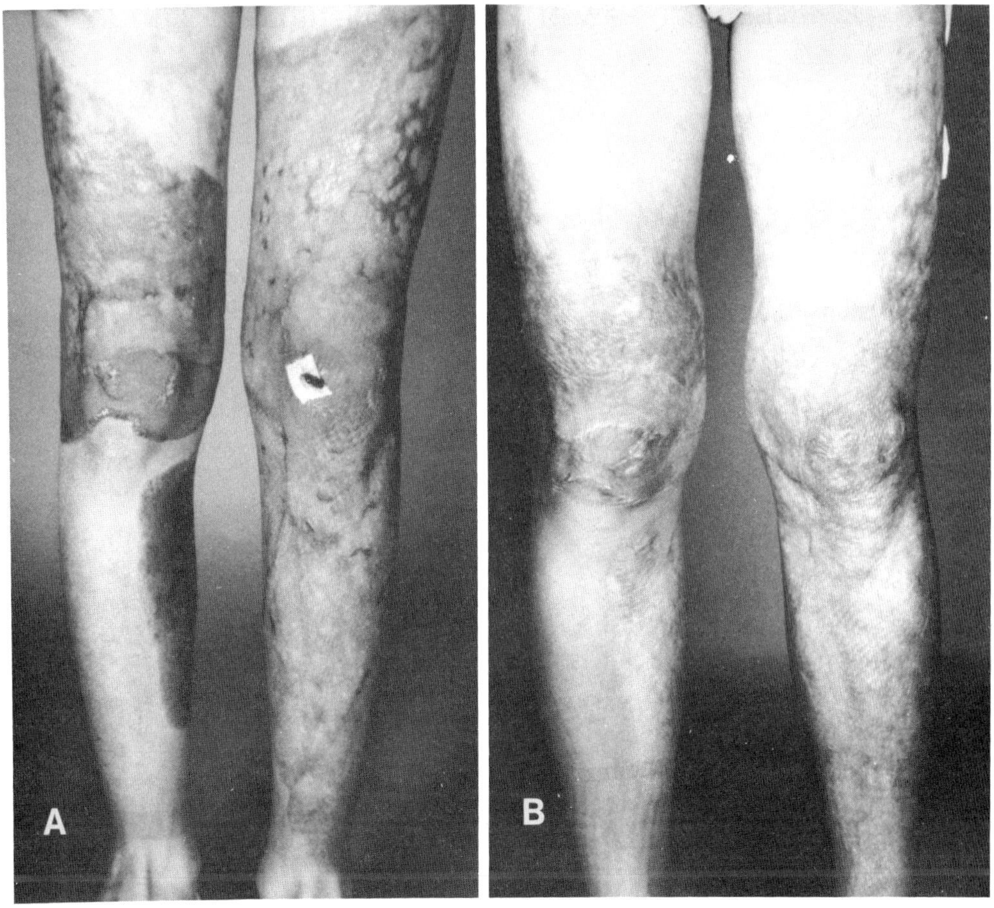

FIGURE 14–6. (*A*) Active scar formation on patient's lower extremities 4 months following burn injury. (*B*) Mature scar on same patient 14 months later.

cation should begin within 2 weeks of wound closure or skin grafting.[33,36,61,65] Leung and Ng[66] used pressure garments as a means of minimizing hypertrophic scarring and noted that application of pressure garments within 1 to 2 months post burn produced better results than treatment that was delayed longer than 6 months. Early application of pressure prevents vascular pooling, serves to toughen the skin to resist shearing forces, and may minimize itching.[54,67]

The amount of compression necessary to induce scar maturation is controversial. Many researchers have stated that approximately 25 mm Hg capillary pressure is necessary to produce changes in scar tissue, but this value has not been proven absolute.[5,63] Scars treated with pressure greater than 15 mm Hg have been noted to be flatter, smoother, and less erythematous than scars treated with lower pressures.[56,68] However, accelerated remodeling may occur with pressures less than 10 mm Hg. At pressures greater than 40 mm Hg maceration and paresthesia may occur.[56] Cheng and colleagues[63] used a special air-flow measuring manometer to measure garment-scar interface pressure on 50 patients. They found a wide variation of pressures over different parts of the body. These differences were due in part to the compliance of the tissue underlying the scar and in part to the geometry of the area. The average

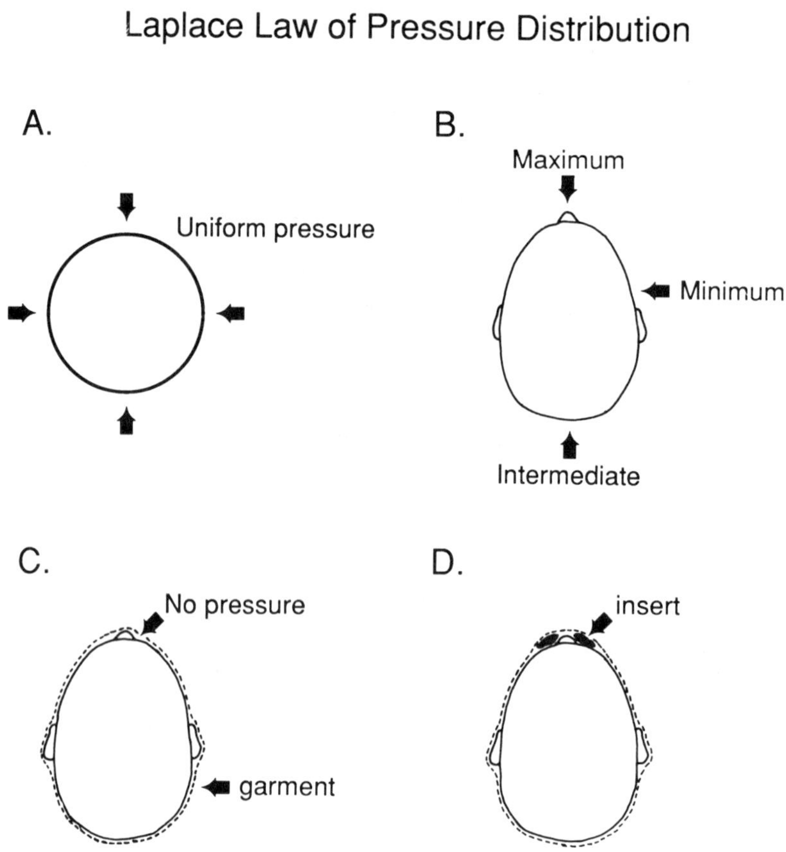

FIGURE 14–7. Illustrations of Laplace law of pressure distribution. (*A*) Pressure is exerted uniformally to a circle. (*B*) Maximum pressure is exerted over convex surfaces with smaller radii, such as the forehead or tip of nose. Minimum pressure is exerted over convex surfaces with larger radii, such as along the side of the head. (*C*) When a pressure garment is applied to the body, no pressure is achieved over concave surfaces such as the nasolabial folds. (*D*) An insert placed under the garment delivers pressure to a concave surface.

garment-scar interface pressure was 5 to 15 mm Hg and only a few had pressures over 20 mm Hg. There was an additional 50 percent decrease in interface pressure after the garments had been worn for 4 weeks. Interestingly, good clinical results of scar tissue remodeling were reported with these patients. Clinically, positive results may be achieved with lower pressures over time. However, higher pressures, in a safe range of 25 to 35 mm Hg, may induce more rapid maturation of hypertrophic scars.

Deitch and associates[31] have outlined four clinical guidelines for compression therapy intervention. Their suggested guidelines for use of compression therapy are outlined in Table 14–4.

Compression therapy must be constant, such that pressure is maintained 22 to 23 hours a day.[6,32,58] Pressure dressings are removed only for personal hygiene, moisturizing the skin, and stretching exercises with massage. However, this relief period should not exceed 30 to 60 minutes at any one time.[6,16,32] Compression therapy is required until the signs of complete scar maturation (pale, planar, pliable) have occurred; otherwise, the scar may reoccur.

TABLE 14–4. Suggested Guidelines for the Use of Compression Therapy

No prophylactic compression therapy is required in any patient whose wounds heal in less than 10 days.
If the burn wound heals in 10 to 14 days, prophylactic compression therapy is advised for noncaucasian patients of all ages.
For patients of any age or race whose burn wound heals in 14 to 21 days, the use of prophylactic compression therapy is strongly suggested.
If the burn wound heals in greater than 21 days, prophylactic compression therapy is mandatory for all patients.

MATERIALS FOR COMPRESSION AND PRESSURE

There are multiple materials available for compression and pressure therapy. The literature advocates many different techniques the therapist can use to apply pressure to a burn scar.[59,67,69–77] Depending on a patient's age, skin or scar status, location of the burn, and cost, different materials may be used. Pressure dressing materials are utilized in a progression beginning with those creating the least amount of shearing force and ending with the use of custom-made garments. A review of these various materials follows.

Elastic Bandage

Elastic bandages often are used early in pressure therapy since they can be applied over burn dressings without creating a shearing force. They serve to control edema, enhance venous and lymphatic drainage,[78,79] and provide early vascular support for new skin grafts or recently healed wounds. They are inexpensive and can be washed and reused if needed. Elastic bandages provide adequate pressure if properly applied. However, with improper application, as in wrapping either too tightly or unevenly, edema, compromised circulation, neuropathy, or pressure sores can occur. Elastic bandages need to be reapplied every 4 to 6 hours due to slippage and loosening of the wraps with movement. Frequent inspection helps ensure that adequate, but not damaging, pressure is being applied. All burn team members involved with pressure therapy should demonstrate skillful bandaging techniques before using an elastic bandage on a patient. In addition, the patient and/or family member should be instructed in proper application of an elastic bandage. Proper application of an elastic bandage includes the following points: (1) the bandage is wrapped in a distal to proximal fashion with more pressure applied distally, (2) one half of the bandage width is overlapped with each successive turn, (3) the application of tension to the bandage is provided on the upstroke turn, and (4) circular wraps on the extremities should be avoided. To determine whether a bandage is applied at an appropriate pressure, two finger widths should be able to slide under each turn of the wrap. If more than two fingers fit under the bandage, then the wrap is too loose. The figure-of-8 wrapping technique has been shown to provide more support than the spiral wrap technique, and should be used when applying compression to the lower extremities[80] (Fig. 14–8). An easy way for a caregiver to remember the sequence of application of a figure-of-8 pattern is to repeat the following after anchoring the elastic wrap: angle up, straight around the back, angle down, straight around the back, and so on. Either a spiral or figure-of-8 pattern can be used with the upper extremi-

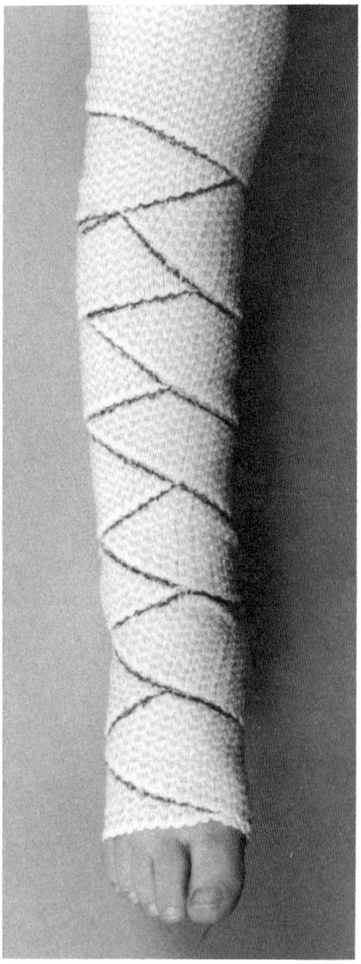

FIGURE 14–8. Figure-of-eight elastic bandage applied to the lower extremity. The crisscross pattern anteriorly is indicative of a properly applied wrap.

ties. However, if the spiral wrap is used, a figure-of-8 pattern should be performed over the elbow to allow greater freedom of movement. Circular or spiral wraps are applied to the trunk. A figure-of-8 or spica wrap can be used for pressure in and around the shoulders and hips (Fig. 14–9). For adults who actively can flex their metacarpalphalangeal joints against resistance, the fingers can be wrapped with an elastic bandage in a "figure-of-8 finger wrap" as outlined by Rivers.[81] Although pressure under an elastic bandage is determined by the tension applied and the area wrapped, Parks[15] stated that each layer of wrap provides approximately 10 to 15 mm Hg pressure on the extremities and 2 to 5 mm Hg pressure on the thorax. Therefore, double wrapping the leg may be needed to prevent venous pooling in patients with deep lower extremity burns and provide greater patient comfort. Providing too much pressure on the trunk may be difficult.

Self-Adherent Elastic Wrap (Cohesive Bandage)

Self-adherent elastic wrap, also called a *cohesive bandage,* can be utilized on hands and feet early in wound healing to prevent or control edema, provide vascular support, and minimize scar tissue formation. This wrap has several trade names and is

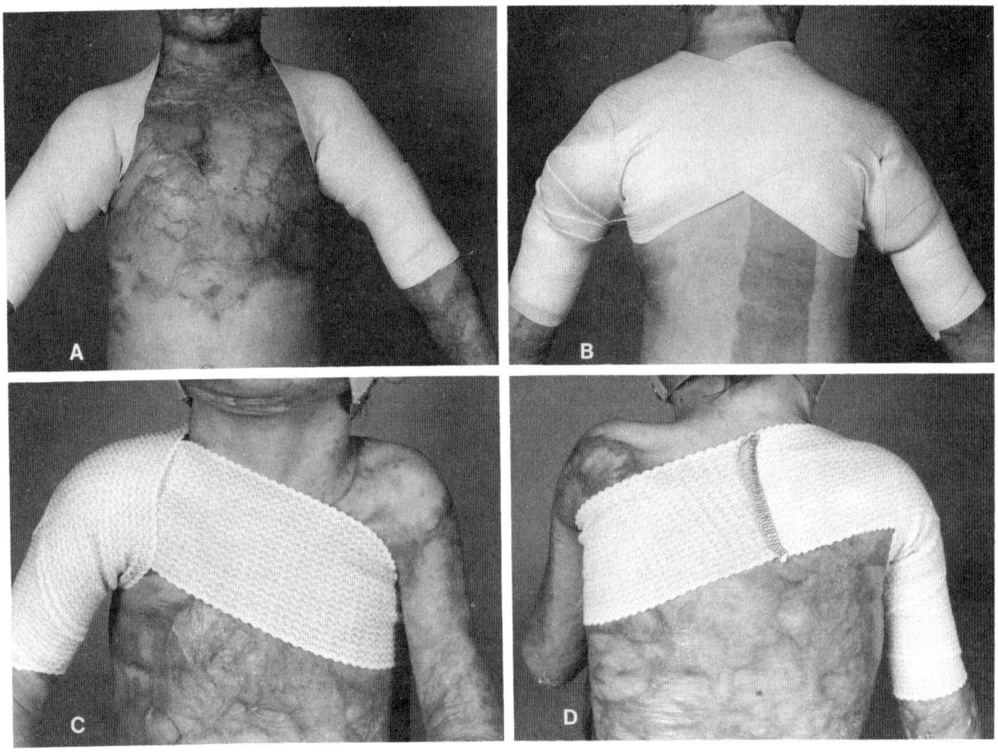

FIGURE 14–9. (*A*) anterior view and (*B*) posterior view of double figure-of-eight wrap to the shoulders. The wrap is spiraled counterclockwise up one arm, under the axilla, and over the anterior shoulder. It then crosses the back and goes under the opposite axilla, returning over the anterior shoulder, and crosses the back again to go under the original axilla. The same process is repeated for the opposite shoulder. This pattern encourages shoulder retraction. Foam can be placed in the axillas, under the elastic bandages, to increase pressure on the anterior and posterior axillary folds. (*C*) anterior view and (*D*) posterior view of a spica wrap to the shoulder. The wrap is started the same as the figure-of-eight, however after coming from under the opposite axilla, the wrap crosses the chest, goes over the top of the original shoulder, and is wrapped under that axilla and up the anterior surface of the shoulder. This wrap applies pressure to the area as well as holds dressings in place.

available in multiple widths and a variety of colors (Appendix J). The cohesive bandage can be applied over dressings and on fragile tissue that cannot tolerate a shearing force. A cohesive bandage interferes somewhat with movement, so minimizing the dressings underneath is helpful. Applying a piece of nonadherent gauze to an open area is sometimes sufficient. With deeper open areas, nonadherent gauze can be covered with a piece of surgical netting prior to application of the wrap. After applying an elastic wrap to a hand, cream can be applied to the wrap between the fingers to prevent the fingers from adhering to each other during activities. As with an elastic bandage, a cohesive bandage is applied in a distal to proximal fashion. While a figure-of-8 technique can be used,[82] the wrap is normally applied in a spiral pattern (Fig. 14–10). A cohesive bandage is an excellent means to apply compression to pediatric or infant hands and feet and may be used as the definitive pressure treatment of choice for children under 2 years of age.

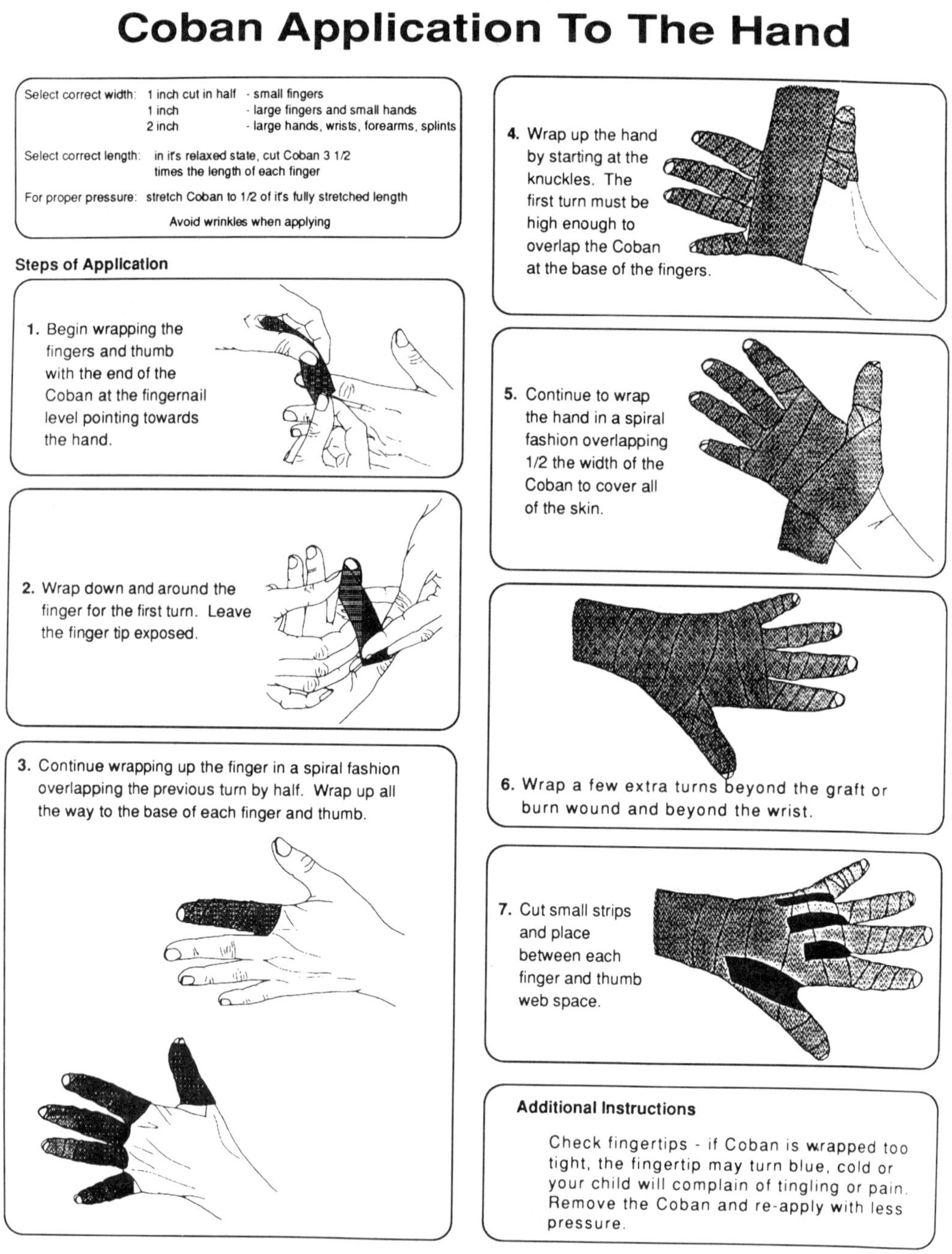

FIGURE 14–10. Guidelines for application of a self-adherent elastic wrap. (Courtesy of Shriners Burns Institute, Cincinnati Unit.)

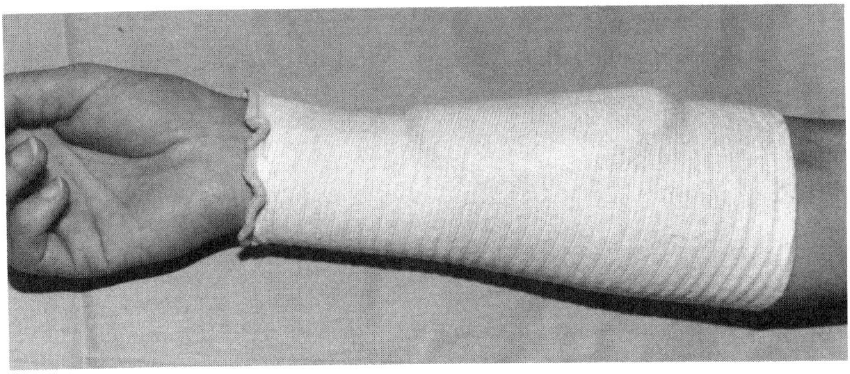

FIGURE 14–11. Tubular support bandage with foam insert applied to the upper extremity for use as definitive pressure on a small isolated burn.

Elastic Tubular Support Bandage

When a healed burn surface is able to tolerate a minimal shearing force, a tubular support bandage (TSB) can be used. The TSB may be an interim compression device used after elastic bandages and before custom-made pressure garments, or may be used as the definitive compression appliance for a patient. These bandages are cotton-based and come in a variety of tubular sizes and prefabricated garments. According to the size chosen, low tension (5 to 10 mm Hg), moderate tension (10 to 20 mm Hg), or high tension (20 to 30 mm Hg) can be achieved.[83] Common trade names of TSB are listed in Appendix J. Several studies have demonstrated the effectiveness of TSB in suppressing hypertrophic scar formation, satisfactory patient compliance, and cost reduction.[83-85] The TSB is easy to apply and works well for the rapidly growing child, less than 3 years of age, as size changes can be made easily. Areas that can be effectively treated with the TSB are the upper and lower extremities and the trunk. A doubled-layered TSB, with or without an insert, works well especially for a smaller isolated burn on an extremity (Fig. 14–11). Because the TSB is the same diameter throughout, and an extremity is tapered, more pressure is delivered to areas of larger circumference. Doubling the TSB distally or using a prefabricated shaped support bandage will help equalize the pressure by providing a graduated distal to proximal compression to the limb.

Ready-Made Elastic Pressure Garments

Several companies now manufacture "off-the-shelf" elastic garments in various sizes for many areas of the body (Appendix K). Because a variety of these garments can be stocked in the burn center, a patient can be fitted with an acceptable compression garment after a few quick measurements. Face masks, chin straps, gloves, finger and arm sleeves, knee-high hose, briefs, and vests are available in ready-made garments. Depending on the desired fit and size of burn, these garments can be used as the definitive pressure garment or utilized on an interim basis until the custom-made garment arrives. Wear and care is similar to a custom-made garment and will be discussed in the next section.

Custom-Made Elastic Pressure Garments

In the early 1970s, the first commercially made pressure garments became available through the Jobst Institute. Currently, there are at least five companies manufac-

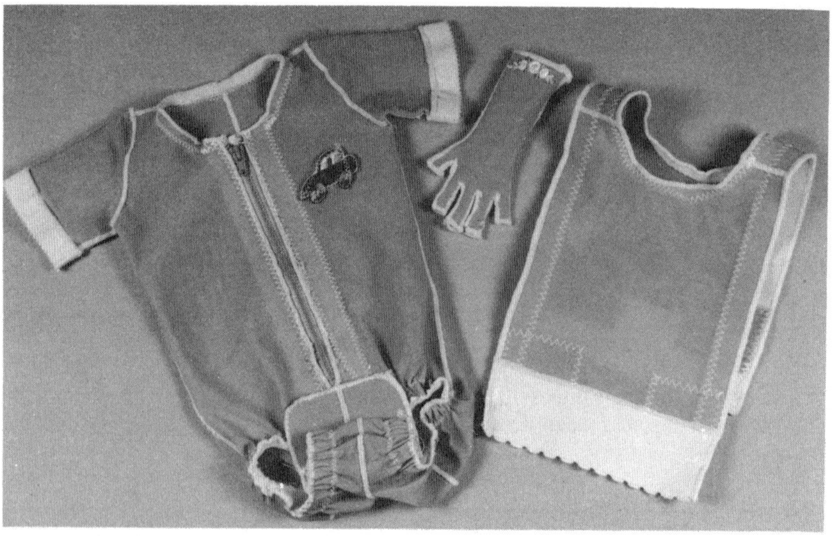

FIGURE 14–12. Examples of pressure garments manufactured at Shriners Burns Institute, Cincinnati. (*Left*) Child's romper with car applique. (*Middle*) Glove with open finger tips. (*Right*) Bib worn to assist with holding waist height garment or panty girdle up when vest is not required.

turing elastic pressure garments for every part of the body, offering multiple options and colors (Fig. 14–12 and Table 14–5) (Appendix K). Ward and colleagues[86] surveyed burn centers in the United States to determine what was important to therapists in selecting a pressure support supplier. They found that accessibility for orders, reliability of fit, ease of measurement, and availability of obtaining nonstandard supports were the most important factors. From this survey it was shown that multiple suppliers for pressure garments in the United States, who can accommodate a wide variety of patient needs, are available.

Measurement for pressure garments is recommended when: (1) a patient's burn wound is almost healed, (2) there are only a few open areas no larger than a quarter, (3) a donor site is expected to heal in 7 to 10 days, and (4) no significant edema is present. A patient with a large-body-surface-area burn usually will have areas that will be skin grafted or healed sooner than other areas. If possible, these healed areas should be measured and fit with garments rather than delay measuring a patient until all of the burn wound is healed. All grafted areas, donor sites, and partial-thickness burn areas requiring greater than 10 to 14 days to heal should be measured for pressure garments. Most companies provide forms with detailed instructions for measuring each body part. Measurements should be taken directly over the skin, not over bandages. However, if a patient wears a diaper, measurements should be taken over the diaper. After recording a patient's measurements, they can be mailed, telephoned, or faxed to a company. If a face, hand, or foot is particularly difficult to measure, such as with a contracture or amputation, a positive plaster mold of the area may be sent to the pressure garment company to ensure a correct fit.[87] Generally, the time from order to receipt of pressure garments is between 1 to 2 weeks, depending on which company is used, whether the order is telephoned, faxed, or mailed and which type of return delivery service is requested. After the first set of garments arrives and is assessed to fit properly, a second set is ordered so the patient has one garment to wear while the other is washed and dried.

TABLE 14–5. Comparison of Pressure Garment Companies

	Barton-Carey	Bio-Concepts	Gottfried Medical, Inc.	Jobst	Medical Z
Types of material	Regular sheer (nylon/Spandex); soft; heavy	Regular (nylon/Spandex); close knit; soft; lining; insert	Regular (Powernet-nylon/Spandex); insert	Regular (Powernet-nylon/Spandex); lining	Regular (Family of Lycra)
Ready-made garments	Unavailable at this time	Multiple styles available from toddler to adult	Soon to be available	Multiple styles available from toddler to adult	Unavailable at this time
Color	35 choices; 6 fluorescent; monogramming; appliques	30 choices; appliques	Beige	Beige; dark brown	Flesh; brown; black
Pressure	25 to 35 mm Hg	25 mm Hg	18–22 mm Hg	15–32 mm Hg	17–24 mm Hg
Turnaround time	Standard—shipped 2 days from when order received; urgent service—24 hours	Standard—2 weeks total turnaround time; UPS next day or 2-day service	Standard—3 to 5 days; hotline—shipped in 48 hr	Standard—shipped 5 days from when order received	Standard—8 working days
Care	Wash—machine, delicate; Dry-machine, low heat; no bleach; mild detergent	Wash—by hand or machine, warm water; Dry—machine, no heat	Wash—machine, delicate; Dry—machine, no heat; no bleach	Wash—machine, warm water, no additives; Dry—lay flat, no heat	Wash—by hand, warm water; Dry—lay flat, no dryer
Cream compatibility	Any cream	Any cream	Any cream	Any cream	Neutral ph creams
Educational materials	Wear and care instructions upon request	Videotape; instruction manual; seminars available	Videotape; measuring instructions	Literature for professionals and patients; videotape; inservices provided	Videotape

A patient essentially should be healed prior to application of a custom-made pressure garment. Open areas should be small and the skin somewhat dry, requiring and tolerating light lubrication. Gauze bandages should never be wrapped around an extremity under a pressure garment. The abrasiveness of a gauze, as well as wrinkles, can cause blisters, and the increased circumference of a part can lead to a constricting increase in pressure to the area. If a garment is fit before the scar or skin has healed sufficiently, blisters or maceration will occur. If fitting is delayed more than 2 months, optimal scar control may not be achieved.[63,88]

When applying a lower extremity pressure garment, the garment is turned inside out to the point where the seam or area that defines the heel is reached. The foot is inserted into the garment and the rest of the material is pulled over the foot and heel. Then, the remainder of the garment is inched up the leg slowly. When applying an upper extremity pressure garment, all the material must pass the hand before the garment is advanced up the rest of the forearm and arm. These procedures decrease shearing forces to the skin and increase the life of the garment. Multiple garments should be donned in a distal to proximal fashion and removed in a proximal to distal fashion. Gloves, for example, should be applied before sleeves and sleeves should be taken off before gloves. This sequencing will prevent congestion or edema in the distal part of the extremity.

Pantyhose worn under a garment is useful to ease application of waist-height garments and to hold small nonadherent gauze patches in place where needed (Fig. 14–13). Nylon kneehighs, with the foot portion cut out, also can be used on the upper extremities to ease application of sleeves or vests. The therapist should inform the patient that the nylon should remain on the arm under the garment. A plastic bag placed over the hand or foot also assists with application of a garment (Fig. 14–14). After all of the garment passes the hand or foot, the plastic bag is removed.

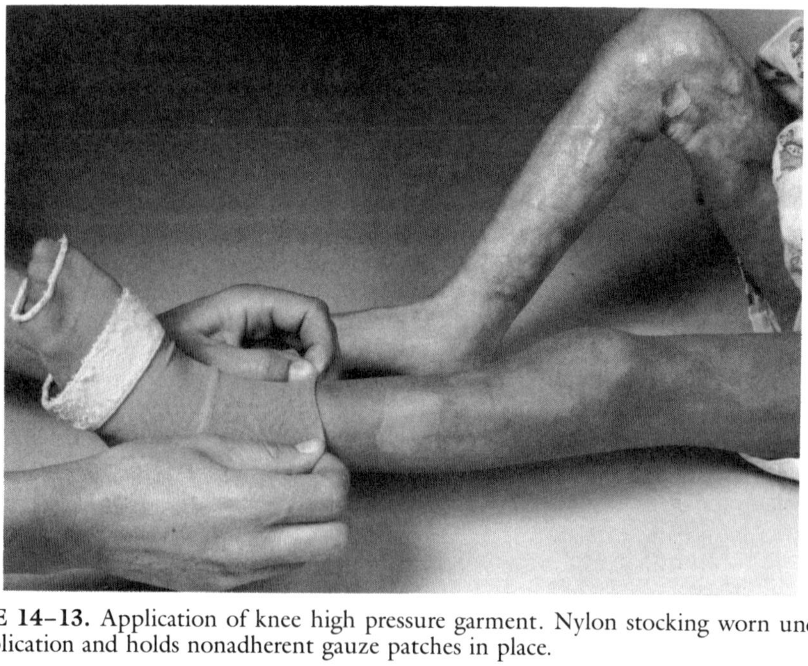

FIGURE 14–13. Application of knee high pressure garment. Nylon stocking worn underneath eases application and holds nonadherent gauze patches in place.

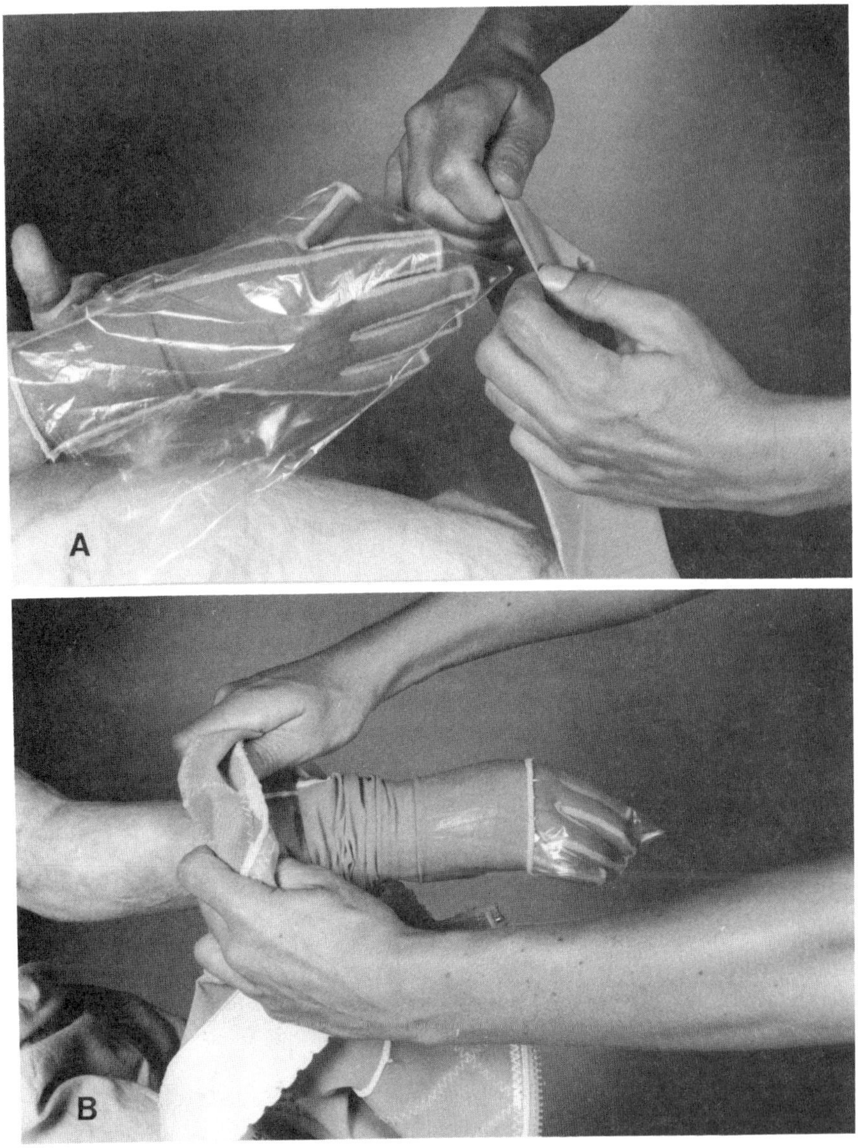

FIGURE 14–14. (*A*) Plastic bag placed over the hand to assist with application of pressure garment. (*B*) After all of the garment passes the hand the plastic bag is removed.

For certain areas of burn scar, alternatives to pressure garments may be more acceptable to some patients. These may include the use of Isotoner gloves, girdles, sport bras, long-line bras or girls' leotards bought in a smaller size.[58]

Pressure Garment Options. Many different pressure garment options exist and these are ordered as necessary for each individual patient. Table 14–6 shows examples of options and when these options might be used. Some companies will apply lace or colorful appliques for children's garments if requested.

Wear and Care of Pressure Garments. Pressure garments should be worn for 22 to 23 hours a day, and only removed for bathing, applying moisturizing cream, and when massaging scars during stretching exercises. They should not remain off longer

TABLE 14–6. Commonly Used Pressure Garment Options

	Application
Material	
Soft material	Decreases shear. Useful over bony prominences that repeatedly break down. Infants. Obese patients.
Insert	Conforms to irregular shape. Decreases wrinkling of material. Relieves pressure on sensitive areas.
Liners	Decrease shear. Useful over elbows or knees.
Gussets	Insert in axilla.
Expansion panels	Assist with donning garments. Decrease shear. Decrease wrinkling in popliteal space. Removes seam from heel and elbow.
Closure	
Velcro	Holds vest down and pants up when used together. With palm burn, dorsal Velcro closure if glove used. Can apply to proximal end of glove and attach to sleeve to make removal difficult for child.
Zipper	Avoid use on extremities if possible. If used in sleeves or waist heights, should be applied laterally. Avoid use in face masks so that hair does not catch.
Front	For adults, if possible, so that additional person not required to apply and remove garment.
Back	For chest burns. For child who will unzip front closure.
Style	
Gloves	
Open fingertips	Allows for tactile stimulation and improved prehension.
Closed fingertips	Prevents distal edema.
Slant inserts	Provides increased pressure to dorsal web space.
Lower Extremity Garment	
Open/closed toes	Patient preference.
Open crotch	Easier to void. Tends to irritate medial thigh. Does not provide pressure to buttocks or pubis.
Closed crotch	Provides pressure to buttocks, pubis, and superior thigh. Does not irritate thighs.
Upper Body Garment	
Turtleneck	For burns on superior chest extending onto neck.
Scoop neck	Increased comfort if area not burned.
Shoulder flap	Assists in holding sleeve in place.
Romper/body brief	Holds upper torso garment in place if pants are not required.

TABLE 14–7. Tips for Proper Care of Pressure Garments

Wearing
1. Rub moisturizing cream completely into skin to minimize build-up in garment.
2. Do not over stretch garments when applying or removing.
3. Always wear socks over the garment when garment covers feet.
4. Alternate use of garments. Have at least two properly fitted garments.

Washing
5. Wash garments daily to avoid build-up of body oil and moisturizing cream.
6. Soak garments one hour before washing.
7. Attach Velcro loop and hook sections together prior to washing.
8. Machine wash, gentle cycle.
9. Place in lingerie bag or pillow case if washing by machine.
10. Do not use chlorine bleach.

Drying
11. Do not use heat.
12. If dryer is used, dry on air fluff only.
13. Lay garment flat to dry; do not hang.

than 30 minutes to 1 hour at any one time. Garments should fit snugly (unable to easily pinch fabric away from body part), but not so tight that circulation is compromised or marks from seams remain indented on the skin for longer than 30 minutes after the garment is removed. Custom-made pressure garments are approximately 60 percent porous; therefore, a sunscreen should be used in conjunction with them if a patient will be out in the sun for any period of time. The pressure garments available today are a combination nylon and spandex material that is compatible with all moisturizing creams. However, vitamin E oil may be absorbed into the garment and degrade the spandex. Regardless of type, the cream must be completely washed out of the garment. Changing garments every 12 hours and carefully cleaning the garments to ensure that body oil and creams have been removed will prolong the life of the garment. Manufacturers include instructions for care with the garments. In general, most garments can be laundered in a washing machine on gentle cycle with cold or warm water and a mild detergent. No chlorine bleach should be used. Garments should be air-dried or dried in the clothes dryer with no heat. Heat will make the fibers brittle (Table 14–7). Although Cheng and associates recommend that patients have a new set of garments every month; realistically, a burn patient's garments should last about 2 to 3 months before requiring replacement. For active patients and those who return to work, gloves may require more frequent replacement. In addition, children may need measurements taken for new garments sooner, particularly during a rapid growth phase. Garments need to be replaced when they lose their resilience, fail to hold their shape and begin to sag, are oily to the touch, have irreparable holes, or become too tight from growth or weight gain.

Complications with Pressure Garments. Despite the clinical effectiveness noted with custom-made pressure garments, there are several hindrances to their use: (1) they must be worn continuously for many months, (2) they do not apply equal pressure to all body areas, (3) they must be altered frequently, (4) they are difficult to don, (5) they can be uncomfortable and hot, (6) they may cause irritation or scar breakdown, (7) they may retard bone growth or alter bony architecture, and (8) they may retard growth of soft tissue.[89] Some specific complications caused by pressure garments follow.

Scar Maceration. A frequent occurrence with pressure garment wear is scar maceration. Clinically, the scar becomes discolored or shiny, blisters occur, and finally an open wound appears. Maceration may be caused by friction between the garment and scar with application or movement, tightness of the garment over joints, perspiration, poor hygiene, or skin sensitivity.[90] These open areas generally occur on healed partial-thickness burns and donor sites where rete pegs are missing.[91]

Friction. Recently healed skin and scar tissue often cannot tolerate the shearing force caused by application of pressure garments or even friction between the garment and skin that occurs with movement. If an open area occurs that is small or superficial, a nonadherent gauze patch is placed over the area and the patient may continue to wear the pressure garment. If the wound becomes larger or deeper, wearing of pressure garments should be discontinued for 1 to 2 weeks to allow healing to occur. The application of pressure should continue with self-adherent elastic wrap and/or elastic bandages, depending on the body part involved. If recurrent open areas become a problem, some garment companies can add inserts of soft material to specific areas. When the wound becomes healed or small and superficial in size, wearing of the garment can be resumed. Use of nylon hose is recommended in this instance to assist with donning the garment over fragile skin and scar.

Tight Fit over Joints. Fit of a garment should be monitored routinely to prevent excessive pressure over joints, which can lead to skin irritation and breakdown with activity. Patients and caregivers are instructed to monitor the garment for material that is stretched too widely and for long-standing marks on the skin from seams, so that improper fit can be avoided.

Hygiene. Proper hygiene must be stressed to patients and caregivers when pressure garments are worn. The garments retain body heat, and when splints or inserts are used, more heat is retained. Excess perspiration alone or in combination with a buildup of cream causes scar maceration. Scar maceration with continued poor hygiene leads to infection and increased healing time. The patient must bathe daily and all garments must be laundered daily. Moisturizing cream should be massaged into the skin and scar without leaving a visible residue on the surface. Adults and some adolescents may need to use an unscented deodorant or antiperspirant to control body odor and wetness if excessive perspiration becomes a problem. Skin beneath splints and inserts should be monitored for breakdown. If necessary, wearing time of these additional appliances is decreased to prevent tissue breakdown. Cornstarch can be applied to an area to help absorb moisture. The skin and insert or splint should be cleansed and thoroughly dried before each reapplication.

Skin Sensitivity. Some patients occasionally develop a rash, or dermatitis, while wearing pressure garments. These conditions may be due to various causes and a physician should examine the patient for an accurate diagnosis. Some dermatitis may be due to a specific soap or cream the patient is using, and simply changing product brands may alleviate the condition. Laundry detergent used to wash garments also may be a source of irritation and changing the detergent as well as ensuring the garments are properly rinsed after washing will help. A patient may develop a superficial *Staphylococcus* infection, scabies, or impetigo, which will require appropriate treatment. Occasionally, a topical steroid is used and the wearing of garments can continue. However, if dressings are needed, elastic bandages are substituted for garments until skin condition improves.

Skeletal and Soft Tissue Growth. Leung and associates[89] reported on regressed skeletal growth of the chin and thoracic cage of four children due to pressure treatment and narrowing of the transverse arch of an adult's hand due to a pressure garment and insert. They discussed padding procedures to distribute pressure more evenly and recommended masks for children be worn for no more than 12 hours per day. For this reason, children under 1 year of age typically are not put in hard face masks. Usually, a soft face mask is used, with or without an insert. In addition to regressed skeletal growth, soft tissue bulk also may be retarded in children wearing pressure garments. Clinically this phenomenon is most noticeable on children with unilateral extremity burns under pressure. Monitoring a child to ensure that garments or masks are not applying excessive pressure, frequently remeasuring for replacement garments, recasting for face masks during growth spurts, and discontinuing garments and face masks as soon as a scar matures will help minimize skeletal and soft tissue complications.

Silicone

Silicone is a term relating to a family of polymers based on the element silicon.[92] The polymers range in viscosity from fluid through gel and solid states. Silicone gel pads, which are inert, clear, and flexible, have been used in Australia, Europe, and the United States since the early 1980s and have become increasingly popular over the past several years.[93-99]

Reported benefits of silicone gel pads include increased range of motion, minimizing pain, preventing shrinkage of skin grafts, minimizing hypertrophic scarring, assisting with softening and smoothing of scars, and increasing pressure over movable areas where pressure is difficult to maintain.[93,95] Although the mechanism of action of the silicone gel is not yet known, pressure, temperature, oxygen transmission, water vapor transmission, and silicone absorption do not appear to be factors.[94,96] A recent study reported that 2 months of wear of a silicone gel pad is adequate for both prevention and treatment of hypertrophic scars.[99] Silicone gel pads may cause skin irritation if left in place for prolonged periods of time, so skin should be monitored closely and wearing time gradually increased to 12 to 24 hours a day. If skin irritation occurs, removal of the pads generally resolves the problem. Silicone pads appear useful for small isolated scars. However, the expense and short lifespan of gel pads over joints or under pressure dressings limit the practicality for use of these pads with larger burn scars.

Inserts

Due to the geometry of the body's surface, inserts are sometimes necessary to achieve adequate pressure in certain areas, especially over concave surfaces. Inserts can be made of assorted materials, including various types of foam, felt, silicone elastomer, and putties[100] (Appendix L). Inserts should be applied with Velcro or attached loosely with a few stitches of thread, rather than sewn into the garment. Sewing an insert in place decreases the overall elasticity of a garment and will affect pressure distribution. Felt and foam are inexpensive and can be used over joints, on flat surfaces, and in finger and toe web spaces. Other materials, such as strips of gauze, elastic straps, splinting material, or pliable rubber tubing also can be used to increase pressure in finger web spaces.[101,102] Silicone elastomer inserts are easy to fabricate and they apply even pressure over an entire scar[103,104] (see Chapter 11). Tracheostomy ties can be embedded into an insert to hold it in place on the hands or feet (Fig. 14–15). Felt, with or without Velcro sewn to it, can be applied to the back of an elastomer mold to decrease movement of the insert under a pressure garment and increase its durability. Elastomer inserts are beneficial for thick, rigid scars that are not located over joints.

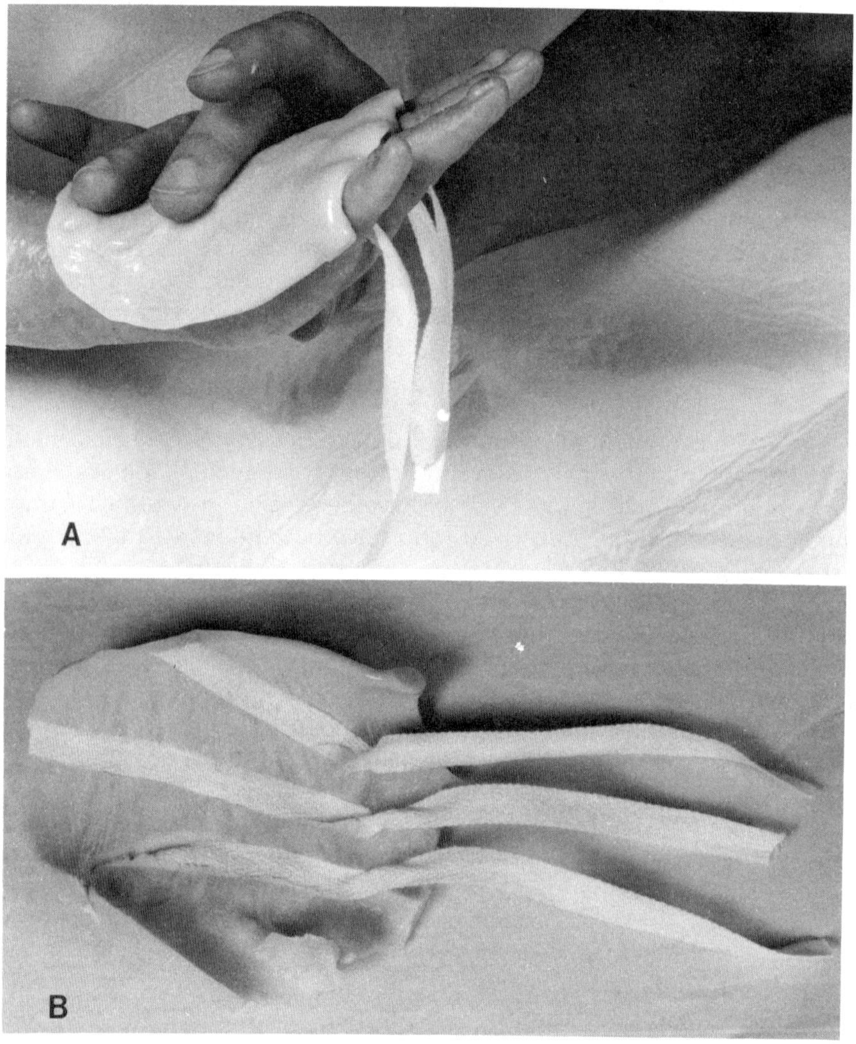

FIGURE 14–15. (*A*) Elastomer insert on dorsum of hand with tracheostomy ties aligned through finger web spaces. These ties are used to hold the insert in place and to increase pressure in the web spaces. (*B*) Underside of elastomer insert with tracheostomy ties embedded in place.

Silicone elastomer putty is a silicone product which, after the putty base and catalyst are combined, provides a smooth, somewhat flexible insert. The putty is even easier and less time consuming to use than regular silicone elastomer. The putty works well for use as finger and toe web spacers, over the dorsum of the foot and toes, in the palm of the hand or for any smaller, rigid scar that requires increased pressure for resolution. Perkins, Davey, and Wallis[105] advocated the use of various "contact media," such as Silastic foam or skin care pads, which can be used with or without pressure or have adhesive properties. These media may reduce maturation time of a scar, reduce shearing forces under garments, and improve the cosmetic appearance of a scar (Appendix L). A contact dermatitis may occur as a result of an allergic reaction to an insert material or due to an insert trapping perspiration against the skin. If a rash occurs, decreasing wearing time, more frequent cleansing, and drying or dusting of the insert with cornstarch may be necessary.

Rigid Transparent Face Mask

The face is one of the most frequently burned areas of the body, most commonly due to a flash burn.[106] Pressure should be maintained on the face until scar maturation occurs to prevent hypertrophic scar formation and deforming contractures, such as eyelid ectropion or lower lip eversion. Usually, this pressure is applied through the use of a custom-made elastic face mask.[107] However, due to the contours of the face, an elastic mask does not provide adequate pressure on the nasolabial folds and adjacent cheek areas or under the lower lip. Inserts of foam, silicone elastomer, or splinting material can be used under the mask to deliver the pressure required for scar remodeling.[64,100,108,109] The elastic mask usually is not well accepted by patients due to its objectionable appearance. In 1979, Rivers and associates[110] reported on improved patient compliance and facial scar management using a rigid, transparent face mask of cellulose acetate butyrate. The mask can exert 33 mm Hg pressure on the underlying tissue and conforms accurately to the contours of the face. A negative mold is made from the patient's face using dental alginate or silicone elastomer and plaster strips. Plaster is then poured into the mold and a positive impression of the patient's face is achieved (Fig. 14–16). A high-temperature plastic is heated and stretched over the positive mold. Straps are riveted to the face mask and secured on the patient's head through the use of Velcro or other strapping techniques (Fig. 14–17). For a patient who does not require a full face mask, a partial rigid mask for either the upper or lower face can be fabricated. In addition, an open elastic face mask or chin strap can be used with a rigid plastic insert over a scarred area. The insert can be secured to the garment with Velcro or snaps if necessary (Fig. 14–18). The face mask is worn at all times except during bathing, meals, and facial massage or stretching exercises. The mask should be cleaned with soap and water and dried prior to reapplication. After an optimal fit is achieved, the patient should be seen monthly so areas of the mask that are not delivering enough pressure can be heated and revised to increase pressure. When scars begin to slow in their maturation, follow-up visits of every 2 to 3 months usually are sufficient.

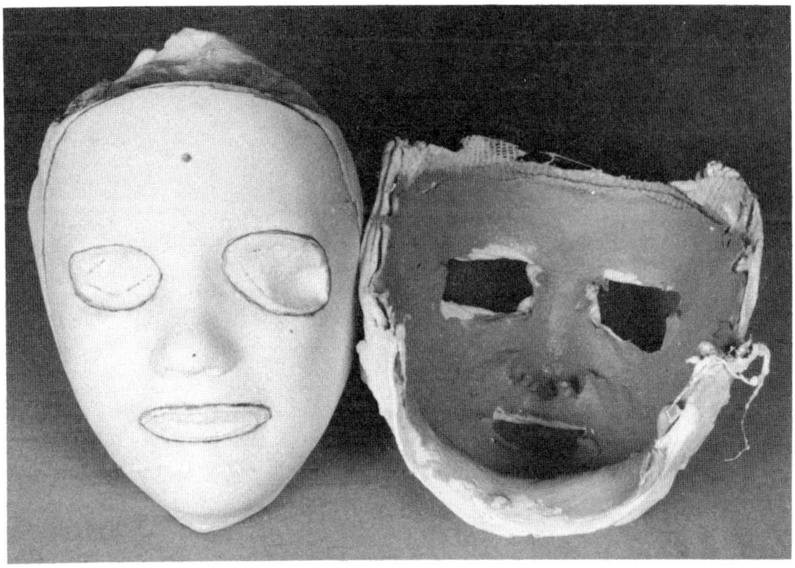

FIGURE 14–16. (*Right*) Negative mold of patient's face made using silicone elastomer and reinforced with plaster strips. (*Left*) Positive plaster mold of patient's face.

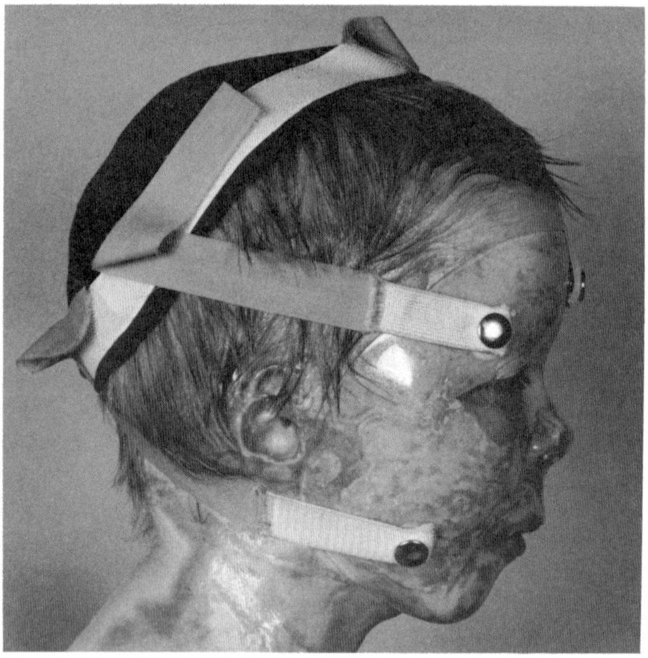

FIGURE 14-17. Hard plastic face mask held in place through the use of straps and a beanie.

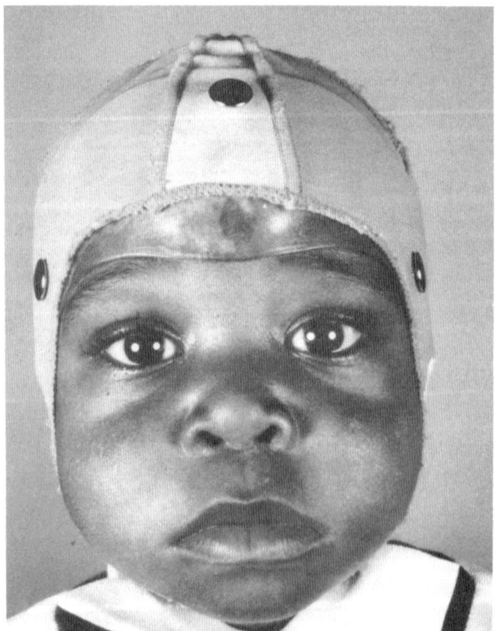

FIGURE 14-18. Spandex open face mask with snaps, used in conjunction with hard plastic insert, provides increased pressure to forehead scar.

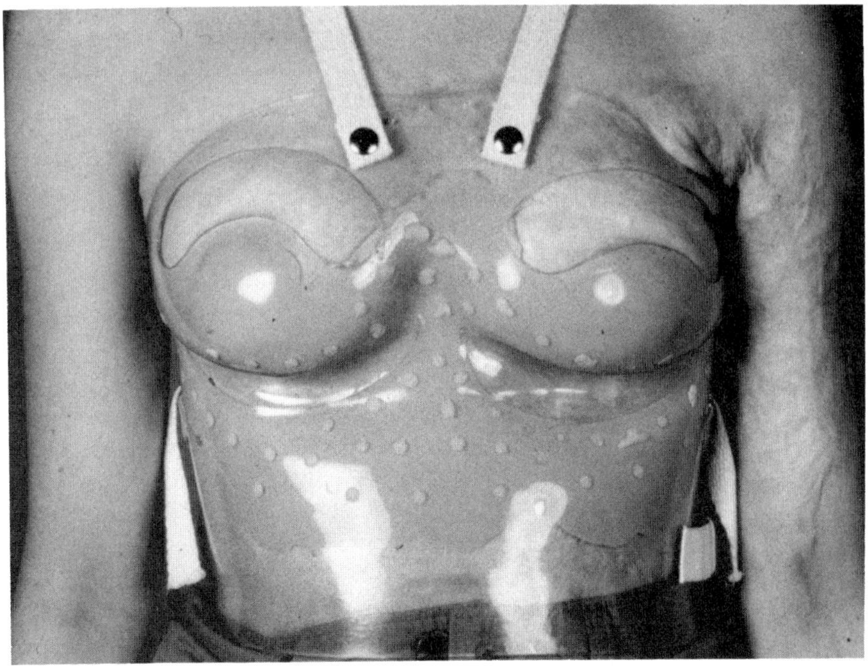

FIGURE 14–19. Hard plastic chest plate with elastomer insert underneath is utilized to apply pressure following breast reconstructive surgery.

Chest Conformers

Because scar tissue following a burn injury does not grow with a child, many girls during puberty require reconstructive surgery to augment their breast development. Following such reconstructive procedures, pressure is required to prevent contracture of the inframammary or intermammary regions. A semirigid transparent chest plate of Surlyn, fabricated similar to a rigid face mask, is useful for larger breast releases[111] (Fig. 14–19). The patient is casted after the sutures or staples are removed from the skin graft and fit with the appliance 1 to 2 weeks later. Until the chest plate can be fit, gauze dressings and figure-of-8 elastic wraps are used to lift and separate the breasts. For smaller releases of the breast, a long-line bra with either a foam or silicone/felt insert provides adequate pressure to the graft. Chest conformers can be fabricated from other materials, such as low-temperature thermoplastics or polyethylene foam.[73,112]

Paramedical Camouflage

Following maturation of burn scars, color and texture changes of the skin still will be evident. This visible scarring can be disturbing, especially to women, if the face and hands are involved. To minimize discoloration and disfigurement of the skin and scars, and to help improve a patient's self-esteem, makeup that camouflages defects was developed. Paramedical camouflage is a process by which the appearance of scars or skin pigment alterations are normalized through the application of proper shades and placement of cosmetics. The patient is instructed in correct application techniques so acceptable results can be achieved at home by the patient (Fig. 14–20). The creams used are opaque rather than translucent, so color correction is possible. They adhere to the skin and are waterproof so the individual can swim or perspire without the cosmetics smearing or being removed. Camouflage cosmetics usually contain a sunscreen and are safe for use on sensitive skin (Appendix M). Also available are procedures that can permanently pigment specific areas so that makeup is not required.

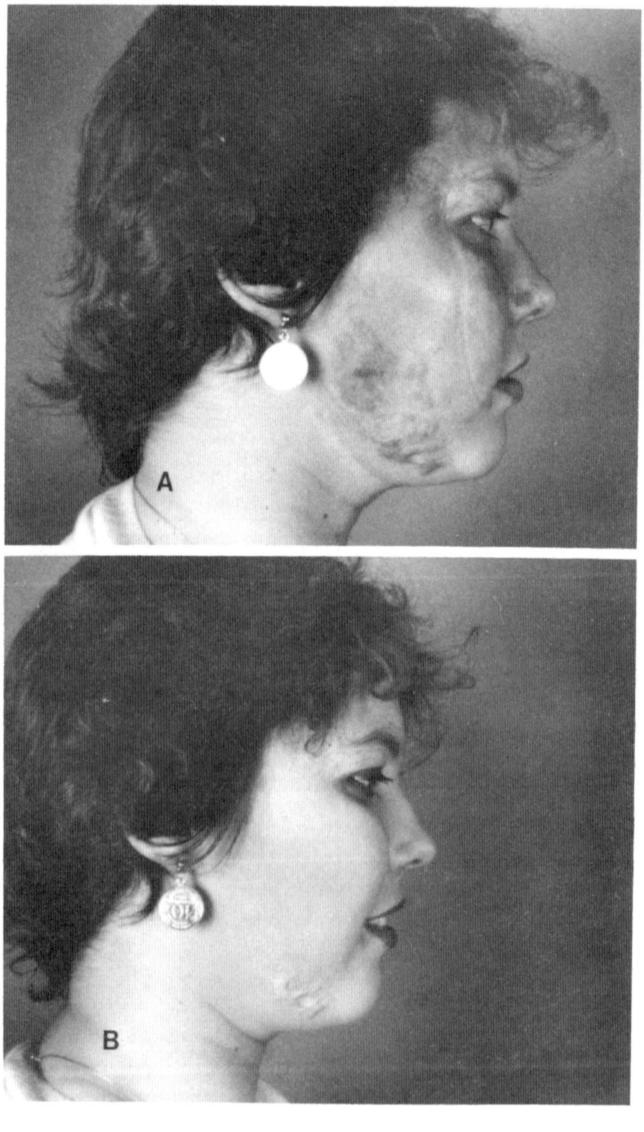

FIGURE 14–20. (*A*) Burn patient with vascular facial scars before application of camouflage makeup. (*B*) Appearance of same patient following application of makeup.

Massage

Massage has been reported to assist with softening scar tissue, possibly through freeing restrictive fibrous bands and increasing circulation,[113-115] although no studies identifying the exact mechanisms by which massage works are available. Massaging lubrication into an area aids in stretching the scar tissue and desensitizes the tissue through tactile stimulation.[116] Patients and caregivers should be instructed to massage rigid, thick scarred areas by pressing hard enough to make the scar blanch, three to six times daily, for 5 to 10 minutes at each session. Rigid sections of scar, usually seen at the edges or seams of skin grafts or on healed partial-thickness burn areas, soften and fade with massage. However, no permanent decrease in thickness of a scar generally is noted with massage.

HOME INSTRUCTION

A responsibility of the burn therapist is education of the patient, family, and/or caregiver. Education of these individuals about the necessity and importance of the scar management program should be stressed. Additionally, instruction in skills necessary for effective performance of this program is essential for an optimal patient outcome. A variety of teaching methods should be used, keeping in mind the emotional and cognitive level of the learner. Methods may include: (1) written programs with written guidelines and pictures; (2) therapist demonstration of technique on the caregiver as well as on the patient and requiring return demonstration on the therapist and patient by the caregiver; (3) use of charts or lists to check off skills when mastered; (4) use of photographs to show application of splints or correct positioning; or (5) videotapes of exercise sessions, donning of all garments, and application of splints.

The following items should be included in a home instruction program:

1. Reviewing changes in the burn wound and scar maturation, including the three Rs and three Ps described earlier. Also, the patient and caregiver should be reminded that the scar usually will get worse before it gets better.
2. Verbal and written instructions in all aspects of scar management. Consistency and persistence should be stressed. The more compliant a patient is with the program, the sooner the results will be achieved.
3. Key points of the pressure program:
   a. Pressure needs to be applied continuously for 22 to 23 hours a day; garments should not be off for more than 30 minutes to 1 hour at a time.
   b. Garments must fit snugly; if they are loose or worn out, the therapist should be contacted.
   c. Garments should not fit too tightly; signs and symptoms should be explained.
   d. Guidelines for proper care of garments should be provided.
   e. The potential for blister formation should be discussed.
   f. Proper patient hygiene should be reviewed.
   g. The patient and/or caregiver should demonstrate correct application and removal of all pressure garments and orthoses.
4. Demonstration of proper scar massage technique.

CASE STUDY

HISTORY

JR was a $2\frac{1}{2}$-year-old oriental male when he sustained a 0.5 percent deep partial-thickness burn to his chest, directly over the sternum, from hot chocolate. The burn wound was allowed to heal secondarily and JR came to the outpatient clinic 8 months later with a raised, red, and rigid hypertrophic scar.

PROBLEM LIST

Raised, red, and rigid scar
Location of scar
Patient unable to participate in scar management program

GOALS

Pale, pliable and only minimally raised scar
Mother independent in massage and application of pressure

INTERVENTION

JR's mother was instructed in the application of a reverse figure-of-8 wrap with elastic bandages to the chest. This wrap crisscrossed anteriorly over the sternum. A silicone elastomer pad with felt backing was applied directly to the scar and held in place by the elastic wrap. His mother also was instructed in scar massage, which was performed a minimum of three times daily.

After 17 months of this program, JR's scar was paler and more pliable but still raised. His mother reported that itching was an occasional problem. A silicone putty insert was fabricated to alternate with the silicone/felt insert and JR's mother was instructed to use cornstarch as necessary on the inserts to help absorb moisture. Massage to the scar was continued.

After 2 years and 6 months of pressure therapy, JR's pressure program was changed to night use only. After 2 years and 9 months of pressure, JR's pressure program was discontinued. The scar over his sternum was light pink and minimally firm in the center. The rest of the scar was pale, pliable and planar. JR's mother was instructed to continue massage three times a day to the center portion of the scar.

RATIONALE

Contributing factors that may have led to the development of JR's hypertrophic scar and long maturation time were his age, race, location of the burn, and prolonged healing time. The sternum is a difficult area to apply pressure due to its concave surface. An elastic wrap with an insert was chosen for treatment, as this combination minimized the amount of extra material the patient had to wear and the insert sufficiently filled the concavity of the chest so that adequate pressure was applied. Alternating the silicone/felt insert with the silicone putty insert helped to decrease the itching that sometimes is associated with use of silicone products.

SUMMARY

Hypertrophic scarring is one of the long-term sequelae of burn injury that occurs following trauma to the reticular dermis and is especially severe in children and dark-skinned individuals. Time from initial injury to wound closure appears to be the greatest predictor of hypertrophic scar formation. Compression is thought to elongate and flatten scars through remodeling of collagen, as well as by creating a state of tissue hypoxia. The overall effect is an accelerated scar maturation process. However, scar maturation may require up to 2 years.

A therapist has several options available for scar management, including compression bandages, custom-made pressure garments, rigid appliances, inserts, and silicone products. Educating the patient and caregiver in all aspects of a pressure program will foster greater compliance and thereby maximize patient outcome.

REFERENCES

1. Stedman's Medical Dictionary. 23 ed, Williams & Wilkins, Baltimore, 1976.
2. Funk & Wagnalls Encyclopedic College Dictionary. Funk & Wagnalls, New York, 1968.
3. Lawrence, JC: The aetiology of scars. Burns 13:S3–S14, 1987.
4. Heimbach, DM: American Burn Association 1988 Presidential Address "We can see so far because. . . ." J Burn Care Rehabil 9:340–346, 1988.
5. Jensen, LL and Parshley, PF: Postburn scar contractures: Histology and effects of pressure treatment. J Burn Care Rehabil 5:119–123, 1984.
6. Ketchum, LD, Cohen, IK, and Masters, FW: Hypertrophic scars and keloids: A collective review. Plast Reconstr Surg 53:140–152, 1974.
7. Linares, HA: Hypertrophic healing: Controversies and etiopathogenic review. In Carvajal, HF and Parks, DH (eds): Burns in Children: Pediatric Burn Management. Yearbook Medical Publishers, Chicago, 1988, pp 305–323.
8. Shakespeare, PG and Renterghem, L: Some observations on the surface structure of collagen in hypertrophic scars. Burns 11:175–180, 1985.
9. Cohen, IK and McCoy, BJ: The biology and control of surface overhealing. World J Surg 4:289–295, 1980.
10. Chvapil, M and Koopmann, CF: Scar formation: Physiology and pathological states. Otolaryngol Clin North Am 17:265–272, 1984.
11. Linares, HA: Proteoglycan-lymphocyte association in the development of hypertrophic scars. Burns 16:21–24, 1990.
12. Kischer, CW and Bailey, JF: The mast cell in hypertrophic scars. Texas Rep Biol Med 30:327–337, 1972.
13. Linares, HA and Larson, DL: Elastic tissue and hypertrophic scars. Burns 3:4–7, 1977.
14. Grooves, AR: The problem with scars. Burns 13:S15–S21, 1987.
15. Parks, DH, Larson, DL, and Houssaye, AJ: Hypertrophic scarring: Pressure dressings. In Feller, I and Grabb, WC (eds): Reconstruction and Rehabilitation of the Burned Patient. NBIE, 1979, pp 20–27.
16. Rockwell, WB, Cohen, IK, and Ehrlich, HP: Keloids and hypertrophic scars: A comprehensive review. Plast Reconstr Surg 84:827–837, 1989.
17. Abston, S: Scar reaction after thermal injury and prevention of scars and contractures. In Boswick, JA (ed): The Art and Science of Burn Care. Aspen Publishers, Rockville, 1987, pp 359–371.
18. Baur, PS, et al: Wound contractions, scar contractures and myofibroblasts: A classical case study. J Trauma 18:8–21, 1978.
19. Nicoletis, C, Bazin, S, and Le Lous, M: Clinical and biochemical features of normal, defective, and pathologic scars. Clin Plast Surg 4:347–359, 1977.

20. Peacock, EE: Wound Repair, ed 3. WB Saunders, Philadelphia, 1984, pp 38–55.
21. Clark, RA: Cutaneous tissue repair: Basic biologic considerations. J Am Acad Dermatol 13:701–725, 1985.
22. Linares, HA and Larson, DL: Early differential diagnosis between hypertrophic and nonhypertrophic healing. J Invest Dermatol 62:514–516, 1974.
23. Linares, HA, et al: On the origin of the hypertrophic scar. J Trauma 13:70–75, 1973.
24. Teich-Alasia, S and Angela, GC: The role of granulation tissue in the formation of hypertrophic scarring in burn lesions. Ann Plast Surg 9:132–138, 1982.
25. Kischer, CW and Shetlar, MR: Collagen and mucopolysaccharides in the hypertrophic scar. Connect Tissue Res 2:205–213, 1974.
26. Kischer, CW: Collagen and dermal patterns in the hypertrophic scar. Anat Rec 179:137–146, 1974.
27. Hayakawa, T, et al: Prolyl hydroxylase activity in human normal skins and post-burn scars. Clin Chim Acta 75:137–142, 1977.
28. Hayakawa, T, et al: The effect of skin grafts on the ratio of collagen types in human post-burn wound tissues. Connect Tissue Res 9:249–252, 1982.
29. Gibson, T and Kenedi, RM: Factors affecting the mechanical characteristics of human skin. In Dunphy, JE and VanWinkle, W (eds): Repair and Regeneration. McGraw-Hill, New York, 1969, pp 87–98.
30. Hayakawa, T, et al: Changes in type of collagen during the development of human post-burn hypertrophic scars. Clin Chim Acta 93:119–125, 1979.
31. Deitch, EA, et al: Hypertrophic burn scars: Analysis of variables. J Trauma 23:895–898, 1983.
32. Ketchum, LD: Hypertrophic scars and keloids. Clin Plast Surg 4:301–310, 1977.
33. Leung, PC and Ng, M: Pressure treatment for hypertrophic scars resulting from burns. Burns 6:244–250, 1980.
34. Larson, DL, et al: Techniques for decreasing scar formation and contractures in the burned patient. J Trauma 11:807–823, 1971.
35. Greenhalgh, DG, Barthel, PP, and Warden, GD: Comparison of back vs. thigh donor sites in pediatric burn patients. Proc American Burn Association 23:33, 1991.
36. Robertson, JC, et al: Pressure therapy for hypertrophic scarring: Preliminary communication. J Roy Soc Med 73:348–354, 1980.
37. Lewis, WHP and Sun, KKY: Hypertrophic scar: A genetic hypothesis. Burns 16:176–178, 1990.
38. Esposito, G, et al: The use of a modified tonometer in burn scar therapy. J Burn Care Rehabil 11:86–90, 1990.
39. Katz, SM, et al: Objective measurement of hypertrophic burn scar: A preliminary study of tonometry and ultrasonography. Ann Plast Surg 14:121–127, 1985.
40. Bartell, TH, Monafo, WW, and Mustoe, TA: A new instrument for serial measurements of elasticity in hypertrophic scar. J Burn Care Rehabil 9:657–660, 1988.
41. Hosoda, G, Holloway, GA, and Heimbach, DM: Laser doppler flowmetry for the early detection of hypertrophic burn scars. J Burn Care Rehabil 7:496–497, 1986.
42. Leung, KS, et al: Microcirculation in hypertrophic scars after burn injury. J Burn Care Rehabil 10:436–444, 1989.
43. Berry, RB, et al: Transcutaneous oxygen tension as an index of maturity in hypertrophic scars treated by compression. Br J Plast Surg 38:163–173, 1985.
44. Sloan, DF, et al: Tissue gases in human hypertrophic burn scars. Plast Reconstr Surg 61:431, 1978.
45. Sullivan, T, et al: Rating the Burn Scar. J Burn Care Rehabil 11:256–260, 1990.
46. Prunieras, M: The biology of healing. In Tubiana, R (ed): The Hand, vol 1. WB Saunders, Philadelphia, 1981, pp 541–551.
47. Peacock, EE: Control of wound healing and scar formation in surgical patients. Arch Surg 116:1325–1329, 1981.
48. Ohura, T, Ariga, A and Sugihara, T: The effect of steroid ointment in preventing keloid formation. Bull Clin Rev Burn Inj 1:19–20, 1984.
49. Apfelberg, DB, et al: Preliminary results of argon and carbon dioxide laser treatment of keloid scars. Laser Surg Med 4:283–290, 1984.
50. Bailin, P: Use of the CO_2 laser for non-PWS cutaneous lesions. In Arndt, KA, Noe, JM, and Rosen, S (eds): Cutaneous Laser Therapy: Principles and Methods. John Wiley & Sons, New York, 1983, pp 187–200.
51. Walker, JJ: Ultrasound therapy for keloids. S Afr Med J 64:270, 1983.
52. Jenkins, M, et al: Failure of topical steroids and vitamin E to reduce postoperative scar formation following reconstructive surgery. J Burn Care Rehabil 7:309–312, 1986.
53. Huang, TT, Blackwell, SJ, and Lewis, SR: Ten years of experience in managing patients with burn contractures of axilla, elbow, wrist, and knee joints. Plast Reconstr Surg 61:70–76, 1978.
54. Fujimori, R, Hiramoto, M, and Ofuji, S: Sponge fixation method for treatment of early scars. Plast Reconstr Surg 42:322, 1968.
55. Jobst Product Catalog, 1990.
56. Reid, WH, et al: Hypertrophic scarring and pressure therapy. Burns 13:S29–S32, 1987.

57. Kischer, CW, Shetlar, MR, and Shetlar, CL: Alteration of hypertrophic scars induced by mechanical pressure. Arch Dermatol 111:60–64, 1975.
58. Johnson, CL: Physical therapists as scar modifiers. Phys Ther 64:1381–1387, 1984.
59. Lamberty, BGH and Whitaker, J: Prevention and correction of hypertrophic scarring in post-burn deformity. Physiotherapy 67:2–4, 1981.
60. Baur, PS, et al: Ultrastructural analysis of pressure-treated human hypertrophic scars. J Trauma 16:958–967, 1976.
61. Kischer, CW and Shetlar, MR: Microvasculature in hypertrophic scars and the effects of pressure. J Trauma 19:757–764, 1979.
62. Law, EJ: Minimizing burn scar and contracture. In Hummel, RP (ed): Clinical Burn Therapy: A Management and Prevention Guide. John Wright, PSG, Littleton, 1982, pp 306–320.
63. Cheng, JCY, et al: Pressure therapy in the treatment of post-burn hypertrophic scar—A critical look into its usefulness and fallacies by pressure monitoring. Burns 10:154–163, 1984.
64. Engrav, LH, et al: Do splinting and pressure devices damage new grafts? J Burn Care Rehabil 4:107–108, 1983.
65. Larson, DL, et al: Contracture and scar formation in the burned patient. Clin Plast Surg 1:653, 1974.
66. Leung, PC and Ng, M: Pressure treatment for hypertrophic scars. Burns 6:224, 1980.
67. Bruster, JM and Pullium, G: Gradient Pressure. Am J Occup Ther 37:485–488, 1983.
68. Naismith, RS: Hypertrophic scar therapy. Pressure induced remodeling and the determinates. PhD Thesis, University of Strathclyde, Glasgow, 1980.
69. Whitaker, J and Lamberty, BH: Pressure garments in the treatment of axillary burns contracture. Physiotherapy 67:5–7, 1981.
70. Zuker, RM, et al: Effective management of deep scald burns to the feet. J Burn Care Rehabil 5:288–290, 1984.
71. Apfel, LM, et al: Computer-drafted pressure support gloves. J Burn Care Rehabil 9:165–168, 1988.
72. Johnson, CL: Bio-concepts. J Burn Care Rehabil 8:325–329, 1987.
73. Becker, BE: Hypertrophic burn scarring: Control of chest deformities with a new device. Arch Phys Med Rehabil 61:187–189, 1980.
74. Angelats, J and Brukardt, B: The use of an elastomer lined neck splint for prevention of neck scarring and contracture. Bul Clin Rev Burn Inj 2:17, 1985.
75. O'Donnell, L: Control of foot contractures: A simple method. Bul Clin Rev Burn Inj 2:26–27, 1985.
76. Fowler, D and Pegg, SP: Early intervention with pressure garments in burn injuries. Bul Clin Rev Burn Inj 2:23–24, 1985.
77. Feldman, AE and MacMillan, BG: The control of scars in different areas by new techniques. Bul Clin Rev Burn Inj 2:21–22, 1985.
78. Fegan, WG: Bandaging the lower limb. Nursing Times 23:1079–1080, 1973.
79. Isherwood, PA, Robertson, JC, and Rossi, A: Pressure measurements beneath below-knee amputation stump bandages: elastic bandaging, the Puddifoot dressing and a pneumatic bandaging technique compared. Br J Surg 62:982–986, 1975.
80. Whitmore, JJ, et al: Bandaging the lower extremity to control swelling: Figure-8 versus spiral technique. Arch Phys Med Rehabil 53:487–490, 1972.
81. Rivers, E: A compression hand wrap. J Burn Care Rehabil 5:291–293, 1984.
82. Byron, PM and Muntzer, EM: Therapist's management of the mutilated hand. In Mackin, EJ (ed): Hand Clinics, vol 2. 1986, pp 69–79.
83. Rose, MP and Deitch, EA: The effective use of a tubular compression bandage, Tubigrip, for burn scar therapy in the growing child. J Burn Care Rehabil 4:197–201, 1983.
84. Judge, JC, May, SR, and DeClement, FA: Control of hypertrophic scarring in burn patients using tubular support bandages. J Burn Care Rehabil 5:221–224, 1984.
85. Kealey, GP, et al: Prospective randomized comparison of two types of pressure therapy garments. J Burn Care Rehabil 11:334–336, 1990.
86. Ward, RS, et al: Investigation of reasons for the selection of particular pressure support suppliers by burn centers in the United States. J Burn Care Rehabil, in press, 1993.
87. Ward, RS, et al: Use of positive plaster impressions to facilitate measurement of anti-burn scar support gloves for severely burned hands. J Burn Care Rehabil 10:351–353, 1989.
88. Malick, MH and Carr, JA: Manual on Management of the Burn Patient. Harmarville Rehabilitation Center Educational Resource Division, Pittsburgh, 1982, p 140.
89. Leung, KS, et al: Complications of pressure therapy for post-burn hypertrophic scars. Burns 10:434–438, 1984.
90. Malick, MH and Carr, JA: Manual on Management of the Burn Patient. Harmarville Rehabilitation Center Educational Resource Division, Pittsburgh, 1982, p 172.
91. Johnson, CL: Wound healing and scar formation. In Covey, MH (ed): Topics in Acute Care Trauma and Rehabilitation: Burn Trauma. Aspen Publishers, Rockville, 1987, 1:1–14.
92. Selmanowitz, VJ and Orentreich, N: Medical-grade fluid silicone—A monographic review. J Dermatol Surg Oncol 3:597–611, 1977.

93. Perkins, K, Davey, RB, and Wallis, KA: Silicone gel: A new treatment for burn scars and contractures. Burns 9:201–204, 1983.
94. Quinn, KJ, et al: Non-pressure treatment of hypertrophic scars. Burns 12:102–108, 1985.
95. Wessling, N, et al: Evidence that use of a silicone gel sheet increases range of motion over burn wound contractures. J Burn Care Rehabil 6:503–505, 1985.
96. Quinn, KJ: Silicone gel in scar treatment. Burns 13:S33–S40, 1987.
97. Kirn, TF: Silicone gel appears inexplicably to flatten, lighten hypertrophic scars from burns. JAMA 261:2600, 1989.
98. Ahn, AT, Monafo, WW and Mustoe, TA: Topical silicone gel: A new treatment for hypertrophic scars. Surg 106:781–787, 1989.
99. Ahn, ST, Monafo, WW, and Mustoe, TA: Topical silicone gel for the prevention and treatment of hypertrophic scar. Arch Surg 126:499–504, 1991.
100. Alston, DW, et al: Materials for pressure inserts in the control of hypertrophic scar tissue. J Burn Care Rehabil 2:40–43, 1981.
101. Quan, PE, et al: Control of scar tissue in the finger web spaces by use of graded pressure inserts. J Burn Care Rehabil 2:27–30, 1981.
102. Gorham, K and Hammond, J: An improved web-space pressure technique to prevent burn syndactyly. J Burn Care Rehabil 12:157–159, 1991.
103. Malick, MH and Carr, JA: Flexible elastomer molds in burn scar control. Am J Occup Ther 34:603–608, 1980.
104. Malick, MH and Carr, JA: Manual on Management of the Burn Patient. Harmarville Rehabilitation Center Educational Resource Division, Pittsburgh, 1982, p 176.
105. Perkins, K, Davey, RB and Wallis, K: Current materials and techniques used in a burn scar management programme. Burns 13:406–410, 1987.
106. Morgan, RF, et al: Management of head and neck burns. J Burn Care Rehabil 6:20–36, 1985.
107. Gallagher, J, et al: Survey of treatment modalities for the prevention of hypertrophic facial scars. J Burn Care Rehabil 11:118–120, 1990.
108. Fader, P: Preserving function and minimizing deformity: The role of the occupational therapist. In Carvajal, HF and Parks, DH (eds): Burns in Children: Pediatric Burn Management. Yearbook Medical Publishers, Chicago, 1988, pp 338–343.
109. Ward, RS, et al: A technique for control of hypertrophic scarring in the central region of the face. J Burn Care Rehabil 12:263–267, 1991.
110. Rivers, EA, Strate, RG and Solem, LD: The transparent face mask. Am J Occup Ther 33:108–113, 1979.
111. Keehnen, J, Daugherty, MB, and Warden, GD: Pressure bracing the inframammary graft. Proc American Burn Association 22:136, 1990.
112. Maclachlan, J: Breast conformers in reconstructive surgery. Proc American Burn Association 22:38, 1990.
113. Bodian, M: Use of massage following lid surgery. Eye Ear Nose Throat Monthly 48:542–547, 1969.
114. Miles, WK and Grigsby, L: Remodeling of scar tissue in the burned hand. In Hunter, JM, et al (eds): Rehabilitation of the Hand, ed 2. CV Mosby, St. Louis, 1984, pp 841–856.
115. Wood, EC: Beard's massage: Principles and techniques, ed 2. WB Saunders, Philadelphia, 1974, pp 48–59.
116. Clarke, HM, et al: Acute management of pediatric hand burns. In Grossman, JAI (ed): Hand Clinics: Burns of the Upper Extremity, vol 6. WB Saunders, Philadelphia, 1990, pp 221–232.

CHAPTER 15

The Use of Physical Agents in Burn Care

R. Scott Ward, PT

Many physical agents are used regularly in typical therapy settings, but not in burn care. Hydrotherapy, which is used mainly for wound care, is the notable exception. Information presented in this chapter will review the theory and physiologic effects, as well as reported uses for various thermal and electrical therapeutic modalities in burn care. For a more detailed review of these therapeutic physical agents, the reader should consult the referenced readings. (See also Appendix N.)

THERMAL THERAPEUTIC AGENTS

The application of heat or cold to tissues causes physiologic changes that affect the outcome of a therapeutic treatment. Rarely, if ever, should a thermal agent, or any physical modality for that matter, be the sole treatment provided. Further, with the exception of hydrotherapy, Fluidotherapy, or laser, heat and cold modalities generally are used only on the healed burn patient.

Physiologic changes resulting from an elevation or decrease in tissue temperature depend on several variables, not all of which can be controlled easily. Some of the variables that affect the magnitude of actual tissue temperature fluctuation are: (1) the intensity of the thermal energy, (2) the rate at which the energy is transferred to the tissue, (3) the impedance of the tissue type to the energy source, (4) the duration of tissue exposure to the energy source, (5) the quantity of tissue exposed to the energy, and (6) the adequacy of blood supply to and from the area.

Physiologic Effects of Therapeutic Heat

EFFECTS ON BLOOD FLOW

Increases in tissue temperature result in vasodilation and increased blood flow to an area.[1,2] The vasodilation is probably due to either an axon or spinal cord reflex, or a reaction to the release of local vasoactive chemicals.[3,4] The most pronounced changes will occur at the site of heat application, but remote vascular changes (reflex vasodilation) also may occur to protect body core temperature. Therapeutic heat should not be used prior to burn wound closure, as heat may lead to an increase in tissue trauma as well as an increase in edema formation resulting from the vascular effects.

EFFECTS ON NERVE AND MUSCLE

Heat can affect muscle spindle and Golgi tendon organ (GTO) firing, nerve conduction velocity, and pain threshold (Figs. 15–1 and 15–2). Mense[5] described a decreased discharge in group II afferents (muscle spindle), which respond to muscle stretch by increasing activity of alpha motor neurons. He also reported an increase in discharge of group Ib afferents (GTO), which respond to increased muscle tension by decreasing alpha motor neuron activity following application of heat.[5] Both of these reactions to therapeutic heat could lead to muscle relaxation due to consequent decreases in alpha motor neuron activity. Gamma motor activity, which is directly proportional to spindle excitability, also has been shown to decrease with superficial heat application.[6] Although the effects of burn injury on the activity of group II afferents, group Ib afferents, and the gamma motor system have not been studied, gamma motor activity may increase with tension or anxiety, both of which are common in burn patients.

Pain relief can occur with the application of heat.[7] In the healed burn patient, therapeutic heat may help to minimize pain associated with passive stretching. Heat is not indicated for pain resulting from the burn wound because the damaged tissue will respond to the modality as an additional pain stimulus.

Burn patients often position themselves in a state of subconscious muscle cocontraction to guard against painful movement. This behavior can lead to muscle-guarding spasms. Anxiety, also common to burn patients, may increase the tension in muscle, further contributing to a muscle spasm. The application of mild heat to burn patients may be valuable in promoting relaxation and decreasing muscle spasm. There are many explanations about the mechanism that leads to decreased spasm from heating tissue superficially. One explanation is that heating of a muscle spindle may decrease the reflex muscle activation, thereby decreasing the spasm.[5] Also, heating of the muscle's GTO may increase discharge, thus leading to an inhibition of the muscle in spasm.[5]

EFFECTS ON CONNECTIVE TISSUE

Favorable alterations in joint stiffness and collagenous structure have been demonstrated with the application of heat. Resistance of a joint to movement is increased with the application of cold and decreased with heat.[8] This change in resistance may be a result of temperature influences on either the viscosity of synovial fluid or the

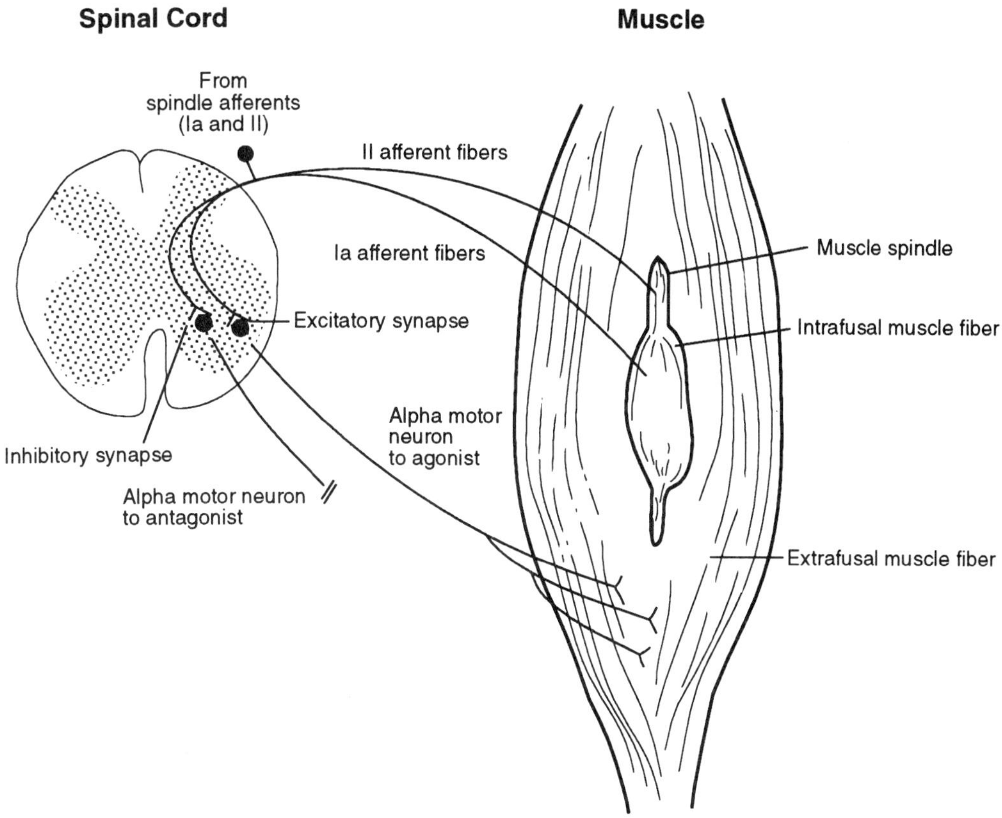

FIGURE 15–1. Representation of the basic components of the stretch reflex. The sensory receptor for this complex is the muscle spindle. Stretching is the primary stimulus which causes the muscle spindle receptor to discharge. This reflex acts to stimulate the agonist muscle to contract as protection from further stretch (contraction of the antagonist is inhibited). The muscle spindle consists of sensory nerve endings that arise from the contractile intrafusal muscle fibers and converge to form two (Ia and II) afferent pathways leading to the spinal cord. Some of the elements of the muscle spindle may be affected by heat and cold.

viscous and elastic properties of capsular structures.[9,10] Lehmann[11] stated that the viscous property of connective tissue prevails over the elastic property when such tissue is either stretched or heated. Connective tissue becomes even more extensible when heated and stretched simultaneously.[11–13] This finding is of particular importance to therapists because heat may permit easier elongation of scar tissue.

OTHER EFFECTS

The physiologic effects of therapeutic heat are depicted in Figure 15–3. Propitious effects of heat have been demonstrated in the resolution of infection and enhancement of the metabolic system. Heat treatments have been used for years on localized infections to hasten the development of an abscess, which then can be drained. Though some data are available on the effects of therapeutic heat on the gram-negative bacterium *Gonococcus*,[14] no data are available on the effects of heat on bacteria common in burn wounds. Therefore, heat-producing modalities are not presently recommended for use in the treatment of burn-related infection.

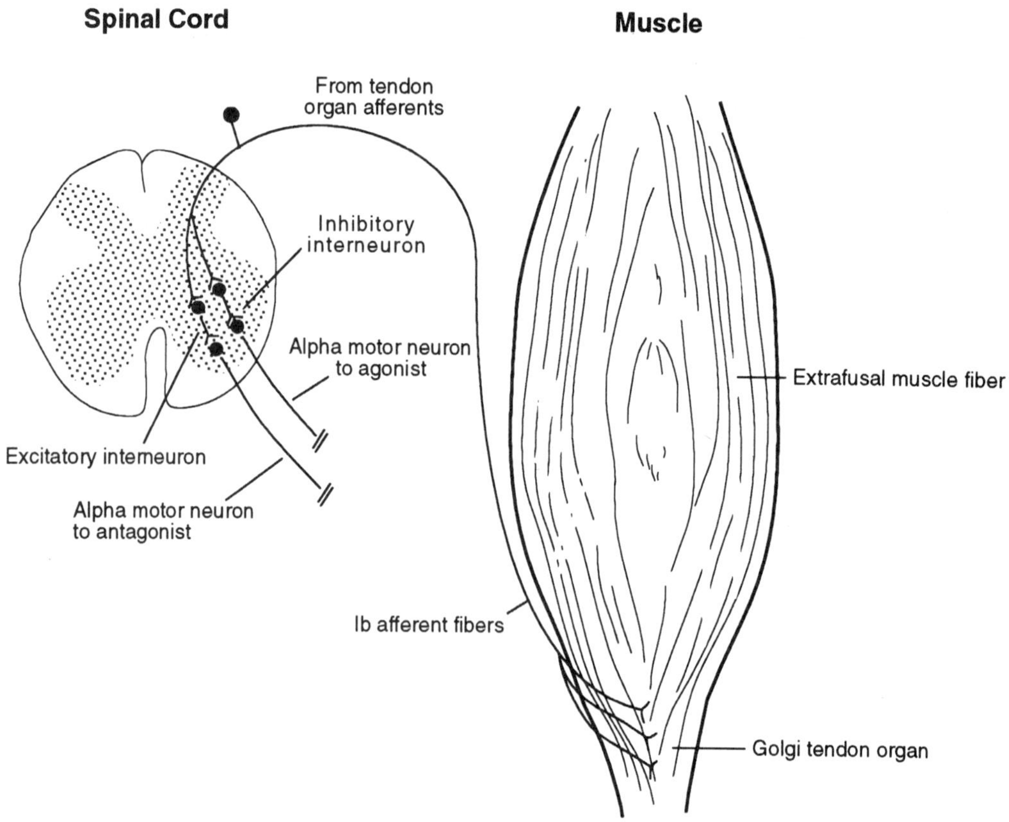

FIGURE 15–2. Schematic diagram of the key elements of the tendon organ reflex. The sensory receptor for this complex is the golgi tendon organ which conveys input along an afferent pathway (Ib fibers) to the spinal cord. The primary stimulus which causes the golgi tendon organ to discharge is tension of muscle. This reflex acts to cause relaxation in the tension producing agonist muscle (contraction of the antagonist is also stimulated). Some of the components of the golgi tendon organ may be affected by heat or cold.

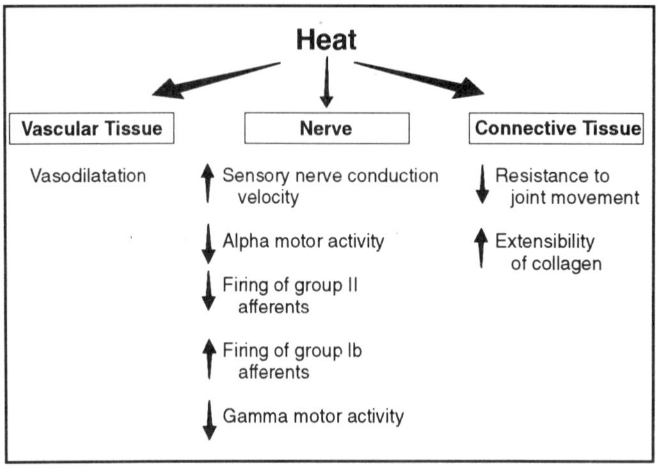

FIGURE 15–3. The physiological effects of therapeutic heat on vascular, peripheral nervous, and connective tissue.

The commonly accepted view of heat application following an injury is that heat should not be used during the acute phase of trauma. Some sources suggest that heat application during the acute phase may increase hemorrhage and edema.[15,16] Fischer[17] stated that an increase in metabolism, which is undesirable during the acute phase of trauma, is seen following the use of heat within therapeutic ranges. Accordingly, therapeutic heat is not recommended for use prior to burn wound closure.

PRECAUTIONS IN THE USE OF THERAPEUTIC HEAT

The most effective temperature range of heat to achieve the aforementioned clinical responses is 40 to 45°C (104 to 113°F).[18] Temperatures below 40°C produce only mild heating effects and essentially are considered ineffective in heating deep tissue structures. Temperatures above this range are liable to be destructive.[18-20] Heat should be used with caution, or may be contraindicated depending on intensity, location (over areas of decreased sensation, gonads, or developing fetus), blood supply, malignancy, or hemorrhagic sites[18-21] (Table 15-1).

A heat modality should be used with caution on a patient with healed skin grafts or burns, as these areas have diminished sensation and a decreased ability to dissipate heat. Diminished sensation is likely due to the destruction and poor regeneration of cutaneous nerves and sensory receptors following the burn injury.[22] Difficulty or the inability to dissipate heat over healed areas is due to lost skin appendages, such as sweat and sebaceous glands, which assist with temperature regulation. Therefore, therapeutic heat may be contraindicated in the patient who has a healed large-body-surface-area burn due to the body's inability to dissipate heat.

TABLE 15-1. General Contraindications for Heat Application*

Areas of anesthesia or cutaneous sensory deficits
(healed skin grafts may exhibit decreased cutaneous sensibility)
Areas with deficient vascular supply
Areas at risk for hemorrhage
Over known or suspected malignancies
Over gonads
Over a developing fetus
Additional contraindications with diathermy:
Presence of metal (internal or external)
Cardiac pacemakers
Areas of high fluid volume
Additional precautions with laser:
Over unclosed fontanels of children
Over or near the cornea

Note: Some heat modalities, such as ultrasound, Fluidotherapy, paraffin, and hot packs, may not be suitable for use over open wounds.

This is not provided as a comprehensive list of contraindications. For a more complete delineation, the reader is directed to applicable physical agent textbooks and references.

* Except hydrotherapy.

Physiologic Effects of Therapeutic Cold (Cryotherapy)

EFFECTS ON BLOOD FLOW

Cold application can control swelling and stop hemorrhage.[3,23] Cold produces a reflex vasoconstriction that is the likely reason for these effects. The vasoconstriction commonly occurs when tissue is exposed to cold for less than 15 minutes. The cold-induced vasoconstriction is often followed by a vasodilative response with prolonged cooling.[24,25] There are several proposed reasons for this vasodilative response, including an axon reflex,[24] depression of smooth muscle activity,[23,26] and protection of the tissue against freezing.[3] Because of these possible responses, the 15-minute period appears to be the most advantageous duration to apply cold for the resolution of edema and inflammation.

EFFECTS ON MUSCLE AND NERVE

Isometric muscle strength is enhanced following cold application.[27] Increased isometric strength may be due to an immediate or delayed effect occurring from a few minutes up to 45 minutes.[28–30] Stimulation of the alpha motor neuron or cold-induced vasodilation are possible explanations for this outcome.

Skilled motor tasks have been shown to be impaired following the application of cold.[31] This particular effect would be detrimental to achieving therapy goals with the burn patient because of the importance of functional exercise in the rehabilitation process.

Myelinated and unmyelinated peripheral nerves are affected by cold. Cold can lead to decreased nerve conduction velocities and impaired neuromuscular synaptic transmission, which results in decreased muscle activity and pain.[32,33] Small, unmyelinated C fibers are less sensitive to cold than myelinated A fibers, and as myelinated A fibers increase in size, they become less sensitive to cold.[34] As a result of cryotherapy, pain control may be due to decreased conduction velocity of those fibers that convey pain information to the central nervous system (Fig. 15–4).

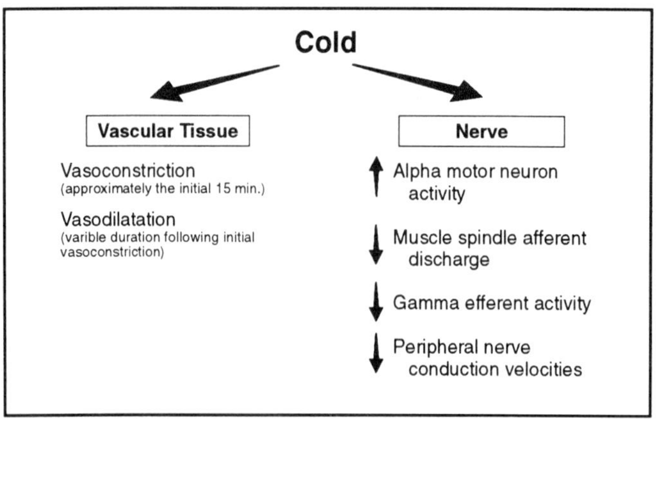

FIGURE 15–4. The physiological effects of therapeutic cold on vascular and peripheral nervous tissue.

TABLE 15–2. General Contraindications for Cold Application

Patients who manifest cold sensitivity (for example; Raynaud's phenomenon, cold intolerance, cold urticaria or cryoglobinemia)
Areas of circulatory compromise
Areas of poor cutaneous sensation
Patients with hypertension
Prolonged application greater than 1 hr
Open burn wounds

This is not provided as a comprehensive list of contraindications. For a more complete delineation, the reader is directed to applicable physical agent textbooks and references.

PRECAUTIONS IN THE USE OF THERAPEUTIC COLD

Exposure time and temperature of cold should be monitored carefully to avoid tissue damage. Standard contraindications to cold treatments include patients with cold hypersensitivity syndromes (e.g., Raynaud's phenomenon, cold urticaria, and cryoglobinemia), hypertension, cutaneous anesthesia and impaired circulation.[35,36] Cryotherapy should not be administered over unhealed burn wounds because the damaged skin lacks protective vascular and sensory tissue. As previously mentioned, burn patients lose normal sensibility, so appropriate sensory testing should be done to determine if a healed burn site is hypersensitive or hyposensitive to cold prior to treatment (Table 15–2).

Cold Versus Heat

A decision about which type of thermal stimulation to use is influenced by several factors, including the therapeutic goal, stage of recovery from a burn injury, medical conditions other than the burn injury, body site to be treated, patient preference or tolerance of cold or heat, and the availability of modalities (in the burn ward, clinic or at the patients home). Table 15–3 provides a summary of the applications of therapeutic heat and cold.

Sources of Thermal Therapy

ULTRASOUND

Clinical ultrasound is used commonly by physical therapists to produce a deep tissue temperature rise within a safe and appropriate therapeutic range. Normal therapeutic settings for application of ultrasound are generally from 0.5 to 2.0 W/cm^2 for variable times depending on the size of the area being treated. Reported advantageous effects of this particular modality include increased extensibility of collagen tissue,[37] including periarticular structures;[38] either increased or decreased motor and sensory nerve conduction velocity;[39–41] increased blood flow;[42,43] and elevation of pain thresholds.[44] These outcomes are due to the thermal effects of ultrasound. There are mechanical (nonthermal) effects produced by ultrasound (e.g., cavitation and acoustic streaming); however, the therapeutic merit of these effects is not known.[45]

TABLE 15–3. General Applications for the Therapeutic Use of Heat and Cold in the Treatment of the Burn Patient

Condition	Thermal Agent	Effect*
Muscle spasm	Heat	Muscle relaxation
	Cold	Muscle relaxation (i.e., muscle spasm)
Pain	Heat	Decreased pain
	Cold	Analgesia
Poor circulation	Heat	Increased blood flow
	Cold	Eventual increase in blood flow
Edema	Heat	Decreased chronic edema
	Cold	Decreased acute edema
Stiff joint	Heat	Decreased joint stiffness
Restrictive scar	Heat	Increased connective tissue extensibility

* Mechanisms of effectiveness are not included. Patient variation, tolerances, and preferences, as well as the etiology of different conditions must be considered in each case.

Ultrasound is indicated for treatment of patients with healed burns because of its influence on collagen and pain. Scar tissue that is more dense than normal tissue is heated preferably by ultrasound. When collagen tissue is heated by ultrasound, the relative increase in tissue temperature allows for an increase in collagen extensibility.[46] Successful use of ultrasound has been described for treating scar tissue that impeded range of motion.[47] Passive stretch is a familiar technique employed by burn therapists in an attempt to elongate collagen, thereby preventing or correcting scar contracture. Combining passive stretch with the application of ultrasound facilitates further tissue elongation.[13,48-50] A decrease in pain during therapy sessions could serve to increase the potential for greater tissue elongation. Ultrasound also is useful in treating joint stiffness resulting from burn-related immobility.[38]

Ultrasound appears to be a safe and effective device for use in resolving range-of-motion limitation and pain in the burn patient. Ultrasound should be used only over healed or grafted areas. Although a coupling agent probably will not irritate healed skin, the skin should nevertheless be monitored for signs of irritation. If irritation occurs, ultrasound treatments should be discontinued until the skin irritation has been resolved. Upon resumption of the ultrasound treatments, another coupling agent should be used. Discomfort of the sound head contacting the healed skin may be a problem because some patients complain of touch-induced paresthesias. Ultrasound can be administered under water, thus alleviating the need for contact between the sound head and the patient.

HYDROTHERAPY

Hydrotherapy in burn care is used in a variety of ways. Cleaning the burn wound for infection prevention and preparation of a burn site for surgery are the most common reasons for using burn-related hydrotherapy.[51,52] Some burn care providers use water as a means of removing burn dressings from a wound.[51] Relaxation, which results from the warmth and buoyancy of the water, may encourage active movement, while the resistance provided by the water allows for active resistive exercise whenever indicated.[53,54]

Exercise during hydrotherapy may begin as soon as a patient is medically stable. Active and passive exercises can be performed in conjunction with wound care, provided the movements do not interfere with or unduly prolong the care during a hydrotherapy treatment session. Extra hydrotherapy sessions for exercise are unnecessary and therefore are not recommended.

Immersion in a standard hydrotherapy tub, showering, or spraying for wound cleansing are common applications of hydrotherapy in burn centers across the United States. Tubbing sessions are routinely performed for a duration of 15 to 30 minutes, one to three times daily.[55] Disadvantages for remaining in the water longer than 30 minutes include an increased possibility for hypothermia and the leaching of electrolytes from the body through the wound.

Hydrotherapy might lead to the spread of waterborne contaminates between patients, or among isolated wounds on the same patient.[56-58] Chlorine, iodine-based additives, detergents, or antimicrobial soaps usually are added to the water before a patient is immersed in an attempt to decrease the likelihood of contamination.[56] Conscientious tub washing and disinfection are necessary after each tubbing procedure to reduce the chance of cross-contamination (see Chapter 7).

FLUIDOTHERAPY

Fluidotherapy is a form of dry heat created by driving hot air through a bed of solid particles. The air and particles assume a fluid-like consistency and provide a heated environment. The temperature of this modality is often set at about 48°C (118°F) and may be varied by the operator. Increases in tissue temperature above that achieved with water or paraffin have been reported with Fluidotherapy.[59-61]

The unit can be used to treat patients with open wounds, but due to the conductive and convective nature of heat transfer from the particles to the area being treated, bulky dressings should be removed prior to treatment. The unit is self-cleaning, and the particles in the unit should be changed about every 6 months. A concern about this modality may be cross-contamination if a burn patient has an open wound. No contamination has been reported in the treatment of open wounds, though no documentation is available that directly assesses the ability of the Fluidotherapy unit to eradicate various common burn flora. If a patient has open wounds, the wound should be lightly covered with gauze, an oversized nonsterile glove, or a long whirlpool plastic glove prior to using Fluidotherapy.

Increases in tissue temperature created by Fluidotherapy have been reported to decrease pain,[60-62] increase range of motion,[60,61] increase blood flow,[60,63] heal superficial wounds, and decrease edema.[60,61,63] In addition, the body part can be exercised while being treated. Because of these benefits, Fluidotherapy can be useful in a burn setting.

PARAFFIN

Paraffin can be used on healed or skin-grafted burn wounds. Paraffin should not be used over open wounds. Head and Helm[64] have empirically suggested the successful combination of paraffin and passive stretch in burn rehabilitation.[64] Beyond

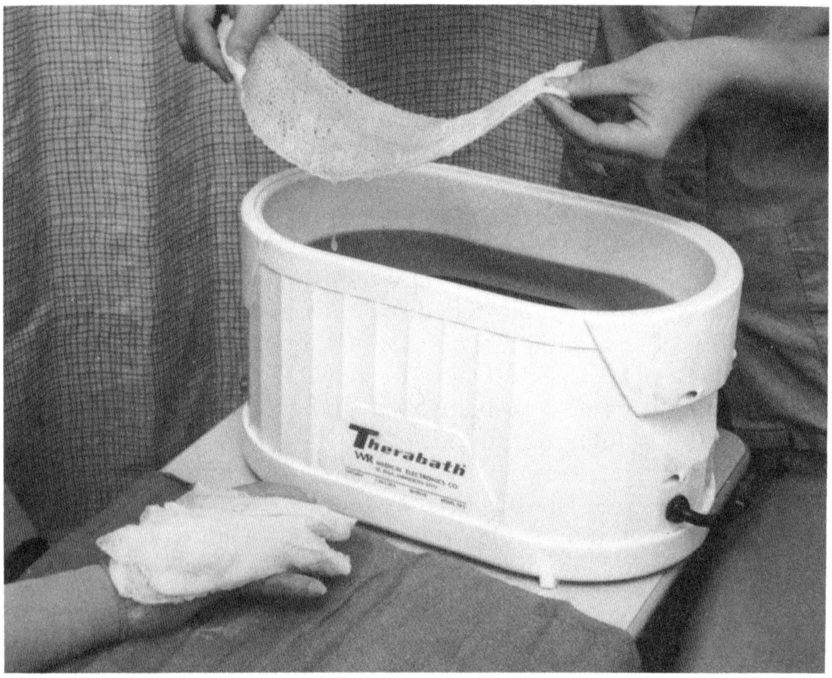

FIGURE 15–5. Application of paraffin by dipping gauze into the heated paraffin and then wrapping it around the grafted, healed fingers and hand. The hand is placed in a plastic bag and covered with a towel for 20 minutes.

the likely effects on collagen produced by the heat, paraffin also may be beneficial because of the softening of the scar by the mineral oil in the paraffin.[64] The most common method of application of paraffin is dipping of the hands or feet. However, wrapping paraffin-impregnated gauze around a joint (Fig. 15–5),[65] and brushing or spooning the paraffin over joints such as the elbow, shoulder, knee, or neck while that joint is being stretched may make this a useful modality for treatment of decreased range of motion. Ideally, the tissue should be placed on a stretch to maximize the effectiveness of this treatment. A paraffin mixture of 2.5 ounces (73.925 milliliters) of mineral oil to 1 pound (373.24 grams) of paraffin will allow the mixture to be liquid at the lower recommended temperature of 46 to 50°C (114 to 122°F) for use with burn patients.[64] Commercially prepared, premixed paraffin blocks, which are acceptable for use with burn patients, are available.

HOT PACKS, HEAT LAMPS, AND DIATHERMY

Hot packs and heat lamps are mild, superficial forms of infrared heat. Because of the shallow depth of heat penetration by these modalities, they may have little effect on deeper layers of scar tissue. These heat modalities may be used on healed tissue to heat the superficial layers and assist with stretching scar contractures. Some burn care facilities use heat lamps to dry out donor sites; however, this technique is contrary to the "moist wound healing" principle (see Chapter 5).

Though the tissue penetration of diathermy produced heat is approximately 3 cm, the application may be difficult. A patient must be comfortably positioned, and little movement by the patient can be allowed for safe application of diathermy.[66]

For most burn patients, maintaining a stretched position, which would be desirable with heat application, is difficult for the length of time required for an effective dose of diathermy. Furthermore, exposing hypertrophic scar tissue to therapeutic doses of diathermy may be damaging.[67] The reason is the vigorous heating produced by diathermy may exacerbate any low-level inflammatory response occurring in the scar tissue and this could result in tissue destruction. The exacerbation of this inflammatory response has not appeared to be a problem with the use of heat modalities, such as ultrasound, on scar tissue, but has yet to be studied with the application of diathermy. Due to the lack of related research, diathermy is not recommended in the treatment of burn patients.

CRYOTHERAPY

Ice or cold packs, cold baths, and ice massage are methods for decreasing tissue temperature. Cold treatment is not prevalent in burn rehabilitation, but may be useful as a possible adjunct in treating problems, such as joint pain, sometimes encountered following stretching, or edema. The primary obstacle in using cold is the possible intolerance of burn patients to extremes of cold.

LASER

Laser is an acronym for light amplification by stimulated emission of radiation. Low-power laser or "cold" laser has been developed with potential rehabilitative uses in pain management and wound healing.[68] In theory, laser treatment is thought to stimulate the return of malfunctioning tissue cells to a normal physiologic state. For example, in treating indolent wounds, laser light stimulates fibroblast cells to increase collagen production while, in treating hypertrophic scars, lasers cause a decrease in scar production by altering the cellular mechanism of overproduction.

Closure of open wounds has been described by Kana and co-workers[69] following application of low-power (helium-neon) laser. Other reported findings include increased collagen formation and blood flow, increases in the intracellular matrix and vascularization, and decreases in numbers of microorganisms and pain.[70-72] One major advantage of low-power laser is the short amount of treatment time required to achieve purported results. Depending on the type of laser used, 10 to 20 seconds for approximately 15 treatments may be effective in wound healing, and 20 to 30 seconds for 10 treatments may result in pain reduction.[73]

At this time, the low-power laser has not been approved for clinical use in the United States by the Food and Drug Administration (FDA). Only a person with an investigational device exemption can use a low-power laser. Given this fact, further information and instruction should be sought if the FDA laser status changes.

Treatment Planning Considerations

Continuous wave ultrasound, hydrotherapy, Fluidotherapy, and paraffin are the most reasonable thermal agent choices available for the burn therapist. Thermal agents standard in therapy settings such as hot packs, diathermy, and some forms of cryotherapy are not explicitly appropriate for burn treatment, but may be useful in treating related musculoskeletal symptoms.

There are many considerations when planning to use a thermal agent in the treatment of a patient. Common regard about the use of thermal agents in burn care should include (1) the presence of painful, open wounds; (2) the potential for cross-contamination; (3) freshly healed wounds that may be fragile to manipulation; (4) diminished cutaneous sensation; and (5) anxiety of the patient toward thermally based treatment modalities. Temperatures produced by modalities should be monitored frequently to protect patients and provide the maximum effect of the desired temperature.

ELECTRICAL THERAPEUTIC AGENTS

The use of electric current has been associated with several physiologic changes that may augment the effect of a coinciding therapeutic treatment (Fig. 15-6). The therapist may observe effects at the treatment site as well as systemic responses to the use of electrical stimulation.

Physiologic Effects of Electrical Stimulation

EFFECTS ON BLOOD FLOW

An increase in circulation has been noted after electrical stimulation, particularly with low frequencies.[74,75] Short on/off impulse intervals (1:1 to 1:2) may be more effective than long impulse intervals in increasing blood flow.[76] This increase may be due to the involvement of the muscle pump or influences on the sympathetic nervous system.[77] Circulation also may improve because of increased metabolism in a stimulated muscle. A corollary to this idea is that intermittent, low-frequency electrical stimulation (i.e., 10 Hz) has been shown to increase the capillary density of stimulated muscle.[78,79] Stimulation of the muscle pump may assist in the resolution of edema.

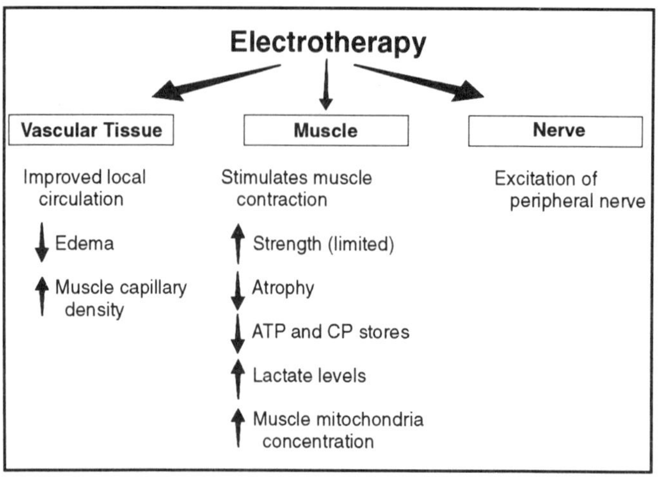

FIGURE 15-6. The physiological effects of electrotherapy on vascular, muscle, and peripheral nervous tissue.

EFFECTS ON NERVE AND MUSCLE

Electrical stimulation results in excitation of peripheral nerves. Under normal conditions, the stimulation of nervous tissue causes contraction of muscle tissue. If denervated muscle is being stimulated, the sarcolemma of the muscle is the likely target for transmission of the electric current.

In healthy, innervated muscle the use of electrical stimulation increases strength and delays atrophy of muscles surrounding an immobilized joint.[80] Combining electrical stimulation with active exercise may further improve strength.[81] In denervated muscle, electrical stimulation may retard muscle atrophy but not with any lasting effects. Biochemical and structural alterations of muscular components, such as decreased adenosine triphosphate and creatine phosphate stores, an increase in lactate levels, and an increase in the muscle concentration of mitochondria also have been described.[82-84]

Maintaining joint motion or correcting contractures with electric current is possible.[85,86] This positive effect is presumably due to stimulation of muscle to contract rather than any direct effect of the current on connective tissue. Hence, connective tissue of burn scar contractures may not be influenced by electric current; however, muscle tissue, which shortens with long-standing burn scar contracture, can be affected. For example, by stimulating muscles that are antagonistic to a contracted muscle, two events occur. First, active muscle action against the contracture is obtained, and second, reciprocal inhibition with subsequent relaxation of the contracted muscle group is achieved. These responses may result in the need for less aggressive stretching of the contracted muscle group.

OTHER EFFECTS

In the treatment of wounds, electrical stimulation may have an influence on the wound healing process. Effects of direct cathodal current on decreasing the growth rate of certain unfavorable microorganisms, such as *Pseudomonas aeruginosa,*[87] *Staphylococcus aureus,*[88] and *Escherichia coli* B,[89] have been reported.[90] Possible mechanisms for this decreased growth rate of microorganisms might include disruption of the homeostatic mechanism of the organism, which leads to death, or interference with the regulatory and/or enzymatic processes of the microorganism.[91,92] Electrical stimulation probably is not practical in treating large-surface-area burn wounds, but may be useful with small infected burn wounds.

The work of Carey and Lepley[93] showed that increases in migration of blood cells and thrombosis of small vessels can be influenced by electrical stimulation. Subsequent to stimulation, the migration of epidermal and dermal cells under the anode has been reported by Harrington and co-workers.[94]

Electrical stimulation also may have an influence on perceived pain. Possible mechanisms to explain resulting pain relief vary. Whether these mechanisms are physiologic or psychologic, electrical stimulation may be able to alleviate pain in some situations. The resolution of pain may result from the effects of electricity on increasing circulation, decreasing edema, or instituting muscle activity. The relief of pain can lead to improved joint motion, hyperstimulation of cutaneous sensory fibers, indirect release of endogenous polypeptides (e.g., enkephalins, beta-endorphins) or neurotransmitters (e.g., serotonin), which can produce analgesia or introduce counterirritation. Pain relief may be the result of a placebo effect.

The parameters of treatment with electrical stimulation include waveform, amplitude, duration, frequency, rise and decay time, duty cycle, and modulation. A discussion of these elements would be lengthy and is beyond the scope of this chapter. The reader is referred to other sources such as Myklebust and Kloth's[95] chapter in *Electrotherapy in Rehabilitation* or Cook's[96] chapter in *Clinical Electrotherapy* on instrumentation. However, there are some general parameters that increase the comfort of electrical stimulation, and increased comfort should be a consideration for patients with burns. Frequency of electrical current is one parameter that influences patient comfort. Generally, the higher the frequency (at least 50 pulses per second) the more comfortable the current feels. Additionally, ramp modulation will provide a more comfortable delivery of electrical stimulation. A gradual increase in the stimulus amplitude (on ramp) allows a gradual recruitment of nerve fibers and muscle contraction, and an off ramp allows a gradual decrease in produced muscle force.

There are various types of electrodes available for use. Some electrodes require a conducting gel and others do not. When using electrodes on burn patients, the conducting medium and the adhesive on the electrode (if any) should be evaluated for their potential to irritate the skin. Possible alterations in skin impedance also should be considered.

Sources of Electrical Therapy

TRANSCUTANEOUS ELECTRICAL NERVE STIMULATION (TENS)

Many patients have experienced pain relief following the application of TENS, although the specific reasons for success with pain control through its use are yet unknown. When setting up a TENS unit, pulse rate, pulse duration, and amplitude are the parameters that determine the characteristic quality and quantity of the stimulation. TENS may be used successfully when the electrodes are placed over the site of pain;[97] in relation to a dermatome,[98] employing trigger, acupuncture, or motor points;[99,100] paravertebrally by identifying a specific spinal cord segment for stimulation;[101] or over a peripheral nerve.[101,102]

TENS has been documented to be effective in acute pain situations apparently by interrupting the pain-spasm-pain cycle.[103] TENS has been shown to be effective on acute pain conditions such as acute tendonitis[104–106] and patellofemoral pain.[107,108]

Chronic pain patients also have been shown to benefit from the use of TENS.[107,108] As with medication, a placebo effect will play a role in some of the success of TENS treatments.[109,110] Whether pain from a burn is treatable by TENS is not well documented. Using auricular acupuncture-like TENS application, Lewis and associates[11] demonstrated some success in the control of burn pain following wound care sessions. Other suggestions for the use of TENS in burn care might be the treatment of pain resulting from donor sites, staple removal from graft sites, small, isolated wounds on extremities, and residual limb pain following burn related amputation.

NEUROMUSCULAR ELECTRICAL STIMULATION (NMES)

According to Baker,[112] NMES can be used in treatment programs to strengthen or maintain muscle mass, maintain or gain range of motion, facilitate voluntary motor control, temporarily reduce spasticity, and substitute for orthoses. In burn care, the most likely of the aforementioned applications are strengthening or maintaining muscle mass, maintaining or gaining range of motion, or facilitating motor control. If cyclical neuromuscular stimulation were to be used over single or multiple burn involved joints, conceivably NMES could provide further range of motion opportunities for the burn patient and thereby increase the efficiency of a therapy session.

Correction of contracture by NMES has been successfully used in patients with muscle contracture or spasticity.[85,86] LeDoux and associates[113] and Peckham and colleagues[114] suggest that the use of NMES may be advantageous by strengthening or facilitating muscles that oppose a contracture. Because range of motion and stretching are major components of burn therapy treatment, NMES may be useful in some instances. Baker and colleagues[115] report that a combination of electrical stimulation and serial casting may be effective in increasing range of motion. No studies have addressed if there is any direct effect from NMES on scar tissue. Apparently, the more severe the joint limitation, the more aggressive the treatment should be to produce the best result.[117]

Apfel and co-workers[116] demonstrated increases in hand range of motion in three burn patients following application of NMES. Each of the patients displayed one or more of the following pathologies: (1) intrinsic muscle tightness; (2) the inability to use the flexor digitorum superficialis (FDS) or the flexor digitorum profundus as an independent unit for proximal interphalangeal joint (PIP) or distal interphalangeal joint flexion, respectively; (3) a soft tissue contracture; (4) decreased hand closure; or (5) the inability of the FDS to continue PIP joint flexion of the joint due to the reciprocal blocking by the intrinsic muscles or ligament tightness.[116]

HIGH-VOLTAGE PULSED CURRENT (HVPC)

There are several devices and protocols for providing treatment with HVPC.[77] HVPC can be used for neuromuscular stimulation and also has been used successfully in treating decreased blood flow, small wounds, pain, and edema.[77] In addition, Newton[77] has made the clinical observation that burn patient range of motion can be increased when using negative-polarity HVPC over scar tissue.

Lindstrom and associates[117] noted improved prevention of deep vein thrombosis with a frequency of 12 to 15 Hz. This work demonstrates that blood flow may be increased by recruitment of the muscle pump or possibly stimulation of the sympathetic nervous system. This increased blood flow may be an important factor in the positive wound healing findings noted by clinicians. Other reasons for wound healing include the effects of current and polarity on microorganisms; blood cell migration; and thrombosis of vessels as previously mentioned.[87-90,93] Im and colleagues[118] showed an improved survival of skin flaps following the application of HVPC presumably due to increased blood flow.

Decreasing edema also may promote wound healing. The resolution of edema by using HVPC is probably due to activation of the skeletal muscle pump or the negative polarity of the stimulation, which may lead to fluid shift from the region. Williams and Carey[119] applied a current of positive polarity to the jugular vein of a dog, which led to clustering of blood cells, while the application of negative polarity reversed the clustering. Albumin, which is the major protein in plasma, normally is negatively charged and hydrophilic. Consequently, if these cells are repelled from an area, a fluid shift from that area also will occur. This same mechanism may cause the shift of other charged proteins and cells that could increase fluid shift.

Short-term and long-term pain relief have been illustrated with the use of HVPC.[120,121] The mechanisms for alleviation of pain are not well understood and may consist of factors such as increasing circulation or decreasing edema, which have been previously discussed.

BIOFEEDBACK

Biofeedback in patient care represents the use of a specific mechanism for making a person aware of some physiologic process in an attempt to teach patients to control their response to a stimulus. For therapists, feedback most commonly consists of alerting a patient to the status of muscle activity. The use of electromyographic (EMG) biofeedback can assist in relaxation or retraining of muscle.[122] Systems can provide either audio or visual feedback, or a combination of the two, to help a patient gain control over the level of activity present in a target muscle. Electrodes are typically placed over the target muscle. If muscle relaxation is the goal of treatment, the patient is trained to reduce activity in the affected muscle. Patients are encouraged to increase the biofeedback input or output manifested when muscle re-education or recruitment is sought. Training of opposing or synergistic muscle groups also may be worthwhile in cases of relaxation or recruitment training.

Biofeedback also may be advantageous in burn therapy to improve range of motion. As previously indicated, burn patients typically have problems achieving normal range of motion. Biofeedback units that can be set to range-of-motion limits are available and patients can be encouraged either to reach, or exceed, these limits. Other reasons for decreased range of motion in burn patients might be muscle-guarding spasm or peripheral nerve injury due to non-burn-related associated trauma, nerve stretch from improper positioning, and edema. If range of motion is limited due to either muscle spasm or lack of muscle activity, EMG biofeedback may assist in the improvement of range of motion by appropriately influencing the related musculature.

Pain management can be another benefit of biofeedback. Biofeedback most commonly is used in the treatment of headache pain,[123,124] but has been demonstrated as practical for other types of chronic pain.[125] Skin temperature, which reflects changes in blood flow (i.e., increased skin temperature indicates increased peripheral blood flow, which should enhance relaxation of peripheral muscles), and electroencephalographic activity are other parameters that can be monitored during pain control sessions.[126]

Biofeedback has promise for use with burn patients. However, increased impedance of healed skin and scar to the feedback signal may occur and decrease the effectiveness of this modality with certain patients. Relaxation training for muscles that are guarding against passive stretch is one possible application. The use of biofeedback for pain control is possibly its most encouraging prospect. Burn patients would be much less distressed if they could be taught to control themselves and their pain during painful burn care events, such as wound debridement, dressing changes, and certain therapy sessions. Although biofeedback seems to be a reasonable modality for use in the treatment of burn patients, the practicality and effectiveness of biofeedback still need to be determined.

MICROCURRENT

Microcurrent electrical neuromuscular stimulation (MENS) is a relatively new physical therapy modality. The "micro" in microcurrent reflects the level of amperage delivered by the unit. In conventional physical therapy electrical modalities, the current is in milliamperes, while microcurrent is at microampere (thousandth of a milliampere) levels. Microcurrents are available in both high- and low-volt devices, although low-volt most frequently is used and usually is delivered below the normal level of sensory perception. The principle supporting the use of MENS is that the current is similar to normal physiologically existing electric currents and can thereby produce beneficial therapeutic effects.[127]

Applications for MENS include treatment of pain, swelling, inflammation, atrophy, and wound healing. Because the current does not produce muscle contractions, decreases in atrophy probably are due to the pain relief afforded, which may allow for increases in activity level.[128] There is evidence that microcurrent is effective in treating nonunion bone fractures,[129] tendon injuries,[130] and skin ulcers.[131] Apparently, negative microcurrents are more effective in repair of nerve and bone, while positive microcurrent stimulation is more effective in healing skin lesions.[132] There is no available research to address the analgesic effects of MENS; however, pain relief following treatment has been documented.[133]

Due to the lack of current sensation, this modality may have application in the burn setting for healing of small wounds or pain control, especially with children or apprehensive patients. Clinical studies must continue to determine suitable application for the burn patient before widespread use of this modality can be expected.

Treatment Planning Considerations

TENS, neuromuscular electrical stimulation, HVPC, biofeedback, and possibly MENS are feasible electrical therapeutic options for use with burn patients. As was the case with thermal modalities, the use of such equipment is not as routine in the burn therapy setting as in other therapy clinics. Nevertheless, these modalities may provide solutions to the healing of small, chronic open wounds or possibly larger surgically treated wounds such as skin flaps, assist with the treatment of range of motion deficits, and provide an alternative to medication for relief of pain.

Caution should be employed with the use of any electrical modality because of the possibility of hypesthesia over a healed burn wound, skin sensitivity, or skin or scar breakdown resulting from heat produced at the electrode site, electrode adhesives, or energy-conducting media. Standard contraindications for these modalities are listed in Table 15-4. Maintenance of the machinery should occur regularly for proper operation to decrease the likelihood of an unnecessary mishap during treatment.

OTHER PHYSICAL AGENTS

Continuous Passive Motion

Salter,[132] as well as Coutts and associates,[133] have illustrated that continuous passive motion (CPM) is valuable in stimulating joint regeneration processes, decreasing

TABLE 15–4. General Contraindications for Electrotherapy

Patients with cardiac (demand) pacemakers (any stimulation across the heart should be undertaken with caution)
Patients predisposed to seizures
Stimulation over the carotid sinus
Stimulation along the pharyngeal region

This is not provided as a comprehensive list of contraindications. For a more complete delineation, the reader is directed to applicable physical agent textbooks and references.

joint stiffness and edema, and maintaining or increasing range of motion. A few reasons for the success of CPM may include the enhancement of joint metabolic activity and nutrition; acceleration of articular and periarticular (tendon and ligament) healing; and, in burn patients, a reduction of immobilization time.[132-134] CPM is a common modality in burn care settings, as over half the major burn treatment centers are using these devices.[135] Covey and co-workers,[136] in a study of 10 hand burns, demonstrated an increase in range of motion in these hands with no increase in pain with the use of CPM. Success with CPM has also been described in increasing range of motion of the knee in a burn patient.[137] CPM can fulfill an important role in supplementing range-of-motion exercises for burn patients during rest periods.[138] Also, CPM can be used with patients unable to independently perform range of motion, such as patients in intensive care settings.[139] A description of the many choices of CPM devices available would be too lengthy for this discussion. Diehm's[140] article provides a very concise review of CPM availability. If there is decreased joint stability, CPM treatment should not be used.

Intermittent Vasopneumatic Compression

Edema is one of several complications that can occur as a consequence of burn injury. Persisting edema can result in pain, decreased wound healing, and diminished function. Extremity edema can be treated by using an intermittent compression device (Fig. 15–7) (Appendix N).

Two types of compression sleeves are available. These include either a single-cell sleeve that delivers equal pressure to an entire extremity or a multiunit sleeve that applies pressure sequentially from the distal to the proximal parts of the limb. The multiunit sleeves can vary as well by either delivering a uniform or a gradient of pressures into each cell. This device, which has been used successfully in treating lymphedema, offers a "milking" action for the removal of fluid.[141]

Pressure is delivered at a time ratio of 3:1 (three time measures on, one time measure off), and is most effective when the pressure of the sleeve is equal to or slightly greater than the patient's diastolic blood pressure.[142] Treatment is contraindicated to an anesthetic extremity. Treatment should be terminated if numbness or tingling occur during the course of the treatment. The treated body part should be inspected for pressure intolerance following treatment.

When an intermittent compression machine is not being used, some form of external compression should be applied, or other treatment provided, to control edema. The alternatives for external compression consist of elastic bandages, taping,

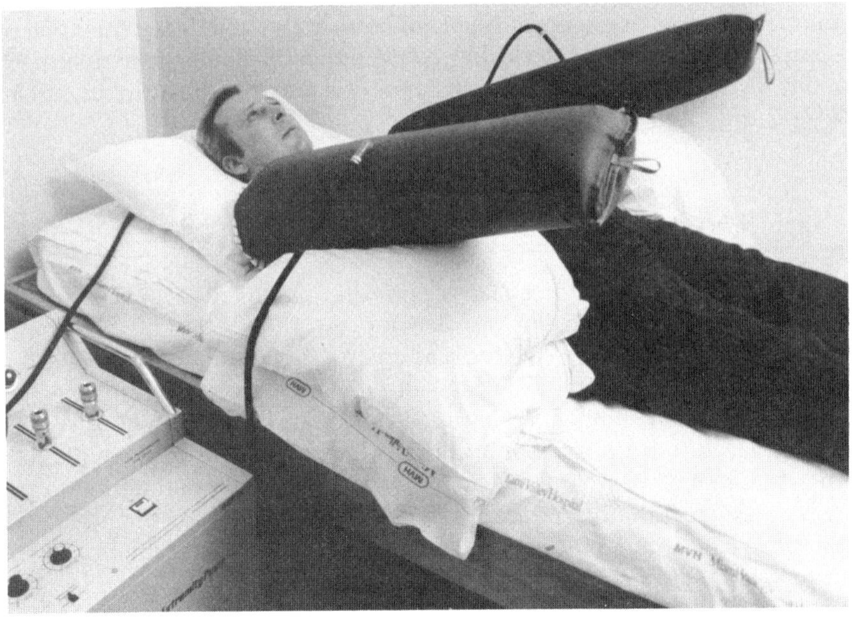

FIGURE 15–7. Intermittent compression device used to decrease bilateral hand edema.

air casts, and pressure support garments. Antiburn scar compression support garments may provide an adequate level of pressure to control edema in the burned extremity. If not, additional pressure can be manufactured into the support. Exercise for recruitment of the muscle pump, positioning, and massage also are important adjuncts in controlling edema. An aggressive treatment approach to extremity edema should provide pain relief and improve wound healing as well as range of motion and function in the burn patient.

Massage

Massage can be useful in helping to reduce edema in a healed burned extremity. In addition, massage may help relax a patient, which may decrease resistance to range of motion exercises. Further, friction massage may loosen scar from underlying tissue, thereby increasing movement when used in conjunction with range-of-motion exercises and stretching.[143]

Friction massage may be performed to a small, specific spot with the palmar surface of the distal phalanx of the thumb, to a wider, but yet small area with the palmar surface of the distal phalanges of the fingers or to a broader area with the base of the palm or the entire palm. Pressure from the massage should be applied so that tension, which can be visualized by a blanching of the tissue, is produced in the scar tissue. Therapists must always keep their hands in firm contact with the tissue surface to avoid friction damage to the scar tissue. When firm contact is applied, the superficial tissue may be moved on the underlying tissue to a limited area in either a circular or linear pattern.[144,145]

When thinking about the use of massage as an adjunct to treatment, the therapist should be attentive to the condition of the skin. Massage should be avoided if the skin, skin graft, or scar tissue is too fragile to be manipulated, since this type of tissue contact may create shearing forces that could either blister or tear delicate tissues. Additionally, if the skin is dry, the application of a suitable moisturizing cream prior to massage is indicated (Appendix C).

Hyperbaric Oxygen Therapy (HBOT)

HBOT utilizes oxygen, which has a pressure greater than normal atmospheric pressure, to treat such problems as decompression sickness, carbon monoxide poisoning, and gas gangrene. The typical chamber in which HBOT takes place is a double-hulled structure of Plexiglass with metal endplates. Either whole-body chambers or extremity chambers are available for treatment with HBOT. A patient, or extremity, is placed into the system and the chamber is pressurized with 100% oxygen. Typical treatments last 90 to 120 minutes plus a 1- to 5-minute initial compression time and a 5- to 15-minute decompression at the end of treatment.[146] What is of interest in burn care is that HBOT also has been used to increase the healing of many different types of wounds.[147]

Necrotic wounds have limited availability of oxygen, which decreases the function of white blood cells. By elevating tissue pO_2, the destructive function of leukocytes may be enhanced.[148,149] If anaerobic bacteria are present in a wound, HBOT may act as an antibacterial agent.[145,150] Further, HBOT may foster wound healing by stimulating collagen synthesis and increasing formation of granulation tissue for earlier wound re-epithelialization.[151]

The use of HBOT in the treatment of burn wounds has been reported to decrease the need for grafting in study subjects,[152,153] length of hospital stay,[147,154] and thus the cost of hospitalization.[147,148] Reported figures on the healing of burn wounds are not statistically significant, but are encouraging.[147,148] The cost and size of the equipment, the need for personnel who are thoroughly trained and experienced in the use of HBOT, as well as the time involved in the treatment may have discouraged burn clinicians from utilizing HBOT for routine treatment of burn wounds.

Some reported complications of HBOT include middle ear barotrauma, sinus squeezes, myopia (usually reversible), claustrophobia, pulmonary oxygen and central nervous system toxicity.[155] These complications usually are not noted when HBOT is applied locally through a single-extremity chamber.

CLINICAL DECISION MAKING AND CASE PRESENTATIONS

Certain factors should be considered when choosing a modality for use with a burn patient. These considerations include the patient's present medical status and past medical history, wound and skin condition, body part to be treated, psychologic state, and ability to learn how to use the modality as a component of a home program. The therapist should understand the rationale for the use of physical agents if treatment plans are to include a thermal or electric modality. As with any other treatment, the results of the modality application should be evaluated to determine whether treatment should continue, be adjusted, or be discontinued.

CASE STUDY 15–1: THERMAL AGENT

PATIENT HISTORY

A 30-year-old female sustained a 22 percent total body surface area (TBSA) flame burn, which included a 10 percent TBSA full-thickness burn to both upper extremities and dorsal hands, and a 12 percent TBSA partial-thickness injury to her anterior chest. The arms and hands were skin-grafted on the seventh day post burn, and all wounds were healed by postburn day 19. No edema was noted. Range of motion (ROM) of the shoulders and elbows was within normal limits. ROM of the wrists was limited in all planes. Flexion of all the digits of the hands was limited slightly. The patient complained of "stiffness" of all affected joints upon active and passive movement.

PROBLEM LIST

Limited ROM in the wrists and fingers of both upper extremities
Feeling of "stiffness" upon movement of the involved joints

GOALS

Full active ROM in wrists and fingers
Decrease patient's reporting of stiffness with movement to just in the morning.

INTERVENTION

Heat modality—paraffin

RATIONALE

Following skin graft adherence on the full-thickness burns, joint stiffness reported by the patient, as well as the decreased ROM, could have been due to either a lack of joint lubrication from immobilization, contraction of the skin graft, or both. Mild pain experienced with stretching and active exercise also limited ROM. Administration of paraffin elevated the temperature of the affected tissues. Heating of the wrists, hands, and fingers might be expected to relax the scar tissue and soften the grafted skin (mineral oil component of the paraffin). Paraffin treatment followed by stretching and active exercise increased joint ROM and decreased joint stiffness.

CASE STUDY 15–2: ELECTROTHERAPY

PATIENT HISTORY

A 42-year-old male sustained a 35 percent TBSA burn, which included full-thickness injuries of the right upper extremity and dorsal hand, as well as the upper chest, and partial-thickness burns to the lower one half of the anterior and posterior trunk, and both anterior thighs. In the days prior to surgery, the patient complained of increased pain "with any activity," and medication "did not seem to help." The patient described his pain as being a 6 on a scale 1 to 10 (1 = no pain; 10 = worst possible pain). ROM was decreased by approximately 25 percent in all planes over all directly or indirectly affected joints and gait deviations were noted. The patient was not compliant in carrying out an active exercise program or activities of daily living (ADLs).

PROBLEM LIST

Pain
Limited ROM
Abnormal gait
Not performing ADLs

GOALS

Decrease pain perception to a level of 3 on a pain scale.
Increase active ROM to within 80 percent of normal limits.
Normal gait pattern.
Independent in ADL's

INTERVENTION

Transcutaneous electrical nerve stimulation (TENS)

RATIONALE

Pain appeared as the major limiting factor for this patient in achieving his therapy goals. An increase in pain medication would have rendered the patient even less capable, or willing, of performing his outlined exercise, ambulation, and ADL program. Acupuncture-like TENS has been shown to be effective in decreasing burn-related pain. The TENS stimulating electrodes were placed over related somatic acupuncture points at areas that were not burned. The TENS stimulation current was direct, positive polarity, which was delivered at a frequency of 1 Hz. The stimulation began at a minimal threshold level and increased until the patient responded that the stimulus intensity had reached his tolerance level. Acupuncture points were stimulated at this final tolerance level for a period of 60 seconds each.[156] Following 5 days of TENS treatment, the patient reported decreased pain and demonstrated increased ROM and independent ADLs.

SUMMARY

Ultrasound, Fluidotherapy, and paraffin are the thermal agents that are presently the most beneficial for use with the burn patient. The heat produced by these modalities may have an effect on increasing the extensibility of collagen in scar tissue, hence increasing potential range of motion and possibly decreasing pain associated with passive stretch. For the acute burn patient, the use of hydrotherapy is better for wound care than exercise.

Several electrical modalities are useful in treating burn patients. Certain equipment may assist with the healing of small wounds (HVPC), while other modalities may afford some form of nondrug pain relief (TENS). Other useful electrical modalities include NMES, biofeedback, and perhaps MENS, which could be effective in application to movement re-education and pain relief.

Not only can many of these modalities be useful for problems related to the burn injury itself, but they also can be valuable in the treatment of problems, such as muscle spasm, which may be an indirect result of a burn injury. No single modality can solve all the difficulties consequent to burn injury; however, a combination of appropriate modalities, along with additional manual and conditioning techniques, may enhance current burn rehabilitation.

Additional study is imperative for determining the efficacy of the discussed physical agents, as well as other therapeutic modalities in burn care. Inevitably, burn therapists will be compelled to conduct clinical research in order to validate patient care choices. Substantiation of the benefits of physical agents in burn therapy could result in increased efficiency and effectiveness in the treatment of patients with burns.

REFERENCES

1. Greenberg, RS: The effects of hot packs and exercise on local blood flow. Phys Ther 52:273–278, 1972.
2. Abramson, DI, et al: Changes in blood flow, oxygen uptake and tissue temperatures produced by the topical application of wet heat. Arch Phys Med Rehabil 42:305–318, 1961.
3. Ganong, WF: Review of Medical Physiology. Appleton & Lange, Norwalk, 1991, pp 550–561.
4. Fox, RH and Hilton, SM: Bradykinin formation in human skin as a factor in heat vasodilatation. J Physiol 142:219–232, 1958.
5. Mense, S: Effects of temperature on the discharges of muscle spindles and tendon organs. Pfluegers Arch 374:159–166, 1978.
6. Fischer, E and Solomon, S: Physiological responses to heat and cold. In Licht, S (ed): Therapeutic Heat and Cold. Waverly Press, Baltimore, 1965, pp 157–159.
7. Lehmann, JF, et al: Modification of heating patterns produced by microwaves at the frequencies of 2456 and 900 mc. by physiologic factors in the human. Arch Phys Med Rehabil 45:555–563, 1964.
8. Hunter, J, Kerr, EH, and Whillans, MG: The relation between joint stiffness upon exposure to cold and the characteristics of synovial fluid. Can J Med Sci 30:367–377, 1952.
9. Wright, V and Johns, RJ: Physical factors concerned with the stiffness of normal and diseased joints. Bull Johns Hopkins Hosp 106:215–231, 1960.
10. Backlund, L and Tiselius, P: Objective measurement of joint stiffness in rheumatoid arthritis. Acta Rheum Scand 13:275, 1967.

11. Lehmann, JF: Effect of tissue temperatures on tendon extensibility. Arch Phys Med Rehabil 51:481–487, 1970.
12. Warren, GC, Lehmann, JF, and Koblanski, JN: Heat and stretch procedures: An evaluation using rat tail tendon. Arch Phys Med Rehabil 57:122–126, 1976.
13. LeBan, MM: Collagen tissue: Implications of its response in vitro. Arch Phys Med Rehabil 43:461–466, 1962.
14. Randall, LM and Krusen, FH: A consideration of the Elliott treatment of pelvic inflammatory disease of women. Arch Phys Med Rehabil 18:283–287, 1937.
15. Brown, AM: Physical medicine in athletic rehabilitation. Maryland Med J 19:61–64, 1970.
16. Eitner, D: Uses of heat. In Kuprian, W (ed): Physical Therapy for Sports. WB Saunders, Philadelphia, 1981, pp 52–61.
17. Fischer, E and Solomon, S: Physiological responses to heat and cold. In Licht, S (ed): Therapeutic Heat and Cold. Waverly Press, Baltimore, 1965, pp 134–135.
18. Lehmann, JF and deLateur, BJ: Therapeutic heat. In Lehmann, JF (ed): Therapeutic Heat and Cold, ed 3. Williams & Wilkins, Baltimore, 1990, pp 418–420.
19. Michlovitz, SL: Biophysical principles of heating and superficial heat agents. In Michlovitz, SL (ed): Thermal Agents in Rehabilitation. FA Davis, Philadelphia, 1990, p 89.
20. Abramson, DI: Physiologic basis for the use of physical agents in peripheral vascular disorders. Arch Phys Med Rehabil 46:216–244, 1965.
21. Smith, DW, Clarren, SK, and Harvey, MAS: Hyperthermia as a possible teratogenic agent. J Pediatr 92:878–883, 1978.
22. Ward, RS and Tuckett, RP: Quantitative threshold changes in cutaneous sensation of patients with burns. J Burn Care Rehabil 12:569–575, 1991.
23. Folkow, B, et al: Studies on the reactions of the cutaneous vessels to cold exposure. Acta Physiol Scand 58:342–354, 1963.
24. Clarke, RSJ, Hellon, RF, and Lind, AR: Vascular reactions of the human forearm to cold. Clin Sci 17:165–179, 1958.
25. Lewis, T: Observations upon the reactions of the vessels of the human skin to cold. Heart 15:177–208, 1930.
26. Major, TC, Schwinghamer, JM, and Winston, S: Cutaneous and skeletal muscle vascular responses to hypothermia. Am J Physiol 240(Heart Circ Physiol 9):H868–H873, 1981.
27. McGown, HL: Effects of cold application on maximal isometric contraction. Phys Ther 47:185–192, 1967.
28. Oliver, RA, et al: Isometric muscle contraction response during recovery from reduced intramuscular temperature. Arch Phys Med Rehabil 60:126–129, 1979.
29. Johnson, J and Leider, FE: Influence of cold bath on maximum hand grip strength. Percept Motor Skills 44:323–326, 1977.
30. Clendenin, MA and Szumski, AJ: Influence of cutaneous ice application on single motor units in human. Phys Ther 51:166–175, 1971.
31. Teichner, WH: Manual dexterity in the cold. J Appl Physiol 11:333–338, 1957.
32. Zankel, HT: Effect of physical agents on motor conduction velocity of the ulnar nerve. Arch Phys Med Rehabil 47:787–792, 1966.
33. Li, CL: Effect of cooling on neuromuscular transmission in the rat. Am J Physiol 194:200–206, 1958.
34. Douglas, WW and Malcom, JL: The effect of localized cooling on conduction in cat nerves. J Physiol 130:53–71, 1955.
35. Michlovitz, SL: Cryotherapy: The use of cold as a therapeutic agent. In Michlovitz, SL (ed): Thermal Agents in Rehabilitation. FA Davis, Philadelphia, 1990, p 84.
36. Lehmann, JF and deLateur, BJ: Cryotherapy. In Lehmann, JF (ed): Therapeutic Heat and Cold. Williams & Wilkins, Baltimore, 1990, pp 624–627.
37. Gertsen, JW: Effect of ultrasound on tendon extensibility. Am J Phys Med 34:362–369, 1955.
38. Lehmann, JF, et al: Heating of joint structures by ultrasound. Arch Phys Med Rehabil 49:28–30, 1968.
39. Currier, DP, Greathouse, D, and Swift, T: Sensory nerve conduction: Effect of ultrasound. Arch Phys Med Rehabil 59:181–185, 1978.
40. Currier, DP and Kramer, JF: Sensory nerve conduction: Heating effects of ultrasound and infrared. Physiother Can 34:241, 1982.
41. Kramer, JF: Ultrasound: Evaluation of its mechanical and thermal effects. Arch Phys Med Rehabil 65:223–227, 1984.
42. Paul, WD and Imig, CJ: Temperature and blood flow studies after ultrasonic irradiation. Am J Phys Med 34:370–375, 1955.
43. Abramson, DI, et al: Changes in blood flow, oxygen uptake and tissue temperatures produced by therapeutic physical agents; I. Effect of ultrasound. Am J Phys Med 39:51–62, 1960.
44. Lehmann, JF, Brunner, GD, and Stow, RW: Pain threshold measurements after therapeutic application of ultrasound, microwaves and infrared. Arch Phys Med Rehabil 39:560–565, 1958.
45. Dunn, F and Frizzell, LA: Bioeffects of ultrasound. In Lehmann, JF (ed): Therapeutic Heat and Cold. Williams & Wilkins, Baltimore, 1990, pp 403–404.

46. Gertsen, JW: Ultrasonics and muscle disease. Am J Phys Med 33:68–74, 1954.
47. Bierman, W: Ultrasound in the treatment of scars. Arch Phys Med Rehabil 35:209–214, 1954.
48. Kottke, FJ, Pauley, DL, and Ptak, RA: The rationale for prolonged stretching for correction of shortening of connective tissue. Arch Phys Med Rehabil 47:345–352, 1966.
49. Lehmann, JF, et al: Effect of therapeutic temperatures on tendon extensibility. Arch Phys Med Rehabil 51:481–487, 1970.
50. Warren, CG, Lehmann, JF, and Koblanski, JN: Heat and stretch procedures: An evaluation using rat tail tendon. Arch Phys Med Rehabil 57:122–126, 1976.
51. Marvin, JA: Perioperative care of the burn patient. In Boswick, JA (ed): The Art and Science of Burn Care. Aspen, Rockville, 1987, pp 93–100.
52. Roberts, ML and Pruitt, BA: Nursing care and psychological considerations. In Artz, C, Moncrief, J, Pruitt, B (eds): Burns: A Team Approach. WB Saunders, Philadelphia, 1979, pp 370–389.
53. Edlich, RF, et al: Bioengineering principles of hydrotherapy. J Burn Care and Rehabil 8:580–584, 1987.
54. Nothdurft, D, Smith, PS, and LeMaster, JE: Exercise and treatment modalities. In Fisher, SV and Helm, PA (eds): Comprehensive Rehabilitation of Burns. Williams & Wilkins, Baltimore, 1984, pp 96–127.
55. Thomson, PD, et al: A survey of burn hydrotherapy in the United States. J Burn Care Rehabil 11:151–155, 1990.
56. Devlin, PM, et al: Automated hydrotherapy pool water treatment system. J Burn Care Rehabil 10:74–78, 1989.
57. Edlich, RF, et al: Water treatment of hydrotherapy exercise pools. J Burn Care Rehabil 9:510–515, 1988.
58. Richard, RL, et al: Autocontamination of the burn patient by hydrotherapy. Bull Clin Rev Burn Inj 1:40–41, 1984.
59. Valenza, J, et al: A clinical study of a new modality: Fluidotherapy. J Am Pod Assoc 69:440–442, 1979.
60. Borrell, RM, et al: Fluidotherapy: Evaluation of a new heat modality. Arch Phys Med Rehabil 58:69–71, 1977.
61, Borrell, RM and Henley, EJ: Fluidotherapy in a hand clinic. Arch Phys Med Rehabil 60:536, 1979.
62. Alcorn, R, et al: Fluidotherapy and exercise in the management of sickle cell anemia. Phys Ther 64:1520–1522, 1984.
63. Borrell, RM, et al: Comparison of in vivo temperatures produced by hydrotherapy, paraffin wax treatment, and fluidotherapy. Phys Ther 60:1273–1276, 1980.
64. Head, M and Helm, P: Paraffin and sustained stretching in treatment of burn contracture. Burns 4:136–139, 1977.
65. Gross, JD and Stafford, FS: Modified Method for Application of Paraffin Wax for Treatment of Burn Scar. J Burn Care Rehabil 5:394, 1984.
66. Kloth, L: Shortwave and microwave diathermy. In Michlovitz, SL (ed): Thermal Agents in Rehabilitation. FA Davis, Philadelphia, 1990, pp 170–199.
67. Lehmann, JF, Warren, CG, and Scham, SM: Therapeutic heat and cold. Clin Orthop 99:207–245, 1974.
68. Seitz, LM and Snyder-Mackler, L: Therapeutic uses of lights in rehabilitation. In Michlovitz, SL (ed): Thermal Agents in Rehabilitation. FA Davis, Philadelphia, 1990, pp 207–208.
69. Kana, JS, et al: Effect of low-power density laser radiation of healing of open skin wounds in rats. Arch Surg 116:293–296, 1981.
70. Yew, DT, Ling Wong, SL, and Chan, Y: Stimulating effect of the low dose laser—A new hypothesis. Acta Anat 112:131–136, 1982.
71. Kovacs, IB, Mester, E, and Gorog, P: Laser-induced stimulation of the vascularization of the healing wound: An ear chamber experiment. Experentia 4:341–343, 1974.
72. MacMillan, JD, Maxwell, WA, and Chichester, CO: Lethal photosensitization of microorganisms with light from a continuous-wave gas laser. Photochem Photobiol 5:555, 1966.
73. Seitz, LM and Kleinkort, JA: Low-power laser: Its applications in physical therapy. In Michlovitz, SL (ed): Thermal Agents in Rehabilitation. FA Davis, Philadelphia, 1986, pp 209–219.
74. Wakin, KG: Influence of frequency of muscle stimulation on circulation in the stimulated extremity. Arch Phys Med Rehabil 34:291–295, 1953.
75. Folkow, B and Halicka, HO: A comparison between "red" and "white" muscle with respect to blood supply, capillary surface area and oxygen uptake during rest and exercise. Microvasc Res 1:1–14, 1968.
76. Currier, DP: Electrical stimulation for improving muscular strength and blood flow. In Nelson, RM and Currier, DP (eds): Clinical Electrotherapy. Appleton & Lange, Norwalk, 1991, pp 188–191.
77. Newton, R: High-voltage pulsed galvanic stimulation: Theoretical bases and clinical applications. In Nelson, RM and Currier, DP (eds): Clinical Electrotherapy. Appleton & Lange, Norwalk, 1991, pp 201–220.
78. Hudlicka, O, et al: The effect of different patterns of long-term stimulation on contractile properties and myosin light chains in rabbit fast muscles. Pfluegers Arch 393:164–170, 1982.

79. Myrhage, R and Hudlicka, O: Capillary growth in chronically stimulated adult skeletal muscle as studied by intravital microscopy and histological methods in rabbits and rats. Microvasc Res 16:73–75, 1978.
80. Booth, FW: Time course of muscular atrophy during immobilization of hindlimbs in rats. J Appl Physiol 43:656–661, 1977.
81. Lainey, CG, Walmsley, RP, and Andrew, GM: Effectiveness of exercise alone versus exercise plus electrical stimulation in strengthening the quadriceps muscle. Physiother Can 35:5, 1983.
82. Greathouse, DG, et al: Effects of electrical stimulation on ultrastructure of rat skeletal muscles. Phys Ther 64:755, 1984.
83. Eisenburg, BR and Gilai, A: Structural changes in single muscle fibers after stimulation at a low frequency. J Gen Physiol 74:1–16, 1979.
84. Eriksson, E and Haggmark, T: Comparison of isometric muscle training and electrical stimulation supplementing isometric muscle training in the recovery after major knee ligament surgery. Am J Sports Med 7:169–171, 1979.
85. Munsat, TL, McNeal, DR, and Waters, RL: Preliminary observations on prolonged stimulation of peripheral nerve in man. Arch Neurol 33:608–617, 1976.
86. Baker, LL, et al: Electrical stimulation of wrist and fingers for hemiplegic patients. Phys Ther 59:1495–1499, 1979.
87. Rowley, BA, et al: The influence of electrical current on an infecting microorganism in wounds. Ann NY Acad Sci 238:543–551, 1974.
88. Barranco, SD, et al: In vitro effect of weak direct current on staphylococcus aureus. Clin Orthop 100:250–255, 1974.
89. Rowley, BA: Electrical current effects on E. coli growth rates. Proc Soc Exp Biol Med 139:929–934, 1972.
90. Kincaid, CB and Lavoie, KH: Inhibition of bacterial growth in vitro following stimulation with high voltage, monophasic, pulsed current. Phys Ther 69:651–655, 1989.
91. Wheeler, P, et al: Neural considerations in the healing of ulcerated tissue by clinical electrotherapeutic application of weak direct current: Findings and theory. In Reynolds, DV and Sjoberg, AE (eds): Neuroelectric Research. Charles C. Thomas, Springfield, Illinois, 1971, pp 83–96.
92. Pilla, AA: Electrochemical information transfer and its possible role in the control of cell function. In Brighton, CT, Black, J, and Pollack, SR (eds): Electrical Properties of Bone and Cartilage. Grune & Stratton, New York, 1979, pp 455–485.
93. Carey, IC and Lepley, D: Effect of continuous direct electric current on healing wounds. Surg Forum 13:33–34, 1955.
94. Harrington, DB, Meyer, R, and Klein, RM: Effects of small amounts of electric current at the cellular level. Ann NY Acad Sci 238:300–306, 1974.
95. Myklebust, BM and Kloth, L: Electrodiagnostic and electrotherapeutic instrumentation: Characteristics of recordings and stimulation systems and principles of safety. In Gersh, MR (ed): Electrotherapy in Rehabilitation. FA Davis, Philadelphia, 1992, pp 51–100.
96. Cook, TM: Instrumentation. In Nelson, RM and Currier, DP (eds): Clinical Electrotherapy. Appleton & Lange, Norwalk, 1991, pp 11–34.
97. Loeser, JD, Black, RG, and Christman, A: A relief of pain by transcutaneous stimulation. J Neurosurg 42:308–314, 1975.
98. Mannheimer, JS: Electrode placements for transcutaneous electrical nerve stimulation. Phys Ther 58:1455–1462, 1978.
99. Melzack, R: Prolonged relief of pain by brief intense transcutaneous somatic stimulation. Pain 1:357–373, 1975.
100. Melzack, R, Stillwell, DM, and Fox, EJ: Trigger points and acupuncture points for pain: Correlations and implications. Pain 3:3–23, 1977.
101. Picaza, JA, et al: Pain suppression by peripheral stimulation, Part I. Observations with transcutaneous stimuli. Surg Neurol 4:105–114, 1975.
102. Sweet, WH and Wepsic, JG: Treatment of chronic pain by stimulation of primary afferent neuron. Trans Am Neurol Assoc 93:103–107, 1968.
103. Barr, JO: Transcutaneous electrical nerve stimulation for pain management. In Nelson, RM and Currier, DP (eds): Clinical Electrotherapy. Appleton & Lange, Norwalk, 1991, pp 261–316.
104. Roeser, W, et al: The use of transcutaneous nerve stimulation for pain control in athletic medicine: A preliminary report. Am J Sports Med 4:210–213, 1976.
105. Ersek, RA: Relief of acute musculoskeletal pain using transcutaneous electrical neurostimulation. J Am Coll Emerg Phys 6:300–303, 1977.
106. Myers, RA, Woolf, CJ, and Mitchell, D: Management of acute traumatic pain by peripheral transcutaneous electrical nerve stimulation. S Afr J Med 52:309–312, 1977.
107. Long, D: Cutaneous afferent stimulation for relief of chronic pain. Clin Neurosurg 21:257–268, 1974.
108. Kirsch, WM, Lewis, JA, and Simon, RH: Experiences with electrical stimulation devices for the control of chronic pain. Med Instrum 9:217–220, 1975.

109. Thorsteinsson, G, et al: The placebo effect of transcutaneous electrical stimulation. Pain 5:31–41, 1978.
110. Loeser, JD: Nonpharmacologic approaches to pain relief. In Ng, LKY and Bonica, JJ (eds): Pain, Discomfort and Humanitarian Care. Elsevier, New York, 1980, pp 275–292.
111. Lewis, SM, et al: Effects of auricular acupuncture-like transcutaneous electric nerve stimulation on pain levels following wound care in patients with burns: A pilot study. J Burn Care and Rehabil 11:322, 1990.
112. Baker, LL: Clinical uses of neuromuscular electrical stimulation. In Nelson, RM and Currier, DP (eds): Clinical Electrotherapy. Appleton & Lange, Norwalk, 1991, pp 143–170.
113. LeDoux, J and Quinones, MA: An investigation of the use of percutaneous electrical stimulation in muscle reeducation. Phys Ther 61:737, 1981.
114. Peckham, PH, Mortimer, JT, and Marsolais, EB: Alteration in the force and fatiguability of skeletal muscle in quadriplegic humans following exercise induced by chronic electrical stimulation. Clin Orthop 114:326–334, 1976.
115. Baker, LL, Parker, K, and Sanderson, D: Neuromuscular electrical stimulation for the head-injured patient. Phys Ther 63:1967–1974, 1983.
116. Apfel, LM, et al: Functional electrical stimulation in intrinsic/extrinsic imbalanced burned hands. J Burn Care and Rehabil 8:97–102, 1987.
117. Lindstrom, B, et al: Electrically induced short-lasting tetanus of the calf muscles for prevention of deep vein thrombosis. Br J Surg 69:203–206, 1982.
118. Im, MJ, Lee, WPA, and Hoopes, JE: Effect of electrical stimulation on survival of skin flaps in pigs. Phys Ther 70:37–40, 1990.
119. Williams, R and Carey, L: Studies in the production of standard venous thrombosis. Ann Surg 149:381–387, 1959.
120. Anderson, SA and Holmgren, E: Pain threshold effects of peripheral conditioning stimulation. In Bonica, JJ and Able-Fessard, D (eds): Advances in Pain Research and Therapy. Raven, New York, 1976, pp 761–768.
121. Sohn, M, Weinstein, MA, and Robbins, RD: The levator syndrome and its treatment with high voltage electrogalvanic stimulation. Am J Surg 44:580–582, 1982.
122. Wolf, SL: Electromyographic biofeedback: An overview. In Nelson, RM and Currier, DP (eds): Clinical Electrotherapy. Appleton & Lange, Norwalk, 1991, pp 361–384.
123. Chapman, SL: A review and clinical perspective on the use of EMG and thermal biofeedback for chronic headaches. Pain 27:1–43, 1986.
124. Turner, JA and Chapman, CR: Psychological interventions for chronic pain: A critical review. I. Relaxation training and biofeedback. Pain 12:1–21, 1982.
125. Jessup, BA: Biofeedback. In Wall, PD and Melzack, R (eds): Textbook of Pain. Churchill Livingstone, Edinburgh, 1984, pp 776–786.
126. Fields, HL: Nondrug pain control. In Fields, HL (ed): Pain. McGraw-Hill, New York, 1987, pp 307–334.
127. Picker, RI: Current trends: Low-volt pulsed microamp stimulation, Part I. Clin Manag Phys Ther 9:10–15, 1989.
128. Picker, RI: Current trends: Low-volt pulsed microamp stimulation, Part II: Clin Manag Phys Ther 9:28–33, 1989.
129. Brighton, CT: Current concepts review: The treatment of nonunion with electricity. J Bone Joint Surg (Am) 63:847, 1981.
130. Owoeye, I, Speilholz, N, and Nelson, AJ: Low-intensity pulsed galvanic current and the healing of tenotomized rat achilles tendons: Preliminary report using load-to-breaking measurements. Arch Phys Med Rehabil 68:415–418, 1987.
131. Carley, PJ, and Wainapel, SF: Electrotherapy for acceleration of wound healing: Low intensity direct current. Arch Phys Med Rehabil 66:443–446, 1985.
132. Salter, RB: The biologic concept of continuous passive motion of synovial joints. Clin Orthop 242:12–25, 1989.
133. Coutts, RD, Toth, C, and Kaita, J: The role of continuous passive motion in the rehabilitation of the total knee patient. In Hungerford, D (ed): Total Knee Arthroplasty. Williams & Wilkins, Baltimore, 1984, pp 126–132.
134. McGough, CM: Introduction to CPM. J Burn Care Rehabil 9:494–495, 1988.
135. Johnson, CL: PT/OT Forum (editorial). J Burn Care Rehabil 9:396, 1988.
136. Covey, MH, et al: Efficacy of continuous passive motion (CPM) devices with hand burns. J Burn Care Rehabil 9:397–400, 1988.
137. McAllister, LP and Salazar, CA: Case report on the use of CPM on an electrical burn. J Burn Care Rehabil 9:401, 1988.
138. Covey, MH: Application of CPM devices with burn patients. J Burn Care Rehabil 9:496–497, 1988.
139. Richard, RL, Miller, SF and Staley, MJ: The physiologic response of a patient with critical burns to continuous passive motion. J Burn Care Rehabil 11:554–556, 1990.
140. Diehm, SL: CPM devices. J Burn Care Rehabil 9:498–503, 1988.

141. Richmand, DM, O'Donnell, TF, and Zelikovski, A: Sequential pneumatic compression of lymphedema. Arch Surg 120:1116–1119, 1985.
142. Ellingham, C: Mechanical agents: external compression. In Scully, RM and Barnes, MR (eds): Physical Therapy. JB Lippincott, Philadelphia, 1989, pp 909–914.
143. Falkel, JE: Burns. In O'Sullivan, SB and Schmitz, TJ (eds): Physical Rehabilitation: Assessment and Treatment. FA Davis, Philadelphia, 1988, pp 515–541.
144. Wood, EC and Becker, PD: Beard's Massage. WB Saunders, Philadelphia, 1981, pp 49–50.
145. Tappan, FM: Healing Massage Techniques, ed 2. Appleton & Lange, Norwalk, 1988, pp 83–85.
146. Holcomb, JR, Matos-Navarro, AY, and Goldman, RW: Critical Care in the Hyperbaric Chamber. In Davis, JC and Hunt, TK (eds): Problem Wounds: The Role of Oxygen. Elsevier, New York, 1988, p 200.
147. Kravitz, S: Use of Hyperbaric Oxygen in Wound Healing. In Kloth, LC, McCulloch, JM, and Feedar, JA (eds): Wound Healing: Alternatives in Management. FA Davis, Philadelphia, 1990, pp 302–320.
148. Babior, BM: Oxygen-dependent microbial killing by phagocytes. N Engl J Med 298:659, 1974.
149. Lucca, M, Unger, HD, and Devenny, AM: Treatment of Fournier's gangrene with adjunctive hyperbaric oxygen therapy. Am J Emerg Med 8:385, 1990.
150. Nelson, EW, Jr, Bright, DE, and Villar, LF: Closure of refractory perineal Crohn's lesion. Integration of hyperbaric oxygen into case management. Dig Dis Sci 35:1561, 1990.
151. Hunt, TK and Pai, MP: The effect of varying ambient oxygen tensions on wound metabolism and collagen synthesis. Surg Gynecol Obstet 135:561, 1972.
152. Grossman, AR: Hyperbaric oxygen in the treatment of burns. Ann Plast Surg 1:163, 1978.
153. Cianci, P, et al: Adjunctive hyperbaric oxygen therapy reduces length of hospitalization in thermal burns. J Burn Care Rehabil 10:432, 1989.
154. Cianci, P, et al: Adjunctive hyperbaric oxygen in the treatment of thermal burns: An economic analysis. J Burn Care Rehabil 11:140, 1990.
155. Davis, JC, Dunn, JM, and Heimbach, RD: Hyperbaric Medicine: Patient Selection, Treatment Procedures, and Side-Effects. In Davis, JC and Hunt, TK (eds): Problem Wounds: The Role of Oxygen. Elsevier, New York, 1988, p 230.
156. Lein, DH, et al: Comparison of effects of transcutaneous electrical nerve stimulation of auricular, somatic, and the combination of auricular and somatic acupuncture points on experimental pain threshold. Phys Ther 69:671–678, 1989.

CHAPTER 16

Discharge Planning and Follow-up Burn Care

Cheryl J. Leman, MA, OTR/L, FAOTA
Nanci Ricks, PT

Open communication among burn team members is necessary to adequately prepare a burn patient for discharge from the hospital. Wound healing status is an important determinant in deciding the day of discharge but not the only factor that must be considered. Knowledge of the home environment, distance between the home and hospital, and support systems available are other considerations the team must investigate prior to setting a discharge date. To provide a smooth transition from the hospital to home, information gathering should start as soon as possible following hospital admission. Regardless of the team member who obtains this information (e.g., the social worker, physical or occupational therapist, or nurse) effective discharge planning can occur only through a coordinated team effort.[1-3] The purpose of this chapter is to familiarize the therapist with the discharge planning process, items to include for a successful home program, and issues to address with outpatient therapy and follow-up of a burn patient.

DISCHARGE PROCESS

Family Structure

The family structure is important in both adult and pediatric burn cases. Determining how a family functions must be established early to plan a home care teaching program. Who will be the primary caregiver, who will provide moral support for independent self-care function, and who will be responsible for assuring that appropriate home therapy occurs are key questions to answer. Consideration must be given to whether the primary caregiver in the home is capable of providing adequate post-burn care or if alternative placement is needed.

If a child is to go home with foster parents, the involvement of the child's biological parents must be clarified.[4] Often natural parents are required to attend therapy sessions even if their child is in foster care. The responsibilities of the natural parents must be determined in terms of home programming. If the child is going to a temporary foster placement, the type of recordkeeping needed for the courts about parental participation also must be decided. Social services personnel are helpful in this situation.

Payment Method

A vital piece of information that must be obtained at the beginning of hospitalization is whether an individual has insurance, and if he or she does, what is the extent of coverage. The limitations in services covered can affect greatly discharge plans. Although some institutions have means of obtaining funds for acute care, outpatient care plans can be affected seriously if insurance coverage is unavailable. Lack of funding does not mean that care may not be obtained, rather that creative discharge planning must be implemented early. Cases that are covered by worker's compensation generally are easier to plan. With worker's compensation, however, the team must ensure that a patient's needs are communicated and that requirements for documentation are followed. In cases in which there is no insurance, application for medical assistance or Medicaid must be implemented immediately. For patients covered by a health maintenance organization (HMO), approval for outpatient services must be obtained prior to the date of service. Depending on the HMO plan, a patient may not be able to return to the primary treatment facility following discharge.

Home Situation

Because many burn injuries occur in the home with resultant house damage, information about the status of the home is important. Many adult burn patients may need to find alternative housing when discharged. In the case of pediatric burn patients whose parents also have been injured, other nearby family members may provide housing. If a child's burn was the result of abuse, arrangements for foster housing may need to be initiated with an appropriate agency. Adults, especially the elderly, also can be the victims of abuse, so evaluation of the home environment for these individuals may be indicated.

Another consideration is whether there are architectural barriers in the home that will impede independent function. If a patient's limitations are going to be long term, home adaptation plans and adaptive equipment training may need to be implemented. Adequate bathing facilities are necessary for proper wound and skin care.

Senior citizens often are burned in the home while doing normal activities of daily living such as cooking or bathing. Many times an injury occurs because the individual has a disability or marginal functional skills as a result of dementia or physical deterioration. In these situations, alternate living environments may need to be considered or home care assistance will need to be arranged.

Home Location

If a patient needs to travel a distance to the primary care facility, the means of transportation must be considered. The driver of a family may have to work or may be the one injured, requiring alternate transportation arrangements. Although public transportation may be available, the patient may lack the physical skills to use it safely. Facially disfigured patients also may not be ready to use public transportation. In cases in which appropriate public transportation is not readily available, special-needs transportation services may be purchased. For persons whose cost of care is being compensated, purchased services generally can be arranged.

When the distance between the home and hospital is too great to travel daily, referral to home care agencies or alternate living arrangements may be needed. When a patient requires continued intensive therapy, referral to an in-patient rehabilitation facility may be the only solution.

Community Resources

There are numerous community resources available, and they should be considered in discharge planning. Visiting nurses can assist in providing home wound care. Home health therapists should be consulted for home adaptations. Therapists also may assist in teaching self-care and exercise activities. Referral to a burn support group should be considered when adjustment problems are apparent. The social worker generally can arrange these services with the patient, but the therapist usually identifies the need. Rehabilitation nurses also can organize community resources when assigned a specific patient's case.

Other Disciplines

In addition to occupational and physical therapy, there are other disciplines that can help burn patients adapt and achieve optimal function. These disciplines include vocational counselors, social workers, psychologists, chaplains, recreational and speech therapists, orthotists, and cosmetologists. Depending on a patient's needs, referral to any of these professionals will augment the rehabilitation process.[3,4]

DISCHARGE EVALUATION AND DOCUMENTATION

A burn injury can affect function in many ways. Even if the total body surface area burn is limited, the entire patient must be evaluated to assure that there is a complete record for future reference. The patient and family should understand the evaluation information and how the data will be used to assess progress. Using the information to set goals for a home program can give the patient a focus for treatment and provide feedback during subsequent follow-up visits and therapy. For example, if a patient requires 150° of shoulder flexion to reach glasses in a cabinet, this measurement can be used as a goal to achieve through home exercises.

The following information should be included in a complete discharge evaluation for a burn patient. Some of the items are specific for pediatric patients; however, most of the information should be obtained on all patients.

Physical Function

A patient's range of motion (ROM), posture, strength, and endurance should be monitored throughout hospitalization. Precisely measuring ROM or strength is sometimes difficult during the acute wound healing phase due to dressings and pain, but obtaining an objective record at the time of discharge usually is possible.

A goniometric evaluation of ROM should include all motions of any involved area and a generalized total body ROM assessment. On subsequent measurements, the motions of the involved area should be evaluated the same way to assure that the proximal and distal joints are in the same position. For example, when assessing shoulder flexion, the position of the elbow and forearm and trunk posture should be closely controlled to fully assess the effect that scarring can have on shoulder motion. Documentation includes whether the elbow was flexed or extended and whether the forearm was supinated or pronated.

Whenever possible, strength should be assessed using a system that can be calibrated to assure that the results are objective and reproducible. When strength is poor, a manual muscle test (MMT) is appropriate. When strength is fair to good on a MMT, an isokinetic dynamometer or another functional strength test can be used.

Burn patients' cardiopulmonary endurance can be lower than normal at hospital discharge. Decreased cardiopulmonary endurance can occur because of decreased activity levels during hospitalization, an inhalation injury, or even the effect of trunk scarring on chest expansion and posture. Although the patient has been encouraged to walk during hospitalization, function at home requires a greater level of endurance than what is maintained in a hospital. A baseline record of endurance easily can be obtained by recording heart rate, blood pressure, and respiration responses to an established amount of aerobic exercise. A standardized cycle ergometer, treadmill, or the Step Test are examples of activities that can be used.[5]

In addition, the burn patient should be evaluated in terms of: (1) postural symmetry, (2) scoliosis, (3) kyphosis, (4) decrease or increase in lordosis, (5) leg length, and (6) ability to maintain correct alignment over time.

Developmental Level

A record of a child's developmental level at discharge is vital information. This information can be compared to admission or future evaluations to document progression or regression and in determining therapy frequency. A standardized test is useful but not imperative. Whatever approach is used, the therapist should include all of the child's highest developmental skills. During an interview with the parents, the child's development prior to hospitalization should be documented.

Kinesthetic Awareness

Generally defined as a person's awareness of where his or her body is in space, kinesthetic awareness can encompass sensation, body image, and spatial awareness. Prolonged bed rest, hospitalization, and injury to the skin and underlying tissue can affect a patient's kinesthetic awareness. A valid standardized test to measure kinesthetic awareness in burn patients presently is unavailable. However, there are several ways to assess kinesthetic awareness, such as opposite extremity placing and movement or tactile sensation tests. Another less objective assessment includes observing whether the patient looks at, uses, and touches most areas of the body. The therapist should determine if there is behavior that may indicate a decreased proprioceptive or tactile sense and whether the patient moves in a manner that depicts an internal awareness of his or her body in space.

Neurologic Status

A burn injury or its treatment can cause damage to peripheral nerves.[6] There also can be central nervous system damage. This damage can be due to smoke inhalation, chemical toxicity, or other brain injury at the time of burn trauma. Many times, the therapist is one of the few members of the burn team who has the knowledge to identify subtle signs of neurologic involvement during the acute care phase. If neurologic complications have occurred during hospitalization, the extent of deficit should be noted at discharge. This documentation can serve as a baseline for monitoring recovery and developing an appropriate treatment plan.

Scar Tissue

Every burn patient will scar differently. Scar activity may be affected by factors such as: (1) race, (2) age, (3) depth of burn, (4) infections during wound healing, (5) skin care, and (6) compliance with pressure therapy. At discharge, an accurate description of a patient's scar tissue should be obtained to use as a basis for comparison in the future.

Three characteristics used to describe scar are color, contour, and texture.[7] The color intensity of the scar should be documented. If scar tissue is elevated, the location and height should be noted. The pliability of the scar should be recorded to indicate whether the scar is rigid or soft when pinched gently. How the scar feels when massaged and appears when pressure is applied and then removed should be described. Skin-grafted areas and those allowed to heal spontaneously should be noted, as well as the appearance of any remaining open wounds.

Pressure Therapy

Patients usually are discharged from a hospital with some form of pressure therapy (see Chapter 14). Their pressure program, including type and location of insert materials, should be documented. If a patient has been measured for custom garments, the style of garment ordered should be noted. Skin condition should be described in terms of fragility (e.g., translucent, shiny, or thin) and ease of blistering, or durability to resist shearing forces of custom garments.

Functional Skills

Assessment of activities of daily living skills should include whether the patient can eat, dress, and perform bathing and grooming skills independently or the amount of assistance that is needed. The time the patient requires for these activities and any adapted motions or equipment should be documented. The patient's ability to perform transfers (e.g., bed, chair, tub) as well as the pattern and speed of ambulation should be recorded. Assessment of kitchen skills is important with patients who were injured while cooking. If hand strength and dexterity are affected, the patient's limitations and kitchen safety techniques should be reviewed and documented.

Documentation

A discharge summary must be entered in a patient's medical record to comply with hospital standards, assure reimbursement, support quality assurance programs, provide evidence for chart audits by insurance companies, and to indicate the patient's condition and level of function. The summary note should include the types of treatment administered, frequency, and the patient's functional status at the time of discharge. The amount of patient education provided and the patient's level of understanding of his or her condition should be included. The date of any return appointment or where the patient is to receive further treatment also should be noted.

If the patient is transferred to another hospital or will receive outpatient therapy at another facility, a discharge report should be prepared (Table 16–1). This report is independent of the hospital chart summary but contains the same evaluation data. For a successful referral, the receiving therapist must have a complete review of the patient's physical condition and response to previous treatment. In areas without a burn unit, the therapist may have limited experience in burn rehabilitation and may

TABLE 16–1. Items to Include in a Discharge Evaluation

1. Physical function
   a. ROM
   b. Strength
   c. Endurance
   d. Posture
2. Developmental level
3. Kinesthetic sense
4. Neurologic involvement
5. Scar tissue
6. Pressure therapy
7. Functional skills

require extensive information about the patient. If video equipment is available, discharge video tapes of the patient are useful in place of written reports.[8]

HOME PROGRAM

The patient and family must be well educated about the home care process prior to discharge.[9] Home care booklets, classes, and video tapes are the primary means that many burn care facilities use to convey this information.[10-13] Pictures are effective means of education with patients from various ethnic groups and socioeconomic backgrounds to overcome language differences. If the family has access to a video cassette recorder, video cassettes are an excellent way of documenting function, evaluation results, therapy sessions, home exercises, pressure therapy, and skin care.[10-12] Once completed, a video tape can be used for family education or as information for a home care or outpatient therapist.

Regardless of the teaching method used, adequate time must be allowed for patient and family education. Throughout the patient's hospital course, open communication about what can be expected following discharge can aid the learning process.[14] A family conference prior to discharge will help to assure that everyone involved has an opportunity to have questions answered and participate in making decisions. Compliance following discharge is achieved when the patient and family have a thorough understanding of the necessary home care procedures and activities. A method for testing patient and family understanding, either through question and answers or demonstration of techniques, should be established. The basic components that should be covered in every home care program follow (Table 16-2).

Wound Care

Many times a patient is discharged with small wounds requiring continued care. Wound care instructions should include how to cleanse the wound, how to remove and apply dressings, frequency of care, and signs and symptoms of complications. The dressing usually is a nonadherent gauze that is thin enough to use under a pressure garment.

TABLE 16-2.
Topics to Include in a Home Program

1. Wound care
2. Skin care
3. Exercise regimen
4. Activities of daily living
5. Pressure program
6. Splints and orthotics

Skin Care

A burn patient usually will use a lubricating cream on healed areas of scar prior to discharge. The home program instructions should include type of cream to use and technique and frequency of application. The lubricant used depends on the quality or dryness of the skin or sometimes on the preference of a burn center staff.

Recently healed burn skin is more susceptible to sunburn, so the patient should always wear sunscreen when outside. The importance of avoiding sun exposure and the type of sunscreens that can be used should be explained.[15] Methods of bathing, whether in a shower or tub, should be covered in terms of length of time, frequency, and type of soap to use. Unscented soaps are preferred, but the specific brand is usually the preference of the physician. Techniques for dealing with sebaceous cysts, ingrown hairs, blisters, and itching also should be explained; however, instructions should be confirmed by the attending physician. Pigment changes and maturation should be addressed, in addition to the changing appearance of scars.

Exercise Regimen

The home exercise program should be explained clearly. What exercises are necessary, how to do them, the number of times they should be done throughout the day, repetitions per session, and how to judge progress should be included. Low-cost exercise equipment can be fabricated easily for home use[16] (Appendices O, P, and Q). Home exercise records, which include number of repetitions and frequency, help patients keep track of their daily exercise program. These records are also a good way of reporting to the therapist. A patient should understand clearly the need for exercises and what can occur if they are not performed correctly. A patient must be taught that without specific stretches or exercises, scars contract and can impair joint motion and function. The signs of progressing scar contracture and the need to seek immediate assistance if this occurs must be emphasized.

Methods to enhance a patient's overall physical well-being at home should be discussed. Examples of some activities to consider are aerobics, running, walking, cycling, swimming, dance, martial arts, and domestic activities such as woodworking, gardening, cooking, and cleaning.[17] The idea of going home with so many suggested activities and required exercises can be overwhelming to a patient. A patient may benefit from developing a daily activity schedule with advice from the therapist.

Activities of Daily Living

Although a patient may be able to perform independently self-care skills at discharge, continuing them independently at home must be emphasized. Many times the patient will seek assistance from a family member because this approach is easier or more time efficient. There also are times when family members, wanting to be helpful, will assist with self-care that the patient is able to do. To avoid this conflict, a summary of self-care activities the patient can perform independently and those requiring assistance should be provided. When needed, the use and purpose of adaptive equipment should be understood by the patient. This summary is reviewed and updated as the patient progresses through follow-up.

Pressure Program

During hospitalization, a patient usually is educated about long-term care needs, which may include the use of pressure garments. Various types of interim pressure garments may be in use by the time of discharge. Regardless of the amount of predischarge training, the need for pressure, the type of garments a patient will wear, and garment care techniques should be included in the home program. The therapist should explain to a patient that pressure on active scar tissue is the most effective way to achieve optimal results. How garments should fit, when they should be replaced, and how long a patient should wear them must be described. Problems that can arise with incorrect fit, who to call when problems occur, and how to reorder must be explained and given to a patient in writing to assure appropriate follow through with the prescribed program.

Splints

Conforming or dynamic splints may need to be used at home.[18] Many times they only are used when resting or at night. Sometimes a splint may need to be used during the day to increase function. Regardless of the types of splint used, splint application, wearing time, and care must be reviewed with a patient and family. Precautions include avoiding exposure of a thermoplastic splint to heat and not placing a pad under a splint to relieve pressure. Anytime a patient is discharged with a splint, a minimum 2-week follow-up appointment for splint recheck should be made due to changes in limb size or ROM that may occur. Educating the patient about these changes should help to prevent skin problems due to rubbing, shearing, or inappropriate pressure.

OUTPATIENT TREATMENT

A patient's appearance should be noted and functional baseline assessed at the first outpatient appointment. The discharge evaluation is reviewed and compared with the patient's presenting status. This comparison helps to assess adaptation to home and ability to follow through with home program instructions. Additionally, the patient's perception of progress, skin condition and pressure program compliance are factors to assess. A burn injury experience can affect patients emotionally and can have an affect on compliance and motivation. Ultimately, a patient (or caregiver of a child) is responsible for success of the outpatient program. Being aware of perceptions and attitudes helps in determining the need for other services such as counseling.

Determining the physical demands of a patient's job, if not done during hospitalization, must be determined during the outpatient treatment assessment. The physical demands of the job, tools used, strength requirements, and working environment should be identified. These are important factors for program planning that also help to determine whether vocational rehabilitation services will be needed. Many of the activities used to restore function can have a dual purpose by providing return-to-work conditioning.

Once the assessment is completed, the outpatient treatment plan can be developed, including short- and long-term goals. The therapist, in conjunction with the patient, determines the goals to be accomplished in 3 to 6 months and how to progress to that point. In most cases, goals should be directed toward a normal life-style, including self-care independence, return to work, and school. One must consider how the rehabilitation goals fit into a patient's life-style and how treatment can be included in the patient's normal daily routine. Taking the time to develop goals and a plan with a patient will encourage compliance with the outpatient treatment program.

Frequency

Initially, the number of times a week patients require formal rehabilitation depends on the extent of their needs and the support available at home. The treatment plan should prioritize activities to make the best use of the therapist's available time. Activities a patient can do without the therapist prior to the actual treatment time, such as removing garments, applying skin moisturizer, and beginning stretching exercises, should be identified to maximize the treatment session. As function improves, the number of visits per week can be decreased, with patients assuming greater responsibility for their own progress.

Treatment Intervention

Most outpatient rehabilitation treatments for burn patients use the same techniques as with other types of patients. The purpose may be the same, such as to increase strength, but the technique may vary depending on a patient's skin condition and age. The focus of any treatment activity should be to improve the patient's functional abilities in order to resume a normal life, which includes returning to work and school as soon as possible. For example, rather than having patients focus on doing shoulder exercises to increase range, the treatment should be directed toward reaching over head to grasp an object.

Sequencing the order of treatment activities is necessary to prevent tissue injury and minimize patient discomfort. Skin lubrication, massage, and stretching should precede strengthening exercises. This order is important to ensure optimal scar pliability. Maintaining consistency in the sequence of treatment activities teaches patient a program plan that can be followed at home, which may lead to improved compliance.

Skin Conditioning

Various activities can be used to improve skin tolerance for touch and the shearing forces of custom-made pressure garments. To increase skin tolerance for garments, interim types of pressure bandages and presized garments can be used.[19]

Massage and exercise while wearing the interim garments also can help to increase skin tolerance. Hypersensitivity is a problem with areas that heal spontaneously and with donor sites. These areas usually are hyperemic and very fragile during the early stages of wound maturation. Although interim pressure bandages and garments are helpful, some areas may require more attention in terms of desensitization. Activities requiring touch and use of different textures, graded from fine to coarse, can help increase skin tolerance and decrease sensitivity.

Stretching

Stretching is necessary to elongate scar tissue. Skin and scar lubrication and massage should precede stretching activities to prepare dry or tight skin for increased motion and to prevent skin rupture. Massage should be done gently to avoid friction, using creams that are not water-based.[20] The purpose of stretching to increase flexibility is so a patient can perform activities of daily living more fluidly.

If a patient lacks full ROM, stretching should be performed before initiating other types of exercise. When planning a stretching program, the following points should be remembered: (1) caution should be taken to avoid injury due to forceful, dynamic stretch; (2) slow, sustained stretching should be done first; (3) each stretch is held from 30 seconds to 5 minutes, depending on patient tolerance; and (4) effective stretching requires attention to the position of adjacent joints.

Instructing a patient to stretch at home in the morning should allow greater movement throughout the day. As children go through growth spurts and require more intensive therapy, stretching will play an essential part in their exercise regimen.

Flexibility Exercises

Flexibility exercises for a burn patient are essentially ROM exercises that involve combined joint movements. For example, elbow flexibility requires attention to changing positions of the shoulder, forearm, and wrist. In designing flexibility exercises for a patient, the focus is directed toward complete movement and the effect of the scar complex on the limb, rather than on a specific joint. Flexibility exercises are a form of active stretching.

Modalities

PARAFFIN

Paraffin is a modality used in outpatient burn treatment when flexibility, joint pain, and skin dryness are problems. Paraffin frequently is applied in conjunction with stretching because of the inherent heat and skin-lubricating effects. Paraffin can be used on any joint area where the skin is tight and extremely dry[20-22] (see Chapter 15).

CONTINUOUS PASSIVE MOTION

Continuous passive motion (CPM) devices can be used as an adjunct to a home program when the patient has difficulty with maintaining ROM. Since function is the goal, a CPM unit should be used only when the patient is resting or as a precursor to the daily exercise routine. CPM is beneficial for patients who cannot attend therapy on a regular basis but are reliable enough to use the device at home. Upon prescribing a CPM device, settings should be re-evaluated at least every 2 weeks.

Strengthening Exercises and Endurance Training

A myriad of exercise equipment is available for strength and endurance training. The choice of equipment used with a burn patient depends on what is available in the specific clinic. Free weights have been the basic strengthening modality used in the past; however, electronic and computerized equipment has become more popular. With decreased mortality occurring with burn patients, the goal of burn rehabilitation has progressed from independent self-care to return to a normal life, including work and school activities. Although burn wound maturation may cause functional limitations for a period of time, the use of equipment for strength and endurance training can improve the recovery process.

FREE WEIGHTS

Free weights such as dumbbells and cuff weights commonly are used in outpatient burn rehabilitation for strengthening or augmenting stretching and ROM exercises.[23] Because of the sensations and discomfort a burn patient may experience with certain movements, attention should be given to the time needed to perform a set of repetitions and the posture or position a patient assumes during exercise. Although free-weight exercises are something a patient eventually should be able to do unsupervised, the exercises must be performed in a consistent manner to be effective. Patients should be taught to monitor their posture during an exercise session. Once a patient can do exercises independently, the number of sets, repetitions, and weight should be progressed as the patient's performance improves.

ISOKINETIC DYNAMOMETER

The isokinetic dynamometer has been used for strengthening and ROM exercises with burn patients during various phases of recovery.[24] The protocols used during outpatient burn therapy vary slightly from standard treatment protocols. Because of the slow and sometimes rigid movements a burn patient exhibits following discharge, the speed of exercise generally is decreased until the patient's speed of movement improves. Velocity spectrum training is effective for decreasing rigid movement in addition to gaining strength; however, the spectrum initially consists of lower speeds and less repetitions per speed than those recommended for orthopedic-type injuries.[25] Midrange or end-of-range training protocols are useful when there are limitations in ROM.[25] They allow strengthening to occur despite range limitations and often may increase motion. A patient's performance can be assessed using the objective data the equipment provides. Assessing the need for a change in protocol should be done after every five to eight treatments initially. As the patient progresses, the speeds and repetitions can be changed, depending on the patient's specific needs, with assessments being done every 10 to 15 treatments.

BALTIMORE THERAPEUTIC EQUIPMENT WORK SIMULATOR

The Baltimore Therapeutic Equipment (BTE) Work Simulator can be used for upper extremity exercise during various phases of burn recovery[26] (Appendix R). Although many rehabilitation programs use the BTE Work Simulator as an evaluation instrument, a number of exercise attachments can be used for fingertip desensitization, functional upper extremity strengthening, and ROM activities for a burn patient. The device provides information regarding resistance level, time, and distance of an exercise bout. Although protocols for its use vary, monitoring time and resistance level are effective in burn therapy to progress a patient through the rigid, slow movements that often are used to perform activities. One approach to exercise progression for a burn patient is to use 60 seconds as a baseline time unit, increasing to 3 or 5 minutes, depending on the attachment used. Once a patient's power level stabilizes, the resistance level and time can be increased.

ENDURANCE

Activities to increase endurance in adults should be graded by monitoring the patients heart rate, blood pressure, and respirations. Cycle ergometry and paced walking are methods commonly used for endurance training. The appropriate heart rate can be determined using either the individual's age or cardiopulmonary response to a graded exercise bout.[5] Whichever approach is used, attention should be given to monitoring a patient's response while maintaining a prescribed work rate for an established amount of time. Patients should learn how to monitor their response to continue their aerobic training when they are home.

Decreased endurance in children can affect them in many ways. They may not interact with other children energetically, and they can lose spontaneity in their play and generally have lethargic attitudes. Including endurance training concepts when treating children is important, although younger children probably will not cooperate with an aerobic exericse program. The therapist should select several activities a child can do at home and encourage performing the activities one after another on a daily basis. A child's attention span may limit the aerobic benefit of an activity, so creativity in designing a program will facilitate participation. Activities such as running around the block, cycling, swimming, continuous obstacle courses, or play on extensive playground equipment generally can keep a child active for longer than 15 minutes.

Work Conditioning

The physical demand of a job has three components: strength, flexibility, and endurance. Additionally, specific job skills require gross or fine motor skills or both. For a burn patient, physical limitations may pose potential barriers for successful return to work. Table 16-3 identifies some of these potential barriers.[27] Significant factors used to predict the length of time a burn patient will remain off work are the

TABLE 16–3. Potential Barriers for Return to Work

Heat/cold intolerance
Sensory impairment
Decreased standing tolerance
Decreased ROM and strength specific to burn area
Decreased cardiovascular endurance
Questionable tolerance for an 8-h work day
Safety issues relating to sensory loss or sensory changes
Fear of reinjury
Decreased grip/pinch strength
Decreased dexterity
Decreased functional capacity
Improper body mechanics
Questionable skin integrity

Adapted from Zeller et al.[27]

percent of total body surface area burned, depth of burn, and whether the hands were involved.[28]

The similarity between work skills training and burn therapy is the emphasis of basic physical skills such as reaching, stooping, pushing, lifting, and hand manipulation. Identifying the skills a patient will need to return to work and integrating them into basic treatment goals can be simple.[26] For example, a patient's job may require frequent reaching and manipulation of small objects at or above eye level. Many functional activities require the same skills. If a patient has upper extremity burns that involve the shoulder, arm, and hand, initial treatment goals include full shoulder, elbow, forearm, and hand ROM. As part of therapy, the patient performs hand activities overhead that mimic home care activities. By integrating specific work tasks into an outpatient program, the objectives of improved functional ability and beginning work skills acquisition are reached simultaneously.

There is a variety of equipment designed for work capacity training. Work-conditioning equipment from companies such as Valpar and WEST can be used for both acute and outpatient burn rehabilitation[26] (Appendix R). Knowledge of specific work skills and creative treatment planning are requisites for effective work conditioning during outpatient therapy (Table 16–4).

TABLE 16–4. Work-Conditioning Activities

Work Demands*	Equipment/Activities
Lifting, pushing, pulling	West 2, Isokinetics, BTE Work Simulator
Climbing, walking	Bicycle, flexibility exercises, Isokinetics, BTE Work Simulator
Stooping, kneeling, crouching	Valpar Component Work Samples; flexibility exercises; West 2, 4, and 7
Reaching, handling, manipulating	Valpar Component Work Samples, Pennsylvania Bi-manual, Minnesota Rate of Manipulation, BTE Work Simulator

*As found in Dictionary of Occupational Titles, ed 3, US Department of Labor, Government Printing Office, 1965, vol 1.

Casting

Plaster casts are used frequently in place of a splint during outpatient burn rehabilitation.[29] By using casts, small grafting procedures can be done on an outpatient basis. A decrease in the number of physical therapy treatments, improved wound closure, and a decrease in healing time in children has been reported with the use of casts following skin grafting to the lower extremity.[30]

Serial casts can be applied in an outpatient setting to a joint with decreased ROM[18,20,29,31] A cast is applied with the joint stretched to its maximal ROM. The cast either remains in place for 3 to 10 days or is wedged after 24 to 48 hours to change the joint angle. When wedged, the cast is reinforced with plaster strips to maintain the stretched position for another 24 to 48 hours. Both methods can be repeated serially until full ROM is achieved (see Chapter 11).

Healing casts are generally applied to outpatients over areas that have not healed for a long period of time. The plaster is applied over a dressing on the wound. The cast can remain for 3 to 10 days before removal. The wound is then inspected and an additional cast applied if necessary.

Splints

Dynamic splints generally are used in outpatient therapy; however, conformer-type splints can be used at night. The splints that are used should provide pressure or stretch and still allow motion whenever possible. The outpatient therapist should monitor the patients splinting program and alter the splints when necessary to ensure proper fit.

Developmental Therapy

Simply ensuring full ROM is not sufficient therapy for a child recovering from burn injuries. Often times a child can have full ROM but still not move correctly. Integration of movements is essential for fluid motion. Children recovering from burns may need to develop the following components of movement:

1. Balance
2. Equilibrium
3. Trunk control
4. Bilateral integration
5. Proximal stability for distal mobility
6. Rotational components in all movements

Incorporating a developmental treatment approach into a child's burn rehabilitation program can enhance ROM while improving mobility. This approach can accomplish a broad spectrum of goals while focusing primarily on the underlying issue of how the child moves. Massage, stretch, and flexibility exercises should precede developmental therapy to achieve overall goals more effectively.

Home Activities

Although the extent of injury for some patients requires intensive outpatient treatment, the ultimate goal should be to direct the patient toward improving ROM and function through normal activity at home.[17] Many patients are anxious to decrease the number of outpatient treatments per week, while others rely on outpatient therapy to improve their function. Those patients who rely solely on the therapist for exercise frequently do not follow through with home activities and eventually require reconstructive surgery.

BURN-RELATED ISSUES

Despite a comprehensive team approach, extensive home care education, and progressive rehabilitation, functional or psychologic problems can occur during the outpatient phase of recovery. The functional problems usually are related to skin condition, scar and contracture development, or the physical condition of the patient. Psychologic problems have numerous contributing factors and usually are demonstrated by depressed, unmotivated, or noncompliant behaviors. In many instances, one type of problem leads to another. For example, when patients are noncompliant, they frequently do not follow through with home program instructions, and scar contractures frequently result. Scar contractures can limit functional skills, which can frustrate patients and cause them to be even more unmotivated.

There are numerous methods that can be used to manage both physical and psychologic problems when they occur. However, early identification of the specific problem with prompt intervention is the preferred method. When the therapist becomes aware of behaviors indicative of disturbances in physical or mental status, more frequent follow-up assessments and referral to appropriate supportive services can limit the extent of disability acquired.

Altered Skin Integrity

The integrity of a patient's skin plays a major role in its ability to withstand external forces. Areas that heal spontaneously, donor sites, and grafted areas with a greater than 3:1 mesh are initially fragile and prone to abrasions. The skin integrity of burn patients will influence the frequency and types of activities in which they can be involved.

Frictional forces that also can lead to skin abrasion include

1. *Pressure garment friction:* Donning a pressure garment or improperly fitting garments can cause blistering.
2. *Functional friction:* A patient may do the same repetitive motion throughout the day, which can cause abrasion in a particular area. For example, a child who crawls for locomotion is likely to have knee abrasions.
3. *One-time incident:* A patient may rub against an object, fall, or forcefully stretch a particular area and cause sloughing of the skin in a specific area.

An open area must be kept clean. An antibacterial ointment may be applied to prevent infection. High-risk areas can be protected by applying rubberized or gel-like pads that absorb friction, or adding extra linings in garment areas of high stress, such as the knees. Areas easily traumatized with activity also can be protected with a thin dressing or using a nylon interface or undershirts beneath a pressure garment.

Skin Function

SWEAT AND OIL GLANDS

Partial- and full-thickness burns can decrease or destroy the sweat and oil glands in the dermis. Due to the destruction of these glands, patients may be able to perspire only from their uninjured skin. The injured skin also may be extremely dry and constantly peel or crack. Consequently, attention should be paid to burn patients' body temperature so that they do not become overheated. Creams also may need to be applied frequently throughout the day, depending on the climate, to add moisture to the skin.

ITCHING

Injured skin will undergo an active itching stage during healing.[32] Itching also is associated with dry skin. The patient should be cautioned to pat the area to relieve itching and avoid scratching to prevent tissue injury. In most cases, the more a patient scratches, the more he or she itches. Itching can have a dramatic impact on the patient's life, causing sleep and mood disturbances if the problem is severe. Oral medications and topical creams should be prescribed for the patient to minimize the effects of itching.[33]

SENSATION

Injured skin may not have intact sensory nerves or sensory receptors, causing decreased sensation.[34] Patients should be aware of the hazards of decreased sensation and learn to compensate. They should be taught to check with their noninjured skin the temperature of bath, shower, and dish waters; car seats; and cooking utensils and even be aware of the temperature of sand on a beach. Decreased sensation also can play a role in kinesthetic awareness. Sensing where the patient's body is in space without normal sensory feedback to the brain is difficult. Injured sensory nerves can cause pain. Applying deep pressure to an area or pressure garments may help decrease this pain.

EXPOSURE

Injured skin can be sensitive to ambient temperatures.[34] Sunscreens should be applied any time a patient is in the sun, even if simply riding in a car. The burn patient will need to be more cautious of the sun,[16] especially at higher altitudes. Although heat is a problem because of altered sweating, frostbite can be an issue that warrants education about proper clothing to prevent exposure. Suggestions may include the use of gloves, hats, thermal socks, and proper shoes during cold weather.

Scar Contracture

Not all scarring limits motion; however, scar contracture is the primary cause of functional deficits in burn patients. A contracture is essentially a shortening of a scar over a joint surface, limiting joint mobility. Pressure garments are used to minimize scar proliferation, but continuous activity is necessary to overcome the contractile forces of scar. Flexible inserts, applied over joint surfaces and worn under pressure garments, frequently are used to limit scar contracture development. When a contracture develops, serial casting and dynamic splints can help reverse the problem. There are times, however, when a contracture is so strong that preventing further loss of motion can be the only goal. This type of contracture eventually requires surgical release to restore functional mobility.

Edema

Dependent edema is routinely observed in the lower extremities following full-thickness burns with associated lymphatic damage. Also, the hand commonly is affected by edema, especially when there are circumferential burns to the upper extremity. When edema is present, motion is painful and often limited. The skin becomes fragile and prone to damage due to shearing forces. Chronic edema can lead to fibrosis.[35] Continuous external support in the form of pressure garments helps minimize edema. If the skin is not ready for custom-made garments, interim garments, elastic bandages, and other forms of elastic wraps are effective in managing edema.

When edema is present in the lower extremities, additional external support may be necessary during ambulation and can be provided by doubling the elastic wraps. When a patient is resting, elevation of the lower extremities and frequent active ROM exercises, such as ankle pumps, should be encouraged. Intermittent compression pump therapy often is used to treat chronic edema of the extremities.[36]

Resolving hand edema requires attention to the amount of compression that is applied proximally. If a pressure garment sleeve fits tighter than the glove, the edema will be trapped in the hand. In cases in which edema is the major factor limiting hand function, a custom sleeve should be replaced by an interim sleeve or tubular elastic support until an edema dissipates. Self-adherent elastic wraps or progressively decreasing the size of glove worn are commonly used techniques to overcome hand edema.[20] These techniques usually are done in conjunction with frequent or daily retrograde massage and hand activities emphasizing ROM.

Weight Changes

Throughout hospitalization, patients are constantly told they need to eat to heal their wounds. In many instances, this idea stays with the patient after discharge from the hospital. Unfortunately, metabolism normalizes and weight gains occur because of the patient's increased caloric intake or decreased activity level.[37] Occasionally, patients lose weight due to depression or an inability to eat a variety of foods because of oral burns, scarring, or limited upper extremity mobility. Changes in weight also can be closely related to a patient's changing body image. A significant weight change can be psychologic in origin or can add to the difficulty in dealing with a changing body scheme. Regardless of the cause, weight changes have a detrimental effect on scar control because garments become too loose or too tight before they are worn out. When garments are too tight, distal edema or paresthesias can occur, which causes the patient to discontinue wearing the garment. If a garment is loose, pressure on the scar decreases, making the garment ineffective. Patients should receive instruction about proper nutrition and what to do when garment fit changes.

Psychologic Problems

There are innumerable causes of psychologic problems following a burn injury.[38–40] Although patients may appear capable of caring for themselves and comfortable with their home program, they may have adjustment problems that they do not communicate. Reports from family members are helpful; however, the only sign of psychologic problems that a therapist may have is a change in the behavior of a patient. Noncompliance with exercise instructions and poor therapy attendance are indicators that a patient is experiencing psychologic problems. Typical signs of depression, such as lethargy and poor self-care, also are symptoms. Postural changes need to be observed to determine if they are due to scarring or possibly related to a poor self-concept. Another type of behavior that may be seen in the injured worker is malingering. The individual will appear to be trying to adhere to the therapy program but fails to demonstrate progress. Regardless of the sign or symptom, the patient should be seen by a counselor who is capable of assessing what services the patient needs. Group sessions with other burn patients are helpful in providing support.

RE-EVALUATION AND TREATMENT TERMINATION

The outpatient therapy program should be re-evaluated periodically. Frequency of treatment, program progression, and return to work or school status are factors to consider during the re-evaluation process. There are times when return to work or school part time can have a positive effect on recovery while the outpatient continues with therapy on a less frequent basis. Once patients achieve full active ROM, independence in their exercise program, as well as the skills needed to function at home independently and return to school or work full time, they can be discharged from their outpatient therapy program. Outpatient therapy may be discontinued during the recovery period, which means the patient still may be required to exercise, wear pressure garments, and use splints at night. Burn scar maturation can take up to 18 months following injury. To prevent unforeseen problems during this time, a schedule of follow-up care is needed.[2]

Outpatient Clinic

Outpatient clinic visits start when a patient is discharged from the hospital. During these routine medical checkups, the burn team evaluates the individual's functional status, skin condition, and scar maturation. Initially, the patient is seen every 1 to 2 weeks for approximately 1 month. The visits then are scheduled less frequently if continued improvement is demonstrated. During a clinic visit, the therapist should evaluate the individual for: (1) ROM, (2) posture, (3) gross strength, (4) endurance, (5) functional skills, (6) skin integrity, (7) garment fit, (8) splint needs, and (9) present exercise regimen. Decisions should be made concerning any reconstructive surgery needs and new pressure garments.

For the adult burn patient who has returned to work, return appointments for follow-up care should occur every 2 to 3 months until the wearing of pressure garments is discontinued. Children who have survived a burn injury should be followed until they are full-grown. For example, a child can be perfectly well adjusted to a burn injury, have full ROM, and not have any problems with scars or open sores at the age of 7 years. By age 12, the child could have developed severe problems in any or all of those areas. Following scar maturation, the child may need to be seen only every 1 to 2 years, depending on the severity of the burn, growth spurts, and the ability of his or her primary caretaker to manage problems that arise.

SPECIAL PROGRAMS

There are a wide variety of programs available directed toward enhancing a person's life after a burn injury. The therapist's role in these programs depends on community need, financing, and the time available to contribute to a program. Beginning any program can be a large undertaking, and therapists must be certain they are committed to completing the task.

When deciding to initiate a program, there are several key questions that must be answered.

1. *Community need:* Are there individuals who have requested this service? The absence of a program does not constitute a need.
2. *Financial support:* What will be the source of financial support? Can the hospital or local fire stations assist? Will insurance provide some financial coverage? If there will be fund raising activities, who will manage them?
3. *Administration and organizational structure:* Who will run the program? Will there be burn team involvement? Will it be run by volunteers?
4. *Referrals:* How will persons be entered into the program? Who is eligible? Who will answer their questions? Who can refer, e.g., fire stations, hospital personnel, schools, and/or social services?
5. *Goals:* What is expected to be accomplished in 6 months as well as 6 years?

Prevention Programs

A variety of prevention programs are available for the public. They are targeted toward special age groups or the public in general.[41,42]

FIRE-SETTERS' PROGRAMS

Fire-setters' programs are designed to educate and counsel people who have demonstrated fire-setting tendencies. A program like this often models the Big

Brother/Sister Association. A trained volunteer is assigned one person to educate and counsel in order to find alternative activities to fire-setting.

SCHOOL PROGRAMS

School programs are designed to educate children about fire safety. These programs visit schools in the community and provide classes with individual instruction. They can consist of lectures, slides, movies, group role-playing, or even an obstacle course that mimics getting out of a burning building.[43,44]

PUPPET PROGRAMS

Puppets are used to educate preschool children about the basics of fire safety. These programs can go to local libraries, preschools, day care centers, and churches. They use a combination of group word play, singing, and dancing to enhance young children's memory of the concepts.[45]

HEALTH DAYS

Health days can be a short-term way of disseminating information about fire safety. A combination of the previously mentioned activities can be used during health fairs, fire safety month, or physical therapy or occupational therapy week.

Camps

Burn camps provide an overnight, outdoor setting where children with the common experience of surviving a burn injury can gather. There are approximately a dozen camps in North America that cater to child burn survivors[46] (Appendix S). Camps are scheduled once a year and last anywhere from a weekend to a week. Physical and occupational therapy can have a significant impact on the lives of these children during burn camp. The goals of therapy at camp can be threefold: (1) to provide treatment to those children who would regress if they did not receive therapy for a week; (2) to adapt physically challenging activities to the individual needs of the child, and (3) to provide an atmosphere that physically challenges children while allowing them to be successful. This experience can improve a child's self-confidence toward physical activity and encourages an enthusiasm for a healthy body.

To date, there are no camps available for adult burn survivors, although the concept is of value.

School Re-entry

A school re-entry program is designed to prepare teachers and children for the return of a classmate who has survived a burn injury. These programs generally are initiated by the burn team because of the need to explain the hospital experience to the class members. The child can help decide what the program consists of and possibly choose who presents the program. This empowerment can give a child the feeling that needs are being addressed. Presentation options are: (1) slides, (2) a

TABLE 16–5. Topics to Include in a School Re-entry Program

1. How injury happened
2. Details of hospitalization
3. Wound care and dressing changes
4. Physical and occupational therapy
5. Splints, garments, face masks
6. Exercises
7. Care of injured skin

video tape of the child or another burn patient, (3) lecture, (4) group role playing, and (5) garment and splint samples.[47,48] Table 16–5 depicts topics usually covered during a school re-entry program.

In the midst of all the medical information, the audience should see what the child has experienced while describing the normal aspects of the child. The audience should learn that a burned individual needs to be treated like any other human being.

Support Groups

The purpose of a support group is to provide a setting in which former burn patients can meet to discuss their experiences. These discussions can lead to a better understanding of where they have been and acknowledgment of where they are headed. These groups can meet weekly, bimonthly, or monthly and can be directed toward adolescents, young adults, adults, families of burn patients, or even the health professionals that work in the field of burn care.

CASE STUDY

HISTORY

OM, a 39-year-old electrician, suffered a 40 percent total body surface area thermal burn when an electric panel exploded where he was working. He sustained deep partial-thickness burns to the chest, right lateral trunk, and bilateral upper extremities, including the dorsum of both hands and superficial partial-thickness burns to his face and neck. OM underwent three operative procedures for excision and skin grafting of his burn wounds. All donor skin was taken from his legs. Total length of hospitalization was 34 days. Transportation to therapy, three times a week, was arranged by a rehabilitation nurse assigned to his case by his insurance carrier.

At his initial outpatient visit, ROM measurements were within normal limits. However, OM reported discomfort during right shoulder flexion and abduction at the end of range. Initial bilateral grip strength on a dynamometer was 50 lb with the right hand and 55 lb with the left. Overall strength was rated normal by a manual muscle test, but OM reported fatigue during the day. His scars were hyperemic and soft except for a band of scar extending from the right hip to the right shoulder. This band was slightly firm to touch and blanched with full shoulder flexion and abduction. Although OM's face burns healed in less than 2 weeks, his facial scars were hyperemic, and he was very concerned about his appearance.

PROBLEM LIST

Pain at end range of right shoulder flexion and abduction
Decreased grip strength bilaterally
Poor endurance
Active scarring
Right axillary band with shoulder flexion and abduction
Patient concern of facial scars
Unable to perform necessary work activities

GOALS

Eliminate pain at end range of right shoulder flexion and abduction
Increase grip strength bilaterally to within normal limits
Increase endurance by 10 percent a week until OM is able to tolerate the activity of an 8-hour work day
Avascular, pliable, flat scars
Eliminate right anterior axillary scar band with shoulder flexion and abduction
Satisfactory reintegration with peers
Return to previous job

INTERVENTIONS

Paraffin was applied for 20 minutes to the right shoulder and lateral chest wall followed by massage and stretching exercises for the first 5 weeks of treatment. After 5 weeks, paraffin was discontinued and scar massage and active, slow sustained stretching was performed followed by strengthening exercises. Cuff weights and an isokinetic dynamometer were used for strengthening exercises. A stationary bike provided endurance activity; the BTE Work Simulator was used for hand ROM and strengthening and desensitization training, and the Valpar Small Tools Work Sample, O'Connor's Tweezer Test, and Pennsylvania Bi-Manual Test assisted with hand dexterity training. Specific BTE tools and lifting practice on the WEST II were used to prepare OM for return to work.

OM wore a custom-made long-sleeved vest, waist-height pants, gloves, and face mask for scar control. To apply additional pressure on his anterior axillary scar band, a silicone gel sheet was used under the garment.

OM attended a burn support group to assist with his adjustment to his perceived disfigurement. Total length of outpatient therapy was 7 weeks. OM returned to light duty at work at that time and to full duty within 3 weeks following his return to work. He was followed in outpatient clinic every 2 months. At 1 year, compression garments were discontinued and he was discharged from further outpatient follow-up.

RATIONALE

The patient had multiple problems at the time of discharge due to his extent of burn and period of hospitalization. Paraffin was used initially on the right axillary band as heat decreased shoulder pain while the heat and oil increased the scars pliability. Stretching and massage always preceded strengthening exercises so that the tissue was at maximal elongation before strengthening was begun. Stretching and massage were performed with the pressure garments removed so that physical and visual access to the scars was possible. Strengthening exercises were performed while he wore the garments to improve the skin's tolerance to shearing forces and mechanical trauma. All strengthening and endurance exercises were increased gradually over the 7-week period to maximize gains and prevent injury. Specific hand dexterity training and lifting activities were chosen using information from OM's job analysis. These activities provided him with specific agility and strength necessary for return to work.

The pressure garments selected provided compression to all grafted and partial-thickness burn areas as well as donor sites to minimize scar formation. The burn support group provided the patient with a forum for expressing his feelings regarding his burn injury as well as introducing him to individuals who could provide emotional support to him during difficult times. OM was discharged from outpatient follow-up when all goals were achieved.

SUMMARY

From the day of hospital admission through outpatient therapy, the therapist's underlying goal of treatment should be to help the patient return to as normal a life as possible. Discharge planning should begin as soon as the patient is medically stable in the hospital. If planning is initiated early, the therapist will have a better perspective of the patient's family structure, insurance, home situation and location, as well as available community resources when the patient is ready to leave the hospital.

A thorough discharge evaluation should be performed to establish a baseline of function for reference during outpatient therapy. This baseline can be used for charting progress, determining the therapy schedule, documenting functional abilities to insurance companies and employers, and providing feedback for the patient. At the time of hospital discharge, the patient or primary caregiver should be able to independently conduct a home program of wound care, skin care, exercise, activities of daily living, pressure therapy, and splint application as necessary.

As the burn patient progresses to outpatient therapy, a vast array of treatment techniques is available for the therapist. Many of the techniques and equipment used in general rehabilitation settings can be used with burn patients for improving strength, endurance, and flexibility. To prevent complications such as scar rupture, lubrication, massage, and stretching activities should begin any treatment session.

The therapist should develop realistic goals with the patient and determine the treatment strategies to achieve these goals. Although the treatment strategies to achieve physical goals are important, the role of education with the burn patient should not be overlooked. Throughout the course of outpatient therapy, the burn patient should be taught about altered skin integrity, sweat and oil gland function, itching, sensory disturbances, problems with sun exposure, scar contracture, potential edema complications, possible weight changes, and psychologic manifestations.

When patients leave the hospital, they should be referred to an outpatient clinic for follow-up. The therapist and physician monitor the patient's physical and psychologic progress and need for reconstructive surgeries. During clinic visits, the individual's ability to return to work or school should be determined.

There are a number of special programs available to former burn patients or for those working with burn patients. These programs include prevention programs, camps, school re-entry, and support groups.

Rehabilitation of burn patients requires knowledge, skill, commitment, and dedication. Therapists working with this patient population must understand the complications that can occur during burn recovery in order to provide appropriate rehabilitative care. Throughout the treatment process, education for patient and family is essential to help them assume responsibility for recovery.

REFERENCES

1. Parks, DH: Timing of burn therapy in the pediatric patient. Clin Plast Surg 17:65–70, 1990.
2. Petro, JA and Salisbury, RE: Rehabilitation of the burn patient. Clin Plast Surg 13:145–149, 1986.
3. Stern, LM and Davey, RB: A team approach with severely burned children in a multidisciplinary rehabilitation setting. Burns Therm Inj 11:281–284, 1985.
4. Weimer, CL, Goldfarb, LW, and Slater, H: Multidisciplinary approach to working with burn victims of child abuse. J Burn Care Rehabil 9:79–82, 1988.
5. Pollock, ML, Wilmore, JH, and Fox, SM: Exercise in Health and Disease. WB Saunders, Philadelphia, 1984, pp 168–182.
6. Helm, PA, et al: Burn injury: Rehabilitation management in 1982. J Burn Care Rehabil 4:411–422, 1983.
7. Johnson, CL: Physical therapists as scar modifiers. Phys Ther 64:1381–1387, 1984.
8. Gallagher, J, et al: Discharge videotaping: A means of augmenting occupational and physical therapy. J Burn Care Rehabil 11:470–471, 1990.
9. Yurko, LC and Fratianne, RB: Evaluation of burn discharge teaching. Proc American Burn Association 20:5, 1988.
10. Adriaenssens, P, et al: The video invasion of rehabilitation. Burns Therm Inj 14:417–419, 1988.
11. Klepitsch, L, et al: Burn patients' self-education program for physical and occupational therapy. Proc American Burn Association 20:182, 1988.
12. Ridgeway, C, Daugherty, MB, and Warden, G: Instruction for outpatient therapists: Individual burn rehabilitation video tapes. Proc American Burn Association 22:100, 1990.
13. Mason, S and Forshaw, A: Burns after care: A booklet for parents. Your child at home after injury. Burns Therm Inj 12:343–350, 1986.
14. Sampson, LJ: The development of a discharge planning index for use in a pediatric acute burn unit. J Burn Care Rehabil 11:365–372, 1990.
15. Giuliani, CA and Perry, GA: Factors to consider in the rehabilitation aspect of burn care. Phys Ther 65:619–623, 1985.
16. Richard, R, et al: Once a day is not enough: Home exercise equipment for the burn patient. Proc American Burn Association 24:175, 1992.
17. Rivers, EA: Rehabilitation management of the burn patient. Adv Clin Rehabil 1:177–214, 1987.
18. Rivers, EA: Rehabilitation for burn patients. In Kottke, FJ, and Lehmann, JF (eds): Krusen's Handbook of Physical Medicine and Rehabilitation, WB Saunders, Philadelphia, 1990, pp 1070–1100.
19. Bruster, JM and Pullium, G: Gradient pressure. Am J Occup Ther 37:485–488, 1983.
20. Hunter, JM, et al: Rehabilitation of the Hand. CV Mosby Company, St. Louis, 1990, pp 849–854.
21. Gross, JD and Stafford, FS: Modified method for application of paraffin wax for treatment of burn scar. J Burn Care Rehabil 5:394, 1984.

22. Head, MD and Helm, PA: Paraffin and sustained stretching in the treatment of burn contractures. Burns 4:136–139, 1977.
23. Fisher, SV and Helm, PA: Comprehensive Rehabilitation of Burns. Williams & Wilkins, Baltimore, 1984, pp 109–142.
24. Cronan, T, Hammond, J, and Ward, CG: The value of isokinetic exercise and testing in burn rehabilitation and determination of back-to-work status. J Burn Care Rehabil 11:224–227, 1990.
25. Davies, GJ: A Compendium of Isokinetics in Clinical Usage. S&S Publishers, La Crosse, 1984, pp 71–86.
26. Leman, CL: An approach to work hardening in burn rehabilitation. Top Acute Care Trauma Rehabil 1:62–73, 1987.
27. Zeller, J, Sturm, G, and Cruse, CW: Burn patients are successful in work hardening programs. J Burn Care Rehabil, in press, 1993.
28. Bowden, ML, Thomson, PD, and Prasad, JK: Factors influencing return to employment after a burn injury. Arch Phys Med Rehabil 70:772–774, 1989.
29. Jordan, MJ, et al: Dynamic plaster casting for burn scar contracture. Proc American Burn Association 16:17, 1984.
30. Ricks, N and Meagher, D: The benefits of plaster casting for lower extremity burns after grafting in children. J Burn Care Rehabil 13:465–468, 1992.
31. Bennett, GB, et al: Serial casting: A method for treating burn contractures. J Burn Care and Rehabil 10:543–545, 1989.
32. Vitale, M and Luterman, A: Severe itching and the burn patient. Proc American Burn Association 20:46, 1988.
33. Bell, L, et al: Pruritus in burns: A descriptive study. J Burn Care Rehabil 9:305–308, 1988.
34. Ward, RS, et al: Sensory loss over grafted areas in patients with burns. J Burn Care Rehabil 10:536–538, 1989.
35. Salisbury, RE, et al: Postburn edema of the upper extremity: Evaluation of present treatment. J Trauma 13:857–862, 1973.
36. Vasudevan, SV and Melvin, JL: Upper extremity edema control: Rationale of the techniques. Am J Occup Ther 33:520–523, 1979.
37. Ireton-Jones, C, Turner, WW, and Baxter, CR: Nutritional considerations in recovered patients with burns. J Burn Care Rehabil 11:581–582, 1990.
38. Rivilin, E: The psychological trauma and management of severe burns in children and adolescents. Br J Hosp Med 40:210–215, 1988.
39. Browne, G, et al: The psychological adjustment of burn survivors. Burns Therm Inj 12:28–35, 1985.
40. Orr, DA, Reznekoff, M, and Smith, GM: Body image, self-esteem, and depression in burn-injured adolescents and young adults. J Burn Care Rehabil 10:454–461, 1990.
41. Schmeer, S, Stern, N, and Monafo, WW: An outreach burn prevention program for home care patients. J Burn Care Rehabil 9:645–647, 1988.
42. Victor, J, et al: A statewide targeted burn prevention program. J Burn Care Rehabil 9:425–429, 1988.
43. Haney, A, Seh, D, and Krob, MJ: Fire prevention for teenage mothers enrolled in high school. J Burn Care Rehabil 9:648–649, 1988.
44. Varas, R, Carbone, R, and Hammond, JS: A one-hour burn prevention program for grade school children: Its approach and success. J Burn Care Rehabil 9:69–71, 1988.
45. Morrison, MI, Herath, K, and Chase, C: Puppets for prevention: Playing safe is playing smart. J Burn Care Rehabil 9:650–651, 1988.
46. Rosenstein, DL: Camp celebrate: A therapeutic weekend camping program for pediatric burn patients. J Burn Care Rehabil 7:434–436, 1986.
47. Rosenstein, DL: A school re-entry program for burned children. Part I: Development and implementation of a school re-entry program. J Burn Care Rehabil 8:319–322, 1987.
48. Meyer, DO, Barnett, PH, and Gross, JD: A school re-entry program for burned children. Part II: Physical therapy contribution to an existing school re-entry program. J Burn Care Rehabil 8:322–324, 1987.

SECTION IV

The Concerns

Problems have only the size and the power that you give them.

S.H.

CHAPTER 17

Psychologic Support and Pain Management of the Burn Patient

Barry F. Moss, PhD
John J. Everett, PhD
David R. Patterson, PhD

Burn trauma is often a physically painful and taxing experience replete with emotional issues. This chapter explores the varied ways in which individuals psychologically cope with burn injury as well as the psychologic and psychopharmacologic factors involved in treating burn pain. To illustrate the diversity of responses to burn trauma, the following factually based case studies are presented.

CASE 1

TC was an attractive, single, 21-year-old woman who arrived at the medical center with 80 percent total body surface area (TBSA) burns to her torso, neck, lower face, arms, and hands. She had an elevated blood alcohol level upon arrival. Her boyfriend reported that they were fighting, and she had poured gasoline on her shirt and threatened to kill herself if they were to break up. After the couple made up, TC accidentally lit her shirt on fire while attempting to light a cigarette. TC was in the intensive care unit (ICU) for the first month following her injury, during which time it was necessary to amputate two fingers of her left hand. Her mother was quite concerned about her recovery and would regularly visit, often insisting on talking to TC about why she should become more religious. Once TC had medically stabilized and was transferred to the acute burn center, she had several difficulties adjusting to treatment. Despite closely monitored treatment with pain medications, she complained that staff members were causing excruciating pain during procedures, even with procedures that are typically pain free. She often appeared anxious and depressed, complained of frequent nightmares, and was hostile toward some staff while being flirtatious with others. Despite these difficulties, TC's burns healed well with relatively minimal cosmetic impact. After TC was discharged from the hospital, she reported being depressed and having low self-esteem. The first year after discharge was particularly hard for her, as she continued intermittent phases of anxiousness and depression. She attributed these persistent episodes to her burn injury.

CASE 2

AB was a 32-year-old married man who arrived at the medical center with burns to his chest, face, and hands. AB was speeding to his next landscaping job when his car rolled over while AB unsuccessfully negotiated a turn. Considerable time was required to extricate AB from the burning car. Thus, his injuries were quite severe, resulting in considerable facial disfigurement. While in the ICU, it was necessary to amputate AB's right hand. His family members and wife visited him frequently and were consistently supportive and optimistic in his presence. Once physically stable, AB was transferred to the acute burn care unit. Although he was friendly, pleasant, and optimistic about his recovery, staff and family members reported seeing AB become tearful and sad at times. Although AB reported some pain during range-of-motion and wound-cleansing procedures, he felt that pain was generally tolerable. As AB progressed in his therapies and became proficient at using his prosthetic hand, his dysphoric moods became less frequent. He reported feeling concerned about his ability to return to his old job in landscaping because of the nature of his disabilities. However, he felt he was a "survivor" and would find another way to make a living. AB reported that during his inpatient hospitalization he had taken time to re-evaluate his priorities and resolved to spend more time with family and friends upon discharge. The first year after discharge was difficult for AB, and he found himself getting angry over his new limitations. As time progressed, however, these episodes of anger reduced in frequency. He also had difficulty adjusting to people staring at him in public due to his facial disfigurement. After the first year AB reported doing well and only rarely thought about the accident or felt unhappy about his limitations.

As can be seen from these case examples, the psychologic ramifications of burn injuries often can include anxiety, depression, regression, increased hostility, and existential crisis. However, burn trauma also can result in positive changes including a reassessment of one's personal values, a greater commitment to fulfilling goals, and an enhanced appreciation of one's life. To determine how people will adjust psychologically to burn injury, it is necessary to consider the complex interaction between premorbid personality style, extent of injury, and social and environmental contexts. The first section of this chapter explores how these patient factors influence psychologic adjustment at each of four separate time periods: prior to the injury and at the early, intermediate, and long-term stages of recovery. The remaining two sections focus on psychologic and pharmacologic issues related to pain control.

COPING WITH A BURN INJURY

Psychologic Adjustment Prior to Burn Injury

How people cope with burn trauma is strongly influenced by their preinjury psychologic status. If a person is highly dysfunctional before sustaining major trauma, this dysfunction is likely to be amplified after the injury. However, if a person has displayed good coping skills prior to burn trauma, subsequent adjustment to injury often is free of psychologic complications.

A number of epidemiologic studies suggest that people who sustain burns have a higher incidence of psychologic maladjustment than the general population. This finding suggests that "normal" people who sustain burns fail to fully recover psychologically, a notion that is misleading for a number of reasons. First, the causes of many burn injuries indicate that many individuals were psychologically impoverished prior to sustaining burns. For example, a substantial number of burn injuries are the result of suicide attempts,[1-3] assault[4,5], and arson.[6,7] Second, estimates of preexisting psychiatric disorders in burn patients are significantly higher than normal population standards.[2,8-10] Among the most common premorbid disorders diagnosed in burn patients are depression, antisocial personality disorder, organic brain syndromes, and alcohol and drug abuse.[9-14]

The relationship between burn injury and prior psychiatric disorders is complex. In general, individuals with these disorders often are predisposed to carelessness or involvement in dangerous activities. For example, depression, alcohol intoxication, and organic brain syndromes commonly are accompanied by poor concentration, impaired judgment, and slowed motor responses, all of which can contribute to increased risk of accidental burn trauma (e.g., automobile accidents). In contrast, burn trauma sustained by people with antisocial personality disorder is likely to originate from a different set of circumstances. People with antisocial personality disorder are often characterized as thrill-seekers, manipulative, aware of their social environments, socially skilled, egocentric, and lacking in underlying emotionality.[15,16] These "thrill-seeking" tendencies (e.g., reckless driving) most likely contribute to the higher representation of antisocial personality among burn patients. In summary, sustaining a burn injury is an intricate interaction between personal characteristics and environmental factors. The best indicator as to how survivors will cope is often how they were functioning in life prior to their injury.

Stages of Physical Recovery

Three basic stages of burn recovery consistently have been identified for burn survivors.[17-20] As can be seen in Table 17-1, each stage has a relatively distinct set of adjustment issues and consequences for psychologic treatment. These stages refer to the level of physical recuperation the burn patient is experiencing (intensive critical care, acute rehabilitative care, and long-term adjustment), and in turn, correspond to early, intermediate, and later periods of recovery. The duration of each of these stages varies from person to person depending on individual personality and temperament factors, the extent of burn injury, and the treatment environment.

TABLE 17–1. Psychologic Adjustment Difficulties and Modes of Psychologic Intervention for Three Stages of Recovery

	Stage		
	Early	**Intermediate**	**Long-Term**
Environment	Intensive care unit	Inpatient acute and rehabilitation units	Community
Primary patient concern	Day-to-day physical activity	Realizing limitations	Reintegration to society
Identified problem	Delirium, fatigue, anxiety, pain	Depression, posttraumatic stress disorder	Depression, low self-esteem, low quality of life
Psychologic approach	Supportive counseling and comfort measures	Individual counseling and psychopharmacology	Individual counseling, vocational counseling, and family systems counseling
Identified problem	Family grief issues	Sexual acting-out and hostile behavior	
Psychologic approach	Family systems counseling	Behavioral extinction	
Identified problem		Dependency, over-demanding	
Psychologic approach		Behavioral limit setting and assertiveness training	
Identified problem		Noncompliance, creating staff conflicts	
Psychologic approach		Behavioral contracting and selective reinforcement	

THE EARLY STAGE OF RECOVERY

The early stage of burn recovery is the period during which patients undergo critical care. Patients experience significant physiologic changes, and there is uncertainty regarding their physical outcome. Usually, severely burned patients are treated initially in an ICU. During this time, the patient is likely to experience repeated emergency medical procedures and significant physiologic stressors such as anoxia, electrolyte imbalance, infections, and edema.[20] Psychologically, patients usually are focused on issues of immediate survival and comfort rather than past mistakes or future ramifications of their injuries. The most frequently reported psychologic complaints during this stage of recovery are delirium, anxiety, sleep disturbance, and confusion, respectively. Although the symptoms of delirium can be disturbing to family or staff, delirium actually may be a positive coping mechanism that provides patients a means to escape intense pain and physical trauma. If physiologic causes of delirium are excluded, allowing the delirium to run its course often is most appropriate.

In general, direct psychologic intervention during the early recovery stage usually is inappropriate. Many patients are drowsy, disoriented, and intubated, which makes meaningful communication difficult. In addition, memory during this period may be limited. Even when patients are oriented and aware of the extent of their injury, focusing on past or future concerns can be counterproductive. Direct confrontation of the ramifications of the injury (e.g., employability) can overwhelm coping resources that are needed to first facilitate physical survival. Supportive psychologic interventions that focus on immediate concerns and augment whatever coping strategies the patient currently is using (e.g., escapist daydreaming) are effective approaches during the early stage of recovery. An exception is when a patient explicitly requests to confront issues regarding past regrets or future concerns. In this case, allowing the patient to express concerns and solve problems, or in some cases, redirecting the patient to the more urgent issue of survival, can alleviate anxiety and facilitate recovery. In summary, psychologic intervention during this period is based on following the patient's lead. The objective is to strengthen existing coping strategies while avoiding overloading the patient with too many demands or high-level cognitive input.

During the early recovery stage, a patient's psychologic adjustment is often best served by focusing psychologic interventions on familiar people in the burn patient's social system. Because patients at this stage typically have a limited tolerance for processing new information, the presence of family and friends can alleviate anxiety and agitation. In addition, because of reduced information-processing capacities, the patient's coping potential often is highly influenced by the cues received from significant others. As family members often experience high levels of stress and anxiety,[21] the patient potentially can pick up on these cues and act accordingly. However, if individuals close to the patient convey a sense of calm, hope, and support, the patient can assimilate these behaviors as the appropriate course of action. This social influence highlights the importance of working with the patient's family to educate them regarding strategies to alleviate grief issues and to avert premature confrontation with harsh realities. Taking these prophylactic steps with family members can help focus the patient's concentration on physical recovery and prevent overtaxing coping resources.

THE INTERMEDIATE STAGE OF RECOVERY

After a patient has stabilized physically, issues of healing take precedence over those of survival and the patient has entered the intermediate phase of recovery. This phase usually lasts throughout inpatient treatment. During this stage, the patient usually is out of the ICU and surgical procedures are less frequent. Physical status improves, sleep usually becomes more regular, and clarity of thought returns. However, patients frequently experience a considerable degree of pain at rest and often must endure a series of potentially painful procedures. Dressing changes, wound cleansing, exercising, and splinting are common treatment routines, each of which can cause a significant level of physical discomfort and pain.

Psychologically, severely burned patients usually cope during this stage by remaining in a state of psychologic shock, despite their improved physical status, or by beginning to seriously contemplate the ramifications of their burn injury. In the former case, psychologic intervention is not necessary as long as the patient continues to make progress toward recovery. Psychologic shock usually will diminish with time, gradually giving way to coping with pragmatic concerns. In the latter case in which patients begin processing the long-term impact of their injury during their hospitalization, negative emotional reactions can be experienced. The most common psychologic problems experienced by patients in the intermediate stage are depression and post-traumatic stress disorder (PTSD). Other intrapsychic difficulties include nightmares, anxiety, and regression (e.g., behaving in a way that is characteristic of an earlier developmental stage). Behavioral problems also occur and include such interpersonal difficulties as hostility, dependence, or inappropriate sexual behavior.

Depression in burn patients has been related to hospitalizations of over 1 month and the occurrence of unexpected medical setbacks.[22,23] In addition, the severity of depressive episodes has been associated with a patient's level of resting pain and the pressure of family or marital problems.[8,24] Although brief psychologic counseling often is helpful for depression, medications may be necessary with more severe depressive episodes, especially when suicidal ideation is present. A psychologic phenomenon similar to depression is termed the "loss of will to live" or a "death wish" by some investigators.[8,25] This syndrome has been defined as a period of 48 hours or longer in which a patient exhibits apathy, poor grooming and hygiene, passive noncompliance with caregivers, social disengagement, and self-devaluation. Although relatively rare, this syndrome is associated with a high mortality rate. Thus, patients who experience this syndrome must have access to psychologic or psychiatric treatment.

PTSD occurs when patients repeatedly experience a distressing event (e.g., recurrent, intrusive memories of a burn injury), exhibit avoidance of experiences that remind them of their trauma, and appear to be overly aroused. Although PTSD is relatively common, its course in burn patients usually is brief, with symptoms rarely extending beyond discharge from the hospital. However, a combined counseling and medication treatment approach is helpful when symptoms do not abate after a short period.

Psychologic difficulties such as anxiety, nightmares, and regression tend to be less problematic than depression and PTSD. Anxiety is common during the first few weeks of hospitalization but tends to decrease fairly rapidly after approximately 1 month. Nightmares also are common during early hospitalization, and this phenomenon tends to remit after patients adjust to the hospital environment and medication regimens. A minority of burn patients experience a significant degree of regressive behavior,[8,23] such as withdrawal, throwing tantrums, and dependence.

In addition to intrapsychic difficulties, burn patients potentially may exhibit a number of problematic behavioral patterns. Hostility, noncompliance, dependence, sexually acting out, and setting staff against one another are a few of the problematic behaviors medical staff and family have noted during the recovery course of some burn patients. The consistent application of behavior modification techniques is often helpful to reduce these types of behavioral complications.[26-29] Techniques such as behavioral contracting, assertiveness training, selective ignoring of negative communication or behaviors, and limit setting are particularly effective in minimizing these behaviors.

Behavioral contracting has been found effective to decrease noncompliance, promote independence, and prevent patients from inciting conflict among staff members. Behavioral contracting involves clearly specifying in a written agreement, available to both the patient and staff, exactly what behaviors are expected of the patient and what can be expected for complying with the contract. For example, a contract may specify that a patient must achieve a certain level of compliance with the exercise program before a weekend pass would be recommended by the therapist.

Assertiveness techniques and limit setting are useful, especially for dealing with dependent or demanding patients. These strategies involve a gentle yet firm establishment of treatment limits that can be reasonably expected (e.g., politely explaining that scheduling demands only permit a limited amount of time for the therapist to spend with each patient). Finally, selectively ignoring certain patient behaviors, such as hostile or sexual remarks, can be quite effective in eliminating this type of difficulty. Many patients find the negative reactions these behaviors elicit in staff highly reinforcing and will perform these behaviors as long as they achieve some reaction. Consistently ignoring these types of responses while being attentive to the patient when he or she acts appropriately cannot only extinguish the difficult behavior but also may model appropriate methods of social interaction.

Not all of the difficulties that patients encounter during the intermediate stage result in dysfunctional coping. Patients in the intermediate stage often struggle with existential issues. In cases in which the burn is severe or there has been significant disfigurement, patients often have to confront radical changes in appearance or a future in an alternative occupation. For a number of patients, this time is for carefully assessing and restructuring one's value system. This type of internal re-evaluation process often can lead to positive life changes. If patients take the time to contemplate and prioritize personal values and life goals, they may resolve to establish deeper levels of intimacy with family and friends, and they often acquire a deeper appreciation of life. There are also a number of patients who experience burn trauma with no apparent existential crises or difficulties in coping. As will be discussed in a later section, these patients are not necessarily denying difficulties or remaining in a state of psychologic shock but are coping in a healthy and appropriate manner.

In summary, during the intermediate stage of recovery, burn patients have stabilized physically and frequently become more aware of the ramifications of their injury. Although a majority of patients will exhibit adequate coping skills and will not require psychologic intervention, problems with depression, PTSD, anxiety, nightmares, dependency, and hostility can occur during this stage. A combination of psychologic and pharmacologic treatments often are effective in alleviating these difficulties. Brief supportive therapy and behavior modification strategies are commonly implemented psychologic interventions. Group therapies, especially those that are limited to a specific problem domain (e.g., an amputee support group), also can be helpful during this period. Finally, continued intervention with the patient's family can enhance understanding and communication between family members and increase their capacity to offer the burn patient optimal levels of support.

THE LONG-TERM STAGE OF RECOVERY

The long-term stage of recovery begins once a patient leaves the hospital and reintegrates into society. The majority of patients exhibit acceptable psychologic adjustment after hospital discharge, and only a minority of burn survivors report adjustment difficulties.[30,31] The first year following discharge is usually the most difficult for burn patients, with most adjustment issues remitting after this time.[8,31-33] The first year is a period during which a patient slowly regains a sense of competence and the practical limitations of a burn injury (e.g., limited range of motion and adjustment to a prosthetic device) are most salient. In addition, many burn patients continue to have vivid memories of the accident and often experience changes in family and occupational roles.

The most common problems reported during the first year after discharge from the hospital are associated with vocational and emotional adjustment.[8,31,32,34,35] Vocationally, burn patients often must contend with an extended period of outpatient recovery before they are ready to return to work, and many experience undesirable changes in their employment status such as a job reassignment or reduced work time. The most frequently reported emotional problems during the first year are anxiety and depression.[8,32,36–40] Burn survivors commonly experience both of these syndromes. However, depression and anxiety typically diminish markedly in intensity after 1 year. Individuals who experience adjustment difficulties past 1 year often have a history of depression or other psychologic disorders prior to the burn injury. Depression and anxiety may be prolonged if the burn injury was quite severe or the injury involved facial disfigurement or loss of hand function.[32,40]

Problems in long-term adjustment that persist past the first posthospitalization year usually involve perceptions of a diminished quality of life and lowered self-esteem.[30,33,41,42] Burn survivors who express a lowered quality of life are often those with limited range of motion and subsequent decreased functional capacity. Patients who were noncompliant with the medical staff or those who relied primarily on avoidant coping strategies also are more likely to report a lower quality of life. Self-esteem usually recovers to preinjury levels. However, burn disfigurement can cause a decrease in self-esteem for women and social withdrawal in men. One of the strongest buffers against feeling a loss of quality of life or self-esteem after a burn injury is to receive high levels of social support from family and friends.[43]

In summary, whether a burn survivor experiences adjustment difficulties in the long-term stage is determined by a complex interaction of personality, environment, and extent of injury. In general, if an individual had good coping skills prior to the injury, these skills will facilitate adjustment. If a person's prior coping style was brittle and dysfunctional, adjustment problems are far more likely. However, the unique ways in which individuals respond to long-term burn recovery precludes generalized treatment recommendations. Should those who work with burn patients recognize adjustment issues at this stage of recovery, the best recourse is to provide the patient with resources for psychologic assessment and follow-up care.

The Recovery Process

There are many different perspectives about what factors are responsible for the psychologic recovery of burn patients as they pass through the various stages. Some of these perspectives or models for understanding recovery have gained considerable support in the burn care literature. However, some of the models have proven to be misleading and, if psychologic interventions are based on these models, can be detrimental to the mental health of burn patients.

MISLEADING MODELS

There are four perspectives that were originally popular for explaining the early psychologic recovery of burn patients but are currently considered outmoded and misleading: the disease-medical, psychologic stage, catharsis, and undoing-defense models. The disease-medical approach assumes that observable symptoms are caused by some underlying pathogenic agent, much like the symptom of a fever can signal the onset of a viral infection. In the case of a burn patient who complains that range of motion exercises cannot be performed because of pain, this model would view the pain complaints as only a symptom of a much deeper difficulty such as problems with authority figures, self-destructive tendencies, or simply failing to adjust to the burn. In most cases, accepting a patient's complaints at face value will produce far more positive results than attempting to resolve unstated dynamics.

Approaches based on the assumption that patients must progress through psychologic stages also are misleading. Such models assert that all individuals who sustain loss through traumatic injury will pass through a series of psychologic challenges in a consecutive fashion. For example, a psychologic stage model would propose that people first experience denial, then anger, and then depression before they are capable of truly accepting a disability. In actuality, however, these models are not based on reliable research, and people have been found to be variable in how they respond to debilitating injury. Individuals are capable of going from denial to complete acceptance of their condition as well as any other idiosyncratic series of psychologic responses. These types of stage theories are quite different from the stage theory proposed earlier in this chapter. The stage theory proposed in the present chapter is based on the level of a burn patient's physical recuperation and treatment environment rather than the passage through psychologic challenges.

The catharsis and undoing-defense strategies are similar to stage theories in that they propose that a person must confront specific psychologic challenges before adequate adjustment can be achieved. In the catharsis approach, a burn patient would be required to talk about the injury and express feelings of fear or guilt before adequate psychologic recovery could occur. On the contrary, a burn patient consciously can choose never to talk about or express feelings about the injury and still achieve excellent psychologic recovery.

Proponents of the undoing-defense approach assert that a burn patient would have his or her natural psychologic defense mechanisms (e.g., escapist daydreaming, denial, unrealistic optimism) repeatedly challenged until the stark conditions of his or her injury were accepted fully. Adequate adjustment is not reached until reality is directly confronted. The undoing-defense strategy can be the most inappropriately misleading and damaging approach to recovery. Having to confront difficult issues before one feels ready can sabotage coping mechanisms that already are strained to their capacities. As long as a burn patient is making adequate progress toward physical recovery and reacquiring skills of daily living, there is no reason to challenge defense mechanisms. If a burn patient wants to believe that in the future he or she will have complete cosmetic recovery, there is no reason to repeatedly challenge the belief as unlikely or wishful thinking. Such beliefs can motivate the patient to participate fully in treatments and are much more productive than eliciting hopelessness and depression.

STRATEGIES TO PROMOTE ADJUSTMENT

There are numerous strategies that have been found particularly beneficial for facilitating the psychologic recovery of burn patients. Six of these strategies will be briefly outlined: the social-cognitive, behavioral-learning, education, normalizing, providing hope, and waiting-out models. Advocates of the social-cognitive approach propose that psychologic adjustment improves from achieving greater mastery over one's environment. For example, when a burn patient receives physical therapy that increases hand function or improves range of motion, he or she becomes better able to accomplish goals in the environment. The therapist is in effect facilitating psychologic recovery by enabling the patient to attain higher levels of self-sufficiency.

Supporters of the behavioral-learning approach assume that behavior is learned through reinforcement patterns. Behavior that is rewarded increases in frequency, and behavior that is ignored or punished decreases in frequency. According to this model, if a burn patient is provided with praise for performing assigned exercises, those exercises are more likely to be continued. The principles of the behavioral-learning model have received a great deal of scientific support for facilitating recovery from medical complications.

Proponents of the education model contend that psychologic recovery is impeded by lack of information. For example, a burn patient's lack of motivation can be the result of not being fully informed of the benefits and purpose of treatment. Once educated as to the purpose of a treatment plan, a patient might approach recovery with less passivity, and cooperation may improve.

The normalizing and providing-hope strategies are similar to the education model in that they propose that giving information to a patient facilitates psychologic recovery. The normalizing approach focuses on providing patients with information about the normal course of recovery so as to prime defense mechanisms, alleviate unnecessary anxiety over nonthreatening symptoms, and assure patients that they are not alone in their recovery experience. For example, if shortly after the burn trauma a patient experiences repeated nightmares about the injury, informing the patient that dreams are normal and often will subside in approximately a month can allay concerns of abnormality and refocus the patient's mental energy back on other areas of recovery. The information given to the patient in the providing-hope model focuses on allowing the patient to maintain optimism toward the future in order to facilitate recovery in the present. For example, informing a burn patient who has sustained considerable nerve damage that research on nerve regeneration is under way and may be possible in the future, may make the patient's present disability easier to accept.

According to the waiting-out approach, a patient is viewed as resilient to trauma and many psychologic difficulties naturally will remit with time. For example, when a burn patient has experienced a loss of function, a period of grieving over that loss is a natural reaction and usually will remit with time. Allowing patients to experience their grief reactions and work through them without outside interference allows a natural healing process to occur. If the grief reaction is inordinately intense, occurs in the absence of social support, lasts over a prolonged period, or develops into a full depressive disorder, professional attention is required.

In summary, there are many different explanatory models or approaches for how a burn patient is able to achieve psychologic recovery. The model or approach for recovery that one adopts strongly influences the types of psychologic interventions to be implemented with burn patients. Because of the potential influence of these models on treatment course, it is important for therapists to be aware of the basis for the approach one is using with patients to minimize misleading and possibly harmful assumptions.

Psychologic Adjustment of Pediatric Patients

Although children also pass through early, intermediate, and long-term stages of recovery, there are several adjustment differences that separate them from adult burn patients.[44–46] Children respond differently to hospitalization than adults and subsequently require different modes of psychologic attention. A child's response to the hospital environment often is dependent on age. Infants and toddlers (ages 1 and 2) frequently experience separation anxiety while receiving hospital care. School-age children more typically experience difficulties with agitation, anger, and manipulativeness. Finally, adolescents often are sensitive to control issues and can react to treatment demands with either rebellious noncompliance or regressive withdrawal. In addition to reacting to the experience of inpatient hospitalization, children often have a unique set of psychologic responses to a burn injury. The pain induced through wound cleansing and physical rehabilitation often can establish strong fear reactions to staff members and places within the hospital. Burn trauma also tends to have a large guilt and fear component for children, even when they clearly are not responsible for their injury.

In general, there are a number of psychologic interventions that are particularly helpful for children. In the early stage of recovery, frequent visits by the child's mother often facilitates a young child's adjustment.[47] Children rely on parents and other significant individuals to provide cues on how to react to strange surroundings. Treating anxiety in caretakers to avoid transmission of this response style to the child is especially important. As a child's awareness improves and he or she enters the intermediate stage of recovery, additional interventions often are necessary. Providing children with structure can reduce anxiety and fear reactions. For example, structure can be conveyed through adhering to a daily schedule that is posted in the child's room or by having a core of primary caregivers assigned to the child to enhance familiarity and interpersonal rapport. Adjustment also can be facilitated through explaining medical procedures in developmentally appropriate language. Demonstrating medical procedures through play, such as with dolls, can allay a child's anticipatory anxiety about a procedure as well as help the child form positive associations with treatment interventions.

Unfortunately, avoiding performing painful and anxiety-producing procedures on children is impossible. Such procedures should be isolated to a particular treatment area whenever possible. Children often will begin crying simply by seeing a staff member dressed in scrubs, because the clothes become a conditioned stimulus for pain and anxiety. Thus, isolating therapies to specific times and places will reduce the generalization of such anxiety. Ideally, a child's room will remain a "safe area" where no procedures are performed. Because this ideal situation cannot be maintained always, play areas for children are needed so that the majority of their day is as normal and fun as possible.

Providing children with generous levels of reinforcement for appropriately participating with medical treatments is one of the best methods of assuring continued compliance. The choice of reinforcer should be individually tailored to each child. Praise is one of the strongest reinforcers. Other reinforcement methods include awarding stickers that can be posted on an easily visible progress chart, food snacks, or time with a favored game. However, despite the best efforts of medical staff to be reinforcing and sensitive to a child's needs, some children will continue to exhibit compliance difficulties. At this point, firm and consistent limit setting or implementation of a time-out program may become necessary.

Any therapist who has worked in a burn unit likely has had the experience of a child crying and screaming during procedures or therapy. Despite all the pharmacologic and psychologic approaches to make care more tolerable for children, many will continue to demonstrate such behaviors. To a certain degree, crying, screaming, and bargaining must be accepted and ignored by the hospital staff. When children perceive that the therapist is tempering the treatment as a result of their behavior, such escape tactics will intensify. Thus, while therapy should be provided in a loving and compassionate manner, the child also must realize that the therapist will not be influenced by behavior designed to avoid treatment.

After children with burn injuries are discharged from the hospital, their long-term adjustment usually is satisfactory. However, children who have sustained visible burns, especially to the head and hands, tend to have a greater incidence of adjustment problems and depression. Adolescents, in particular, can be affected by these types of observable burn injuries.[48] Providing resources for brief psychologic counseling or support groups often is appropriate in these circumstances. In summary, pediatric patients, like adults, also experience early, intermediate, and long-term adjustment stages. However, for pediatric patients, completing these stages with adequate adjustment often entails a strong degree of social support from caregivers and a sensitivity on the part of medical staff to provide high levels of reinforcement and consistency in care.

PSYCHOLOGIC APPROACHES TO CONTROL BURN PAIN

The foundation for pain control with burn patients should be opioid-based medication. If a patient is in significant pain while at rest between treatments, he or she most likely is undermedicated. However, with wound cleansing and range of motion exercise, burn pain can be so severe that opioid drugs will not be sufficient. Further, medicating patients for each therapy session may not be practical. Therefore, integrating psychologically based pain control into burn rehabilitation procedures often is useful. Various approaches, as listed in Table 17–2, can be combined with other types of pain-relief modalities. For more extensive reading on psychologic approaches to burn pain, the reader is referred to reviews by Everett and colleagues[49] and Patterson.[50]

TABLE 17–2. Psychologic Pain Control Techniques

Technique	Definition	Example
Reappraisal	Cognitive technique of reinterpreting pain sensation	Pain in burn site interpreted as increased sensation associated with healing a partial-thickness burn
Distraction	Cognitive technique of focusing away from pain sensation	Patient imagines beach scene during therapy
Procedural preparatory information	Describing procedural aspects	Each step of dressing change and why it occurs explained to patient
Sensory preparatory information	Describing sensations expected	Patient told what sensations to expect during various stages of wound care
Respondent (classical) conditioning	Reducing adversity of pain stimuli	Pairing cues for pain with deep relaxation
Operant (reinforcement) conditioning	Strengthening behavior with rewards	Reward patient with rest based on successful completion of exercises; graphing progress

Cognitive Interventions

Cognitive interventions in psychology basically view thoughts as behaviors that can be changed. By altering the manner in which a patient thinks about a sensation, the degree to which that sensation causes suffering can be influenced. The cognitive techniques applied to pain control can be divided into reappraisal and avoidance approaches.

With reappraisal techniques a patient is taught to perceive a sensation in a different manner. Suppose a therapist is performing range of motion to the shoulder of a patient with a burn in that area. As the shoulder is flexed, the patient may feel a stretching sensation in the axilla. The therapist is certain no damage has occurred, but the patient believes that the therapist is "ripping tendons from his or her bone." In this case, the patient has the perception that he or she is being "harmed" by the therapist rather than simply being "hurt." By explaining to the patient that exercise will not make the injury worse, even though he or she might feel discomfort in that area, the patient hopefully will reinterpret the meaning of what he or she feels. If patients sense that a therapist is harming them as a result of the treatment, possibly "fight or flight" instinctual mechanisms could be invoked. Therefore, the more therapists are able to enable patients to reappraise the meaning of physical sensations, the better will be their pain control in most cases.

Another example of reappraisal techniques is to help a patient distinguish "good" pain from "bad" pain. Therapists can explain to the patient that, in certain instances, the presence of sensations is a positive sign. In a burn site, for example, the presence of increased nociception often indicates a partial-thickness burn wound that is likely to heal without skin grafting.

Another form of cognitively based pain control techniques involves the use of distraction. Distraction techniques simply enable patients to focus away from unpleasant nociceptive input. When patients are engaged in conversation during a treatment, therapists are making use of this technique. Thus, merely encouraging patients to talk or watch television may increase the amount of pain they are able to tolerate. More extensive application of distraction techniques may involve patients imagining themselves at a relaxing place, performing mathematical problems, composing "rap" tunes, or playing electronic games. Obviously the use of distraction techniques is most effective when matched to the patient's intellectual level, cultural background, and personal history.

How does a therapist determine when to use avoidance versus distraction techniques? The answer to this question is an important one because some patients have a cognitive style whereby they wish to avoid any knowledge or awareness of pain, while others do best if they focus on their sensations in elaborate detail. Therapists can gain substantial information simply by asking patients how they would like to approach therapy. Otherwise, the therapist will have to rely on observation and trial and error.

Preparatory Information

There are a substantial number of studies that demonstrate that the use of preparatory information can reduce pain and anxiety.[49] Preparatory information techniques tell the patient what will be involved in a procedure. There are two types of preparatory information, procedural and sensory. Procedural information techniques help the patient anticipate what will occur during an intervention. Thus, one might explain to the patient that he or she will be instructed to hold his or her arm at a certain angle while the therapist covers the scar tissue with warm paraffin. Sensory information approaches help patients understand what sensory experiences they might anticipate. For example, patients might be told that when walking for the first time, they can expect tightness in the back of their heel and overall stiffness in their legs.

As rudimentary as such information appears, health professionals often fail to tell their patients what to expect. This information may reduce pain and anxiety substantially. Once again it is important to assess whether such approaches fit well with the patient's style of coping. Some patients would rather leave their treatment to the therapist and not be told anything.

Behavioral Techniques

Behavioral techniques can be divided into classical (respondent) and reinforcement (operant) categories. Classical techniques, which pair relaxation with the stimulus of pain, will be discussed in the following section. Reinforcement techniques, which use the consequences of behavior to strengthen it, can be useful, particularly for burn patients.

To understand the application of reinforcement techniques in pain control, therapists must appreciate that treatments often are painful and are essentially an aversive stimuli or punishment. Further, the cessation of a therapeutic procedure often represents rest or reward for a patient. As such, the conditions under which patients rest in therapy often provides a form of contingency management. If a patient is allowed to rest based on the amount of pain they express, then such pain behavior essentially is being reinforced and strengthened. However, if patients are encouraged to work to a preset criterion (e.g., number of exercise repetitions, distance walked) then rest can become a reward for the amount of therapeutic activity completed.

In a classic work on applying behavioral approaches to physical therapy, Fordyce[51] recommended the quota approach to determining how much exercise should occur before rest. When using the quota system, therapists have the patient perform a therapeutic activity for 3 baseline days to a point of fatigue or pain. That baseline level (e.g., distance walked, number of repetitions) is recorded. The therapist then takes the average of the baseline for those 3 days and calculates 80 percent of it. The 80 percent baseline becomes the starting point for therapy. As an example, if a patient walks 75 feet, 125 feet, and 100 feet on 3 consecutive days, the therapist would set 80 percent of the baseline average of 100 feet as the starting point, that is, 80 feet. The patient then increases walking distance by 5 percent each session, and progress is graphed. Whether or not this approach is used, patients must work to preset criteria in therapy rather than pain or fatigue.

An important point to understand about reinforcement techniques is that, at times, a patient's pain behavior must be ignored. If the burn team has done everything to alleviate pain, yet the patient continues to complain of pain, then the caregiver should encourage the patient to focus on other areas and to ignore the pain. While this approach may seem cruel or insensitive, the clinician should explain to the patient that discussing the pain will only make it worse. Just as people salivate when they see food, people feel physical pain more when they focus on it. If this perspective is explained to patients, they may better understand why the therapist is not always attentive when they complain of pain.

Relaxation and Hypnotherapy

To the degree that patients become tense when they feel pain, they will experience pain more acutely. By using deep relaxation techniques, muscle relaxation can be paired with painful procedures to make them more manageable. On the other hand, therapists seldom have the time to practice deep relaxation with their patients. Therefore, relaxation techniques that can be instituted quickly are recommended. The cornerstone of relaxation techniques is breathing and encouraging patients to take slow deep breaths. This technique can work remarkably well to counteract anxiety. If this technique fails, patients can be encouraged to take "balloon breaths" in which they inhale, fill their cheeks, and slowly let air out through pursed lips. Having patients place their bodies in a position where they can relax is another simple step that may facilitate comfort during procedures. The therapist also can suggest relaxation in various areas of the body; for instance, picking up an extremity and dropping it with a suggestion of heaviness ("just let your arm get so relaxed that it drops when I let it go").

A number of studies suggest that hypnosis can facilitate pain control during procedures.[52-54] Again, the issue of time becomes a problem. One approach is to have the psychologist or other mental health specialist hypnotize patients before procedures and then to have the nurse or therapist provide posthypnotic cues for comfort.[55]

Psychologic Pain Control with Children

All of the approaches previously presented apply, in principle, to children. However, this population has some special needs. Young children will have more difficulty grasping the cognitive ramifications of pain sensation. The use of puppets, dolls, and very simple language ("good" versus "bad" pain) can be useful in enabling children to reinterpret sensations. Some children will do well with simple distractions (e.g., television, video games), while many will benefit from participating in their procedures. Allowing children to control their own therapy often is helpful, but limits usually will be necessary. For example, a therapist may tell the child that he or she has 2 minutes to do his or her exercises but, after that, the therapist will do the exercises for the child. A therapist should follow through at that point and do the remainder of the exercises. As mentioned earlier, if children realize they can escape procedures by protesting, crying, or other means, their pain behavior usually will exacerbate. Allowing children time-out cards, which they can use to buy a preset, limited number of rest periods, can be successful.

Some of the strategies discussed earlier that apply to managing the psychologic adjustment of children apply also to pain control. Painful procedures generally should be done outside of the child's room. A pediatric patient's hospital room ideally will be kept as a "safe area" where aversive input is minimally experienced. Whenever possible, therapies should be experienced as "play" rather than treatment.

Pain control will be enhanced if playing catch can be substituted for arm exercise or riding a tricycle can be used as a leg exercise. Finally, reinforcement charts in which children earn a sticker or other reward each time they complete a therapy can be useful. Such charts can be posted on a child's wall so that progress can be seen.

PHARMACOLOGIC INTERVENTIONS FOR PAIN AND OTHER COMPLICATIONS

A basic understanding of pharmacologic options and strategies for the management of burn pain and other complications is of utmost importance for burn therapists. Traditionally, opioid drugs (e.g., morphine and methadone) have been the treatment of choice for burn pain management. Unfortunately, a number of myths regarding the immediate and long-term effects of opioids, colloquially referred to as narcotics, have resulted in a reluctance among many physicians to administer opioids at sufficient dosage levels. Moreover, even with high doses of opioids, burn pain sometimes remains virtually intolerable for many patients.[49,56,57] Thus caretakers need to be aware of pharmacologic agents that can be used safely with opioids for pain management. Additionally, pain is qualitatively and quantitatively different at various stages of healing and during different burn care procedures. Each of these situations requires specific pain management strategies.

The ultimate responsibility for adequate pharmacologic management belongs to the physician. However, other staff members such as nurses and physical and occupational therapists generally have more patient contact than physicians, especially during painful procedures, such as debridement. Thus, they are in an optimal position to assess the efficacy of pain medications and may suggest re-evaluation of the pain management plan. The drugs discussed here do not represent all of the pharmacologic options for burn pain management. Rather, specific examples are provided of drugs representative of the following groups: opioids, nonsteroidal anti-inflammatory drugs (NSAIDS), benzodiazepines, and nitrous oxide. Also described are some of the other types of drugs that might be used with burn patients. Before describing these different drugs, however, one must differentiate the two main types of burn pain to determine optimal management strategies.

Background versus Procedural Pain

Burn patients typically experience two main types of pain: background pain and procedural pain.[49,52,56] Background or resting pain occurs when patients are at rest, relatively motionless, and not actively involved in treatment procedures. Background pain usually has a dull, throbbing quality and relatively low intensity. In most instances, this pain can be adequately controlled with opioids, provided therapeutic levels are maintained continuously. Procedural pain, which occurs during wound debridement, rehabilitation treatments, and other activities, has a much greater intensity and is most commonly described with such adjectives as "stabbing," "severe," and "excruciating."[56] In fact, procedural pain, while of relatively short duration, is often so intense that even high dosages of opioids do not provide sufficient analgesia.[49,56] Although background pain usually can be controlled with steady doses of opioid drugs, procedural pain often requires the use of analgesics that are of fast onset, short duration, and high potency. For procedural pain, the timing of the opioid administration should allow the opioid to reach its therapeutic peak during the burn care procedure and then to clear from the patient's system so sedation will be minimized for the remainder of the day or night.

One factor that cannot be overemphasized is the importance of scheduling pain medication on a regular basis. Traditionally, opioid drugs have been administered on an "as-needed" (prn) basis. Use of this approach requires the staff to wait until the patient complains of pain before providing medication. As-needed strategies should be avoided and a more structured, "regular" opioid schedule should be followed. Regular administration of opioids keeps patients' drug serum level steady in their bloodstream. As such, they are not subjected to the opioid "peaks and valleys" that contribute to emotional vacillation as well as inconsistent pain control. Secondly, consistent medication schedules remove the elements of external reward and bargaining with staff that may otherwise result as a response to pain behavior. If patients receive adequate levels of opioids at regular levels, they will be far less likely to complain of pain and argue with the staff that they need more medication. Thus, background medication should be scheduled every few hours (depending on the serum half-life of the drug) and procedural medication should be administered prior to treatment interventions on a consistent basis.

Opioids

Opioids are clearly the treatment of choice for burn pain. Nonetheless, there exists within the medical profession a reluctance to prescribe adequate dosages.[58,59] This hesitancy is due largely to an unwarranted fear that patients will continue to "crave" opioids and become abusers after they leave the hospital,[60,61] as well as fears of dangerous side effects such as respiratory depression. The impact of these fears in burn care settings is especially damaging, because burn patients often require more than standard dosages of opioids for pain relief. Fortunately, the likelihood of a patient without previous substance abuse history becoming addicted after using opioids for pain management essentially is nonexistent. In one survey involving over 10,000 former burn patients treated with opioids while hospitalized, 22 patients were found to abuse drugs after leaving the hospital. However, all 22 had been abusers prior to being burned.[62] In another study involving 11,882 patients who received opioids, only one patient developed what was referred to as drug dependency.[63]

Whereas opioids are highly addictive when taken for psychologic reasons, (e.g., euphoria, escape from reality), research evidence suggests that this occurrence is not the case for burn patients who receive opioids for a physical reason, that is, pain relief. As pain subsides with healing, most patients no longer feel the need to continue using opioids.[64] In fact, even patients who self-administer opioids with patient-controlled analgesia (PCA) pumps reduce their dosages as pain diminishes.[65]

Another contributing factor to undermedication is the fear of respiratory depression. As is the case with addiction, these fears generally are unwarranted provided minimal efforts are made to visually monitor a patient's physiologic status.[66] Moreover, there are several opioid antagonists (e.g., naloxone) that can rapidly rescind respiratory depression. Table 17–3 lists several opioids commonly used for burn pain, their duration of action, and their peak effect in hours.

TABLE 17–3. Commonly Used Opioids for Burn Pain, Duration of Action, and Peak Effect

Drug	Duration of Action (hours)	Peak Effect (hours)
Morphine	3–6	0.5–2
Hydromorphone	4–5	0.5–2
Oxycodone	4–6	1
Methadone	4–6	0.5–1.5
Meperidine	2–4	1–2
Fentanyl	1–2	—

Data from American Pain Society,[73,76] Foley, KM;[74] and Roxane Laboratories.[75]

TABLE 17–4. Opioids—Relative Side Effects

	Respiratory Depression	Emesis	Constipation
Morphine	High	Moderate	High
Hydromorphone (Dilaudid)	Moderate	Low	Low
Oxycodone (Percodan)	Moderate	Moderate	Moderate
Methadone (Dolphine)	Moderate	Low	Low
Meperidine	Moderate	Moderate	Low
Time-release oral morphine (MS Contin)	Moderate	Moderate	Moderate

Data from American Pain Society;[73,76] Foley, KM;[74] and Roxane Laboratories.[75]

With the exception of sustained-release morphine tablets, which are a long-acting, oral form of morphine particularly suited for background pain, little difference is found among the other opioids with regard to recommended uses and duration of action. Although the effects of opioids are theoretically similar, each patient may react differently. Potential side effects are listed in Table 17–4. Monitoring a patient's response to this form of pain medication is important. For example, a burn patient with compromised respiratory function due to smoke inhalation or perhaps some preexisting condition, may not be a good candidate for morphine, which has the highest potential for respiratory depression.

In summary, opioids are an effective, safe means of burn pain control, and the physician can select from a wide variety of opioids depending on the type of burn pain, as well as various patient characteristics. Unfortunately, a number of myths and misconceptions have resulted in undermedication and unnecessary patient suffering. In reality, serious side effects and addiction rarely occur. Thus burn caretakers should advocate aggressive pain management strategies. Staff and patients should be educated to understand and promote this form of patient care.

Nonsteroidal Anti-inflammatory Drugs

NSAIDS are a group of drugs that are effective for managing mild to moderate pain. Some of the more commonly used NSAIDS are acetylsalicyclic acid (aspirin) and ibuprofen. NSAIDS can be used in combination with opioids and in fact have demonstrated to have an additive effect when used as adjuncts to opioids.[67-69] This approach is useful particularly when patients fail to respond adequately to opioids or in instances when opioids need to be reduced due to undesirable side effects. NSAIDS also are useful as hospital discharge approaches, when some patients must be weaned from opioids. Some patients require pain medications for up to several weeks after being discharged, and NSAIDS are an effective means of pain management that can be safely administered at home.

Some precautions with NSAIDS are warranted. NSAIDS can cause abdominal pain and gastrointestinal (GI) bleeding.[70] Also, NSAIDS result in prolonged bleeding, which can be dangerous particularly for patients with large wounds. Finally, all NSAIDS decrease temperature, which can make it especially difficult to detect infections in patients with low white cell counts or immunosuppression.[71]

Benzodiazepines

After pain, anxiety is the most frequent complaint expressed by burn patients.[72] While controlling anxiety in itself is important for increasing patient comfort, high levels of anxiety can intensify pain, and vice versa. Thus the likelihood exists for patients with untreated anxiety to become affected by a "vicious cycle" of pain and anxiety. This cycle is most likely to occur just prior to and during dressing changes, because at this time anxiety levels tend to be at their highest. Fortunately, there are a number of drugs available in the benzodiazepines class that may be very useful to reduce anxiety during medical procedures. Moreover, benzodiazepines are useful particularly for burn care since they generally can be used safely in conjunction with opioids. Selected benzodiazepines are presented in Table 17–5.

As with opioids, the differential side effects of benzodiazepine and individual patient characteristics are important considerations for drug selection. For example, geriatric patients tend to require benzodiazepine dosages at approximately half the normal adult dosage.

Nitrous Oxide

The inhalant nitrous oxide (N_2O) is another pharmacologic agent that can be used during dressing changes. A recommended dosage for analgesia is 25 to 50 percent N_2O with oxygen. For maximum benefits, the patient should be instructed to

TABLE 17–5. Selected Benzodiazepines

Drug	Uses	Half-life, $t_{1/2}$ (hours)
Lorazepam (Ativan)	Anxiety/sedation, alcohol withdrawal	10–18
Alprazolam (Xanax)	Anxiety/sedation, alcohol withdrawal, panic	12–15
Chlordiazepoxide (Librium)	Anxiety/sedation, alcohol withdrawal	5–30
Diazepam (Valium)	Anxiety/sedation, alcohol withdrawal	20–50
Midazolam	Anxiety/sedation, alcohol withdrawal	

Data from American Pain Society;[73,76] Foley, KM;[74] and Roxane Laboratories.[75]

take deep breaths while inhaling N_2O. In some cases, particularly for highly anxious patients, having the patient begin N_2O for a few minutes prior to beginning the dressing change is useful. This approach allows the patient to experience analgesia as well as increasing relaxation simply by virtue of deep breathing. A minority of patients experience nausea from N_2O, but other side effects associated with temporary use are infrequent.

Other Pharmacologics

Some other drugs commonly administered and their side effects are listed in Table 17–6. Neuropathic pain, which often is secondary to some form of nerve damage, typically does not respond well to opioid medications. Examples of neuropathic pain include that found in amputation sites, brachial plexus and avulsion injuries, and various neuralgias. Both antidepressant and anticonvulsant drugs can be useful to treat this type of pain. Antidepressant drugs also can be useful for treating depressive symptoms and sleep problems.

TABLE 17–6. Other Drugs Used with Burn Patients

Type of Drug	Name	Use	Side Effects
Antidepressant	Amitryptline, nortryptline, desipramine, imipramine, doxepin	Neuropathic pain (i.e., phantom limb pain), major depression, sleep problems	Sedation, dry mouth, memory impairment, urinary retention, orthostatic hypotension, weight gain
Anticonvulsants	Carbamazepine, phenytoin, valproic acid, clorazepam	Trigeminal neuralgia/ post-herpetic neuralgia, phantom pain	Ataxia, diplopia, dysarthria, nystagmus
Antihistamines	Diphenhydramine, hydroxyzine cyproheptadine	Anxiety, itch, sedation	Constipation, oversedation, dry mouth
Neuroleptics	Haloperidol	Neuropathic pain, anxiety/agitation	Dystonia, sedation, movement disorders with long-term use
Neuromuscular blockers	Pancuronium bromide, vecuronium	Paralyzing agents	Respiratory collapse (patient must be intubated)
		Miscellaneous	
Psychostimulants	Dextroamphetamine, methyphenidate	Lethargy, depression	Insomnia, change in personality, cardiac toxicity
Muscle relaxants	Baclofen, dantrolene, methocarbane	Trigeminal neuralgia/ muscle spasms	
Benzodiazepines	See Table 17–5	Anxiety reduction, muscle relaxant (spasticity), some analgesia	Sedation, respiratory depression, ataxia, lethargy; confusion

Data from American Pain Society;[73,76] Foley, KM;[74] and Roxane Laboratories.[75]

A number of other drugs can be useful for various problems that arise for the burn patient. An anesthetic, such as ketamine, can be useful for procedures that children cannot tolerate in a fully conscious state. Antihistamines (e.g., hydroxyzine) can be useful for treating itching, anxiety, and sleep problems. Neuroleptics (e.g., haloperidol) can be used for severe agitation, and occasionally anxiety and neuropathic pain. Neuromuscular blockers (e.g., pancuronium bromide) are used as paralyzing agents when a patient is on a ventilator, and it is essential that the patient not move. Psychostimulants (e.g., dextroamphetamine) may be administered when the patient is lethargic and depressed. Muscle relaxants (e.g., baclofen) may be used to treat muscle spasms. Finally, benzodiazepines (e.g., midazolam) often are used to treat anxiety and procedural pain as stated previously.

A Typical Pain Medication Protocol

The following protocol from Harborview Medical Center describes a typical pharmacologic approach that might be used for treating a burn patient experiencing pain.

Step 1: PCA is used as a means for patients to self-determine their opioid requirements for the first 48 hours. If a patient does not want to use a PCA pump (usually because of the intravenous access requirements), then the response to pain medication should be carefully monitored and medications should be titrated accordingly for at least the first 2 days of care.

Step 2: The patient is converted to oral medication if possible. For background pain, the patient should receive regularly scheduled, long-acting opioids such as time-release morphine. For dressing changes, more potent, short-acting opioids, such as hydromorphone, should be administered 45 minutes before the procedure.

Step 3: If opioids fail after adjusting to the patient's needs, then adjunctive approaches should be attempted. Such medication failures usually will occur during procedures. The use of benzodiazepines, such as ativan; inhalants, such as nitrous oxide; or psychologic and pharmacologic interventions should then be attempted.

This approach is oversimplified and does not account for the myriad of complications that can occur when treating burn patients. At the same time, however, research findings have indicated that, provided adequate doses of opioids are administered, the above plan will be successful for most patients.

SUMMARY

This chapter has provided an overview of the psychologic and pharmacologic issues involved in the treatment of burn trauma. Three common stages of physical recovery have been reviewed (early, intermediate, and long-term) along with the possible psychologic and pain complications associated with each stage. During the early stage, patients are not well-focused, and psychologic adjustment is best facilitated by working indirectly through the burn patient's family and friends. Direct intervention becomes beneficial once the patient enters the intermediate stage where physical stability and awareness of limitations occur. Intervention also can be necessary during the long-term stage, which begins once the patient leaves the hospital and returns to community life.

A number of psychologic reactions to burn injury that can occur during the stages of recovery including depression, posttraumatic stress disorder, anxiety, nightmares, regression, and existential crisis have been reviewed. In addition, behavioral difficulties such as hostility, dependence, or sexually acting out also have been found to occur. Psychologic interventions beneficial for treating these difficulties include behavior modification; psychopharmacology; and individual, family, group, and vocational counseling. Pain control also is an issue during the recovery stages. Pharmacologic agents considered to be helpful to modulate burn pain include opiates, nonsteroidal anti-inflammatory drugs, benzodiazepines, and nitrous oxide. Finally, psychologic interventions outlined as helpful adjuncts to pain control medication include cognitive and behavioral techniques, relaxation strategies, hypnosis, and patient education.

Throughout this chapter the many psychologic difficulties burn patients encounter have been emphasized. One must note that only a minority of patients exhibit significant adjustment difficulties. A number of burn patients may experience a natural grieving process over physical losses; however, most will exhibit acceptable long-term adjustment. Those patients who have a particularly poor psychologic adjustment to a burn injury tend to have had poor coping mechanisms before the burn trauma. For many burn survivors, the injury can be a catalyst to re-evaluate personal goals and values and form closer bonds with family and friends. How a person reacts to burn trauma is determined by a complex interaction of the burn patient's personality, environmental context, extent of injury, and social support system. Decisions regarding psychologic and pharmacologic interventions with burn patients must be flexible enough to take this diversity in individual response into account.

REFERENCES

1. Andreasen, NC and Noyes, R: Suicide attempted by self-immolation. Am J Psychiatry 132:554–556, 1975.
2. Davidson, TI and Brown, LC: Self-inflicted burns: A 5-year retrospective study. Burns 11:157–160, 1985.
3. Skully, JH and Hutcherson, R: Suicide by burning. Am J Psychiatry 140:905–906, 1983.
4. Hight, DW, Bakalar, HR, and Lloyd, JR: Inflicted burns in children. JAMA 242:517–520, 1979.
5. Krob, MJ and Johnson, A: The burned-and battered adult: An unrecognized syndrome. Proc American Burn Association 18:103, 1986.
6. Gruber, AR, Heck, ET, and Mintzer, E: Children who set fires: Some background and behavioral characteristics. Am J Orthopsychiatry 51:484–488, 1981.
7. Heath, GA, Gayton, WF, and Hardesty, VA: Childhood firesetting. Can Psychiatric Assoc J 21:229–237, 1976.
8. Andreasen, NJC, Noyes, R, Jr, and Hartford, CE: Factors influencing adjustment of burn patients during hospitalization. Psychosom Med 34:517–525, 1972.
9. Brezel, BS, Kassenbrock, JM, and Stein, JM: Burns in substance abusers and in neurologically and mentally impaired patients. J Burn Care Rehabil 9:169–171, 1988.

This chapter was written by psychologists for physical and occupational therapists. Because medications are an integral part of burn care, some basic information about pharmacologics was provided. Although a substantial amount of input was received from hospital pharmacists in writing about drugs, it should be stressed that it is outside the realm of competence and practice for either psychologists or therapists to decide on dosages of medications.

We would like to acknowledge Janet Gibbons, H. Richard Miyoshi, and Mary Bordenaue-Birchfield for their generous consultation on the pharmacology of pain control.

10. Noyes, R, Frye, SJ, and Slymen, DJ: Stressful life events and burn injuries. J Trauma 19:141–144, 1979.
11. Doctor, ME and Bernstein, NR: Introduction: The psychological aspects of burn care. J Burn Care Rehabil 13:2–3, 1992.
12. Kolman, PBR: The incidence of psychopathology in burned adult patients: A critical review. J Burn Care Rehabil 4:430–436, 1983.
13. MacArthur, JD and Moore, FD: Epidemiology of burns: The burn patient. JAMA 231:259–263, 1975.
14. Rockwell, E, et al: Preexisting psychiatric disorders in burn patients. J Burn Care Rehabil 9:696–705, 1986.
15. Cleckley, H: The Mask of Sanity. CV Mosby, St. Louis, 1964.
16. Widom, CS: A methodology for studying noninstitutionalized psychopaths. J Consult Clin Psychol 45:674–683, 1977.
17. Berini-Marzouk, B, et al: Behavioral changes in burned adult patients during their stay in hospital. Burns 8:365–368, 1981.
18. Jorgensen, Z and Brophy, JL: Psychiatric treatment of severely burned adults. Psychosomatics 14:331–335, 1973.
19. Patterson, DR: Psychological management of the burn patient. Top Acute Care Trauma Rehabil 1:25–39, 1987.
20. Steiner, H and Clark, WR: Psychiatric complications of burned adults: A classification. J Trauma 17:134–143, 1977.
21. Shelby, J, et al: Severe burn injury: Effects on psychologic and immunologic function in noninjured close relatives. J Burn Care Rehabil 13:58–63, 1992.
22. Andreasen, NJC and Norris, AS: Long-term adjustment and adaptation mechanisms in severely burned adults. J Nerv Ment Dis 154:352–362, 1972.
23. Hamburg, DA, Hamburg, B, and deGoza, S: Adaptive problems and mechanisms in severely burned patients. Psychiatry 16:1–20, 1953.
24. Choiniere, M, et al: The pain of burns: Characteristics and correlates. J Trauma 29:1531–1539, 1989.
25. Tempereau, CE: Loss of will to live in patient with burns. J Burn Care Rehabil 10:464–468, 1989.
26. Wernick, RL, Brantley, PJ, and Malcom, R: Behavioral techniques in the psychological rehabilitation of burn patients. Int J Psychiatry Med 10:145–150, 1980.
27. Zide, B and Pardoe, R: The use of behavior modification therapy in a recalcitrant burned child. Plast Reconstr Surg 57:378–382, 1976.
28. Cox, MD: Treatment and management of a case of self-burning. Behav Res Ther 14:382–385, 1976.
29. Simons, RD et al: Behavioral contracting in a burn care facility: A strategy for patient participation. J Trauma 18:257–260, 1978.
30. Browne G, et al: Psychosocial adjustment of burn survivors. Burns 12:28–35, 1985.
31. Blades, BC, Jones, C, and Munster, AM: Quality of life after major burns. J Trauma 19:556–558, 1979.
32. Chang, FC and Herzog, B: Burn morbidity: A follow-up study of physical and psychological disability. Ann Surg 183:34–37, 1976.
33. Sheffield, CG, III, et al: Suicide by burning. Am J Psychiatry 140:905–906, 1983.
34. Helm, PA and Walker, SC: Return to work after burn injury. J Burn Care Rehabil 13:53–57, 1992.
35. Korloff, B: Social and economic consequences of deep burns. In Wallace, AB and Wilkinson, AW (eds): Research in Burns: Transactions of the 2nd International Congress on Research in Burns. Livingstone, Edinburgh, 1966, pp 229–234.
36. Adler, A: Neuropsychiatric complications in victims of Boston's Coconut Grove disaster. JAMA 123:1098–1101, 1943.
37. Andreasen, NJC, Norris, AS, and Hartford, CE: Incidence of long-term psychiatric complications in severely burned adults. Ann Surg 174:785–793, 1971.
38. Tucker, P: Psychosocial problems among adult burn victims. Burns 13:7–14, 1987.
39. Ward, HW, et al: Prevalence of postburn depression following burn injury. J Burn Care Rehabil 8:294–298, 1987.
40. White, AC: Psychiatric study of patients with severe burn injuries. Br Med J 284:465–467, 1982.
41. Blumenfield, M and Reddish, PM: Identification of psychologic impairment in patients with mild-moderate thermal injury: Small burn, big problem. Gen Hosp Psychiatry 9:142–146, 1987.
42. Bowden, L, et al: Self-esteem of severely burned patients. Arch Phys Med Rehabil 61:449–452, 1980.
43. Bernstein, NR, O'Connell, K, and Chedekel, D: Patterns of burn adjustment. J Burn Care and Rehabil 13:4–12, 1992.
44. Bernstein, NR: Emotional Care of the Facially Burned and Disfigured. Little, Brown, Boston, 1976.
45. Knudson-Cooper, MS: Emotional care of the hospitalized burned child. J Burns Crit Care 3:109–115, 1982.
46. Wilkins, TJ and Campbell, JL: Psychological concerns in the pediatric burn unit. Burns 7:208–210, 1981.
47. Woodward, J: Emotional disturbances of burned children. Br Med J 1:1009–1013, 1959.
48. Bogaerts, F and Boecks, W: Burns and sexuality. J Burn Care Rehabil 13:39–43, 1992.
49. Everett, JJ, Patterson, DR, and Chen, ACN: Cognitive and behavioral treatments for burn pain. Pain Clin 3:133–145, 1990.

50. Patterson, DR: Practical applications of psychological techniques in controlling burn pain. J Burn Care Rehabil 13:13–18, 1992.
51. Fordyce, WE: Behavioral Methods for Chronic Pain and Illness. CV Mosby, St. Louis, 1976.
52. Patterson, DR, Questad, KA, and Boltwood, M: Patient reports about their health and physical functioning three months after a major burn. J Burn Care Rehabil 8:274–280, 1987.
53. Patterson, DR, Questad, KA, and deLateur, BJ: Hypnotherapy as an adjunct to narcotic analgesia for the treatment of pain for burn debridement. Am J Clin Hypn 31:156–163, 1989.
54. Patterson, DR, et al: Hypnosis for the treatment of burn pain. J Consult Clin Psychol 60:713–717, 1992.
55. Barber, J: Rapid induction analgesia: A clinical report. Am J Clin Hypn 19:138–147, 1977.
56. Perry, S, Heidrich, G, and Ramos, E: Assessment of pain by burn victim patients. J Clin Behav Res 2:322–326, 1981.
57. Perry, SW, Cella, DF, and Falkenberg, J: Pain perception vs. pain response in burn patients. Am J Nursing 87:698–699, 1987.
58. Angell, M: The quality of mercy. N Engl J Med 306:98, 1982.
59. Perry, SW: Undermedication for pain on a burn unit. Gen Hosp Psychiatry 6:308–316, 1984.
60. Hill, CS: Clinical issues: Achieving balance in national drug control policy: The use of analgesia. In Wilford, BB (ed): Balancing the Response to Prescription Drug Abuse: Report of a National Symposium on Medicine and Public Policy. AMA Department of Substance Abuse, Washington, DC, 1990, pp 37–49.
61. Melzak, R: The tragedy of needless pain. Sci Am 262:27–33, 1990.
62. Perry, S and Heidrich, G: Management of pain during debridement: A survey of US burn units. Pain 12:267–280, 1982.
63. Porter, J and Jick, H: Addiction rare in patients treated with narcotics. N Engl J Med 302:123, 1980.
64. Twycross, RG: The management of pain in cancer: A guide to drug and dosages. Oncology 2:35–43, 1988.
65. Hull, CJ and Sibbald, A: Control of perspective pain by interactive demand analgesia. Br J Anaesth 53:385, 1981.
66. Miller, RR: Analgesics. In Miller, RR and Greenblatt, DH (eds): Drug Effects in Hospitalized Patients. Wiley, New York, 1976, pp 133–164.
67. Beaver, WT: Aspirin and acetaminophen as constituents of analgesic combinations. Arch Intern Med 141:293–300, 1981.
68. Beaver, WT, Wallenstein, SL, and Houde, RW: Clin Pharmacol Ther 9:303–313, 1968.
69. Sunshine, A, et al: Analgesic efficacy of two ibuprofen-codeine combinations for the treatment of postepisiotomy and postoperative pain. Clin Pharmacol Ther 42:374–380, 1987.
70. Insel, PA: Analgesic-antipyretics and antiinflammatory agents: Drugs employed in the treatment of rheumatoid arthritis and gout. In Gilman, AG, et al (eds): The Pharmacological Basis of Therapeutics. Pergamon Press, New York, 1990, pp 638–653.
71. Hill, CS: The NSAIDs: When and why to use them for pain control. Reprinted from Primary Care & Cancer, Primary Care Handbook: Pain Management. Dominus, New York, 8:41–46, 1988.
72. Patterson, DR, et al: The psychological effects of severe burn injuries. Psychol Bull 113:362–378, 1993.
73. American Pain Society: Special Features: Principles of analgesic use in the treatment of acute pain and chronic cancer pain. Clin Pharmacol 9:601–611, 1990.
74. Foley, KM: The treatment of cancer pain: New Engl J Med 313:84–95, 1985.
75. Roxane Laboratories: 3-Step Analgesic Ladder for Management of Cancer Pain. McMahon Group, New York, 1991.
76. American Pain Society: Principles of Analgesic Use in the Treatment of Acute Pain and Cancer Pain, 3d ed. American Pain Society, Skokie, Ill, 1992.

CHAPTER 18

Management of the Pediatric Burn Patient

Sandra Utley Reeves, OTR/L
Glenn Warden, MD, FACS
Marlys J. Staley, MS, PT

Management of the pediatric patient with a major burn presents many complex problems to members of the health care team. Burns are the leading cause of non–motor-vehicle deaths in children 1 to 4 years of age and are the second most common cause of death in children 5 to 14 years of age. Scald injuries represent approximately 40 to 50 percent of all burns, with the highest incidence seen in the toddler age group. Because children sustain a large number of burn injuries, the clinician should be aware of the major differences between the pediatric and adult burn patient. The purpose of this chapter is to describe some of the differences between a child and adult and to provide suggestions on properly managing the child with a burn injury.

NORMAL PEDIATRIC PARAMETERS

The normal child is not just a "small adult" but rather a dynamic human, progressing through a series of predictable developmental landmarks. From infancy (not speaking) through nubility (of marriageable age) the child undergoes extensive changes in all body systems. To appropriately manage the burned pediatric patient, one must have a working knowledge of some of the more common physiologic parameters and developmental levels under which a child operates at different ages. From infancy until adulthood pulse rate decreases from an average 120 beats per minute to 70 beats per minute, blood pressure increases steadily from an average 80/45 to 120/80 mm Hg, and respiratory rate decreases from approximately 40 breaths per minute to 12 breaths per minute. Tables 18–1 through 18–3 illustrate normal

TABLE 18–1. Normal Ranges and Averages for Pulse Rate for Ages 0 to 18 Years

Age	Normal Range		Average Pulse Rate (beats/min)	
Newborn	130–170		120	
1–11 mo	80–160		120	
1 yr	80–140		120	
2 yr	80–130		110	
4 yr	80–120		92	
6 yr	75–115		85	
8 yr	70–110		78	
10 yr	70–110		74	
	Males	**Females**	**Males**	**Females**
12 yr	65–105	70–110	85	90
14 yr	60–100	65–105	80	85
16 yr	60–100	60–100	75	80
18 yr	55–90	55–95	70	75

From Nelms, BC and Mullins, RG[1] p. 759, with permission.

TABLE 18–2. Normal Ranges and Averages for Blood Pressure for Ages 0 to 18 Years

Age	Range		Average Blood Pressure (mm Hg)	
0–6 mo	64/30–96/62		80/45	
6 mo–1 yr	60/50–118/70		89/60	
2 yr	74/40–124/89		99/60	
4 yr	79/55–110/85		99/60	
6 yr	80/46–118/64		94/62	
8 yr	89/48–121/66		105/60	
10 yr	94/52–128/85		111/66	
	Male	**Female**	**Male**	**Female**
12 yr	92/58–135/86	94/59–132/86	115/72	115/75
14 yr	98/60–142/90	98/62–138/90	120/75	118/76
16 yr	102/60–148/90	100/62–142/90	125/76	122/76
18 yr	105/62–152/90	102/62–144/90	128/77	122/77

From Nelms, BC and Mullins, RG[1] p. 761, with permission.

TABLE 18–3. Normal Ranges and Averages for Respiratory Rate in Breaths per Minute for Ages 0 to 16 Years

Age	Normal Range	Average
Newborn	30–80	40
1–6 mo	30–60	35
6 mo–1 yr	22–60	35
1 yr	22–40	30
2 yr	22–34	28
4 yr	20–28	26
6 yr	18–28	24
8 yr	18–26	22
10 yr	18–26	20
12 yr	16–24	18
14 yr	12–20	16
16 yr	12–20	16

From Nelms, BC and Mullins, RG[1] p. 760, with permission.

ranges and averages for pulse rate, blood pressure, and respiratory rate at various ages. In addition, Tables 18–4 through 18–6 describe gross motor, fine motor, and self-care behaviors or tasks that occur at differing ages.

INTEGUMENTARY SYSTEM

In contrast to the child's rapidly changing physiologic and physical status, the integumentary system undergoes a slow maturation process.[1,2] During infancy (0–18 months) the epidermis is loosely connected to the dermis and may blister readily. Only small amounts of sebum and sweat are produced, and the skin is dry and susceptible to chafing and rashes. Evaporation of water through the thin epidermis is great, and the infant has increased fluid needs. The thin stratum corneum, limited secretion of sebum and sweat, and alkaline skin composition make the infant vulnerable to thermal and chemical contacts in the environment.[1] Infant skin problems continue through early childhood, and increased contact with the outside world exacerbates some of these. The secretion and evaporation of the sebum and sweat, along with body water, keeps the child's skin alkaline (as opposed to acidic in the adult, which is somewhat bactericidal) and prone to skin infections.[1] When children get burned, their immature integumentary systems sustain a greater insult than adults.

PRINCIPLES OF BURN WOUND MANAGEMENT IN THE PEDIATRIC PATIENT

Although the principles of burn wound management in a pediatric patient are similar to those for adults, there are major differences in regard to the management of a pediatric patient less than 5 years of age. Moreover, in pediatric burn patients less than 2 years of age, burn management is a clinical challenge even in a minor or moderate burn injury.

TABLE 18–4. Developmental Sequence of Gross Motor Skills

Age	Mobility/Gross Motor Skills
0–2 mo	When prone, raises head to 45° and turns head to both sides. When supine, alternately kicks feet, rolls from back to side-lying. When upright, head "bobs" but remains erect.
3–5 mo	Has integration of Moro reflex. When prone, raises chest and head to 90° propping with forearms, can prop on extended arms, has integration of tonic labyrinthine reflex and symmetrical tonic neck reflex and rolls to supine. When supine, has integration of tonic labyrinthine reflex and asymmetrical tonic neck reflex. When upright, aligns head with trunk, bears a small portion of weight on feet.
6–8 mo	When prone, Landau reflex is exhibited, reaches for items, assumes quadruped position, pivots, and crawls. When supine, rolls to prone, sits unsupported for at least 30 sec, can sit propping self with hands. When standing, extends legs and bears larger portion of weight on lower extremities and pushes body up and down. Pulls self to sitting.
9–11 mo	Creeps, pulls to standing, and cruises holding onto furniture, walks with one hand held, can lower self to the floor and stand alone.
12–15 mo	Walks alone, creeps up stairs, squats and stands up independently to recover a toy, walks backward, throws ball awkwardly with some projection.
16–19 mo	Runs awkwardly, walks sideways, walks upstairs with one hand held, creeps backward downstairs, climbs up onto adult-sized furniture, seats self onto small chair, can balance on one foot with support.
20–23 mo	Walks downstairs with one hand held, jumps in place, kicks a ball forward.
24–27 mo	Independently goes up and down stairs, nonreciprocally; jumps with feet together and/or from bottom step of stairs; stands on balance beam with both feet, attempts to step; throws ball overhand.
28–31 mo	Walks on tiptoes, throws a ball vertically, rises from sitting to standing smoothly, takes a few alternate steps on balance beam.
32–36 mo	Goes up stairs alternating feet, balances on one foot 1 to 2 sec, begins heel-toe gait, swings arms when walking, runs.
3 yr	Walks with reciprocal arm swing with arms free of shoulder height balance position, hops on one foot two to three times, runs well, climbs stairs independently one foot per tread, walks down stairs two feet per tread, rides tricycle using pedals, catches large ball with arms extended, stands in place and shifts weight when throwing a ball, climbs three rungs on ladder.
4 yr	Stands on one foot 3 to 4 sec, climbs up and down stairs independently with one foot per tread, broad jumps, hops, gallops, skips with one foot, bounces ball awkwardly.
5 yr	Stands on one foot 6 to 8 sec, goes down stairs alternating feet without support, heel to toe walk, starts to roller skate, jumps rope and catches large ball on bounce.
6 yr	Skips alternately, throws ball stepping with foot opposite of throwing arm, standing broad jump of 3 ft.

Data from Frankenburg, WK and Dodds, JB;[13] Roger, S and D'Eugenio, DB[14,15] and Kauffman, NA: Occupational Therapy with Children: The School Setting. In Hopkins, HK and Smith, HD (eds): Willard and Spackman's Occupational Therapy, ed 6. JB Lippincott, Philadelphia, 1983, p 683.

TABLE 18–5. Developmental Sequence of Perceptual/Fine Motor Skills

Age	Perceptual/Fine Motor Skills
0–2 mo	At 4 wk has reflexive grasp, initiated by touch, immediate involuntary release.
3–5 mo	Reaches for dangling objects, at 3 mo uses ulnar-palmar prehension with sustained voluntary grasp on contact only, at 4 mo fingers own hands at midline and uses primitive squeeze grasp against body or other hand, at 5 mo uses palmar grasp with thumb abducted, swipes at and grasps rattle placed in hand.
6–8 mo	Uses radial-palmar grasp with thumb in opposition to grasp small cube and inferior-pincer grasp on raisin, transfers toys from hand to hand, rakes or scoops up small items, pulls peg out of pegboard, at 8 mo uses radial-digital grasp on cube and scissors grasp on raisin.
9–11 mo	Pokes with isolated index finger, drops items with crude voluntary release, uses inferior-pincher grasp with small items. By 10 mo uses true pincer grasp and three-jaw chuck grasp, holds crayon to paper in adaptive grasp.
12–15 mo	Turns pages of cardboard book, imitates scribbles, uses fine pincer grasp, supinated grasp developing with wrist extended, good release, places one or two pegs in pegboard, makes tower of two cubes, places objects in and out of containers, scribbles spontaneously using simian pencil grasp with fist clenched.
16–19 mo	Independently places six pegs in pegboard, makes three-cube tower, places round form in three-piece formboard, imitates crayon stroke using palmar-supinate grasp, turns pages in book (two or three at a time).
20–23 mo	Puts six pegs in pegboard within 34 seconds, imitates vertical and circular scribbles after demonstration, completes three-piece formboard, builds six-cube tower, holds crayon with fingers, attempts to imitate folding paper.
24–27 mo	Hand preference begins, draws vertical and circular strokes imitatively, completes reversed formboard, aligns two or more cubes horizontally for train, builds tower of six to seven cubes, unscrews jar lid, scribbles with circular motion, begins to use digital-pronate grasp of pencil.
28–31 mo	Builds eight-cube tower, aligns three cubes for train with smokestack, imitates paper folding, imitates drawing a horizontal stroke.
32–36 mo	Begins to use static tripod pencil grip and copies a circle already drawn, cuts with scissors, strings large beads, pours well from glass to glass.
3 yr	May shift handedness, builds tower of 9 to 10 cubes, turns a doorknob with forearm rotation, imitates a three-cube bridge, can imitate drawing a cross.
4 yr	Copies a cross (+), builds a six-block pyramid, at 4½ yr copies square, tries to cut with scissors on straight line.
5 yr	Uses a dynamic tripod pencil grip, copies diagonal lines and triangle, can perform sequential finger opposition slowly with visual regard, imitates a 10-block pyramid.
6 yr	Copies diamond, by 6½ yr hand dominance is established.

Data from Frankenburg, WK and Dodds, JB[13]; Roger, S and D'Eugenio, DB[14,15]; and Kauffman, NA: Occupational Therapy with Children: The School Setting. In Hopkins, HK and Smith, HD (eds): Willard and Spackman's Occupational Therapy, ed 6. JB Lippincott, Philadelphia, 1983, p. 683; and Erhardt, RP: Erhardt Developmental Prehension Assessment. In Erhardt, RP: Developmental Hand Dysfunction: Theory Assessment Treatment. Ramsco Publishing, Laurel, Maryland, 1982, p. 48.

TABLE 18–6. Developmental Sequence of Activities of Daily Living Skills

Age	Activities of Daily Living/Self-Care Skills
3–5 mo	Sucks pureed foods from a spoon, holds own bottle.
6–8 mo	Drinks from a cup with help, picks up spoon.
9–11 mo	Feeds self small finger foods.
12–15 mo	Feeds self with spoon (spillage), picks up and drinks from a cup (spillage), cooperates with diapering and dressing by extending or moving limbs, removes socks, attempts to brush hair.
16–19 mo	Drinks from cup independently, feeds self entire meal with spoon, purposefully removes socks.
20–23 mo	Attempts to wash face and hands, cooperates with brushing teeth, attempts to put shoes on, zips and unzips large zipper, begins toilet training.
24–35 mo	Sucks through a straw, spoon feeds without spillage, begins using fork, removes all clothing except those with small or back fastenings, unfastens snaps, shoelaces, medium-sized buttons, puts on simple clothes without assistance, washes and dries hands independently, toilets independently except for wiping.
3 yr	Puts on underpants, socks, shoes, teeshirt; unbuttons accessible buttons.
4 yr	Laces shoes, fastens large-sized buttons.
5 yr	Fastens medium-sized buttons, dresses self except for bows and small-sized buttons.
6 yr	Ties bows and shoelaces, fastens small-sized buttons.

Frankenburg, WK and Dodds, JB[13]; Roger, S and D'Eugenio, DB[14,15]; and Kauffman, NA: Occupational Therapy with Children: The School Setting. In Hopkins, HK and Smith, HD (eds): Willard and Spackman's Occupational Therapy, ed 6. JB Lippincott, Philadelphia, 1983, p. 683.

The major differences in a young pediatric patient compared to older children or adults include:

1. Body surface areas differ from adults, with the head and neck accounting for 21 percent of the total body surface area (TBSA) (<2 years). In addition, the body surface area to body weight ratio is larger in the pediatric age group.
2. The skin is much thinner so that lower temperatures or shorter exposures to heat or chemicals may create deeper burns in a young child. Therefore, many wounds that initially appear superficial may eventually require skin grafting.
3. Scald injury initially appears "cherry red," thus frequently is mistaken for a superficial injury when in reality it is a full-thickness injury.
4. Dehydration is a frequent postburn complication due to diarrhea, evaporative water loss, and increased fluid requirements.
5. Burns greater than 10 percent TBSA require formal fluid resuscitation.
6. Temperature control is more difficult, and hypothermia is a common operative complication.
7. Burn injury in young pediatric patients has a higher mortality rate.
8. Hypertrophic scarring is more severe and scar maturation is prolonged.
9. Donor sites frequently become hypertrophic.
10. Rehabilitation is more difficult due to the inability of the very young pediatric patient to cooperate.

Minor Burn Injury

In an uncomplicated burn of less than 10 percent TBSA, wounds frequently can be treated on an outpatient basis. Small burns often are due to scalds from spills, and wound depth is difficult to determine. If the wounds do not heal within 2 to 3 weeks, the patient then is readmitted for excisional therapy. As a pediatric patient tends to experience more severe hypertrophic scarring, these small wounds must be excised, with placement of either a closed 1.5:1 meshed graft, or preferably a sheet graft, to achieve the best cosmetic results.

If the burn wound is small and determined early to be full thickness, excisional therapy can be initiated promptly. However, this category of burn injury does not necessitate that the patient go to the operating room immediately for excisional therapy but can allow for a period of stabilization.

Moderate Burn Injury

The second category of injury is moderate burn injury, characterized by 10 to 20 percent TBSA involvement. In this category, the cause of the burn is frequently a scald injury from submersion. This injury is deeper, with the depth more easily determined. These patients require burn shock resuscitation. Wound coverage generally can be achieved with one grafting procedure; however, an experienced surgical team is mandatory.

Major Burn Injury

Burns of 20 to 40 percent TBSA comprise a difficult group of patients and in the age range of less than 3 years can have significant morbidity and mortality. These patients require management in burn centers with clinicians experienced in treating the young pediatric patient. If there is no concomitant inhalation injury and there is mixed partial- and full-thickness burns, then operative procedures are begun, usually after resuscitation of burn shock and stabilization. If there is concomitant inhalation injury and the wounds are full thickness, then the approach of prompt removal of nonviable tissue is followed. In general, the removal of all dead tissue within the first 7 days following injury is preferred.

Massive Burn Injury

The very young pediatric patient with burns greater than 40 percent TBSA usually will have associated inhalation injuries, and early removal of nonviable tissue is imperative for survival. Herndon and colleagues[3] have used the philosophy of massive early excision in the first 24 hours with excellent results. These patients are similar to a group with burns greater than 70 percent TBSA in older children and adults.

Operating Room Techniques

PREOPERATIVE PREPARATION

A pediatric burn patient without an intravenous line or nasogastric tube should not be taken off food and water after midnight prior to surgery. Instead, the surgical procedure should be planned so the patient has nothing orally for only 3 to 4 hours. A pediatric burn patient can become dehydrated easily. Consequently, in all but the smallest burns, an intravenous line should be in place the night before the surgical procedure to prevent this complication.

ANESTHESIA

In the pediatric patient with a small burn injury, ketamine is an excellent anesthetic agent for excision and skin-grafting procedures. In more extensive procedures, which require more time to perform, inhalation agents may be required. To become expert with the use of ketamine and the use of adjuvants such as nitrous oxide and/or diazepam requires practice. In addition to monitoring of blood pressure, monitoring patient oxygenation with oximetry has made procedures under ketamine much safer.

TEMPERATURE CONTROL

The pediatric burn patient will experience a major problem in temperature control both in the operating room (OR) and on the ward. The OR should have the highest room temperature and humidity that the operating team can tolerate. A patient's temperature during the operative procedure should be monitored carefully. Other methods to maintain body temperature, including warming intravenous fluids, use of warm solutions, placement of heating pads under the patient, and covering exposed areas, should be routine OR procedures.

BLOOD LOSS

A study of blood loss in the pediatric age group has shown a loss of approximately 2 percent of the circulating blood volume for each percent area excised and grafted.[4] Use of this formula can standardize blood requirements for excisional procedures. Careful monitoring of blood with replacement is essential in the very young pediatric burn patient.

Surgical Approach

The surgical approach to wound coverage in the pediatric age group depends on the severity of injury, which includes extent of injury, depth of injury, location of injury, age of patient, presence of inhalation injury, concomitant injury, and comorbid diseases.

WOUND EXCISION

As in an adult patient, wound excision may be performed to the fascial layer or as a tangential excision. In a pediatric patient, a true tangential excision with viable dermis is rare, as the dermis is very thin. Excision down to fascia in a pediatric patient, although technically easier and associated with less blood loss, results in marked cosmetic deformities as well as difficulty in reconstructive surgery that frequently is required secondary to subsequent growth.

DONOR SITES

The ideal donor site in a pediatric patient is the back.[5] The use of thighs, buttocks, abdomen, and chest frequently results in hypertrophic scarring of the donor sites; however, the back usually heals without hypertrophic scarring and with only a skin texture alteration. If very thin skin is used for a graft, the cosmetic result in the recipient site is not acceptable, and if the skin is too thick, donor site scars are at greater risk for hypertrophy. In the very young pediatric patient, a donor site should be treated as an initial partial-thickness burn wound with an antibiotic ointment. The use of thin films or synthetic dressings to cover buttock and thigh donor sites is difficult because patients in this group are not toilet-trained.

SKIN-GRAFTING PHILOSOPHY

A pediatric burn patient demonstrates marked hypertrophic scarring, so minor and moderate burns should be grafted with a sheet skin graft in which drain holes have been made with a scalpel. Sheet grafts result in a marked improvement in cosmesis and function.[6,7] Although sheet grafts require more expertise and careful placement than meshed skin grafts, the results are worth the extra time and effort.

REHABILITATION OF THE PEDIATRIC PATIENT

The course of a child's rehabilitation is directly affected by certain factors. In the acute phase, these factors include the severity of injury, occurrence of life-threatening or secondary complications, immediate postburn management, period of time to wound closure, age, and premorbid health of the child. In the rehabilitative phase, factors include a child's genetic tendency for hypertrophic scarring, speed of scar maturation, need for reconstructive or cosmetic surgery, availability of postdischarge rehabilitation services, the child's growth and development, the psychological adjustment of the child and family, and compliance with the recommended treatment.

A knowledgeable, well-coordinated team can make a difference in a child's quality of life. Each team member brings to a child special skills with the team goal of returning the child to a healthy, active life.[8]

The Family

The family plays a major role in the rehabilitation of a burned child. The family may include mother and father, siblings, relatives, close friends, or foster parents.

Whoever has the distinction of being "family" for a child should be given special attention by the therapist, because they will be responsible for providing care and support to the burned child following discharge. Beginning with the initial interview, a rapport should be established early with the family, which then sets the stage for ongoing interaction and family compliance with the rehabilitation program. A therapist should build on the family's strengths, while respecting individual coping mechanisms, and promote a normal interaction between family and child. The family should be recognized as a constant entity in the child's life, and the therapist should be both instructor and partner during the entire course of the child's recovery.

Early and frequent family education regarding all aspects of a child's care will foster the family's trust and respect for the therapist and increase the probability of compliance following discharge. Pacing the family's involvement with the child's rehabilitation should be individually tailored to the patient and family's level of comfort to avoid frustrating or overwhelming them. Written instructions with illustrations, frequent observation of therapy sessions combined with participation, and reciprocal demonstration of rehabilitation techniques, all help to ensure successful skill acquisition by a family member.

Positioning

Proper positioning of a burned child is a challenge due to small body size, usually high level of activity, and inability to cooperate with a positioning program. An infant's normal flexion posturing encourages the contracture position. "Passive" positioning techniques, which may involve use of restraints, traction, or splinting, usually are necessary with the young pediatric patient as well as adolescents who are unresponsive, incoherent, or uncooperative. This approach is useful especially following skin grafting to prevent graft disruption by a child moving or scratching. For small active children, air band splints may be used to reduce edema, protect the burned area from trauma, prevent or decrease scar contractures, and they can be applied over low-profile splints[9] (see Chapter 11). "Active" positioning techniques such as the use of arm supports, pillows, or footboards are ideal for adolescents or children who can cooperate with nonrestrictive forms of positioning.

Exercise and Activities of Daily Living

The initiation of an exercise program with a burned child usually begins within the first 24 to 48 hours following burn injury. Although contractures generally do not develop during the first 48 to 72 hours postburn, joint range of motion often is limited by acute edema or restrictive eschar. Exercise should include gentle, repetitive active or active-assistive range of motion. As the child becomes stabilized medically, a more aggressive, individually customized exercise program can be instituted.

PASSIVE EXERCISE

Passive sustained stretching and massage to healed burn tissue is routinely performed with the pediatric patient to elongate tight scar bands or to lengthen shortened soft tissues, such as the Achilles tendon. Combining these techniques is useful for all body areas, but especially for the face, axillary folds, flexor creases, and web spaces of the hand or foot. Massage is especially important when treating the scars of infants because their small size and rapid growth makes the proper fit of scar compression garments difficult and therefore less effective.

Stretching and massage requires the use of two hands, so a child should be stabilized on a mat on the floor or between the therapists legs, so both hands will be available. The family also may assist by either holding the child or massaging while the therapist stretches. Following instruction, passive exercise and/or massage may be performed by a family member or, depending on the age of the child, by the patient. Cuff weights can be used to gently stretch a tight extremity while the child's attention is diverted with an activity that uses the other extremities. *Gentle* passive stretching also can be performed under general anesthesia to evaluate true range of motion in an uncooperative child or to stretch resistant contractures without pain.[10]

When passively exercising a child with an acutely burned extremity, precautions are similar to those for adults. However, because the skin over the dorsum of the fingers is much thinner than that of adults or adolescents, they are at greater risk for boutonnière deformities. Extra care must be taken when passively exercising the dorsally burned pediatric hand to avoid excessive force to an already compromised extensor hood mechanism. Lost degrees of flexion due to dorsal skin tightness can be regained later through exercise, and if necessary with surgical release. However, once a boutonnière deformity occurs, especially in the pediatric hand, permanent functional loss almost always results.

Because an infant grows rapidly, clinicians should recognize that scars should be kept flexible so that normal growth is not adversely affected, especially in the hands and feet (Fig. 18–1). Frequent massage and sustained stretch is the most effective means to accomplish this. However, if the scars compromise growth, the burn team should consider surgical intervention.

ACTIVE AND ACTIVE-ASSISTIVE EXERCISE

Active and active-assistive exercises are used with all children as soon as they can actively participate in an exercise program. To encourage active participation, developmentally and age-appropriate recreation/play activities should be incorporated into therapy sessions.[11,12] These play activities can and should be modified to meet desired therapeutic goals. For example, to encourage active stretching of an axillary scar band, playing basketball, with the hoop gradually elevated, can be used with an older child, or reaching up to hit a balloon or to pop bubbles for a younger child. The therapist should be creative and flexible during therapy sessions to provide as many choices to the child as possible. As time allows, structured exercise sessions are followed by therapeutic but fun activities of the child's choice. This opportunity gives children a sense of control in a setting where they are allowed very few options. These activities also give children the psychological benefit of participating in their own physical recovery, which in turn increases trust, cooperation, and interest in the therapy program.

STRENGTHENING ACTIVITIES

Resistive exercises and extended periods of activity are initiated as a pediatric patient's strength improves. Graded exercise devices and play activities used for

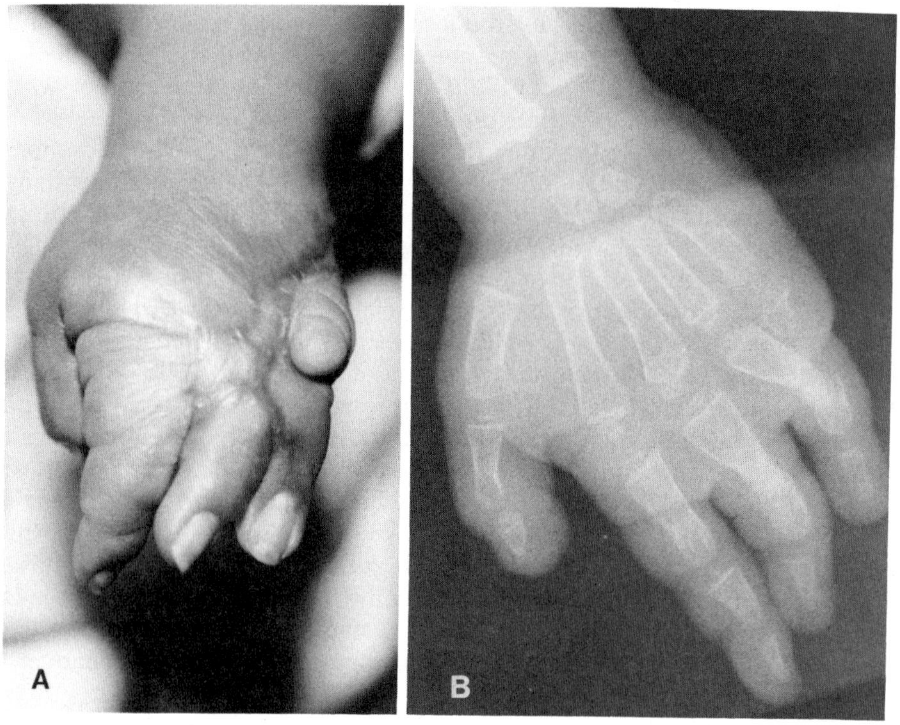

FIGURE 18–1. (*A*) An example of how scars interfere with normal growth is seen in this full-thickness burn to the dorsal metacarpal area of the left hand sustained when the child was 6 days old. The force of the scar on the fingers prevented growth of the little finger and stunted normal growth in the middle and ring fingers. (*B*) A radiograph of the same patient reveals fusion of the middle and ring proximal interphalangeal joints due to the linear pull of scar tissue.

strengthening and increasing endurance include graded foam exercise sponges; therapy putty; Thera-band; stacking cones (that stick together slightly); gross motor games (ball toss, "Simon says," kick the balloon); or bicycling and tricycling (Fig. 18–2). Board games, crafts, puzzles, and small toys are good activities for developing fine motor coordination. The therapist should keep an inventory of activities with known therapeutic value; that can be easily graded in complexity or physical requirements; are safe and appropriate for various age and culture groups; and can be adapted for use in bed, when sitting, or for the ambulatory patient (Tables 18–7 and 18–8).

SELF-CARE ACTIVITIES

Age-appropriate self-care activities such as feeding, helping with dressing changes, bathing, applying cream, and dressing are ways to increase physical activity. Self-feeding is encouraged as soon as a child is allowed food by mouth (Fig. 18–3). Whenever possible, children should assist with their own burn care to decrease fear and foster interest in recovery. Bathing and dressing oneself helps to increase range of motion, flexibility, and endurance. Except when the burn has resulted in a

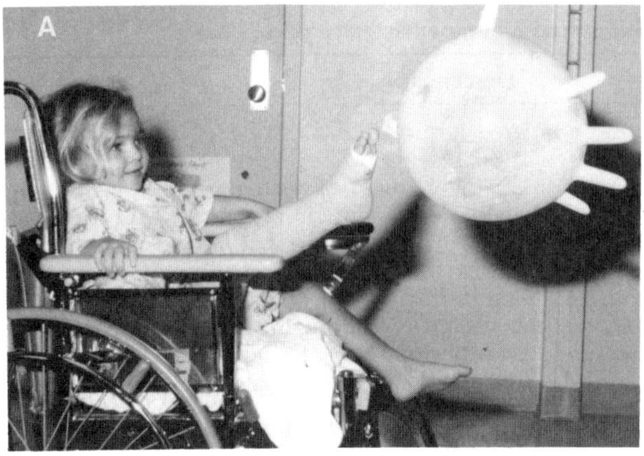

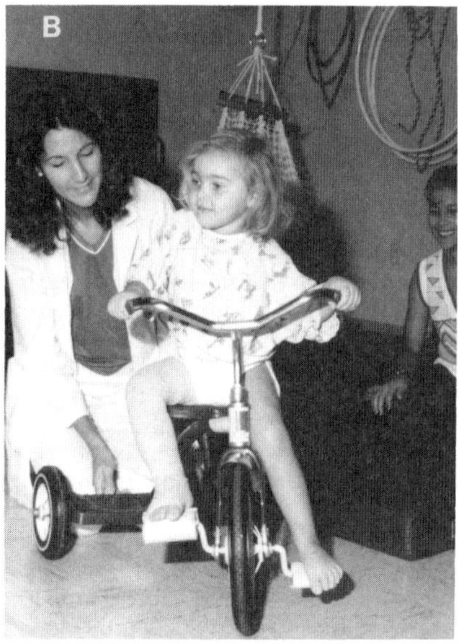

FIGURE 18-2. (*A*) Therapeutic activities, such as kicking a balloon, are used to encourage active range of motion of a burned extremity beginning with an activity that provides joint mobility. (*B*) As a child feels less anxious and mobility improves, activities are progressed to provide more joint range of motion and resistive exercise such as riding a tricycle.

permanent functional loss, any use of adaptive devices, such as built-up handles, should be considered temporary and kept at a minimum to prevent dependency on special equipment.

DEVELOPMENTAL SCREENING

Children often regress emotionally and developmentally during the acute phase of burn recovery, but these usually are temporary responses to a very stressful situation. However, if an appropriate developmental recovery is not made as the acute stage draws to a close, a formal, in-depth developmental assessment should be considered. The child can be screened for developmental problems during play and activities of daily living. The Denver Developmental Assessment and Reference Chart by Frankenburg and Dodds[13] are useful, quick references when observing a child for developmental milestones. These tests screen children from birth to 6 years of age for developmental delays. Children can be assessed in the areas of gross motor development, language, fine motor development, adaptive behaviors and personal-social behaviors. The Developmental Programming for Infants and Young Children—Early Intervention Developmental Profile and Preschool Developmental Profile by Rogers and D'Eugenio[14,15] can be used to assess children from birth to 60 months of age. The six areas of development addressed by these assessments are perceptual and fine motor, cognition, language, social and emotional, self-care, and gross motor. These evaluation tools can be adapted for use with normal, high-risk, and handicapped populations. Information from these assessments should be shared with the treatment team, who can then modify their treatment goals to foster skills where deficits were noted.

TABLE 18–7. Suggested Therapeutic Activities

Activity	Description
Gross motor activities	Foam Nerf balls, balloons, or inflated surgical gloves can be used for a variety of gross motor games and activities. Hitting or kicking these items provides low-resistance range of motion for the extremities while unlikely to cause trauma to burn sites or healed grafts. Maximum effort is needed for the patient to make the ball or balloon travel very far so it is a good activity for increasing strength and endurance. A string can be attached to the balloon and hung from the ceiling keeping it off the floor and saving the therapist from spending too much time chasing the balloon. Nerf basketball is a good activity for upper extremity range of motion. Scooter boards, tricycles, hoola hoops, the game Forward Pass, drawing on a large mirror or paper hung on the wall are all beneficial as gross motor activities. *Precautions:* Small children should not be allowed to mouth ballons or play with them unsupervised due to danger of choking if the balloon deflates. Children should not be allowed to inflate surgical gloves because they may inhale the powder from inside the gloves. Foam balls are difficult to clean and may be a contamination risk to a child with exposed, unhealed burns.
Fine motor activities	Board games, puzzles, dominos, plastic-coated playing cards, peg games, and other commercially available games can be used to increase fine motor coordination, sitting tolerance, and social interaction. *Precautions:* Such games and activities must be age-appropriate for the child. Games with minimal small, loose pieces are recommended. Paper play money may need to be laminated or sealed in clear contact paper so it can be cleaned between patients.
Computer games	Good for eye-hand coordination and for cognitive awareness. A variety of computer games are available for patients from age 3 and up. "Nintendo time" can be a positive reinforcement for appropriate behavior in the "difficult" adolescent or older child. *Precautions:* Unlimited use of computer games may interfere with other therapy goals. The noise may be distracting to others, but the equipment still needs to be in an area supervised by staff to prevent inappropriate or excessive use.
Arts and crafts	A variety of craft activities can be physically therapeutic while enhancing self-esteem. Therapeutic benefits include eye-hand and fine motor coordination, upper extremity range of motion and strengthening, general endurance and sitting tolerance, cognitive stimulation and opportunities for creativity. *Precautions:* Craft activities should be analyzed for therapeutic benefits, age appropriateness, and the potential for contaminating or traumatizing a healing graft or burn wound.
Expressive play activities	A doll with a bed and a variety of "doctor things" is helpful when teaching a small child about medical procedures and for allowing the child to express their anxieties through play. A doll house with a family of dolls is also beneficial for expressive play especially if the burn occurred at home, involved other family members, or if the child was abused.
Toys	Parallel, associative, and cooperative play should be encouraged between children if cross-infection is not a concern. Toys are the tools of childhood and therefore a variety of washable toys should be available, especially for the younger child, in order to encourage normal play activities. These toys could include rattles; busy boxes; activity boards; pounding bench; musical toys (drum, toy piano, xylophone); plastic puzzles; nesting/stacking toys; building blocks; Bristle or Duplo blocks (or for older children, Lego blocks); hand puppets; toy farm with animals; inflatable punching toy and beach ball; drawing paper and plastic crayons; a magnetic board with letters and numbers; a large chalk or dry marker board; a Velcro dart game; a variety of books; a record or tape player with an assortment of recordings for various ages; a variety of balls, dolls, cars, planes, trains, trucks, hats for dress-up, several toy telephones; scooter toys; a rocking horse, tricycle, or Big Wheel; wagon; and, if space allows, a set of child-size table and chairs; a playhouse or play kitchen with dishes and plastic food. A separate play area where absolutely *no* medical procedures of any kind are allowed is essential.

TABLE 18–8. Suggested Toys for Various Age Groups

Up to $2\frac{1}{2}$ Yrs	3–4 Yrs	5–7 Yrs	8–10 Yrs
Rattles	Crayons and coloring books	Bean bags/balls	Jigsaw puzzles
Squeak toys	Musical toys	Construction sets	Models
Nesting toys	Building blocks	Snap-together models	Erector sets
Hand puppets	Play Dough	Jump rope	Horse shoes; Jarts; ring toss
Picture books	Tricycle	Bicycle	Table games

Pediatric Splinting Considerations

A splinting program frequently is indicated following a burn injury that involves the face, neck, or extremities. Decisions regarding the duration and frequency of splint wear should depend on the original depth of the burn, presence of grafts, location of the burn, and anticipated potential for contracture formation. In addition to the small size of children, the therapist must consider other anatomic differences, such as thinner, more fragile skin and hypermobile joints. Also, parents have difficulty being aggressive enough in stretching a contracture due to the pain they may cause their child. Anticipated or actual patient and family noncompliance affects the decisions that are made regarding the type of splint fabricated and the splinting schedule.

For infants and small children, splinting is initiated at the first evidence of skin tightness prior to any loss of range of motion. Unlike older children or adolescents, they do not have the understanding or the physical strength to exercise against a

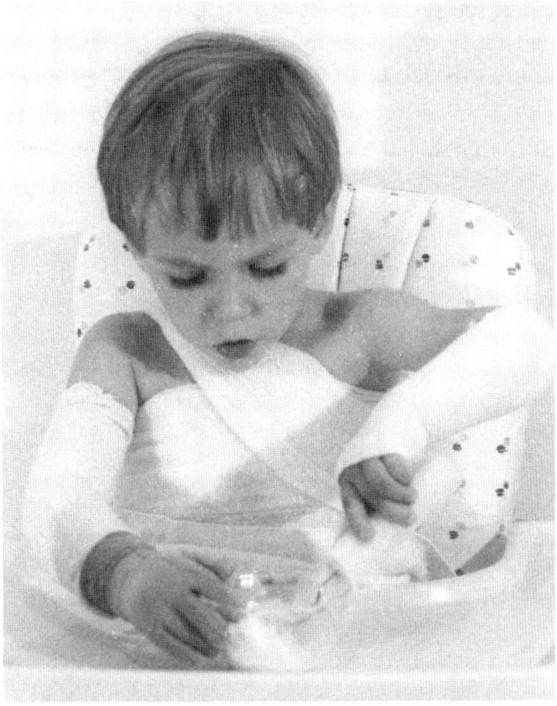

FIGURE 18–3. Pediatric patients should be encouraged to participate in such age-appropriate activities of daily living as self-feeding.

tightening scar. Therefore, splinting them as soon as initial edema subsides or stabilizes is advised. Unless there is deep tissue damage, such as a ruptured tendon or fracture, splints should be used only during naps and at night so that active use of the extremities during play can be encouraged. If range of motion decreases, the wearing time is increased to 24 hours a day except for exercise and activities such as dressing changes or bathing, eating, and supervised play. Unlike adults and adolescents, small children do not tend to lose strength or joint mobility when immobilized in splints for extended periods, providing the splints are removed for regular exercise or activity sessions.

Some splints that work well with larger children or adolescents are not as effective with small children, and minor problems may require a large splint. For example, dynamic splints can be used with adolescents or older children, but they are not recommended for small children because they often are difficult to keep in place. Clinically, adjustable three-point elbow or knee extension splints and dynamic ankle splints are of benefit to children over the age of 3. However, serial static splints or casts may be more practical and effective with smaller children. Since no dynamic force is applied and adjustments are made only by the therapist, there is less chance of a maladjusted splint that may result in pain, pressure areas, or other problems. Another example is the individual finger splint for correcting interphalangeal joint flexion tightness. These small splints tend to fall off, rotate, and are easily lost. Even if only one finger is affected, especially if it is the fifth digit, a hand splint may be necessary for the small child to effectively correct a contracture. A finger splint may correct a flexion contracture but will not prevent or correct the external rotation contracture that often occurs in this type of burn.

Because of a young child's small size and the presence of "baby fat," foot and hand splints may have to be made longer so they can be anchored to the leg or an extended wrist. Otherwise, the splint will tend to slide distally and actually place the extremity in a deforming position. Two foam straps applied in an X pattern over the ankle or back of the hand retain volar splints in place more effectively and comfortable than one strap crossing the wrist or ankle. In addition, adding extra straps or applying the splint with an elastic bandage or self-adherent wrap may be necessary. Heavy or contour foam padding assists to secure a small hand or foot into a splint and to keep the fingers extended or the toes flexed. Cotton socks over the splint may prevent the child from removing the splint. However, they also make "spot checking" of the splint's fit by staff or family difficult and may result in the splint being worn improperly for extended periods.

When a child's hand has multiple contractures or problems, treatment priorities should be decided on and approached in stages. Trying to correct all the problems at once with one splint, especially with children, is not practical and could result in pressure areas, skin breakdown, joint inflammation, unnecessary pain, and delay in healing that could contribute to increased scarring. Focusing splinting efforts on increasing metacarpalphalangeal joint flexion and thumb palmar abduction, which are critical to function, sometimes is best. After functional gains in the larger joints are made, then emphasis can be placed on improving motion in the interphalangeal joints.

Following surgery, "guardrails," made of thermoplastic material attached to the splint, can be used to protect graft sites that are being treated with open exposure rather than being wrapped in a dressing (Fig. 18–4). The guardrails keep a child

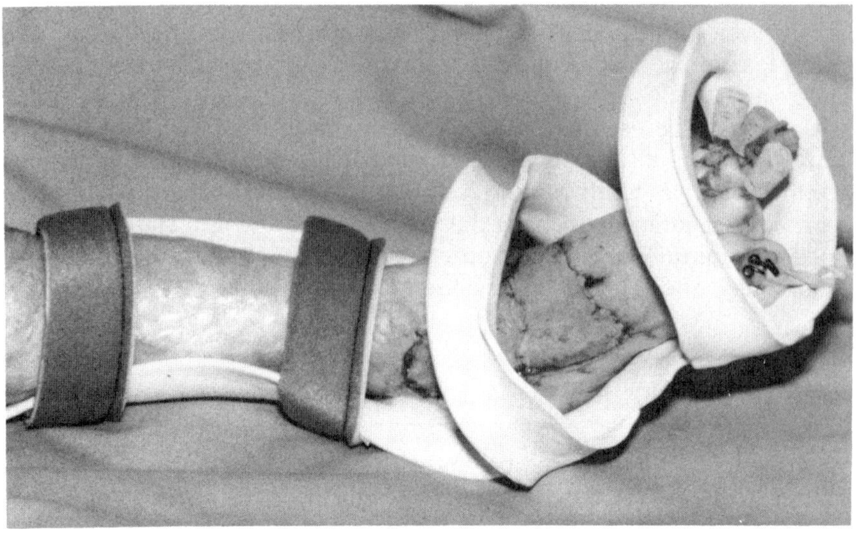

FIGURE 18–4. A postoperative foot splint with guard rails used to immobilize and protect sheet grafts on the dorsal surface of the foot.

from rolling over onto the graft site or can be used to prevent the child from touching the graft.

Providing and displaying written instructions and whenever possible, writing instructions directly on the splints using a permanent marker or indelible pen, is advisable. Specific instructions help make all persons involved with a child's care more aware of how, when, and why a splint should be applied.

Physical Agents

With severely burned pediatric patients, long-term exercise programs continue following discharge and may require the use of additional physical agents such as paraffin, Fluidotherapy, or ultrasound to treat scar contractures (see Chapter 15). When using surface heat modalities, the therapist must first evaluate the child's tolerance to heat both physically and psychologically. Newly healed burned skin often is hypersensitive to heat, and children also may be frightened by modalities that use heat, depending on the cause of their original burn. Dipping a hand or foot into a paraffin bath may frighten a child, while applying paraffin with a paint brush or gauze may be less intimidating.

Fluidotherapy delivers heat more efficiently than paraffin because higher temperatures are better tolerated in the dry environment[16] and can be used to help decrease a child's skin hypersensitivity. A game can be played by placing small objects of various sizes, shapes, and densities into the chamber and having the child capture them. Because children cannot easily see the objects, they must be located by sense of touch and by repeatedly grasping and digging through the granular material. Therefore, Fluidotherapy provides heat and facilitates active exercise. In addition, children may be less anxious and more cooperative with therapy because they are being entertained. Active-assistive and passive exercises also can be performed during Fluidiotherapy. However, because the dry heat of Fluidotherapy can cause excessive evaporative water loss of the skin and scars, care should be taken to moisturize the skin following treatment.

Ultrasound can be used to soften connective tissue and assist with mobilization of tight joint capsules in children. Ziskin and Michlovitz[17] advise against overexposure of epiphyseal plates to ultrasound, but therapeutic intensities are considered safe. They warn against intensities above 3.0 W/cm^2 when using a stationary transducer for periods of 3 minutes or greater, otherwise demineralization of bone, damage to epiphyseal plates, and retardation of bone growth could result.

Scar Management Techniques

Scar management in children begins with assessing the child's potential for hypertrophic scarring and/or contractures. If a child has had previous injuries that required sutures or sustained a deep dermal abrasion, these scars may offer evidence as to the type of scars that may develop. The child may or may not develop the same types of scars as the parents, but if both parents develop hypertrophic scarring or either parent has formed a keloid scar, the child will have a higher potential for excessive scarring. When compared to adults, young children appear to have a higher incidence of hypertrophic scarring and scar band formation, especially if the wound takes longer than 2 weeks to completely heal.

WOUND AND SKIN CARE

Itching can be a serious problem with newly healed burns if scratching results in excoriation of the new epithelium. Most of the damage from scratching is due to trauma by the fingernails or from a shearing force caused by rubbing. Even with the fingernails cut very short, a small child cannot be expected to refrain from trying to rub or do something to relieve discomfort. However, even very small children can be taught to gently "pat" the irritated areas, which usually brings relief without damaging the skin. Oral antihistamines can relieve some itching but may cause drowsiness during school or playtime hours, so they usually are recommended for use at bedtime. Itching also can be relieved by keeping the newly healed tissues well moisturized with a water-based lotion. Covering fragile healed areas for protection at night or during rough play is advisable.

The pores of surviving sweat and sebaceous glands often are obstructed by scar tissue, resulting in an accumulation of secretions. These secretions appear as scattered "whiteheads" or water-filled pustules in areas of healed deep partial-thickness burns and at graft sites. This condition may occur in burned children of all ages but especially with adolescents who are already at risk for acne and other skin conditions that result from increased perspiration and oil production. These pustules usually resolve by spontaneously opening to make new pores. Adolescents should be warned not to squeeze them or infection could occur. Children of all ages should avoid use of 100 percent polyester or nylon fabric clothes because these fabrics are nonabsorbent and do not "breathe," leading to increased perspiration and moisture buildup. A child or adolescent should use cotton socks and ventilated shoes, because foot and toe burn scars are susceptible to fungal infections.

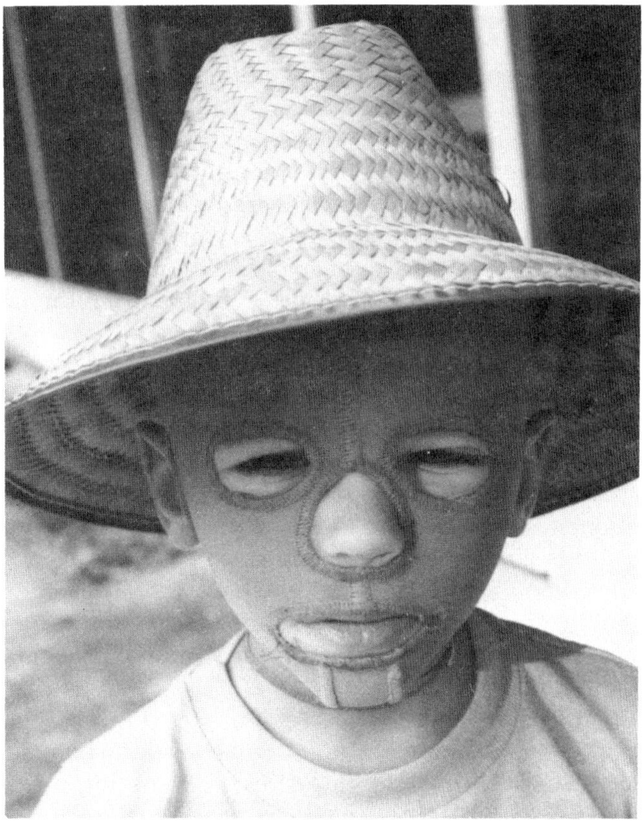

FIGURE 18–5. A young patient wearing a broad-brimmed hat to protect his face from the sun.

Newly healed burns and immature scars are very susceptible to sunburn and hyperpigmentation if sun exposure is allowed. All burns should be covered with soft, lightweight cotton (or at least a cotton polyester blend) clothing. For children with face and neck burns, a hat with full brim (not a cap) is recommended (Fig. 18–5). Children should refrain from activities that expose them to direct sunlight or strong reflected glare for at least a year after their burn injury or last surgical procedure. Nongreasy sunblock lotions with a sun protection factor (SPF) rating of 15 or higher (Appendix C) have been found to be effective in protecting against reflected sunlight but should be applied hourly even if labeled "waterproof." Lotions that contain padimate O (octyl dimethyl PABA) or PABA ester, are not recommended since they may irritate a child's hypersensitive skin or scars.

SPECIAL COSMETICS

When a burn involves the face or hands, special cosmetics may be of interest, especially to adolescents. Makeup consultations should be offered to both sexes; however, use of cosmetics is ultimately the patient's choice. Females routinely use cosmetics to enhance their appearance for social acceptance and peer approval. Males tend to use cosmetics for special occasions, such as for photographs, proms, and graduation ceremonies. The makeup is used to correct uneven pigment after the burn scars are mature and the texture has been flattened out by compression therapy (see Chapter 14).

COMPRESSION THERAPY

Children require pressure on their burn scars to minimize scar hypertrophy and contractures and to speed scar maturation. Rapid growth of a child dictates close monitoring of the scar management program for garment revision or remeasuring.

Scar compression often begins with the use of elastic bandages or temporary, tubular compression bandages and garments. Elasticized cotton tubular bandages can be used to make inexpensive, temporary compression garments for use until custom compression garments can be tolerated over fragile, newly healed tissue. However, if the therapist makes garments from the tubular dressings, a double layer of the material should be used, similar to the way that a tubular ready-made garment is constructed. A single layer tends to wear out rapidly, does not give even pressure, and actually may cause bruising of a child's newly healed burns beneath the elastic fibers in the fabric. Padding may be necessary beneath garments especially over fragile areas. If corrugation of the burned skin occurs under the elastic fibers of a tubular compression bandage, elastic bandages should be used instead. Tubular dressings also tend to wear out with repeated laundering and may no longer provide adequate compression if not replaced regularly. Tubigrip makes temporary gloves that may fit adolescents and older children. However, because these gloves typically run small in the fingers, a larger than recommended size may be needed for newly healed hand burns, even if tightening the wrist portion of the glove is required.

Compression Garments

There are numerous options to consider when measuring and ordering garments for children. When ordering a vest or body suit, the zipper for small children should be in the back to prevent them from unzipping the garment and disrupting the pressure. For older children and adolescents who are expected to dress themselves, the garments should have front zippers regardless of burn location. Zippers in extremities should be used only in the initial garments to prevent trauma during donning, not to make it easier for the parents to apply. Zippers prevent lengthwise elasticity and may ruffle after laundering, resulting in uneven scar compression.

Superior shoulder or torso burns require a body brief garment with sleeves, not a vest, to provide adequate pressure to these areas, especially in the active child. Snap crotch openings can be designed in garments to help facilitate diaper changes and toilet training.

For children in a growth spurt, expansion panels should be included in the trunk and extremities. When measuring for garments, care must be taken not to pull the measuring tapes too tight, especially in obese children. However, when measuring over diapers, the tapes should be pulled snugly. Multiple garments should be ordered for children in diapers or those who have been recently toilet-trained. New garment measurements should be taken every 3 to 4 months or as needed to accommodate for growth and development.

Small hands and feet are a challenge to measure and fit properly with pressure garments. When measuring hands or feet, length measurements are more accurately obtained from a photocopy of the palmar surface of the child's hand or sole of the foot than from an outline of the hand or foot. The photocopy is sent to the garment company to confirm the accuracy of the measurements recorded. All gloves, gauntlets, and anklets should be measured to at least $1\frac{1}{2}$ inches above the wrist or ankle, regardless of the location of the burn, to make removal more difficult for small children and to ensure proper pressure over the dorsum of the foot or hand. For infants, better pressure on the hand may be achieved through the use of self-adherent elastic wrap with foam in the web spaces. If a child's hand is burned only in the midpalm and does not involve the web spaces, a compression glove alone may be contraindicated. Gloves tend to pull the thumb into adduction and fold the palm. Instead, an insert of open-cell foam padding or silicone putty is recommended under a glove or secured with self-adherent elastic wrap. Except in the case of partially amputated fingers, fingertips should be left open so that caregivers can better monitor the circulation of a child's fingers. Closed fingertips also may interfere with proper compression in web spaces.

Inserts

Silicone putty, silicone gel sheets, or skin care pads work well as inserts for children because they are gentle on fragile skin. Narrow strips of Velfoam padding, worn between the fingers or toes under compression gloves or footgloves, work well to preserve web spaces and do not macerate the skin or interfere with hand or toe function. Wider pieces of Velfoam padding also work well to protect sensitive scars over flexion creases from abrasion by the garments.

Aquaplast splinting material $\frac{1}{16}$-inch thick can be used for thin, flexible conformers that fit well under a fabric face mask garment (Fig. 18–6). This material conforms especially well around the eyes, nose, nasolabial folds, and chin. The fabric face mask with an Aquaplast splinting material conformer appears to give adequate multidirectional compression. However, school-age children and adolescents may prefer to wear a Uvex face mask when out in public (see Chapter 14).

Special Areas of Concern

HANDS AND FEET

Two types of burns common to small children are contact burns involving the palmar surface of the hand and fingers and dorsal foot burns involving the toes. With a palmar burn (Fig. 18–7), the hand should be splinted in wrist extension, finger extension and abduction, with the thumb in radial abduction (Fig. 18–8). Use of fingernail traction should not be used, especially with small children under 5 or 6 years of age, to avoid damage to the nail beds or displacement of the nails, which may have been compromised by the initial burn injury. In addition to the essential massage and stretching of the palm and digits into extension, weight-bearing activities (e.g., crawling on all fours, pushing a large heavy ball or roll) will assist in minimizing palmar contractures and in desensitizing the area.

The dorsally burned foot should be splinted in full, combined ankle and toe plantar flexion regardless of whether the ankle was burned (Fig. 18–9). This position puts a full stretch on skin surfaces, which tend to contract rapidly in deep partial or grafted full-thickness burns. Silicone putty, secured to the dorsum of the foot with an elastic self-adherent wrap, is a practical, better-fitting alternative to using a hard thermoplastic material for splinting the dorsally burned infant foot in plantar flexion. Similarly, when splinting infant hands, either full-contact "sandwich" splints[18] or splints lined with antipressure contour foam padding (see Appendix L), or a mixture of elastomer and prosthetic foam is useful.

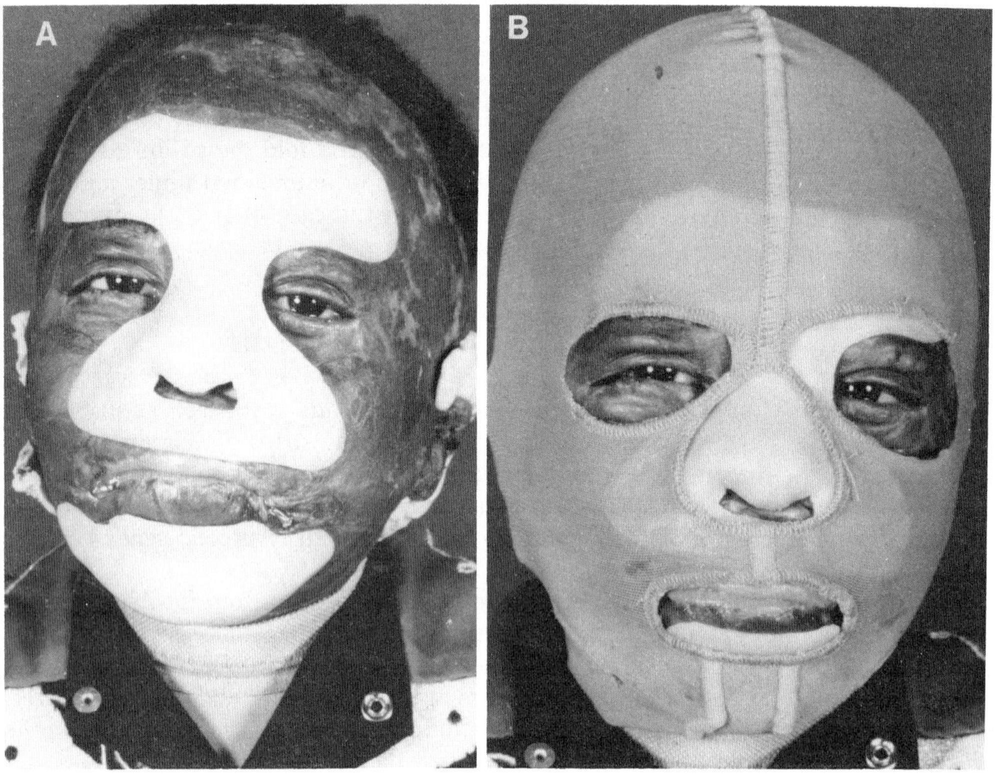

FIGURE 18–6. (*A*) Thermoplastic splinting material facial conformers ($\frac{1}{16}$-inch thick) are used to compress the contours of the chin, nose, and nasolabial folds. Silastic conformers, behind the ears, are used to preserve the skin fold. (*B*) These conformers are held in place using a scar compression garment.

Once palmar hand or dorsal foot contractures begin to develop, they are very difficult to correct nonsurgically. Everyday functional use puts the extremity in the position of contracture, and the child's musculature is not sufficient to resist the steady force of contracting scar tissue. However, splints cannot be worn continuously without the potential for loss of function (e.g., lengthening of the finger flexor and toe extensor tendons or Achilles tendon tightness). As stated previously, splints should be worn all night and at naptime unless joint range of motion is decreasing.

FACIAL BURNS

Electrical burns to the mouth, due to biting an electrical cord, occur with small children. These burns usually involve a full-thickness skin loss in one or both commissures. If allowed to contract, microstomia results, which interferes with eating and oral hygiene and is cosmetically disfiguring. Since these wounds are often allowed to heal by contraction, maintenance of maximal mouth opening is essential. As with all burns, initiation of mouth exercises should begin before wound healing is complete. During this period the child and family are instructed how to perform active and passive mouth-stretching exercises. The mouth opening size should be monitored closely. The maximum lateral stretch size of the mouth is measured by using two rigid, washable rods of $\frac{1}{4}$-inch diameter (acrylic straws, temperature probe covers,

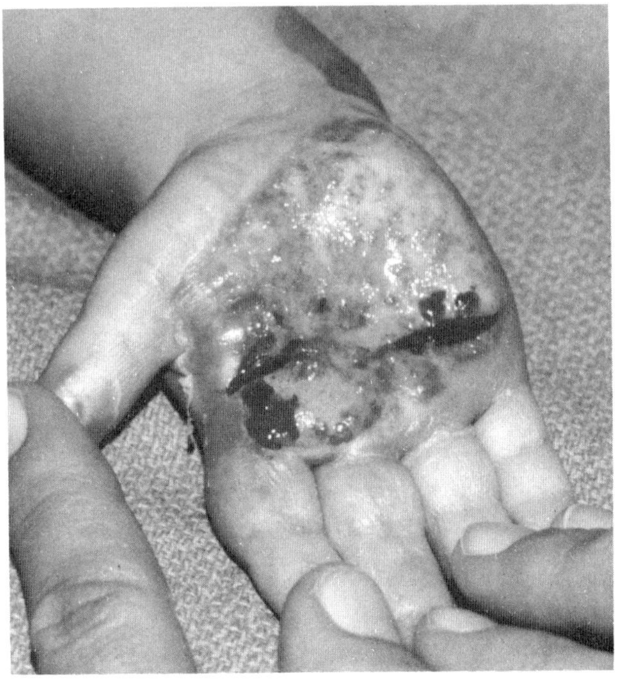

FIGURE 18–7. An example of a typical deep partial- and full-thickness palmar contact burn acquired from a hot surface, such as an oven door or clothing iron.

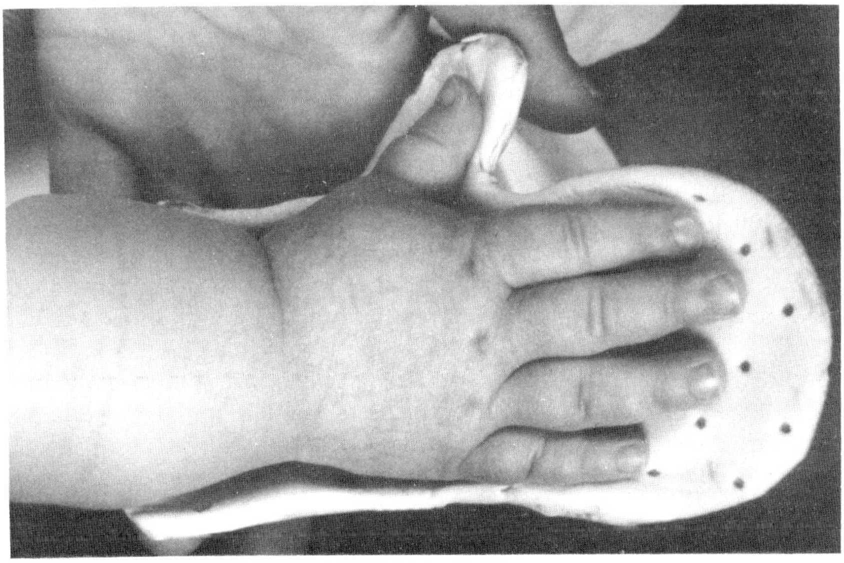

FIGURE 18–8. A palmar stretch splint with the wrist extended, fingers fully extended and the thumb radially abducted.

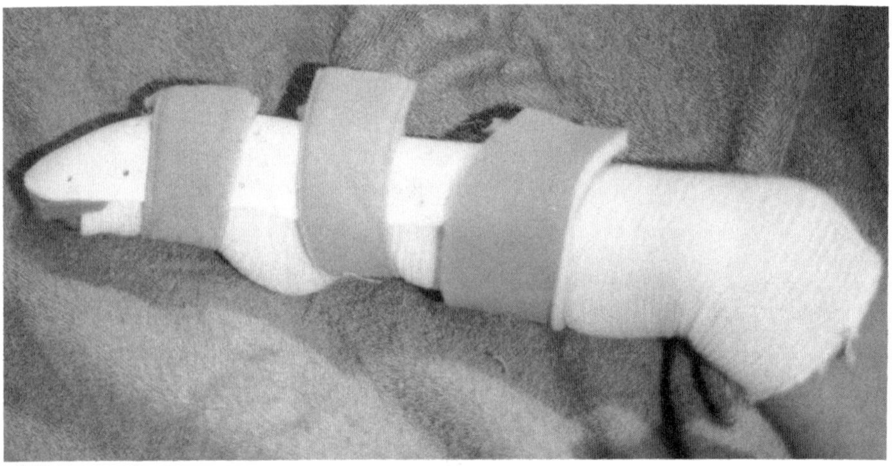

FIGURE 18–9. A splint to stretch a dorsal foot burn with the ankle and toes both in full plantar flexion.

ballpoint pen casings, or plastic dowels). The rods are placed well into the mouth between the teeth and cheeks where they should be positioned parallel and spread horizontally to the maximum tolerated passive stretch. The distance between the outer surfaces of the rods at the commissures of the mouth are then measured with a measuring tape attached to one of the rods. Mouth size during full lateral stretch with the teeth together should be approximately the same size as the distance measured between the lateral canthi of the child's eyes. These rods also are used to passively stretch the mouth for at least 5 minutes, four to eight times throughout the day (Fig. 18–10). In addition to horizontal stretching, vertical stretching and "yawning" encourage further elongation of the commissure. Passive vertical stretching of the mouth can be achieved using a stack of tongue blades or a cone. After a burn is completely healed, massage is recommended to soften and thin the commissure in order to promote mouth symmetry (Fig. 18–11). This same treatment regimen can be used with any facial burn involving the mouth, regardless of the initial cause of injury.

To achieve scar compression on the face, a fabric face mask with an insert or a Uvex face mask are used most frequently. Advantages of the Uvex face mask are that it is all one piece and the child's face and hair can be seen when it is worn. The main disadvantage is that the device is occlusive, and moisture buildup requires frequent removal for those children who develop heat rashes or for adolescents with a tendency toward acne. A Uvex face mask also may crack or break if treated roughly by the child. For infants and children under the age of 5, a fabric mask may be safer than a Uvex face mask. A rigid face mask may restrict facial growth unless frequent revisions are made to accommodate the rapid growth rate of this population. In addition, babies require frequent feedings and often drool, which would necessitate continuous removal of a Uvex mask to clean and dry the accumulation of moisture and oil. Often a combination of facial scar compression devices is best for a child. The therapist needs to be flexible and realistic when designing and fabricating scar compression garments and devices to be worn by an individual child.

NECK AND AXILLA BURNS

The neck and axilla are two locations where preventing the loss of skin surface area is especially difficult in children. Traditionally, these areas have been treated

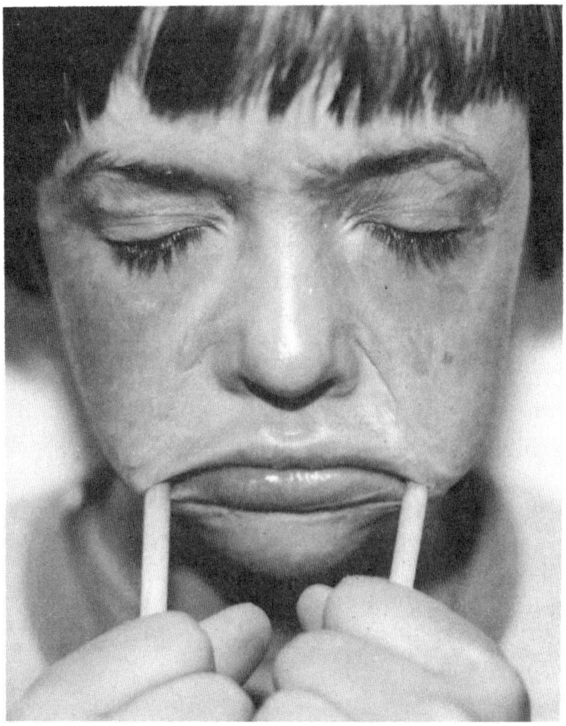

FIGURE 18–10. Patient performing lateral stretch mouth exercise using acrylic rods.

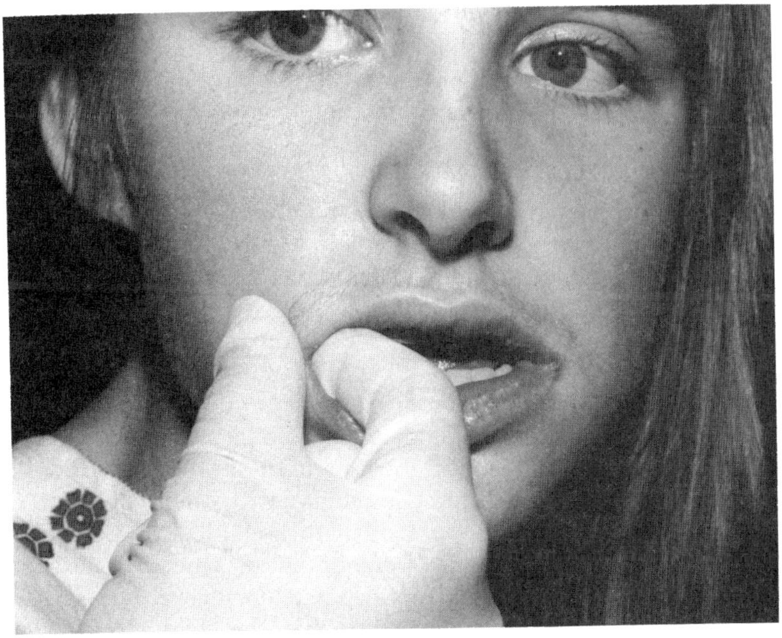

FIGURE 18–11. Massage to a scar nodule at the right commissure.

with rigid splints made of thermoplastics. Neck splints and "airplane" splints are very difficult to keep in place, limit function, and rub during play activities, which can cause blisters and skin breakdown. Airplane splints may fit while a child is in bed, but tend to slide downward when a child is up, regardless of the number and placement of straps. Splint slippage is more of a problem if a patient is obese or an adolescent. Thermoplastic neck conformers may not conform precisely to the neck. If made when the child is supine, the conformer may not fit when the child sits up, and vice versa. If made with the neck extended, the child cannot see his or her feet when walking, and safety becomes an issue.

A custom-made, U-shaped, 2- to 3-inch thick foam collar covered with multiple layers of stockinette and snugly wrapped around the child's neck allows most neck movements except flexion. The collar uses compression rather than neck extension to preserve the flexibility and contour of the anterior and lateral neck. The absorbent cotton stockinette is nonabrasive and allows the skin to breathe. Because the collar is like a circumferential pillow attached around the neck, neck extension is maintained as the patient sleeps without the discomfort of a rigid neck splint or neck roll.

Soft foam conformers wrapped snugly into the axillas with a figure-of-8 elastic wrap or clavicular strap can help prevent tightness of axillary skin folds. These conformers can be worn day and night and interfere less with exercise and play than an airplane splint. If needed, the airplane splint still can be worn over the axillary conformers at night.

Psychosocial Aspects

Sometimes a burn team member can forget how terrifying burn care procedures are to children and families. Fear and anxiety lower patients' pain threshold, making dressing changes, therapy sessions, and other procedures more difficult for them to tolerate.

One way to decrease anxiety of both the patient and the parents is to communicate in advance what can be expected as a result of a burn injury. A child and his or her family will be less overwhelmed by the sight of facial swelling the day after a burn if they are informed ahead of time that this is an expected part of a burn injury. Medical, nursing, and therapy procedures should be explained to a patient and family in understandable terms prior to initiation of the procedures. Technical descriptions are not as necessary as explaining why the procedure is being performed, how long it will take, will it hurt or cause discomfort, and if so, to what extent and for how long. With children, one must relate the procedure to the child's senses and familiar experiences. Some examples might be "your donor site will be right here when you wake up. It will sting for a couple of days like a bad scrape on your knee when you fall off your bike," or "I'm going to get this yucky stuff off your hand and then I'll be done. This cream is going to feel real cold like ice cream when I put it on your burn." Caregivers should focus all their attention on the child, by talking to the child throughout the procedure and not socializing with others in the room.

An effective way to obtain cooperation with a child during a procedure is to demonstrate the procedure on a family member first or, whenever possible, to allow the child to participate in some way. Painful procedures should be scheduled when medications are most effective and when possible, the child should be allowed to determine in what sequence the most unpleasant activities are performed. A child should be able to see and/or handle all materials before they are used, especially if they are warm or cold, and should be given a choice of a pleasant activity to engage in after unpleasant ones are finished. This participation gives children some reassurance and sense of control in a setting where procedures are usually "done to" them instead of "done with" them.

Caregivers should always be truthful with a child. Statements such as "this will only hurt a little," "I'm almost done . . . ," "Mommy will be right back," that were said to decrease short-term anxiety will only foster distrust and subsequently cause greater anxiety later if the truth is stretched. In addition, caregivers should not invade a child's personal space, even for a hug, without permission.

These suggestions cannot guarantee a cooperative child, and the burn team should understand that crying is appropriate. The child who does not protest painful procedures should be viewed with concern. Children's emotional behavior usually regresses during their stay in a hospital and they may whine, cling to parents or staff, or display other behaviors inappropriate for their age. Behavioral limits can be established that allow appropriate expression of emotion without compromising care. Screaming, squealing, biting, and kicking should be discouraged, but a child should never be reprimanded for crying. Physically restraining children during treatments should be avoided unless their behavior poses a major obstacle to safely accomplishing a procedure. Physical restraint can result in frightening a child even more and cause increased negative behaviors. Children should never be made to feel guilty or told that they are "bad" regardless of their behavior. Instead, the behavior should be identified as wrong or inappropriate. This approach helps to preserve a child's self-worth while teaching acceptable behaviors. Desirable behaviors should be reinforced consistently with verbal praise and individual attention.

Adolescent males often are one of the most difficult groups to motivate. They frequently procrastinate with their exercise program, fail to wear compression garments, and may seem oblivious to developing scars and contractures. The "that won't happen to me" immunity attitude is difficult to dispel. "Scare tactics," such as showing adolescents photographs of scars or contractures, may help to develop compliance in some cases, but a better approach for the stubborn adolescent seems to be to have a previously burned adolescent visit and share his experiences. Sometimes the most difficult patient becomes your best advocate for compliance after "graduation" from the scar management program. Whenever possible, a patient should be visited by a recovered burn patient who had a similar burn injury.[19] Also, scheduling adolescents in groups for outpatient therapy is helpful so that they can socialize and support each other.

Family members, especially parents, also need a great deal of support. They frequently need reassurance from the staff to help them cope with their feelings of guilt, helplessness, and concern for their child. The early support that families receive from the burn team can have a positive impact on their compliance with long-term follow-up after discharge. Early involvement of family members in a child's care is beneficial for all persons concerned.

Discharge Planning

Prior to discharge, a child's rehabilitation program should be well-established without daily changes. Caregivers should be independent in wound care, proper application of splints, pressure garments and devices, and with the exercise and scar massage programs.

A school-aged child should be prepared for return to school and association with old friends, especially if functional loss or disfigurement has occurred. School re-entry programs involving teacher and classmates facilitate a child's adjustment by helping the class understand what has happened to the burned child and how they can be of support.[20,21] This program also prevents unnecessary restriction of a child's activities by the school due to misconceptions associated with physical appearance or functional limitations. All children, from preschool age children in day-care centers to adolescents, benefit from this intervention. Such re-entry programs involve communication with the involved teachers and if available, with community therapists working in the school system. Contact with the school should be initiated at least 2 weeks prior to discharge or re-entry into the school. With prior parental permission, written information and instructions are provided to appropriate school personnel. A therapist or burn team member may visit the school to explain to the burned child's classmates and teachers what has happened and help answer any questions they might have regarding compression garments, splints, the child's physical abilities, and need to stay out of the sun. The goal is to return the child to school as soon as possible with the least amount of disruption of normal routines and with the least emotional trauma (see Chapter 16).

Outpatient Follow-up

Long-term outpatient follow-up is necessary with a burned child to ensure maximum function and minimal cosmetic defect over the multiple growth periods between infancy and adulthood. Following discharge, a child should return to the burn care facility in 1 to 2 weeks to be fitted for scar compression garments (if not already done) and to assess the transition from hospital to home for both the child and parents. Early intervention affords the opportunity to answer questions and reinstruct the child and family in key treatment areas, which helps to prevent subsequent difficulties. A child should be seen at 1- to 3-month intervals depending on the number of garments and appliances used and family compliance with the program. Changes in scars should be re-evaluated every outpatient visit for response to compression therapy, repigmentation (which may be an indication of sun exposure), evidence of contracture, and early signs of maturation. The family should be reminded to bring all appliances with them to clinic, because revisions may be necessary. Garments, face masks, and splints will need to be remeasured and revised as growth occurs and scars mature.

A child should be monitored for normal motor and functional development. Over a period of years, scars may interfere with normal growth, and a child may require additional surgery and therapy even after the scars are mature. Therefore, annual visits are advised until a child has completed physical development.

RECONSTRUCTIVE SURGERY

Burn reconstruction of a pediatric burn patient can be divided into two areas. The first is the need for reconstructive surgery to return a child to normal physiologic function. The second, and very important area, is the need for reconstructive surgery associated with growth. Skin grafts and scar tissue do not stretch as a child grows, and the need for reconstructive procedures across joints is a frequent occurrence. Any joint may be involved; however, the major areas of concern are the neck, axilla, antecubital area, wrist, popliteal area, and dorsum of the foot. A full-thickness burn in any of these areas during early childhood may necessitate two or three reconstructive procedures during growth of a child up to adulthood. The general principle that guides the need for growth reconstruction is that as long as a child has normal range of motion, the surgical procedure is delayed even though scar bands may be present. With early loss of range of motion, a scar contracture release with placement of a split-thickness or a full-thickness autograft in the involved area or a Z-plasty is performed. A Z-plasty with placement of normal skin across a scar band may be preferred, because normal skin will stretch as a child grows.

The frequency of reconstructive procedures depends on an individual's growth pattern. Children who grow in "spurts" may require two or three releases in the same area before they reach adulthood. After a child has reached adult height, tight contracture bands should be released even though there may be normal range of motion.

A special consideration in the female pediatric patient is the breast. Breast reconstruction should be delayed until approximately one year after menstruation begins; however, if breast development is abnormal due to axillary contractures, a release of this area should be performed earlier.

CASE STUDY

HISTORY

PL, a 5-day-old female, received 30 percent total body surface area deep partial- and full-thickness burns to her scalp, face, thorax, abdomen, hands, perineum, and left lower extremity, reportedly from a steam vaporizer. Subsequent information revealed that the child was a victim of abuse by her mother, and the child was placed in custody of a local court.

During her acute burn care, PL underwent three surgical procedures involving excision and split-thickness skin grafting to the thorax, abdomen, dorsum of the right hand, left thigh, and left hand. Hand deformities began to occur by 3 weeks postburn, and a radiograph of the left hand revealed dysplasia of the three ulnar fingers. Her scars began to flatten the transverse arch of the hand and deform the joints of the digits. PL's developmental level was delayed slightly in gross motor activities, and she became increasingly delayed for her age in fine motor tasks. She was referred for therapy at 4 weeks postburn at which time exercise, splinting, and compression therapy programs were initiated. PL was placed in a foster home at discharge and the foster mother was instructed in range of motion exercises, scar massage, skin care techniques, and application of her pressure garments and splint.

At 5 months postburn, PL had reconstructive surgery to release the dorsal hand contracture utilizing a flap created from the stunted, dysfunctional little finger. Syndactyly of the index web space was released and skin-grafted, the metacarpophalangeal (MCP) joints were pinned in flexion, and the hand was put in a cast. Three weeks later the cast and pins were removed. One week later, outpatient therapy was resumed

At 28 months postburn, PL had a tenolysis of the extensor digitorum communis (EDC) tendon. At $3\frac{1}{2}$ years postburn, PL required a repeat tenolysis of the EDC tendon and a capsulotomy of the MCP joints of the left hand. PL wore scar compression garments and a left hand sandwich splint.

At $5\frac{1}{2}$ years postburn, PL exhibited functional use of her left hand with only a slight decrease in grip strength and was appropriate for her age emotionally and developmentally.

PROBLEM LIST

Patient unable to assist with therapy program
Rapid growth immediately following burn injury
Severe contraction of wound margins
Distorted palmar arches, decreased passive and active range of motion of left hand
Vascular scars
Slight developmental delay

GOALS

Foster mother independent in home therapy program
Active and passive range of motion of left hand within functional limits
Restore palmar arches of left hand to normal
Avascular, pliable, flat scars
Age-appropriate gross and fine motor developmental level

INTERVENTIONS

PL received outpatient therapy three times per week immediately following discharge. Therapy consisted of massage, passive stretching, and splinting in a sandwich splint. Gross and fine motor activities also were performed. Gross motor activities were discontinued at approximately 10 months postburn, and the foster mother was instructed as to how to perform these at home. PL wore her splint at all times except during therapy, meals, and supervised play periods. After each surgical release, PL's left hand was placed in a cast for 2 to 3 weeks. Following tenolysis surgery, range of motion exercises were re-initiated again after the cast was removed. The sandwich splint was changed to a resting hand splint and worn at night while a dynamic MCP flexion splint was used for short periods of time during the day. Scar massage, active and passive range of motion exercises to the hand, and fine motor activities were continued.

Formal outpatient therapy continued approximately 6 months following her last surgery. Treatment included the use of moist heat, passive and active-assistive range of motion exercises, functional and play activities, and continuous dynamic splinting.

Initially, to minimize scar formation, a romper, waist-height pants, open-faced hood, and bilateral gloves made from soft compression garment material were used due to the age of the child. At approximately 1½ years of age, all garments were discontinued except for the left glove, which was continued for approximately 2 years.

RATIONALE

Since PL was so young, she was unable to actively participate in her burn rehabilitation program. Therefore, a caregiver had to perform her therapy program independently at home. Even with outpatient therapy, full functional recovery with minimal disfigurement can be expected only if a home program is followed. Massage, stretching, and splinting were used to help counteract the contracting forces of the burn scar. However, when these interventions did not succeed, surgical intervention was necessary. Intense outpatient therapy followed each surgical procedure to maximize the patient's outcome. The perseverance and patience of multiple services, therapy teams, and the foster mother who worked with PL was a major factor in this child's regaining functional use of her left hand.

SUMMARY

Burn injuries are tragic events, especially for children. Children do not possess the physical, emotional, or cognitive skills to assist themselves to cope with subsequent treatment and injury sequelae. Physically, their skin and physiologic systems are immature and do not tolerate stress like an adult. Emotionally, children do not possess adequate coping mechanisms to manage the pain and disfigurement associated with a burn. Cognitively, they have limited ability to understand what is occurring or what is expected of them. Burn wound management techniques and the surgical approach to the pediatric patient vary according to whether the burn is minor, moderate, major or massive. Rehabilitation techniques for children are somewhat similar to adults; however, a successful approach requires knowledge of the patient's developmental and cognitive level. The therapist who can address patients verbally, visually, and physically at their current level of functioning and understanding will achieve program goals more easily. Also, because the family plays a pivotal role in the eventual outcome, rapport with and education of the family are fundamental to achieving a successful result.

REFERENCES

1. Nelms, BC and Mullins, RG: Growth and Development: A Primary Health Care Approach. Prentice-Hall, Englewood Cliffs, 1982, pp 262–482.
2. Schuster, CS and Ashburn, SS: The Process of Human Development, 2 ed. Little, Brown, Boston, 1986, pp 131–201.
3. Herndon, D, et al: Determinants of mortality in pediatric patients with greater than 70% full-thickness total body surface area thermal injury treated by early excision and grafting. J Trauma 27:208, 1987.
4. Housinger, TA, Lang, D, and Warden GD: A prospective study of blood loss with excisional therapy in pediatric burn patients. J Trauma 34:139–141, 1993.

5. Greenhalgh, DG, Barthel, PP, and Warden, GD: Comparison of back versus thigh donor sites in pediatric burn patients. J Burn Care Rehabil 14:21–25, 1993.
6. Warden, GD, et al: Excisional therapy of facial burns. J Burn Care Rehabil 7:24–28, 1986.
7. Housinger, TA, et al: The use of sheet skin grafts in pediatric burn patients. Proc American Burn Association 23:32, 1991.
8. Salisbury, R, et al: Manual of Burn Therapeutics, An Interdisciplinary Approach. Little, Brown, Boston, 1983.
9. Barnett, PH and Stafford, FS: Use of plastic air bands for edema and scar contracture. J Burn Care Rehabil 5:469–473, 1984.
10. Blassingame, WM, et al: Range of motion of the shoulder performed while the patient is anesthetized. J Burn Care Rehabil 10:539, 1989.
11. Walls, DL: Infant and/or toddler stimulation program for pediatric burn patients. J Burn Care Rehabil 6:335–340, 1985.
12. Gordon, MD: Burn care protocols: Pediatric recreational therapy after thermal injury. J Burn Care Rehabil 8:336–340, 1987.
13. Frankenburg, WK and Dodds, JB: Denver Developmental Screening Test, rev ed. La Doca Foundation, Denver, 1990.
14. Roger, S and D'Eugenio, DB: The Developmental Programming for Infants and Young Children: Early Intervention Developmental Profile, ed 2, vol 2. University of Michigan Press, Ann Arbor, 1990.
15. Roger, S and D'Eugenio, DB: The Developmental Programming for Infants and Young Children: Preschool Developmental Profile, ed 2, vol 5. University of Michigan Press, Ann Arbor, 1990.
16. Borrell, RM, et al: Comparison of in vivo temperatures produced by hydrotherapy, paraffin wax treatment, and Fluidotherapy. Phys Ther 60:1273–1276, 1980.
17. Ziskin, MC and Michlovitz, SL: Therapeutic ultrasound. In Michlovitz, SL (ed): Thermal Agents in Rehabilitation. FA Davis, Philadelphia, 1986, pp 141–176.
18. Ward, SR, et al: Have you tried the sandwich splint? A method of preventing hand deformities in children. J Burn Care Rehabil 10:83–85, 1989.
19. Andreasen, NC, et al: Management of emotional reactions in seriously burned adults. N Engl J Med 286:65–69, 1972.
20. Rosenstein, DLW: A school reentry program for burned children. Part I: Development and Implementation of a school reentry program. J Burn Care Rehabil 8:319–322, 1987.
21. Meyer, DO, Barnett, PH, and Gross, JD: A school reentry program for burned children. Part II: Physical therapy contribution to an existing school reentry program. J Burn Care Rehabil 8:322–324, 1987.

CHAPTER 19

Management of the Burned Hand

Julianne Wright Howell, PT, MS, CHT

Hands are the most frequent site of thermal injury, and thermal injuries rank second among upper extremity injuries requiring hospitalization.[1] The skin covering the hand comprises less than 5 percent of the body's cutaneous surface, but it represents a highly specialized organ essential to hand function. Thermal injury involving the hand, at any depth, is significant enough to be recognized as a severe burn by the American Burn Association. Although timely wound closure is important, successful management of the burned hand does not result simply from closing the wound. Foremost, the clinician must remember that the hand is an organ that, when one of its parts is injured, the entire organ is likely to suffer.[2] The thin, highly mobile dorsal skin, the sensory-enriched palmar skin, and the delicately balanced musculotendinous systems are all at risk when burned. Also, the therapist must have a thorough understanding of wound healing, hand anatomy and kinesiology and therapeutic modalities, as well as be able to maintain an open dialogue with the attending physician.

This chapter has four general objectives for the therapist: (1) to provide an overview of commonly encountered burned hand problems; (2) to outline factors the therapist should consider during evaluation and assessment of an acute, postacute, and reconstructed burned hand; (3) to offer guidelines for therapy management, and (4) to use the case studies about the burned hand as an opportunity to apply one's didactic knowledge and clinical decision-making skills.

PROBLEMS TO BE ANTICIPATED

An understanding of how the hand normally responds to thermal injury is important. Conditions such as postburn edema and damage to tendons, muscles, periarticular structures, and sensory organs can make the status of a burned hand worse if not properly managed. However, a therapist who has a thorough understanding of the effect of thermal injury on the anatomic structures of the hand will be able to anticipate and minimize or even avoid many burn-related problems. Some of the more commonly encountered complications after thermal hand injury include postburn edema, compartment syndrome, joint deformities, sensory impairment, loss of skin stability, and restricted functional use of the hand.

Postburn Edema

An increase in vascular permeability coupled with a shift of fluids to the extravascular space should be anticipated following thermal injury. In superficial partial-thickness (SPT) burns, minimal fluid is leaked into the extravascular space, and edema is minor and transient. In deep partial-thickness (DPT) and full-thickness (FT) burns edema is more severe and prolonged.[3]

As edema increases during the first 72 hours postburn, so may the pressure within the compartments of the hand. Consequently, excessive intracompartmental hand and forearm pressures will impair arteriovenous and lymphatic function.[4] To ensure that the hand is adequately perfused, the radial, ulnar, and palmar arch pulses should be monitored routinely by direct palpation or a Doppler ultrasound flow meter.[4] Therapists involved in the treatment of these hands during the first 72 hours postburn must be aware of the early signs and symptoms of vascular insufficiency so the condition does not advance into a compartment syndrome. Some of the signs and symptoms of vascular insufficiency are: (1) loss or weakened ulnar, radial, or digital pulses; (2) deep tissue pain and paresthesia indicative of carpal tunnel syndrome; (3) decreased capillary filling of the nail beds; (4) uncontrollable swelling with rapid loss of motion; and (5) intrinsic muscle contracture.[4,5] If vascular insufficiency is suspected, Peacock[6] suggested the hand be elevated with the elbow extended, the dressings and splints removed, and the surgeon notified immediately. If blood flow is not immediately improved by these actions, incising the eschar or fascia by surgical escharotomy or fasciotomy may be required.[4] In this situation, compression dressings and pneumatic compression devices are contraindicated to avoid further occlusion of the vascular pathways. In a vascularly challenged hand, use of any form of compression will increase interstitial pressures within the anatomic compartments such that the rigid eschar surrounding the hand acts as a tourniquet.

Uncontrolled edema must be monitored carefully in the first 72 hours postburn. The clinician will find in many burned hands that edema control following the initial 72 hours should remain a priority in order to minimize stiffening of the soft tissue and loss of tendon glide and joint mobility. A description of methods for managing postburn edema is presented later in this chapter.

Common Burned Hand Deformities

METACARPOPHALANGEAL JOINT HYPEREXTENSION DEFORMITY

Another immediate consequence of postburn edema is hyperextension of the metacarpophalangeal (MP) joints and flexion of the proximal interphalangeal (PIP) joints, commonly referred to as a *claw hand deformity*. The severity of these positions

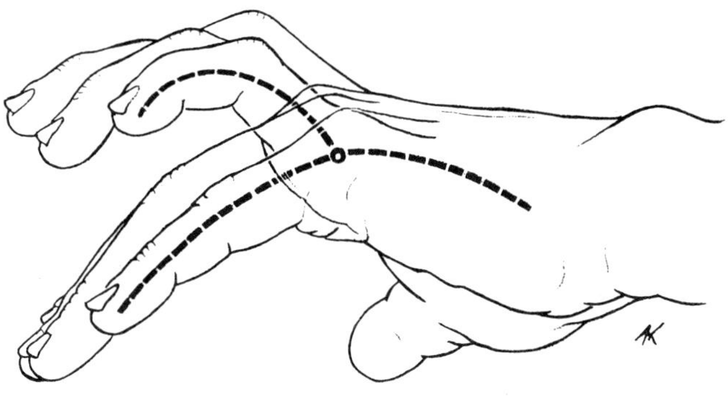

FIGURE 19–1. Metacarpophalangeal joint hyperextension deformity with concurrent flexion of the proximal interphalangeal joints. (From Tubiana, R, Thomine, JM, and Mackin, E (eds): Examination of the Hand and Upper Limb, WB Saunders, Philadelphia, 1984, p 12, with permission.)

appears to be edema-dependent. Hyperextension of the MP joints occurs as the dorsal skin is drawn taut by the fluid shift into the extravascular tissues and as the palmar arches flatten. Flexion of the PIP joints follows as a result of this edema-imposed tension on the common digital extensor tendon system and concurrent hyperextension of the MP joints (Fig. 19–1).[7,8] The predisposition for the MP joint hyperextension deformity to occur is intensified when the dorsal surface of the hand also is burned. Because the dorsal surface of the hand frequently is burned, the likelihood exists for MP joint problems to occur until scar maturation.

Despite early surgical and well-planned hand therapy intervention, hyperextension contractures of the MP joints do develop. Recently, Graham and associates[9] described three types of pediatric MP joint hyperextension contractures. Although this classification system was designed as a preoperative guide for the surgeon, the therapist can use this scheme for early identification of problems involving MP joint hyperextension. Use of this standard method of classification enables the therapist to identify and monitor advancement of a deformity. The recommended method of examination and classification of the three types of MP joint extension contractures are

Type I: The therapist positions the wrist in maximum extension to place the skin and extensor tendons on slack, then passively flexes each MP joint. If more than 30° of passive MP joint flexion is obtained, the wrist is then positioned in maximum flexion, and passive flexion of the MP joints is repeated. If the MP joints cannot be flexed beyond a neutral joint position, this is a type I deformity (Fig. 19–2). In a type I deformity, the dorsal scar is the restricting structure.

Type II: If less than 30° of passive MP joint flexion can be obtained with the wrist positioned in maximum extension, this is a Type II deformity (see Fig. 19–2). The identified restricting structures are the dorsal scar and deeper joint structures.

Type III: If MP joint flexion beyond 30° of MP hyperextension cannot be obtained regardless of wrist position, this is a type III deformity (see Fig. 19–2). The surgically identified restricting structures include extensive dorsal scar, fibrosed intrinsic musculature, and subluxed or dislocated MP joints.[9]

There was a high incidence noted for the ring and little fingers to develop MP joint hyperextension problems. These two fingers accounted for 65 percent of the problem digits studied.[9] Also highlighted was the importance of timely intervention, since the severity of the extension contracture worsened directly with delays in surgical reconstruction.[9]

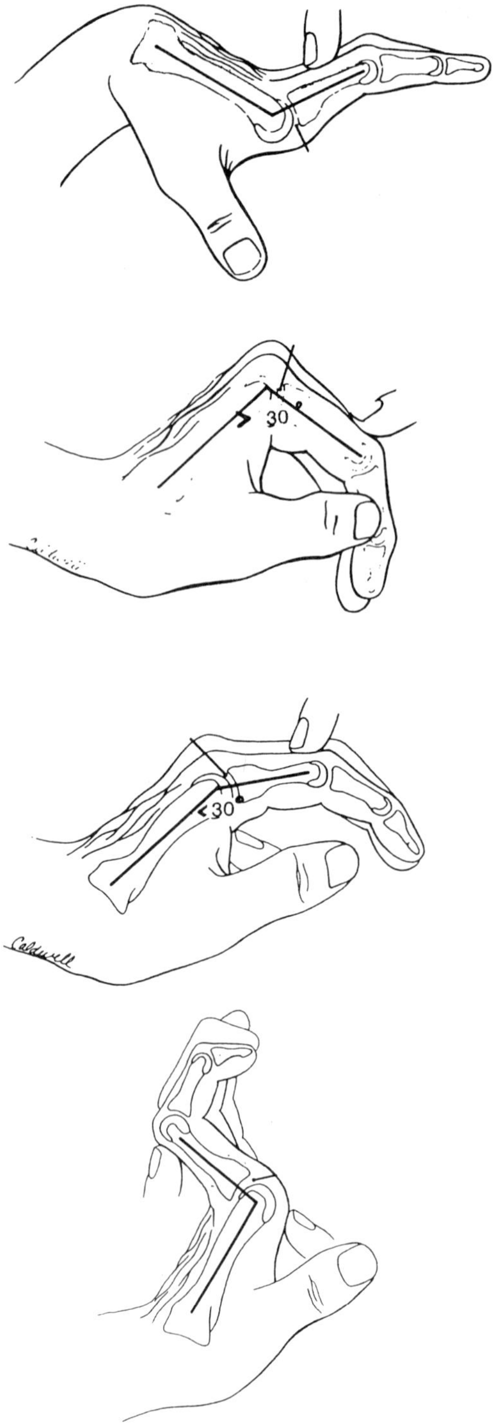

A Wrist Flexion

B Type I

C Type II

D Type III

FIGURE 19–2. Classification of metacarpophalangeal (MP) joint extension contractures. All types of MP extension contractures have restricted passive MP flexion with the wrist positioned in flexion (see *A*). When the wrist is positioned in extension, type I has greater than 30° passive MP joint flexion (see *B*); type II has less than 30° passive MP joint flexion (see *C*); and type III passive MP joint flexion remains fixed (see *D*). (From Graham, Stern, and True,[9]: pp 451–452, with permission.)

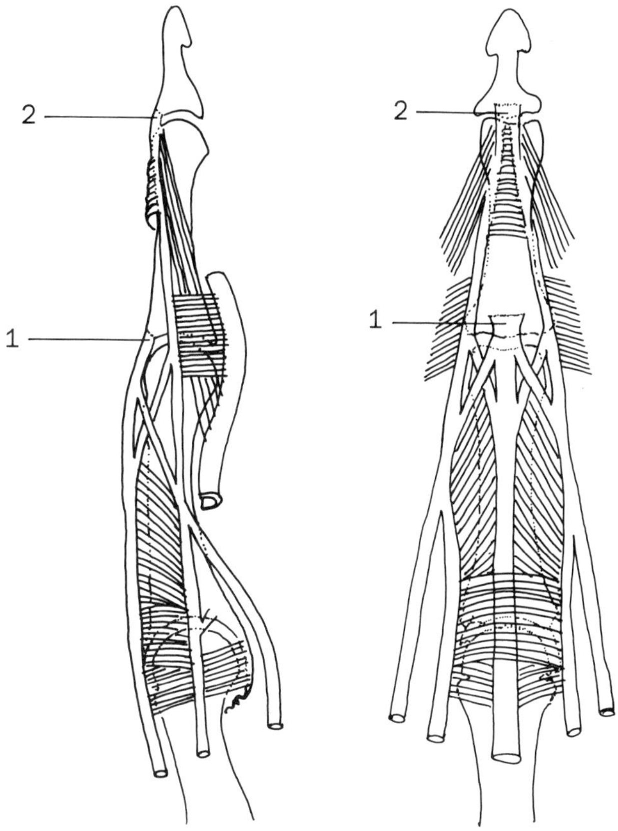

FIGURE 19–3. The extensor apparatus of the finger. (1) Insertion of the central extensor tendon, and (2) insertion of the terminal extensor tendon. (From Tubiana, R, Thomine, JM, and Mackin, E (eds): Examination of the Hand and Upper Limb, WB Saunders, Philadelphia, 1984, p 50, with permission.)

BOUTONNIÈRE DEFORMITY

Therapists should be aware that the potential for a boutonnière deformity exists if an area of burn involves the dorsum of the hand, fingers, or thumb. The potential for this deformity is more likely if the depth of the burn is DPT or FT.

Boutonnière deformity in the fingers involves the extensor apparatus at the PIP joint level (Figs. 19–3 and 19–4). This problem can be the result of direct thermal injury or of tendon ischemia. Tendon ischemia can result when the injured tendon is compressed between the eschar and head of the proximal phalanx as the PIP joint is flexed.[10] The extent of damage to the extensor apparatus often is not known until inspected surgically.[11] Because surgery may not be feasible due to the medical status of the patient or surgeon's choice, involvement of the extensor apparatus should be assumed and protected until viability of the tendon system is known in all DPT and

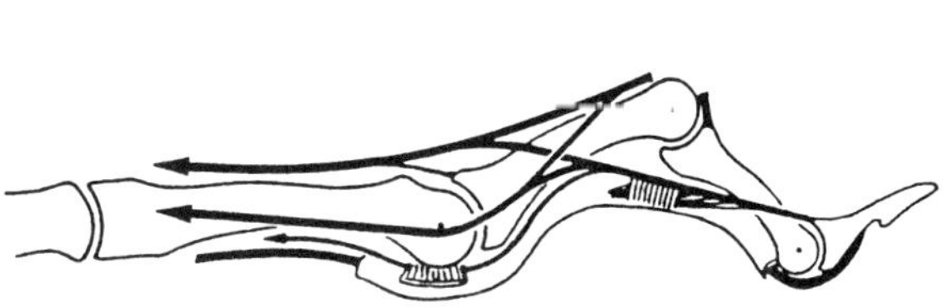

FIGURE 19–4. Boutonnière deformity secondary to thermal injury of the central extensor tendon and/or lateral bands. (From Tubiana, R, Thomine, JM, and Mackin, E (eds): Examination of the Hand and Upper Limb, WB Saunders, Philadelphia, 1984, p 63, with permission.)

FT burns involving the fingers and dorsal hand. Other causes of a boutonnière deformity include flexion of the PIP joint secondary to scar banding volar to the joint axis or secondary remodeling of the volar plate and collateral ligaments in combination with a shortened oblique retinacular ligament attributable to improper immobilization.[12]

The extensor apparatus of the thumb may be directly or indirectly affected by thermal injury. Boutonnière deformity of the thumb manifests as flexion of the MP joint and hyperextension of the interphalangeal (IP) joint. A flexion contracture of the MP joint secondary to a scar band that runs parallel to the thumb MP joint combined with preexisting hyperextension of the IP joint can be one cause. Another cause can be due to a scar band that runs perpendicular to the thumb MP joint and dorsal to the IP joint. The potential for this type of deformity exists if a burn involves the dorsum of the thumb, hand, or wrist, or if the burn surface includes the thenar eminence.

PROXIMAL INTERPHALANGEAL JOINT FLEXION DEFORMITY

Flexion of the interphalangeal joints immediately following injury is a secondary consequence of postburn edema (see Fig. 19–1). Recall that the shift of fluid to the extravascular space in the hand draws the dorsal skin taut, flattens the transverse palmar arch, and disrupts the mechanical balance of the extensor tendon system. This occurrence results in flexion of the IP joints and hyperextension of the MP joints. This situation does not necessarily condemn the IP joints to develop flexion contractures, but if these flexed joints are not carefully monitored and appropriate intervention taken as needed, flexion deformities will ensue.

A therapist should anticipate that flexion deformities are likely to occur when there is persistent edema and/or when the area of burn involvement involves the volar or lateral surfaces of the fingers or palm. The clinician's use of a standardized method to monitor IP joint flexion deformities will only enhance the ability to anticipate problems. The classification scheme suggested by Stern and colleagues[13] is a practical method for a therapist to standardize evaluation of isolated PIP joint flexion deformities. Three types of PIP flexion deformities were described. Type I PIP flexion deformity involves only the scar. To evaluate for type I, the therapist maximally flexes the MP joint, then simultaneously extends the PIP joint passively. If full PIP joint extension is achieved in this position, it is a type I deformity (see Fig. 19–5). Type II PIP flexion deformity involves the articular structures of the PIP joint, such as the collateral ligaments and volar plates. If a type II deformity exists, the PIP joint cannot be fully extended passively by a therapist with simultaneous passive flexion of the MP joint (see Fig. 19–5). Type III flexion deformity is characterized as a fixed deformity of the PIP joint. When the MP joint is held passively in a flexed position, the examiner will not be able to extend the PIP joint (see Fig. 19–5). Usually, the joint surface is irregular or the joint is arthrodesed in a type III deformity. These authors noted that it is often quite difficult to differentiate between a type II and type III PIP joint deformity without the use of radiographs.[13]

Although Stern's method of evaluation was to examine PIP joint flexion deformities, the method can be used to standardize the evaluation of distal interphalangeal (DIP) joint and thumb IP joint flexion deformities. The evaluator passively flexes the PIP joint of the finger or the MP joint of the thumb while simultaneously passively extending the involved distal joint. The type of flexion deformity then can be classified as described previously.

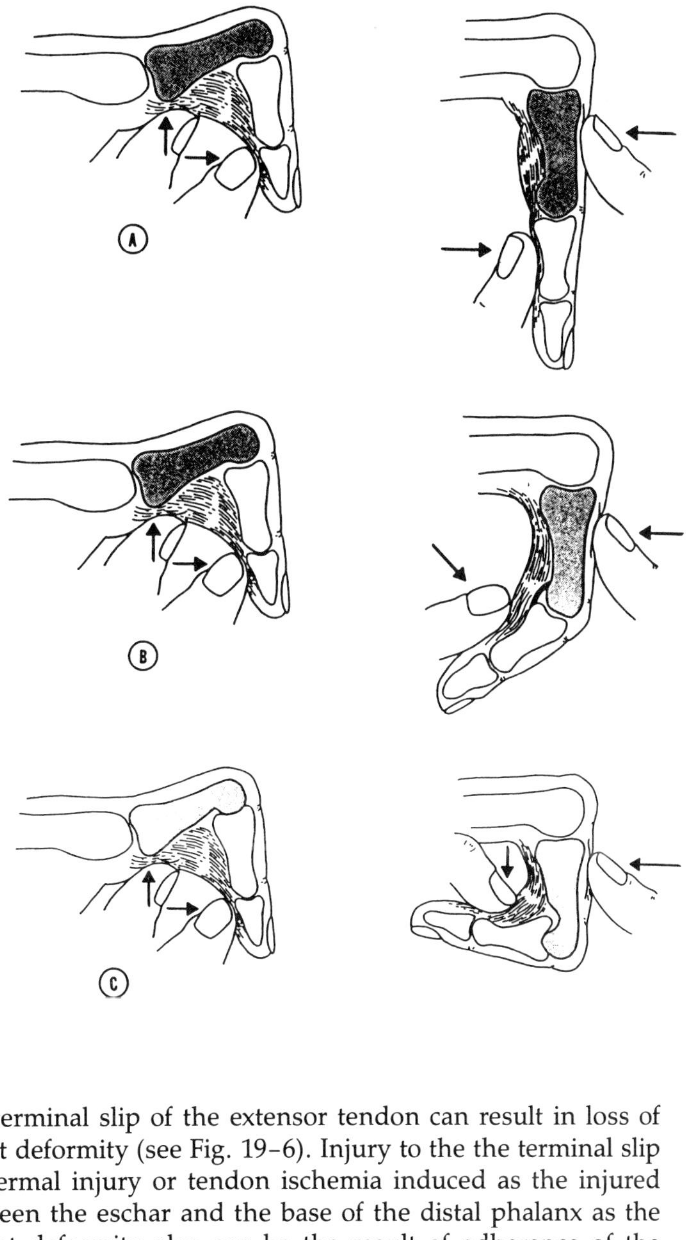

FIGURE 19–5. Classification of proximal interphalangeal joint flexion contractures. A PIP joint flexion contracture exists with MP joint extension in all cases. However in type I, flexion of the MP joint allows full PIP joint extension (see *A*); in type II, flexion of the MP joint does not allow full passive PIP joint extension (see *B*); and in type III, the PIP joint remains fixed regardless of MP joint position (see *C*). (From Stern et al,[20] p 451, with permission.)

MALLET DEFORMITY

Thermal injury to the terminal slip of the extensor tendon can result in loss of DIP joint extension or mallet deformity (see Fig. 19–6). Injury to the the terminal slip can be a result of direct thermal injury or tendon ischemia induced as the injured tendon is compressed between the eschar and the base of the distal phalanx as the DIP joint is flexed. A mallet deformity also can be the result of adherence of the extensor apparatus and lateral bands to the phalanges.[14] Sherif and Boswick[14] suggest that a mallet deformity is the initial presentation of PIP joint hyperextension deformity in the burned hand.

FIGURE 19–6. Mallet deformity secondary to thermal injury of the terminal extensor tendon. (From Tubiana, R, Thomine, JM, and Mackin, E (eds): Examination of the Hand and Upper Limb, WB Saunders, Philadelphia, 1984, p 63, with permission.)

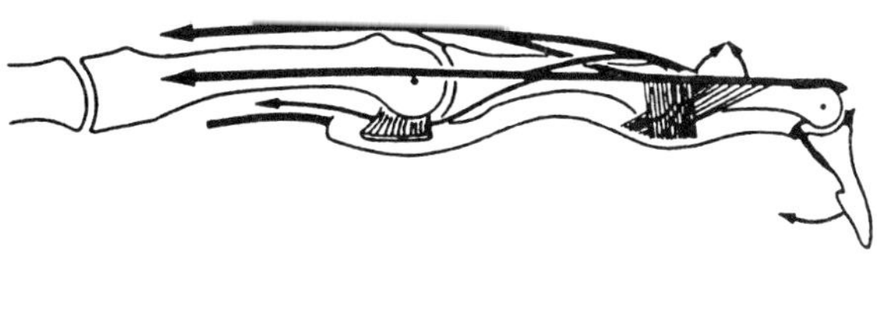

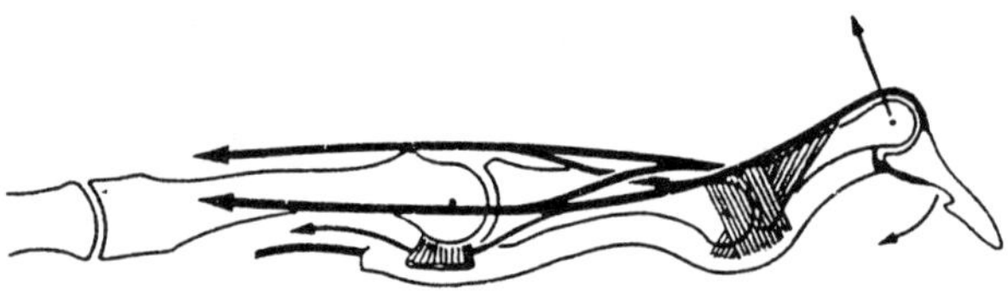

FIGURE 19–7. Proximal interphalangeal joint hyperextension deformity. (From Tubiana, R, Thomine, JM, and Mackin, E (eds): Examination of the Hand and Upper Limb, WB Saunders, Philadelphia, 1984, p 63, with permission.)

A mallet deformity should be anticipated if the burn area involves the dorsal aspect of the finger or thumb distal to the PIP joint or IP joint, respectively. Until the status of the terminal extensor tendon is known, the finger DIP joint or thumb IP joint should be immobilized in extension to prevent any tendon damage or to permit the replacement scar to remodel.

SWAN-NECK DEFORMITY

The swan-neck or PIP hyperextension deformity is characterized by hyperextension of the PIP joint and flexion of the DIP joint (Fig. 19–7). The incidence of swan-neck deformity is most prominent in the middle finger and rare in the little finger. Scarring and contraction of dorsal burn wounds that healed by secondary intention or delayed skin grafting demonstrate a tendency for PIP joint hyperextension burn deformity.[14] Sherif and Boswick[14] hypothesized several causes for PIP joint hyperextension following burn injury. One cause is the presence of dense scar dorsal to the PIP joint axis, which prohibits normal flexion. A second cause is dorsal adherence of the extensor digitorum communis (EDC) tendons at the wrist or hand level so that when the wrist is flexed, a dorsal tenodesis hyperextension of the PIP joint occurs. Other authors[6,15–17] have suggested that ischemic contracture of the intrinsic muscles is responsible for the PIP joint hyperextension deformities seen in the burned hand. Smith[18] cited adhesion of the intrinsic tendons or muscles at the level of the MP joint to be another precipitating factor in PIP joint hyperextension burn deformities. Peacock[19] suggested the cause of a swan-neck deformity is joint stiffness imposed by improper immobilization of the PIP joint in hyperextension.

DORSAL HOODING DEFORMITY

Dorsal hooding or syndactyly is the loss of the dorsal digital web spaces (Fig. 19–8). This deformity can result from inadequate positioning of the fingers or the thumb following a dorsal hand burn. The therapist should anticipate the development of syndactyly in any DPT and FT dorsal hand burn. When splinting a hand with this type of burn, the fingers should be maintained in a position of MP joint flexion of at least 65° to 70° with abduction and the thumb in a position of palmar abduction. These joint positions are optimal for preserving the length of the collateral ligaments and expansion of the web spaces. Initially, postburn edema often prohibits precise positioning of the digital MP joints and thumb. However, as the edema recedes, a therapist should anticipate the need to prevent loss of the digital and thumb web spaces. Appropriate intervention might include application of wound ban-

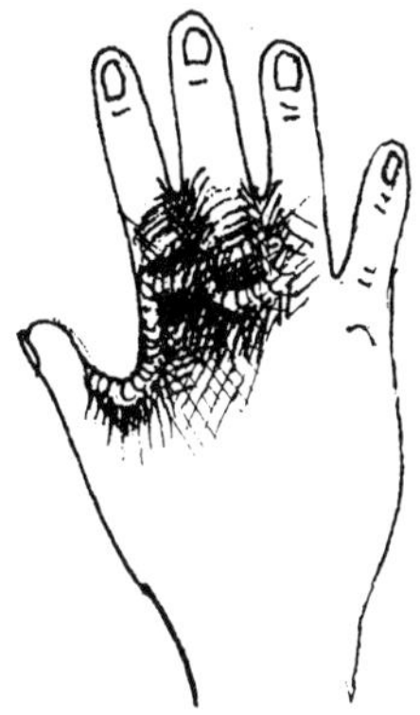

FIGURE 19–8. Dorsal hooding deformity of the thumb, index, middle, and ring digits.

dages to position the web spaces on stretch and web spacers incorporated into the design of a splint.

Loss of web space expansion creates considerable functional impairment. When the span of the first dorsal web space is shortened, thumb palmar abduction and circumduction are limited, and the thumb cannot be positioned away from the plane of the palm for grasp. Four types of thumb contractures have been described.[20] The most common thumb contracture is an adducted thumb toward the index finger with a scar band across the first dorsal web space.

When the span of the web spaces between the fingers is decreased, the breadth of the transverse volar arch is reduced, and MP joint extension and finger abduction is severely restricted. Functionally, spherical grasp and any activities that require a flattened hand are impaired.

Loss of a web space can occur even without being burned. This loss can happen as a consequence of contraction of an adjacent wound or improper immobilization of the web spaces in a shortened position.

CUPPING OF THE PALM DEFORMITY

The concavity of the hand's transverse and longitudinal palmar arches is accentuated in cupping of the palm deformity (Fig. 19–9). Cupping of the palm can be anticipated when a burn is on the palmar surface of the hand, usually as a result of a contact burn. Unless an attempt is made to counteract the process of wound contraction and the reinforcing power of the long finger flexors, cupping of the palm and flexion of the finger joints will result. Precise evaluation of the depth of a palm burn in children often is difficult because the epidermis is very thin compared to the thickened calloused hand of an adult. If the burn conditions are identical for an adult

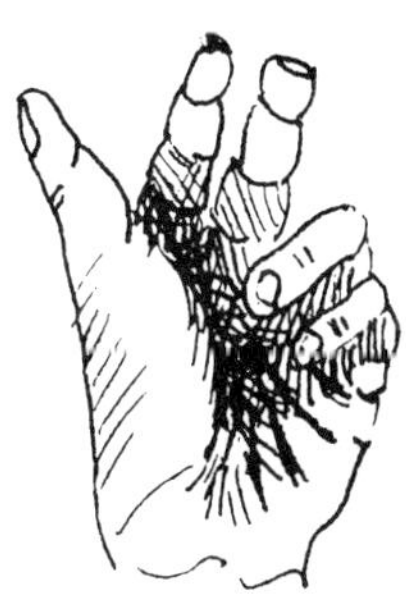

FIGURE 19–9. Cupping of the palm deformity.

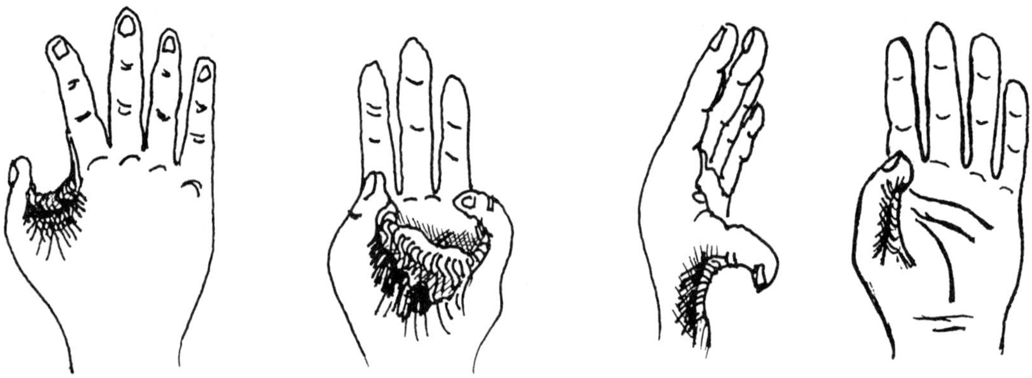

FIGURE 19–10. Nomenclature for scar band deformities of the thumb. (*A*) Adducted; (*B*) Opposed; (*C*) Radially abducted; and (*D*) Flexed. (Adapted from Stern, PJ, Carter, HWN, and MacMillan, BG: Classification and management of burned thumb contractures in children. Burns 11:168, 1985.)

and child, the depth of burn will be much deeper in the child.[21] In addition to the palmar cupping deformity, sensory deficits and loss of the stable grasping surface of the palm should be anticipated. Palmar burns are uncommon, but often require extensive therapy and multiple reconstructive efforts to yield functional results.[21]

SCAR BAND DEFORMITIES

Scar bands develop when wounds cross lines of tension and run perpendicular to the axis of joint motion. These bands frequently cross multiple adjacent joints and are found at the borders of skin grafts and in areas that healed by secondary intention. Examples of common scar bands include the dorsal web spaces, the dorsal-lateral surfaces of the thumb and little finger, and flexor surface of the fingers. In addition to restricting the hand's ability to stretch, scar bands that run across the dorsal web spaces create "skin pockets" that may lead to problems with hygiene.

The thumb commonly develops scar bands that involve the web space and multiple joint axes. Deformities of the thumb created by scar bands, classified from the most to the least common, are: (1) an adducted thumb to index finger with a scar band across the first web space; (2) an opposed, pronated, and volarly adducted thumb with the scar band running across from the thumb MP joint to the midpalm; (3) a volarly flexed thumb with involvement of only the thumb MP and/or IP joints secondary to a scar band running parallel to the thumb MP joint; and (4) a radially abducted thumb with all joints in composite extension with the scar band across the dorsal thumb MP joint proximally to the radial styloid process[20] (Fig. 19–10).

Loss of Specialized Skin Functions

SENSATION

Because of the high density of sensory organs and free nerve endings, and the extent of cortical representation allocated to the skin of the hand, sensory impairment can be functionally devastating. Although studies are limited, permanent sensory deficits following thermal injury regardless of burn depth have been documented.[22,23] Ward and colleagues[23] reported that variables such as age, percent of body surface burned, type of burn, the length of time postburn, or the percent of impairment are not particularly useful in predicting the loss or the recovery of sensation following a burn. Most clinicians agree that burn depth is probably the best predictor of sensory loss and that sensory loss is not averted by closure with a skin graft.[22,23]

In a study by Hermanson and colleagues,[22] three groups of patients with dorsal hand burns were compared to nonburned control groups. The burn groups consisted of patients with superficial dermal burns and subdermal and deep dermal burns that were either excised early and grafted or excised late (2 to 3 weeks) and grafted. Sensory return was measured with Von Frey hairs for light touch, calipers for static two-point discrimination, and the Marstock method for temperature thresholds.

At 5 years postburn, the patients with superficial dermal burns had not recovered normal light touch threshold values. When the control group and patients with early excised and grafted hands were compared, both touch and temperature thresholds were significantly worse in the burned hands. Similarly, the patients with late excised and grafted burned hands demonstrated impaired light touch and temperature thresholds that in later stages remained impaired.

Of all the sensory variables and groups tested by these investigators, temperature thresholds for the deep dermal early excised and grafted group demonstrated the most difference from the nonburned control group. In contrast to the work of Folkerts,[24] who noted that delayed excision and grafting yielded poorer sensation, Hermanson and colleagues[22] found that sensation was not necessarily enhanced with primary excision and immediate grafting. The recovery of sensation in the grafted hands was studied for 2 to 3 years postburn. The final quality of sensation was found to be established at 1 month postgrafting.[22]

Although this information is far from conclusive, therapists should anticipate the probability of impaired sensation, with limited potential for improvement, in all hand burns involving the dermis. Finally, in Hermanson's study,[22] all dorsal hand burns involving the dermis had some degree of permanent impairment to light touch and temperature when compared to normal values.

FINGERNAILS

Because dorsal hand burns are common, fingernails are involved and damaged frequently. The nail is composed of the protein keratin and is therefore only a horny extension of the skin. For nail repair to occur, the germinal matrix of the nail must remain viable. Quite often there may be remnants of the germinal matrix intact, but the nailfold (eponychium) that normally overlies the matrix may be deformed by the forces of wound contraction, which pull the eponychium away from the nailbed. In this situation, if the nail attempts to regenerate, the cells normally contributed by the eponychium to the nailbed are lost, the nail is of uneven texture, creating a "snag nail," or the nail curves downward to grow into the fingertip instead of remaining flat.

Functionally, the fingernail acts as a rigid support against which the fleshy pulp of the finger can stabilize. This stability aids in sensation during pinch activities.[25] Complete or partial loss of a fingernail is not only cosmetically disabling but may interfere with the stability of the fingertip. A burn that involves the surface of the fingertip often limits range of motion of the DIP joint secondary to wound contraction.[26] All these factors may contribute to problems with fine motor dexterity.

The therapist should anticipate questions related to the prognosis of growing a normal nail and the alternatives that are available to enhance function and appearance. There are several surgical procedures to reconstruct the nail; however, obtaining both aesthetic and functional fingernails through surgery is very difficult. Two procedures have been described by McCash:[27] free grafting of an intact toenail unit to the finger or the creation of a nailbed pocket for insertion of an artificial nail prosthesis.[27] Donelan[26] described a proximal release of the nailfold in postburn fingernails to permit the roof of the nailfold to slide distally into its original position. The relief of tension on the nailfold restored normal growth of the nail and range of motion of the DIP joint.[26,28]

An alternative to surgical intervention is the use of commercial self-adhesive fingernails. However, this type of fingernail requires the use of a nonirritant adhesive to apply the nail and can be bulky. A second alternative is the application of an "acrylic nail" by a trained manicurist. This process requires the use of layers of acrylic paste over part of an existing nail. Thirdly, an alternative that can be applied in the acute phase is customizing a nail out of a low-temperature thermoplastic material that is $\frac{1}{16}$-inch thick. Readily bonding materials will stick directly to a nail coated with fingernail polish or can be attached with tape or self-adhesive elastic wrap. The Pillet prosthesis provides a very pleasing result for those patients who require cosmetic improvement, fingertip length, and preservation of sensation. These prostheses are made from silicone and can be slipped over the tip of the finger.[29]

RETE PEGS, NATURAL SKIN LUBRICANTS, AND HAND FUNCTION

Thermal injury into the dermis of the hand destroys the function of the rete pegs along with the sweat and sebaceous glands. The rete pegs contribute to the stability of the skin of the hand, and the sweat and sebaceous glands are necessary for skin integrity.[30]

The absence or interruption of the papillary ridges is evidenced by alteration in the fingerprint pattern. Subsequently, the capacity of these ridges to provide a friction surface for the hand is impaired. The loss of the natural skin lubricants due to thermal destruction of sweat and sebaceous glands also leaves the skin dry and slick. Whereas the palmar aspect of the hand is the primary contact surface for functional activities, the exposed dorsum of the hand routinely endures shearlike frictional forces. Hand burns in which the dermis is injured present the problem of skin that is easily abraded. This problem appears to be related to exposure of the hands to shearing forces during use and the decreased tensile strength of the scar tissue itself. Problems with easily acquired friction blisters, chronic skin abrasion, dry slippery skin, and difficulty with fine motor dexterity tasks reflect the degree of impairment due to the loss of rete pegs, natural skin lubricants, and tensile strength of the skin.

A therapist can anticipate these problems given the depth of burn, time postburn, and the location of the burn. Helping patients understand the reasons for these problems and the role they play in lessening these effects is important. The use of creams to lubricate dry slippery skin is crucial. Patients should be forewarned against bumping their hand and protecting the newly healed surfaces from abrasive, shearlike forces.

TABLE 19–1. Factors for the Clinician to Consider during the Acute, Postacute, and Reconstructive Phase of Management of the Burned Hand

Phase of Management	Factors to Consider
Acute	What is the depth of burn and what tissues are involved? When did the burn occur? Which surfaces of the hand are involved? What course of management has the physician elected to follow?
Postacute	How was the wound closed? Which surfaces of the hand are involved? When did the burn occur and when was wound closure complete? What do measurements and observations reveal?
Reconstructive	What surgical procedures were performed? When was surgery performed? How have the patient's wounds healed in the past? What was the purpose of surgery?

FACTORS TO CONSIDER IN THE MANAGEMENT OF THE ACUTELY BURNED HAND

The acutely burned hand will be defined as the burned hand that has open wounds. There are four important questions that will guide the therapy management of the acutely burned hand, and these are listed in Table 19–1.

What Is the Depth of Burn and What Tissues Are Involved?

The skin of the hand does not have a uniform thickness, so the depth of the wound will vary depending on the surface area burned. For example, the skin covering the dorsum of the hand is considerably thinner than the skin covering the palm. If the entire hand is exposed to the same intensity of heat, the dorsal burn may involve the extensor paratenon and the tendon, whereas only the epidermis may be involved in the palm.

When Did the Burn Occur?

Clinical decisions regarding treatment of the acutely burned hand should be guided by the phase of wound repair. The wound-healing requirements for a patient with a burned hand referred for therapy during the inflammatory phase, 1 to 7 days postburn would differ significantly from the plan for managing a burned hand during fibroplasia (3 to 21 days) or secondary remodeling (>21 days). For instance, management of a hand with dorsal DPT burns at 24 hours postburn may require wound care, elevation for edema control, protective splinting for questionable joint or tendon damage, and gentle intrinsic muscle-pumping exercises for edema reduction. This same hand at 3 weeks postburn may have been primarily excised and skin-grafted. As a result, the hand will now require a more detailed program of exercise to maintain joint capsule integrity and composite flexion and extension flexibility, and

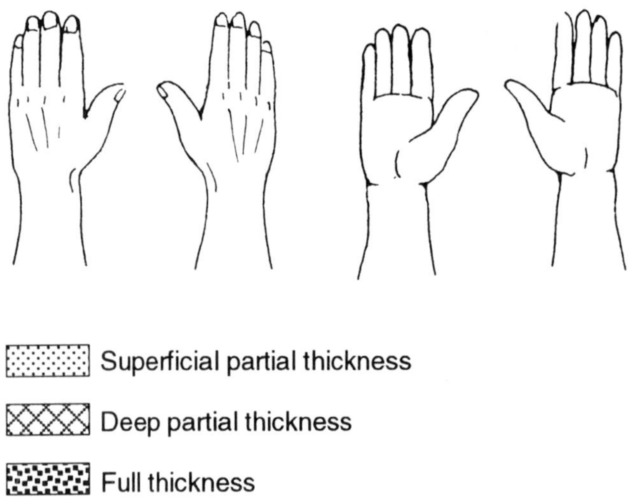

FIGURE 19–11. Area and depth of burn can be recorded on a hand burn chart. (From Howell, JW: Management of the acutely burned hand for the nonspecialized clinician. Phys Ther 69:1077, 1989, with permission.)

splinting also may be required to accomplish these goals. If residual edema remains a problem, the use of a compression wrap or glove would be included in the treatment program.

Which Surfaces of the Hand Are Involved?

A predisposition to contracture has been correlated with the site of DPT and FT burns.[31] The superficial location of the extensor tendons, intrinsic muscles, and joints, as well as the hand's specialized skin functions, make burns involving the hand particularly complex.

The skin covering the dorsum of the hand is thin, elastic, and highly mobile. When burned, there may be a loss of the skin's mobility, which may affect wrist and digital flexion and the span of the web spaces.

When the palm of the hand is burned, the concavity of the palmar arches deepens and loss of the first dorsal web space and joint flexion contractures may follow.

A hand burn chart is especially helpful for sketching the location of burn involvement and recording the depth of the burn (Fig. 19–11). The potential problems can then be reviewed by the therapist and the appropriate treatment planned.

What Course of Management Has the Physician Elected to Follow?

Therapy management of the burned hand will be influenced by the surgeon's plan of care. In most cases, this care will be guided by the patient's medical status, the percentage of total body burn, the depth of the injury, and the surgeon's preference for surgical or nonsurgical management.[4]

In SPT burns, the epidermis retains the capacity to regenerate, so nonsurgical management is followed. The overall goals are to protect the regenerating epithelial cells, reduce edema, control the patient's pain, and maintain active motion and use of the hand. In the SPT hand burn, pain can be a complication if it interferes with active motion and results in stiff joints.[5] When SPT burns are properly managed, they will heal, and hand function rarely is affected.[32]

Because DPT burns retain a limited capacity to regenerate epithelium, surgical options are more numerous. Prior to the introduction of topical antimicrobial agents, control of burn wound infection was difficult. Hand burns were primarily excised and skin-grafted to avoid wound infection.[33] Other treatments for DPT hand burns became feasible with improved topical antimicrobial agents, biosynthetic wound dressings, and the introduction of tangential excision and enzymatic debriding agents.[34-38] The key to successful hand function following DPT burns has been attributed to a well-supervised program of hand therapy, regardless of the method used to close the wound.[39,40]

The capacity for regeneration of the epithelium is lost in FT burns. Therefore, in terms of closing the wound, the treatment of choice favors primary excision and skin grafting, followed by supervised hand therapy. Frequently, in large burns, the patient's medical condition precludes surgery. In this situation, daily wound cleansing, application of topical agents, debridement, and judicious hand therapy are essential for maximal recovery of function.

FACTORS TO CONSIDER IN MANAGEMENT OF THE POSTACUTE BURNED HAND

The postacute burned hand will be defined as the burned hand that has completed wound closure. Wound closure may have been accomplished by secondary wound healing, surgical coverage, or a combination of both. As in the management of the acutely burned hand, therapeutic management of the postacute burned hand can be guided by the four questions listed in Table 19-1. In many cases, this may be the clinician's first encounter with the patient's burned hands, so time should be taken to ask these questions, as the answers will provide a framework for sound management.

How Was The Wound Closed?

The DPT or FT burned hand that is primarily excised and covered with a skin graft, biosynthetic, or biologic dressing offers an ideal situation for the therapist, because expedient wound closure results in fewer problems associated with wound contraction, scar production, and hypertrophy. Unless the wound is *very* small and located on the fingertip, palm, or dorsal phalanges, wound contraction is not a desirable mechanism for closing the DPT and FT wounds of the hand. Early wound coverage also is ideal because tissues of the hand must be elastic and mobile for movement of the hand to be restored.

The ideal situation of immediate wound closure and acute hand therapy is not always a priority for a patient who has extensive or complicated total body burns. Nevertheless, knowing how the wound was closed will help a therapist to anticipate potential problems that may result secondary to the effect of delayed wound closure and wound contraction. Intervention may take the form of splinting to counteract the forces of wound contraction.[41]

Which Surfaces of the Hand Are Involved?

The hand burn chart can be used during the postacute phase of management to sketch the area healed by secondary intention and surgical coverage and to make special notations regarding the location of scar bands and involvement of anatomic structures (see Fig. 19–11).

Because the managing therapist during the postacute phase may not be the same therapist who was involved during the acute phase, carefully inspecting the hand and knowing where and how deep the burn was before initiating treatment are important. For example, at 4 weeks postburn, the wounds may be closed, but the fact that the terminal extensor tendon was damaged and weakened will not be apparent. If a therapist were to initiate a vigorous splinting or exercise program to regain DIP flexion without regard to the status of the tendon, a rupture or attenuation of the terminal extensor tendon might occur. Therefore the therapist should balance gentle flexion exercises and intermittent extension splinting of the DIP joint until sufficient tensile strength is attained.

When Did the Burn Occur and When Was Wound Closure Complete?

Just as clinical decisions regarding treatment of the acutely burned hand are guided by the phase of wound repair, management of the postacute burned hand involves the remodeling phase of wound healing. Clinicians should know the date of injury and the length of time required to heal the wound. In DPT wounds allowed to heal spontaneously, the new skin will undergo extensive remodeling and gain tensile strength for months after injury.[6] Wounds closed with skin grafts and flaps also remodel, at a faster rate, however. Management problems, such as joint contractures, tendon adherence, chronic skin/scar breakdown, and hypertrophic scarring have been documented to increase in direct relation to the time required to close the wound.[31]

Therapy techniques such as splinting, exercise, modalities, and pressure garments and devices can be used to influence the outcome of the tissue remodeling process. Therapy intervention for an adduction contracture of the first dorsal web space would be different for the hand, which is now 3 months postburn and required 2 months for wound closure compared to the hand that is 2 weeks postburn and 10 days post-primary excision and skin grafting. The first case would require low load-long duration forces in order to have any effect in the late stages of remodeling. Serial casting the first web space would be the choice of treatment. In the second case, exercise consisting of gently stretching the web space and intermittent use of a web space splint would be sufficient to reduce the contracture.

What Do Measurements and Observations Reveal?

Observation, measurement, and listening to a patient are important techniques for the therapist who manages the postacute burned hand. Because the progression of joint deformities often is subtle and occurs gradually over a period of time, routine goniometric measurements are essential. A quick graphic reference of hand status can be achieved with the use of a range of motion flowchart as shown in Figure 19-12. Active and passive motion, joint hyperextension, and first dorsal web space expansion are plotted over time using a visual graph. Goniometric measurement of composite digital range of motion as outlined by the American Society for Surgery of the Hand requires the healing skin and scar to be stretched maximally over multiple joints simultaneously.[42] As a result, scar adherence and skin-scar tightness can be adequately assessed.

Goniometric measurement of digital motion should be done with a flat-sided metal goniometer. Active and passive extension is measured with the MP, PIP, and DIP joints of each digit extended simultaneously with the wrist maintained in a neutral position. Similarly, active and passive flexion is measured with the MP, PIP, and DIP joints of each digit flexed at one time while the wrist is maintained in a neutral position. Total active motion (TAM) or total passive motion (TPM) for each digit is calculated separately by adding the flexion angles of the MP, PIP, and DIP joints together, then subtracting the sum of the extension angles from the total degrees of flexion.[42] Normal TAM is defined as 260°, excellent TAM is 220° to 259°, good TAM is 180° to 219°, and poor TAM is 180° or less.[42] Calculation of TAM and TPM for flexion and extension of a finger is shown in Table 19-2.

When there are deficits in motion, composite goniometric measurements provide only one piece of the puzzle. The burned hand often requires thoughtful assessment before the various etiologies of lost motion can be identified. In the section on common burned hand deformities, some evaluation techniques were reviewed for the clinician to identify whether joint structures, taut scar, or both were restricting range of motion. When using these techniques to classify the type of deformity, the clinician also should measure the specific angle at which the joint restriction occurs in order to re-evaluate the effect of therapy intervention. For example, an articular or taut scar restriction would not be suspected as causing a limitation in motion if the therapist could flex the little finger MP joint to 70° with the wrist in a neutral position. However, if the therapist observed that 70° of MP flexion could not be maintained during cylindrical grasp activities, then Stern's method for classifying MP joint hyperextension contractures could be used. The wrist would be held in full flexion while the little finger MP joint is passively flexed. Both angles of passive wrist and MP joint flexion then are measured. In this case, wrist flexion measured 55° with 40° flexion at the MP joint of the little finger, indicating a type I deformity due to a mildly taut dorsal scar. The scar tissue restriction could be treated by simultaneously flexing the wrist and MP joints during superficial heat application, exercise, or low load-long duration splinting. From this example clinicians should see clearly the many problems that can be clarified only by integrating methods of assessment.

Instant photographs are useful to assist in documenting factors that are not easily measured such as scar banding and hypertrophy, nailbed problems, and altered pigmentation. The expansion of the web spaces and ability to flatten the arches of the hand can be documented with repeated overlay tracings of the hand. This documentation method is performed by placing the patient's hand on a sheet of paper with the web spaces actively stretched maximally. The therapist then traces the hand using a different color of pen for each subsequent tracing to distinguish different dates of measurement. Key landmarks are noted to reliably repeat the procedure (Fig. 19-13).

Brand[43] advocated the use of a torque angle curve (TAC) to assess the stiffness of tissues. The TAC is the measurement of force in grams plotted against the angle of

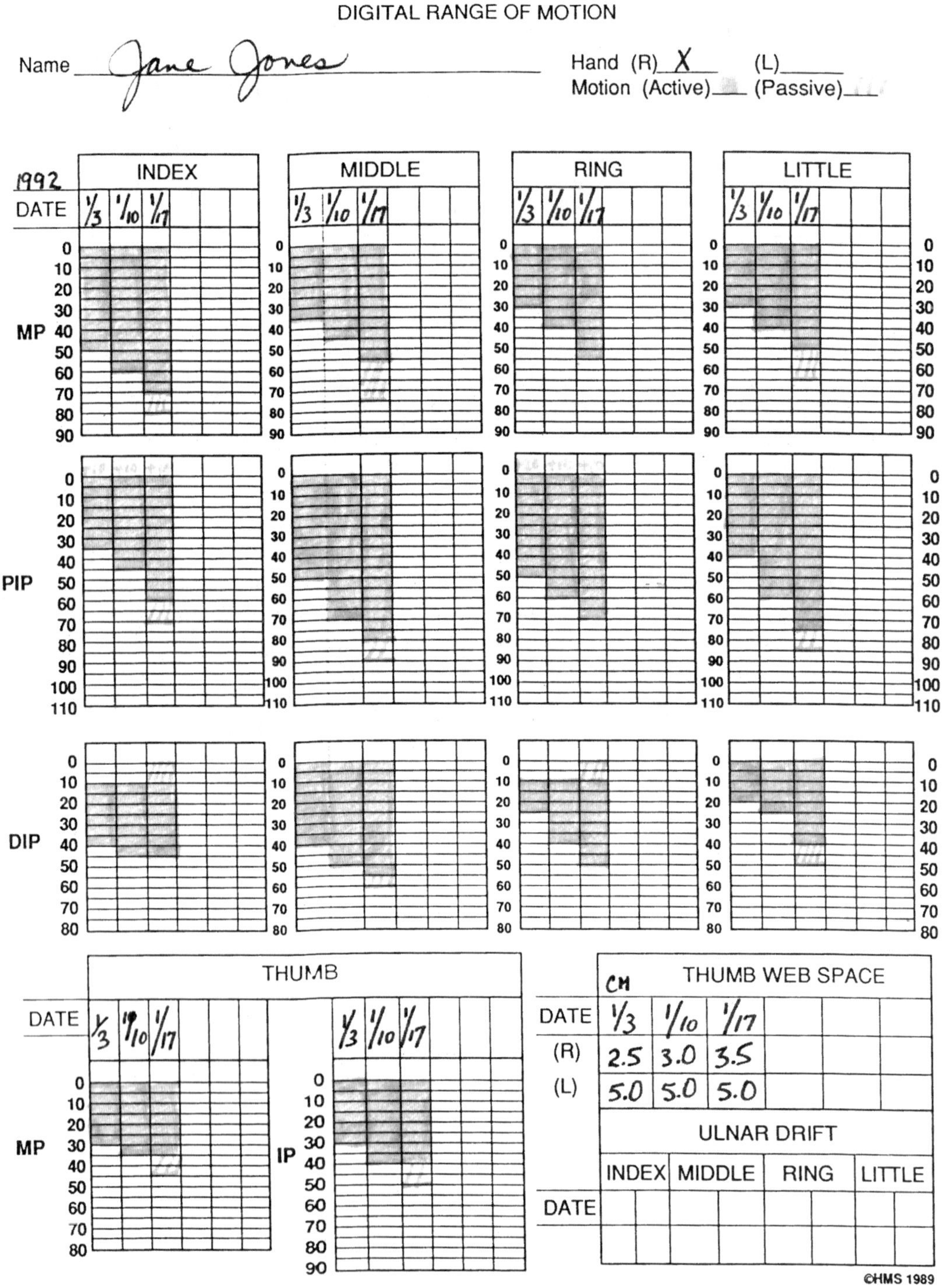

FIGURE 19–12. Range-of-motion flowchart for recording active motion (*solid*) and passive motion (/ / /) of the fingers and expansion of first dorsal web space (in centimeters).

TABLE 19–2. Calculating Total Active Motion (A and B) and Total Passive Motion (C and D)

A. Active Motion		
MP	0° extension to 70° flexion	= 70° total
PIP	+10° extension to 60° flexion	= 70° total
DIP	−10° extension to 45° flexion	= 35° total
B. Total active motion = 70° + 70° + 35° = 175°		
C. Passive Motion		
MP	0° extension to 80° flexion	= 80° total
PIP	+10° extension to 70° flexion	= 80° total
DIP	0° extension to 45° flexion	= 45° total
D. Total passive motion = 80° + 80° + 45° = 205°		

the joint throughout the patient's available passive range of motion (Fig. 19–14). According to Brand and others, the steeper the slope of the TAC, the stiffer the tissues; the more gradual the slope of the TAC, the more pliable the tissues.

Torque angle curves may be used to assess the postacute burned hand's response to therapy intervention. A gentle upward-sloping TAC suggests that remodeling tissues have more potential to respond to therapy methods than does a steeper-sloped TAC.[43] For example, at 6 months postburn, predicting whether surgery or serial casting is the best alternative for improving a flexion contracture of the PIP joint may be difficult. Use of TACs would estimate the amount and nature of the joint's stiffness.

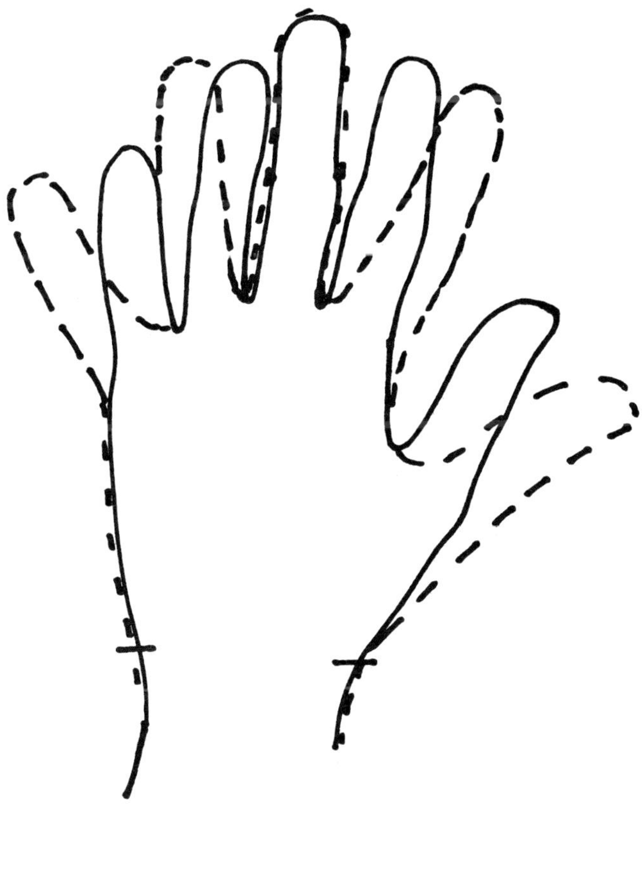

FIGURE 19–13. Tracing of the digital web spaces. The solid line illustrates the initial baseline span of the web spaces and the dotted line represents web space spans following intervention. The middle finger and wrist are used as reference points on subsequent tracings.

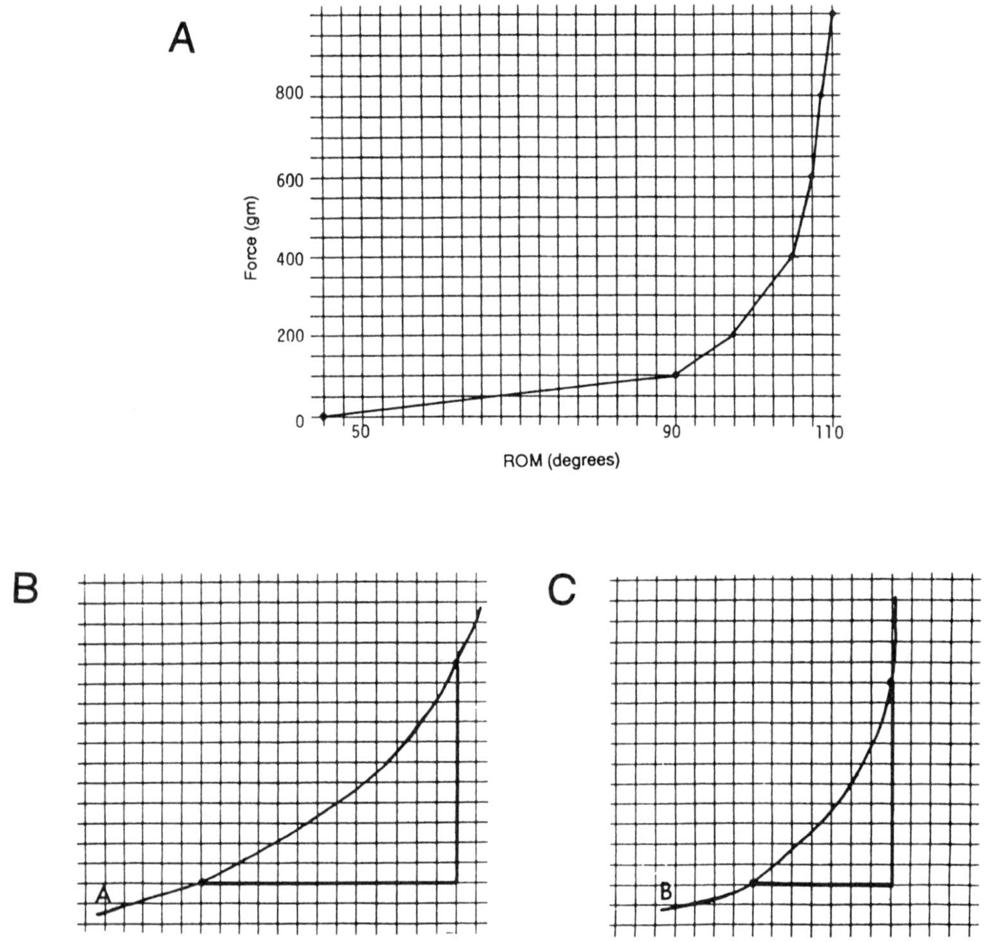

FIGURE 19–14. Torque angle curves (TAC) of normal PIP joint. (*A*) TAC with gradual linear rise in slope; (*B*) TAC with a steeper linear rise in slope. (From Flowers, KR and Pheasant, SD: The Use of Torque Angle Curves in the Assessment of Digital Joint Stiffness. Hand Ther 1:69, 1988, with permission.)

Brand[43] suggests that repeated TACs could be used to predict tissue compliance and to anticipate the response of the tissues to various therapeutic interventions. For example, if the TAC of a PIP joint flexion contracture had a linear slope, a short trial of plaster serial casting could be performed and the TAC measurements repeated. Follow-up measurements will either demonstrate an eventual resolution of the contracture or produce a more vertically sloped TAC, indicating an end to the tissue's compliance. If the latter is true, therapy has been maximized and should be discontinued.

Persistent edema is a common problem in the burned hand. Edema can be monitored by volumetrics and circumferential measurements. Standardization of measurement is important so that repeat measurements are dependable in order to assess the effectiveness of the methods used to control edema. Volume of the hand is done with a Volumeter.[43] Circumferential measurements of the hand and digits can be obtained using a flexible tape measure. The reliability of these measurements may be improved if the measurer makes note of the anatomic landmarks used as a reference and if the same person measures each time. A spring-loaded flexible tape measure, such as the Gulick tape measure, helps the therapist apply the same tension during circumferential measurement.

FACTORS TO CONSIDER IN MANAGEMENT OF THE RECONSTRUCTED BURNED HAND

The reconstructed burned hand will be defined as the burned hand with closed wounds that require surgical intervention to improve appearance and/or function. The ideal candidate for reconstructive burn surgery should have mature burn scars and be committed to the postoperative therapy program. Four questions that will guide the therapeutic management of the reconstructed burned hand are listed in Table 19–1.

What Surgical Procedures Were Performed?

A few of the most common surgical reconstructive procedures of the hand include excision of dense burn scar over the dorsum of the hand and coverage with a skin graft or flap; excision and grafting of unstable burn scar; local flaps such as Z-plasties and advancement flaps for release of scar band imposed contractures most commonly involving the MP, IP, and wrist joints and dorsal web spaces; release of the periarticular structures in severely involved joint contractures; and surgical fusion of unstable or devastated joints.

Preoperative planning with the surgeon should be done, and a specific splint can be fabricated for application in the operating room. For instance, if the purpose of the surgery is to release a scar contracture of the first dorsal web space with application of a skin graft, a splint should be designed to maintain the span of the web space and protect the skin graft. There is no contraindication to applying a splint immediately following skin grafting, provided the pressure is dispersed evenly over the graft. Use of bulky bandages between the splint and the graft will help to promote even pressure. The bulk of the dressing can be reduced as adherence of the graft is evident, usually within 5 to 7 days postoperatively, and the splint can be revised as necessary. A bulky postoperative hand bandage can be avoided in many instances simply by devising a splint to perform the desired function. In the previous example, a splint that immobilized the wrist and thumb MP and IP joints and maximally positioned the thumb in palmar abduction would protect the graft and allow the function of the other digits to be impaired minimally.

Joint fusion postburn is considered for positioning of joints that have been severely dislocated by contracting burn scar and for joint instability caused by the loss of the tendons, ligaments, or the articular surface of the joint. The position in which to fuse a joint should be carefully determined preoperatively. The position of fusion is dependent on the patient's functional needs and can be established by performing a functional assessment as described later in this chapter.

When Was Surgery Performed?

Surgical intervention resets the wound-healing time frames for the burned hand. Following reconstructive surgery, the wound-healing response will be less intense and the phases of wound repair less expansive compared to the same phases experienced acutely postburn. Given these factors, optimal results can be obtained by a therapist exercising both knowledgeable and expedient intervention.

How Have the Patient's Wounds Healed in the Past?

Although wound repair usually will be less intense following reconstructive surgery, clinicians must remember that wound healing is unique for each individual. Awareness of the patient's prior healing response can assist the therapist to anticipate postsurgical complications. These problems may include a prolonged inflammatory response, joint and tissue stiffness, pain, and surface overhealing. Excessive edema and erythema, the inability to maintain tissue length without long-term splinting or exercise, and the overbundant production of dense hypertrophic scar may be evidence of these difficulties. For patients who previously experienced a pronounced inflammatory response, several days of elevation and splint immobilization of the hand combined with mild-compression dressings should be performed. If edema and positioning remain a problem following skin graft adherence or suture removal, an intermittent compression device or plastic air bands are useful.[44,45]

What Was the Purpose of Surgery?

The goals for surgical intervention need to be clearly established preoperatively. The therapist can play a central role in helping to evaluate a patient's functional or cosmetic requirements. Collaboration with the hand surgeon will optimize selection of the best surgical procedures to meet the objectives. A therapist should perform a functional assessment to define and prioritize the patient's functional or cosmetic needs, clarify what surgery can improve, and identify the patient's role in commitment to exercise, pressure garments, and/or splints for the reconstructive program to be successful.

A functional assessment consists of asking patients to list the functional activities they are unable to perform and what they do not like about their hands. Usually, most patients are aware of the functional shortcomings of their hands; however, a skilled therapist is needed to observe the patient performing activities to determine the reason a task is difficult. If the list of "can't dos" is lengthy, having the patient prioritize the tasks in order of importance may be helpful. Typical functional problems include the patient's inability to grasp a glass or cup, to apply a glove, or to slide the hand inside a pants pocket. The inability to grasp a container or don a glove can be related to decreased span of the web spaces, which may be associated with IP and wrist joint flexion contractures. Difficulty with flattening the hand or sliding the hand inside a pocket also can result from PIP joint flexion contractures most commonly involving the little finger.

Photographs or videotapes of patients attempting to perform some of their difficult tasks are often the best method to document the need for surgical intervention. Standardized tests also are useful. Functional tests, such as the Moberg pickup or Purdue pegboard tests for assessing fine motor dexterity, can be used to document dysfunction.[46,47]

A functional assessment may demonstrate the need to fuse the PIP joint of the little finger. As a trial, a plaster cylinder cast can be fabricated to stabilize the joint and is worn by the patient for several days. Finger immobilization provides the "experience" of functioning with a temporarily fused joint to determine whether the loss of joint motion creates additional functional problems. The best functional position to fuse a joint also can be determined and shared with the surgeon. Functional assessments are helpful because they require the patient's input and give them a primary role in deciding which reconstructive procedures should be considered. Eventually, this approach may result in a more satisfied and compliant patient.

GENERAL THERAPY MANAGEMENT GUIDELINES FOR THE BURNED HAND

Splinting

Splinting the acutely burned hand should not be performed unless there is a specific purpose for the splint. For instance, most SPT hand burns do not require a splint, because epithelialization will be completed within 3 weeks postburn. Pain that prohibits movement of the hand or an overzealous patient who might aggravate the inflammatory reaction may be indications to splint a hand with a SPT burn. In these cases, splinting optimally would be used to position the joints or to prevent overactivity.

Purposes for splinting the hand with DPT and FT open wounds are to (1) immobilize and protect tendons, joint structures, skin grafts, and fractures; (2) optimally position involved and uninvolved joints; (3) apply a low load–long duration stretch to the burn surface as it heals; (4) apply pressure to limit hypertrophic scarring; and (5) functionally position a hand with an associated peripheral nerve injury.[48,49] Because wound repair is continuous, the purpose for the splint and the type of splint used are subject to periodic re-evaluation.

During the immediate postoperative period, the hand should be immobilized in a position that places the area grafted or released on a "gentle stretch."[50] For instance, if the dorsum of the hand and fingers are surgically excised and grafted, an antideformity splint places the graft on a stretch by flexing the MP joints. The position of the hand in this splint can be refined by attaching adhesive foam or elastomer putty wedges to the pan of the splint to gently abduct the fingers (Fig. 19–15). Splinting the burned hand for various problems that may occur from the acute through the reconstructive phases will be reviewed. Traditional splinting will be described; however, the reader must remember the importance of designing a splint that addresses the problem.

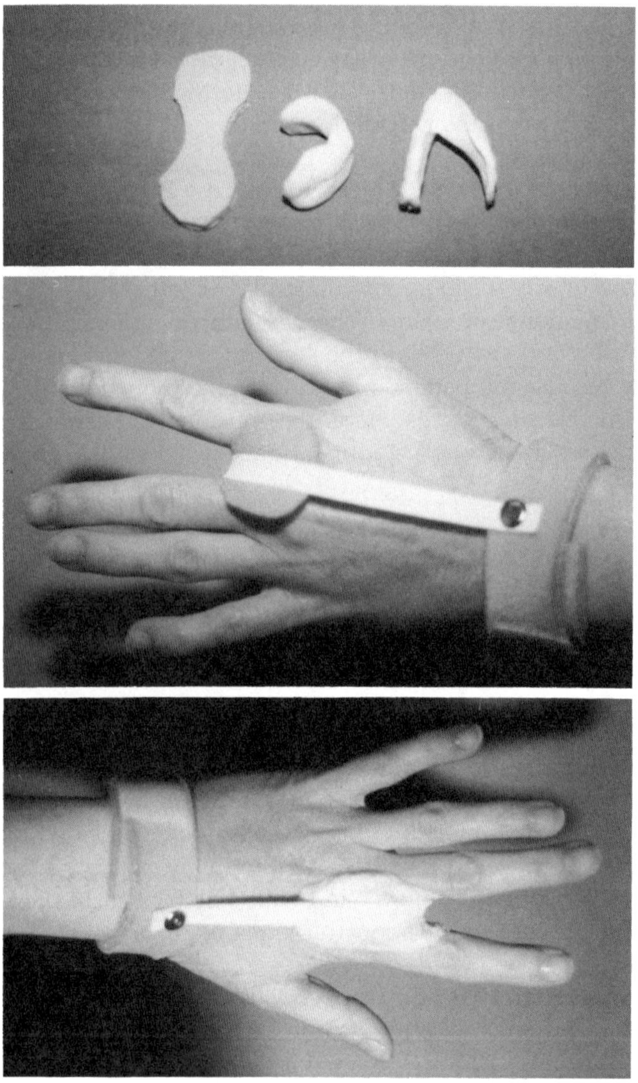

FIGURE 19–15. Web spacer options. (*A*) From left to right, soft splint strap material, putty elastomer, and silicone elastomer; (*B*) dynamic web spacer with soft strap material; (*C*) dynamic web spacer with silicone elastomer.

ANTIDEFORMITY SPLINTS

The antideformity splint positions the wrist in neutral, the MP joints in 70° to 80° flexion, and the IP joints in full extension (Fig. 19–16). This splint is recommended for any acute and postacute burned hand that assumes the edema-imposed claw hand posture or has involvement of the common extensor tendons or extensor apparatus or if the area burned includes the dorsum of the hand and digits (see Table 19–3).

Not all hand burns will be of the same depth or in the same location, hence each splint must be individually tailored. Use of an antideformity splint is not always indicated with dorsal hand burns. For example, in Table 19–4, the burn involves the dorsal and lateral surfaces of the little finger and ulnar side of the hand. The anticipated deformity would be a flexion contracture of the PIP joint, hyperextension of the MP joint, rotation of the little finger, and loss of the fourth web space. Splinting the

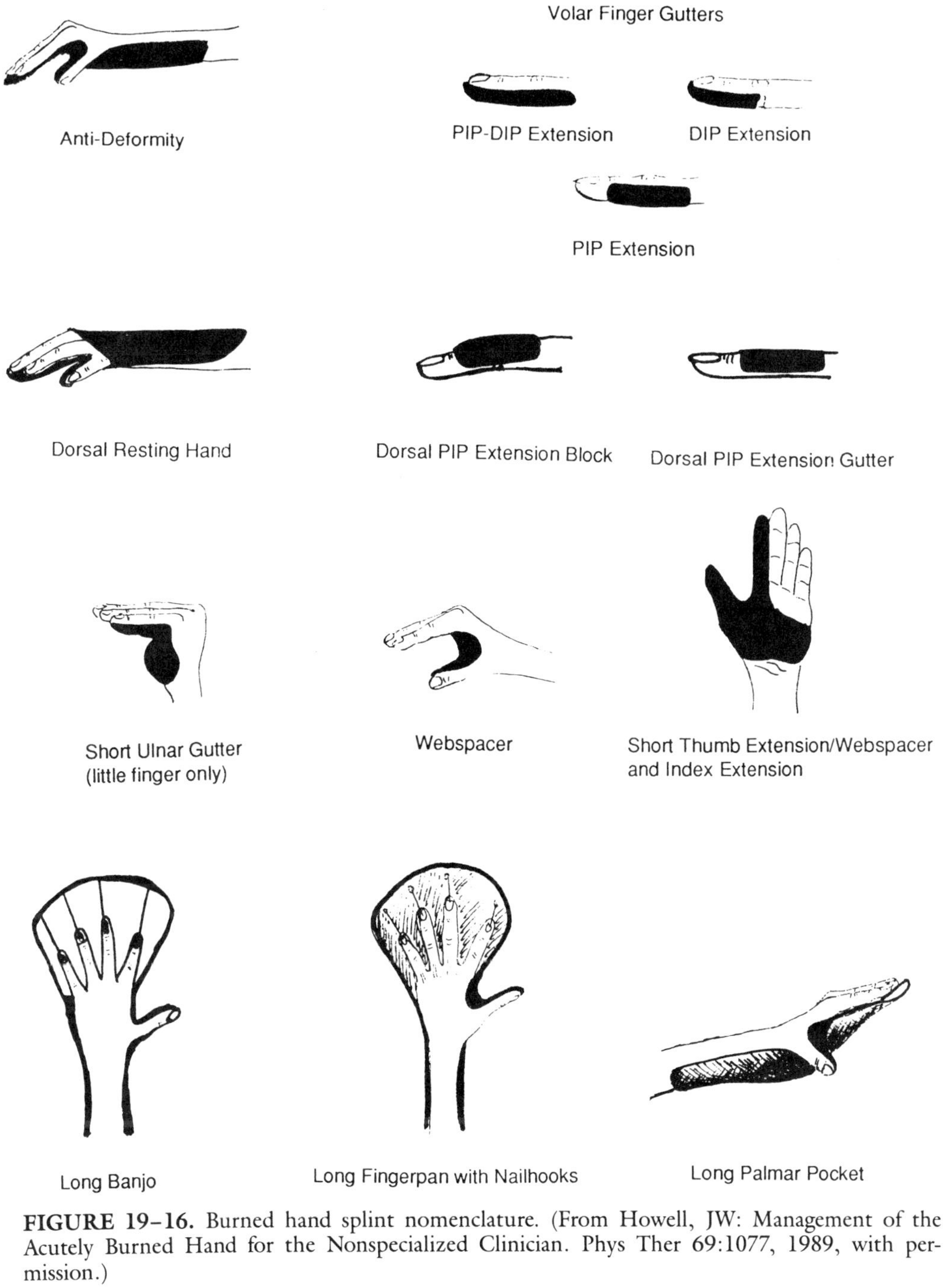

FIGURE 19–16. Burned hand splint nomenclature. (From Howell, JW: Management of the Acutely Burned Hand for the Nonspecialized Clinician. Phys Ther 69:1077, 1989, with permission.)

TABLE 19–3. Area Burned, Problems Anticipated, Suggested Splints, and Exercises for Acute DPT and FT Burned Hand, Case 1

Area Burned	Problem Anticipated	Splint	Exercise
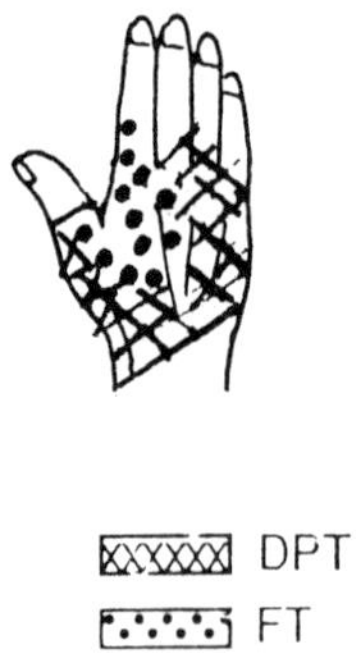	Compartment syndrome Loss of web space MP hyperextension PIP hyperextension Boutonnière fingers and thumb Loss of wrist flexion and deviation	Antideformity Individual PIP extension gutters First dorsal web spacer Individual PIP hyperextension block	Intrinsic muscle pumping Modified fist Digital abduction/adduction Cupping hand Thumb to finger opposition Thumb MP and IP flexion/extension Wrist flexion and deviation

TABLE 19–4. Area Burned, Problems Anticipated, Suggested Splints, and Exercises for Acute DPT and FT Burned Hand, Case 2

Area Burned	Problem Anticipated	Splint	Exercise
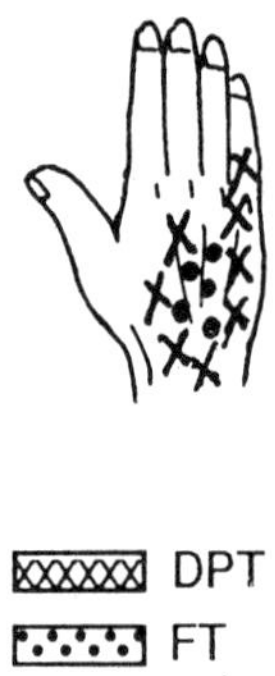	MP hyperextension PIP flexion contracture Loss of web space Rotation of little finger	Short MP flexion—IP extension PIP extension gutter and buddy strap to prevent rotation Web space compression	Isolated MP flexion Adduction little finger Web space stretch Opposition little to thumb Wrist flexion and radial deviation

entire hand in this case would not be appropriate because the task can be accomplished by splinting only the little finger in a position of MP joint flexion and IP joint extension.

During the reconstructive phase of care, an antideformity splint or dorsally based resting hand splint is well suited to position and immobilize the hand. Situations in which these splints would be warranted are following skin grafts to the dorsum of the hand, release of MP joint hyperextension or PIP joint contractures, and reconstruction of the extensor apparatus.

ANTI-BOUTONNIÈRE AND ANTI-MALLET DEFORMITY SPLINTS

A splint to prevent or correct a boutonnière deformity must maintain the PIP joint in extension and prevent DIP joint hyperextension. During the acute and postacute phases, care must be taken to maintain the PIP joint in extension without placing pressure on the thermally damaged extensor apparatus. Often both the PIP and DIP joints will require a volar PIP-DIP extension finger gutter splint as shown in Figure

TABLE 19–5. Area Burned, Problems Anticipated, Suggested Splints, and Exercises for Acute DPT and FT Burned Hand, Case 3

Area Burned	Problem Anticipated	Splint	Exercise
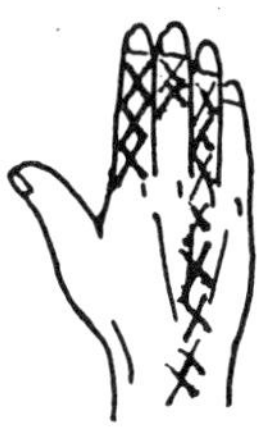 DPT FT	Index: Boutonnière/mallet Middle: Mallet Ring: MP hyperextension Loss of wrist flexion Swan-neck deformity	Index: IP extension gutter Middle: DIP extension gutter Ring: Short MP flexion, −10° PIP extension and DIP extension PIP hyperextension block and DIP extension gutter	Index: MP flexion/extension MP abduction/adduction PIP-DIP extension Middle: MP-PIP flexion/extension Ring: MP flexion/extension Modified fist(?) Wrist flexion

19–16. If the PIP joint cannot be controlled adequately with the volar finger gutter splint, the finger can be positioned between the volar gutter splint and a dorsal PIP joint extension block splint. Finger splints can be fabricated from $\frac{1}{16}$-inch perforated low-temperature plastic or an open-weave low-temperature plastic for wound ventilation. Caution should be taken when attaching the splint to avoid strap-induced ischemia. Pressure can be dispersed more evenly by wrapping roll gauze or self-adherent elastic wrap around the splint. The finger gutter splints can be worn in conjunction with an antideformity splint for additional control of the IP joints. When the terminal slip of the extensor tendon is not involved, movement of the DIP joint should be allowed by using the splint to immobilize the PIP joint only. Flexibility of the DIP joint capsule and oblique retinacular ligament and gliding of the extensor apparatus lateral bands and the flexor digitorum are maintained with DIP joint movement. In lieu of splinting the IP joints, the surgeon may opt to use Kirshner wire fixation to protect the heat-injured tendons.[51]

To prevent or correct a mallet finger, the same splint fabrication principles as stated earlier are used, but the PIP joint is excluded from the splint. A mallet finger should be anticipated if the burn area resembles that shown for the digits in Table 19–5. Until the status of the terminal extensor tendon is known in the acute phase, the DIP joint should be immobilized in a DIP extension splint to prevent further tendon damage. If the tendon has been damaged, splinting should be maintained continuously until adequate tensile strength is attained in the tendon-scar. This process may require 8 to 12 weeks of continuous extension at the DIP joint without permitting flexion of the joint.

ANTI-PIP JOINT FLEXION CONTRACTURE SPLINTS

An individual gutter splint is recommended in the presence of: (1) edema-imposed claw hand posture when the position of the PIP joint cannot be controlled with the antideformity splint, (2) scar banding volar to the axis of the PIP joint and secondary remodeling of the volar plate and collateral ligaments, (3) scar banding that originates in the palm and extends the length of the finger, and (4) surgical release of an isolated joint contracture.

TABLE 19–6. Area Burned, Problems Anticipated, Suggested Splints, and Exercises for Acute DPT and FT Burned Hand, Case 4

Area Burned	Problem Anticipated	Splint	Exercise
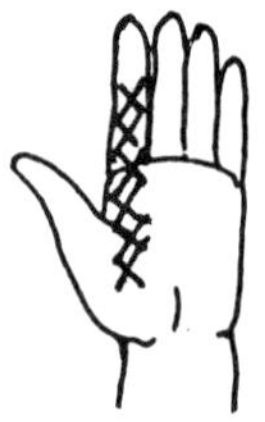 DPT FT	Flexion contractures MP-IP joints Loss of first dorsal web space	Short MP-IP extension and web spacer IP extension gutter	Composite active and passive extension, thumb and index Composite flexion, thumb and index Thumb abduction/extension

Flexion of the PIP and MP joints should be anticipated if the area of burn involvement includes the lateral and/or volar surfaces of the palm or digits (Table 19–6). Often a PIP extension gutter splint will work nicely to resolve a mild PIP flexion deformity provided there is no loss of passive MP joint extension. However, if there is limited composite extension of the PIP and MP joints, a hand-based splint that extends both the MP and PIP joints will be necessary in order to adequately apply a multijoint stretch to the scar band.

The previous information can be used to determine the type of splint needed after surgical release of a scar band volar to the axes of the finger joints. Remembering that the purpose of a splint after surgical release of scar bands is to apply a gentle stretch to the tissues until remodeling and scar maturation occur is very important. Splinting always must be complimented with a balanced program of exercise, pressure, and positioning.[52]

ANTI-PIP JOINT HYPEREXTENSION SPLINTS

The purpose of splinting a PIP joint hyperextension deformity is to prevent or correct hyperextension of the PIP joint. Often this deformity is coupled with loss of DIP joint extension secondary to the imposed mechanical imbalance of the extensor tendon system. This deformity can occur secondary to: (1) positioning PIP joints in hyperextension within a splint, (2) dense scar dorsal to the PIP joint axis, (3) adherence of the extensor digitorum communis tendons to create a tenodesis effect at the PIP joint, or (4) ischemic contracture or shortening of the intrinsic muscles of the hand.[6,14–19] The first goal is to prevent hyperextension of the PIP joint by using a splint to prevent the last 10° of PIP joint extension. The second goal is to maintain gliding of the flexor tendons, the extensor apparatus, and the EDC tendons, if the area of burn permits. The dorsal PIP extension block splint satisfies these requirements (see Fig. 19–16). This splint can be attached with Velcro straps or self-adherent elastic wrap. To flex the PIP joint, the distal strap can be removed. Once edema has stabilized, a figure-of-8 splint can be fabricated that restricts hyperextension but permits flexion of the PIP joint. To use this splint in the acute phase, the figure-of-8

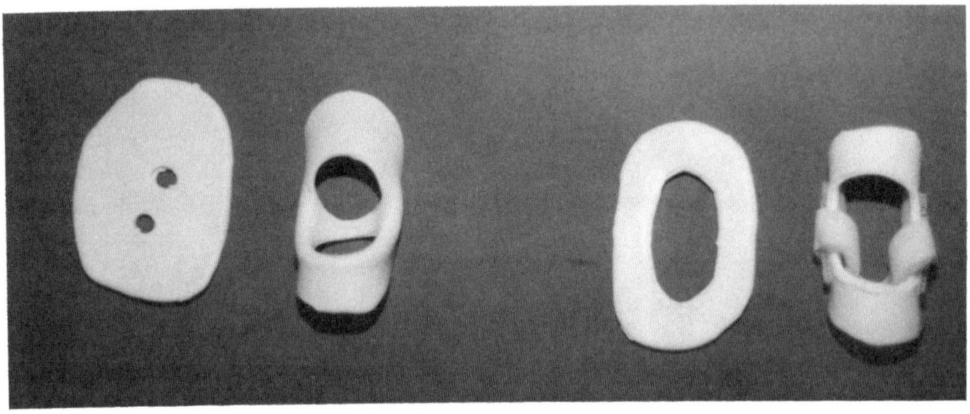

FIGURE 19–17. Figure-of-8 splint (*left*) and modified figure-of-8 splint (*right*) to prevent interphalangeal joint hyperextension.

splint can be modified by excluding the ring portion of the splint and adding an adjustable Velcro strap (Fig. 19–17).

These same splints also can be used to correct the hyperextension-related problems of the finger DIP and thumb IP joints as seen in the boutonnière deformity. Mechanical balance within the extensor tendon system can be restored with the use of either version of the figure-of-8 or dorsal hyperextension block splints (see Fig. 19–17).

ANTI-DORSAL HOODING SPLINTS

Splinting for dorsal hooding should be considered whenever the web spaces and proximal phalanges are involved in the burn (cases 1 and 5 in Tables 19–3 and 19–7). In the acute phase, a gentle stretch to each involved web space can be accomplished when applying wound bandages (Fig. 19–18). Placement of an open-mesh gauze bandage into the web spaces abducts the thumb and fingers, thereby increasing the

TABLE 19–7. Area Burned, Problems Anticipated, Suggested Splints, and Exercises for Acute DPT and FT Burned Hand, Case 5

Area Burned	Problem Anticipated	Splint	Exercise
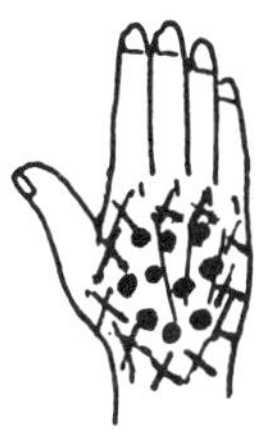 DPT FT	Compartment syndrome MP hyperextension Dorsal hooding Loss of palmar arches Little finger claw deformity Loss of wrist flexion/deviation Loss of composite digital flexion Loss of thumb opposition	Short antideformity splint with finger MPs flexed and abducted; finger IPs extended; thumb abducted and MP-IP extension Separate thumb web spacer	Modified fist only No composite digital flexion Thumb abduction/extension, opposition/flexion Finger abduction/adduction Wrist flexion/extension/deviation Cupping of hand

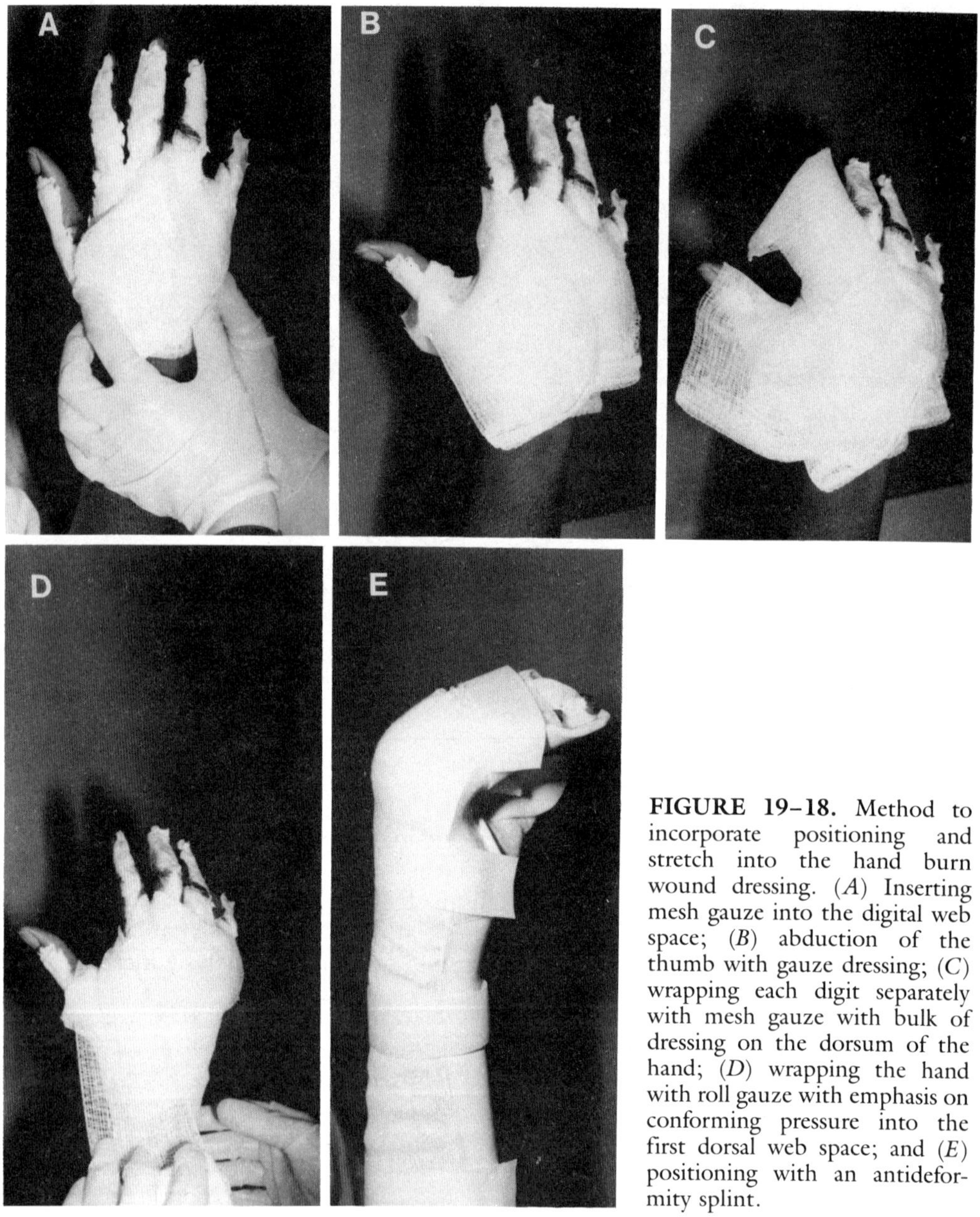

FIGURE 19–18. Method to incorporate positioning and stretch into the hand burn wound dressing. (*A*) Inserting mesh gauze into the digital web space; (*B*) abduction of the thumb with gauze dressing; (*C*) wrapping each digit separately with mesh gauze with bulk of dressing on the dorsum of the hand; (*D*) wrapping the hand with roll gauze with emphasis on conforming pressure into the first dorsal web space; and (*E*) positioning with an antideformity splint.

span of the web space. Although wound contraction cannot be eliminated by wound dressings or splinting, the potential for web space contracture can be reduced by applying tension to the wound, which equals the tension within the wound.[6,53] The antideformity splint then can be applied to assist with finger abduction while maintaining MP joint flexion.

If the first web space is involved, the thumb is positioned in abduction and the MP and IP joints in extension. A web spacer splint is appropriate for cases 5 and 6 in Tables 19–7 and 19–8. A common complication is burn scar contracture that limits both the first web space span as well as composite extension of the index finger. If

TABLE 19–8. Area Burned, Problems Anticipated, Suggested Splints, and Exercises for Acute DPT and FT Burned Hand, Case 6

Area Burned	Problem Anticipated	Splint	Exercise
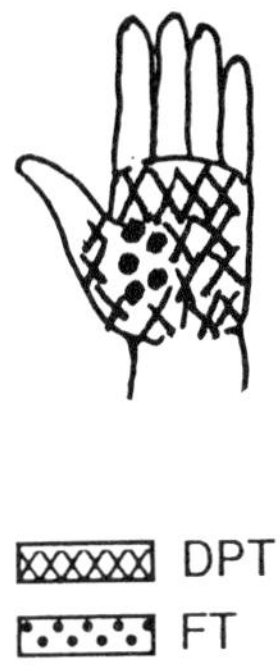	Compartment syndrome Cupping of palm deformity Loss of first dorsal web space Thumb MP flexion contracture Fingers MP flexion contractures Wrist flexion contracture	Palmar pocket Dorsal resting with finger MP-IP joints extended, thumb abducted and extended, wrist extension Web spacer first dorsal	Composite digital extension and abduction Flattening palmar arches Composite thumb flexion Wrist extension combined with composite digital extension

this situation occurs, the splint must be designed to address both problems. Proper positioning can be accomplished with a short thumb extension-web spacer and index finger extension splint that applies a multijoint stretch to overcome both contractures (see Fig. 19–16).

ANTICUPPING OF THE PALM SPLINTS

Cupping of the palm deformity occurs when the area of burn involves the palm of the hand and volar wrist such as in case 6 (Table 19–8). To successfully apply a low load-long duration stretch to the healing burn scar, a splint should flatten the palmar arches and extend the digits. This position, however, places the MP joint collateral ligaments at their shortest length. In this situation, exercises to maintain collateral ligament length should be balanced with splinting to stretch the palmar scar or wound. There are two methods to fabricate a splint to stretch a palmar scar. One method is to fit the forearm trough of the splint dorsally over the forearm and the finger pan volarly under the fingers. Another method is to use a modified gutter splint with a palmar pocket[54] (Fig. 19–16). The palm of the hand drops into the palmar pocket to flatten the cupped arches while volar support is given to the wrist and digits. This splint also can be used to immobilize the hand after skin grafting in this area because the palm will not contact the palmar pocket. For inspection of the graft or wound care, the pocket can be cut out, exposing the palm of the hand. This type of splint may require fingernail hooks or the addition of a banjo outrigger to extend the IP joints and maintain proper positioning (Fig. 19–16).

Pressure Therapy for the Burned Hand

Pressure therapy is used throughout all phases of burned hand management. This section will highlight interventions in the management of hypertrophic scar affecting the hand. Initially, pressure is used in the acute phase for edema control if a compartment syndrome is not present. In wounds healing by secondary intention, pressure also is used to control hypertrophy of granulation tissue.[41,50,55]

The entire burn wound does not close at once. Even after skin grafting there may be small open areas that must heal secondarily. However, pressure can be initiated before full wound closure is obtained. External pressure can be applied directly over wound bandages, during the interim period, with a self-adherent elastic compression wrap. The wrap is applied in a spiral fashion around each individual digit and continued onto the hand and forearm if necessary. To apply pressure in the digital web spaces, a piece of compression wrap can be placed into the web space between each digit. The self-adherent elastic wrap should not be pulled too tight during application as it has a tendency to shrink. This type of wrap works well because it stays in place and does not wrinkle or create a shearing force against the new skin. The elastic wrap also can be applied to leave the fingertip exposed, giving a friction surface for grasp. A strip of adhesive tape applied lengthwise along the ulnar side of the index, middle, and ring fingers will keep the self-adherent elastic wrapped fingers from sticking to one another.

An additional benefit of using a compression wrap is to protect new fragile skin. Many times abrasion of new skin occurs as a result of pulling a pressure glove on and off over the hand. The compression wrap method gives a scar more time to mature and allows additional time for hand size to stabilize before measuring for custom-made gloves. Pressure inserts, such as silicone elastomer, elastomer putty, silicone gelsheets or skin care pads can be used in combination with a self-adherent elastic wrap.

In the postacute and reconstructive phases, pressure is applied to minimize scar hypertrophy. Because scar maturation is a dynamic process, the clinician must periodically review the need for pressure therapy, type of pressure, and physical condition of the gloves and inserts. A therapist must remember that the therapeutic intervention should not interfere with the mobility and function of the hand in the quest for scar control.

Pressure gloves are available commercially as either custom-made or presized.[56] If the need for a custom-made glove is unclear, then an Isotoner, Tubigrip, or presized elasticized nylon fabric glove can be used initially.

Advantages of Isotoner gloves include: (1) availability in wrist and forearm lengths, (2) choice of light to dark colors, (3) low cost, (4) ease of purchase at department stores, (5) stretchy fabric making application easy, (6) stretchy fabric exerting less pressure and less restriction to movement, (7) machine washable, and (8) lack of fraying if fingertips of the glove are removed. Isotoner gloves are ideal for the burned hand that does not tolerate pressure well, for use in the final phase of scar control when less pressure is required to keep the scar flat, or for the sole purpose of holding pressure inserts, such as web spacers, in position (Table 19–9).

Tubigrip gloves are the thickest and most durable of compression gloves, yet these characteristics also make them more difficult to slide over fragile scar. The fingertips can be removed without fraying, and although the sizes run small, there are more sizes (1 through 8) from which to select. The only measurement needed to size the glove is the circumference of the hand over the MP joints with the fingers extended. The manufacturer states that a constant pressure of 25 to 35 mm Hg is applied by the Tubigrip gloves and that the glove is universal, fitting either hand (see Table 19–9).

TABLE 19–9. Clinical Advantages and Disadvantages of Pressure Therapy Gloves

			Elastic Nylon Fabric	
	Isotoner	**Tubigrip**	**Pre-sized**	**Custom-made**
Length variety	X		X	X
Color variety	X			X
Inexpensive	X	X	X	
Expensive				X
Restrictive		X		X
Pliable	X		X	
Easy application	X		X	
No fraying	X	X	X	X
<25–35 mm Hg	X			
>25–35 mm Hg		X	X	X
Sizing easy	X	X	X	
Sizing hard				X
Durable > 6 wk		X	X	X
Durable < 6 wk	X			

Commercially available presized pressure gloves can be ordered from several companies. Generally these gloves are made from an elasticized nylon fabric, are sized small through extra-large, and require only a circumferential measurement at the MP joints. Some of the presized gloves have optional Velcro closure and open or closed fingertips. However, the therapist can cut off the fingertips of these nylon elastic gloves without fear of fraying (Table 19–9). Often presized gloves provide adequate pressure, but their use also is beneficial to discern the need for a custom-made glove or to use until the size of the hand has stabilized and custom-made gloves purchased.

Pressure applied to hypertrophic scar by a garment may not be adequate because garments often do not conform well to all areas. Areas that most often require a pressure insert are digital web spaces, the palm, and volar and dorsal wrist creases. Pressure inserts to control syndactyly are numerous, which is a clue to therapists that this is a difficult area to obtain satisfactory scar control. Individual web spacers can be fabricated from elastomer putty, silicone elastomer, soft splint strapping material, low-temperature plastic or rubber tubing and held in place with a pressure glove (see Chapter 14).

Another alternative is to run strips of elastic over an elastomer putty web spacers and rivet the elastic to a strap anchored around the wrist (see Fig. 19–15). Using this method, a glove is not necessary because the elastic provides dynamic pressure to maintain good contact between the putty and the scar. This technique also works well following surgical release of web spaces, when pressure is needed only in this area versus the entire hand.

Pressure in the palm of the hand cannot be achieved adequately with only a glove or self-adherent dressing. Unfortunately, to apply conforming pressure to the palm, the mobility of the palmar arches will be limited. A scar pad can be fashioned out of silicone elastomer or elastomer putty. The elastomer must be applied thick enough to afford good contact with the glove. An alternative method is to attach a piece of soft-density open-cell contour foam to the scar pad itself. The open-cell contour foam will expand to fill in the space between the glove and the scar pad.

Pressure therapy and splinting can be combined to provide a low load–long duration stretch to a scar band. For example, in case 4 (Table 19–6), the short MP-IP joint extension web spacer splint could be lined with elastomer putty to apply a more conforming pressure. To make this splint, a perforated splinting material should be used. The desired amount of putty is applied over the scar band or hypertrophic scar. Immediately before the putty hardens, the splint is molded over the putty in the desired position. The elastomer putty should be soft enough to fill in the holes of the splint. This process keeps the scar pad in proper position and makes them one unit. As the scar responds to this treatment, additional putty can be added over the original mold for better conformity.

FACTORS TO CONSIDER WHEN USING PRESSURE THERAPY ON THE BURNED HAND

Once the clinical decision has been made that pressure therapy is necessary, the therapist should take the time to ask the questions in Table 19–10. As scar maturation progresses, these questions should be reviewed and the pressure therapy program modified to fit the needs of the patient.

Has the Size of the Hand Stabilized?

If a custom-made glove is necessary, the glove should be measured when edema has resolved. Measuring prematurely can cause an improper fit later. A helpful method to assess if the hand size has stabilized is to measure a few of the circumferences needed for a custom-made glove and then repeat these measurements again in 5 to 7 days. If there is a difference of $\frac{1}{4}$ inch or greater, the glove will not fit properly. If fluctuations in hand size persist, edema control efforts are continued and an Isotoner or presized glove should be used until the size of the hand stabilizes.

Is the Self-Adherent Wrap or an Interim Glove Applying Adequate Pressure?

If scarring appears well-controlled with the use of a self-adherent wrap or an interim glove, these should be continued. However, if a scar begins to hypertrophy, a pressure insert should be added under the wrap or glove. If this intervention does not provide good results, a custom-made glove probably will be necessary.

With isolated finger burns, an entire glove is not warranted. A self-adherent elastic wrap can be applied to a digit, or individual elasticized nylon digital sleeves can be used. This type of treatment would be indicated for burns such as those in case 3 involving the index and middle fingers (see Table 19–5).

TABLE 19–10. Factors for the Clinician to Consider When Using Pressure Therapy on the Burned Hand

Has the size of the hand stabilized?
Is the self-adherent wrap or interim glove applying adequate pressure?
Is a glove and/or insert needed?
What modifications are needed in a custom-made glove?

Is a Glove and/or Insert Needed?

A glove can be used to apply direct pressure to a scar, keep a pressure insert in position, or protect the delicate scar from shearing forces. If the dorsum of the hand, multiple fingers and thumb, or palm require pressure therapy, a glove should be considered (see Tables 19–3, 19–4, 19–7, and 19–8). When the digital web spaces are involved, a glove may be required to keep pressure inserts positioned in the web spaces. When the dorsum of the hand is involved, a glove may be used alone or in combination with a skin care pad to protect the fragile scar from abrasion. The palmar and web space burn has additional requirements (see Table 19–8). For scar control, a glove with open fingertips distal to the PIP joints can be used to hold a scar pad in place. For contracture control, a palmar pocket–web space splint lined with elastomer putty or silicone elastomer can be worn.

What Modifications Are Needed in a Custom-Made Glove?

A custom-made glove is tailored specifically for a patient's individual needs. A variety of options are available that include, but are not limited to (1) closed or open fingertips, (2) zippers and zipper location, (3) color, (4) length of individual fingers, (5) length of the glove, and (6) gauntlet versus glove style.

Closed fingers on a glove make fit more difficult and generally is unnecessary because scar hypertrophy around the finger tips is infrequent. Leaving the finger tips exposed enhances the fit, especially in the web spaces, and permits tactile sensation during pinch and grasp activities.

The need for a zipper often is determined by the fragility of the scar tissue over which the glove will be applied and the dexterity of the patient's hands. If scar tissue is particularly fragile, a zipper will decrease the shearing forces sustained by the dorsum of the hand during application. Zippers make donning a glove easier if mobility and strength of one or both hands are restricted; however, closure of the zipper may require assistance. When a zipper is added, there is an interruption of the elastic pressure applied to the surface over which the zipper is located. Therefore, the location of the zipper should be well planned in terms of the areas requiring pressure and ease of closure.

In recent years, gloves have become quite colorful. Patients can choose a color similar to their skin tone, color-coordinate outfits, or go with a more sporty look. Color does not affect the performance of the glove, and if given a choice, a patient may find the glove aesthetically pleasing, which will encourage regular wear.

The length of the fingers and glove is dependent on the location(s) in need of pressure. As a rule, the length of the finger sleeve should extend at least $\frac{3}{8}$ inch beyond the most distal area of scar. A glove that ends at the wrist is acceptable if there is no need for pressure over the carpal bones. To provide pressure over the carpal bones, the glove should be extended above the distal end of the radius.

Exercise and Activities of Daily Living

The indications for exercise and use of the burned hand for activities of daily living (ADL) vary depending on the depth and location of the burn, the extent of tendon and joint involvement, the phase of wound healing, and the patient's compliance with instruction. For the most part, exercise and ADL must be individually prescribed using these factors and the results of objective measurements.

Exercise during the inflammatory phase is used in a controlled manner to activate the muscle pump to decrease edema. The technique used to reduce edema should be selected carefully to avoid an inflammatory reaction or unnecessary injury of fragile tissues. For example, brief episodes of active composite finger flexion and extension can be encouraged safely in SPT hand burns. However, there is a risk of extensor tendon damage with active composite flexion in deeper hand burns, such as those illustrated in cases 1, 3, and 5 (Tables 19–3, 19–5, and 19–7). In these cases, the exercises outlined by Tanigawa and colleagues[57] for isolated active or passive MP joint flexion combined with active or passive IP joint extension, will impose less stress on this fragile extensor tendon system (Fig. 19–19). Repetitive finger abduction and adduction requires contraction of the dorsal and palmar interosseous muscles, which assists in edema reduction and generally is indicated for burns of all depths. During the inflammatory period, the goal of treatment for burns of all depths is to assist healing of the wound and to avoid prolonging inflammation. The vigor of ADL and the repetition of exercises during this time should be monitored carefully. Frequent exercise, performed four to six times per day with low repetitions (5 to 10), combined

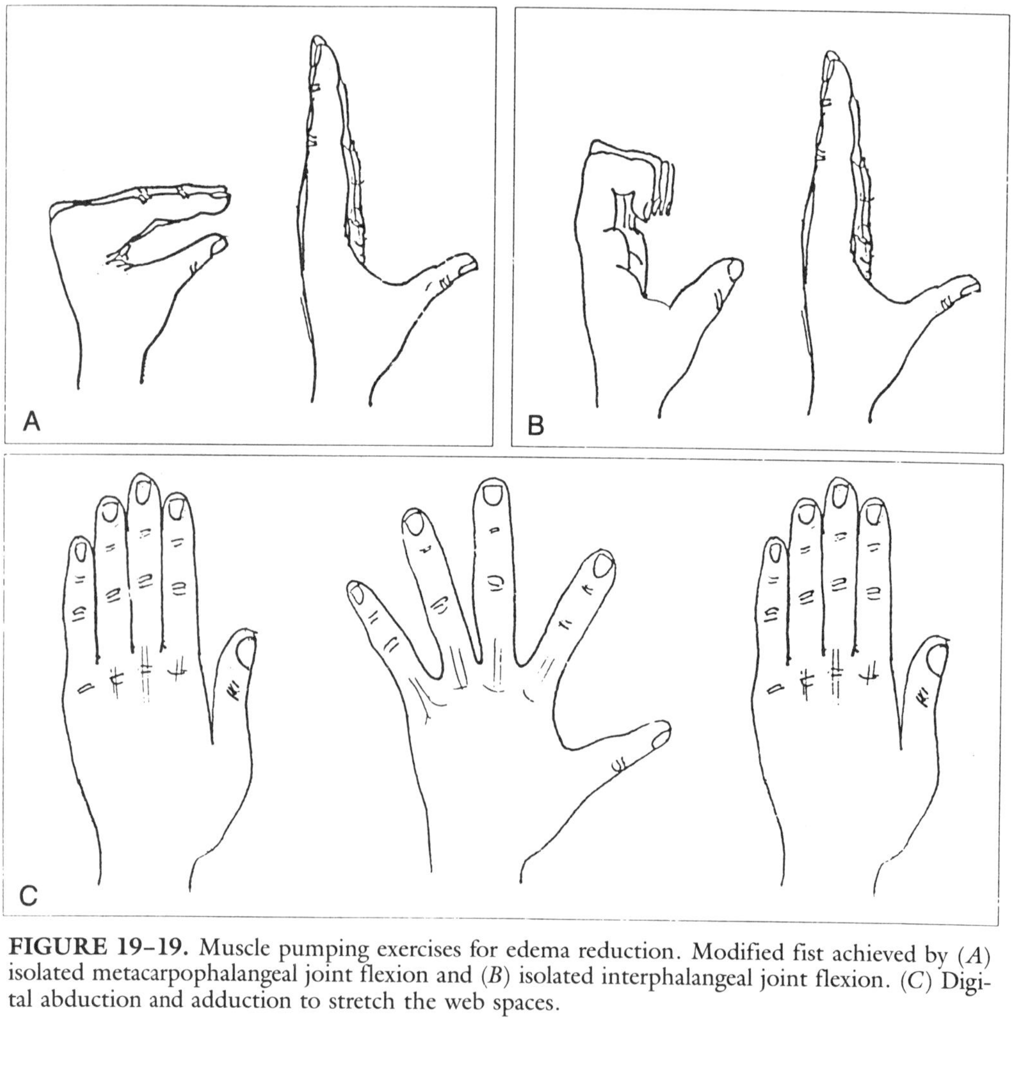

FIGURE 19–19. Muscle pumping exercises for edema reduction. Modified fist achieved by (*A*) isolated metacarpophalangeal joint flexion and (*B*) isolated interphalangeal joint flexion. (*C*) Digital abduction and adduction to stretch the web spaces.

with elevation, compression, and proper positioning, is more beneficial than one intense session.

Exercise during the fibroplastic phase of healing is prescribed to initiate controlled mobilization of the healing tissues while protecting damaged tendons, fractures, and fragile skin grafts and flaps. The choice of exercise should be tailored to the individual needs of the patient. Proper timing of exercise and application of force to oppose the process of wound contraction is a priority during this period. A low load-long duration force will be defined by this author as a gentle force that can be applied to the tissues with adequate duration to effect a measurable biologic change over time without inciting an inflammatory response from the tissues. The mechanisms by which low load-long duration forces can be applied to the tissues can be active and passive exercise, ADL, splints, and pressure therapy. Specific examples of these techniques can be found in case study 7 (Table 19-11). Because the hand consists of many joints, application of a low load-long duration counterforce often is required simultaneously across multiple joints to be effective.

TABLE 19-11. Case Study. Hand Burn Chart with Skin-Grafted Areas Noted (/ / /) and Results of Range of Motion Measurements and Special Tests

Hand Burn Chart

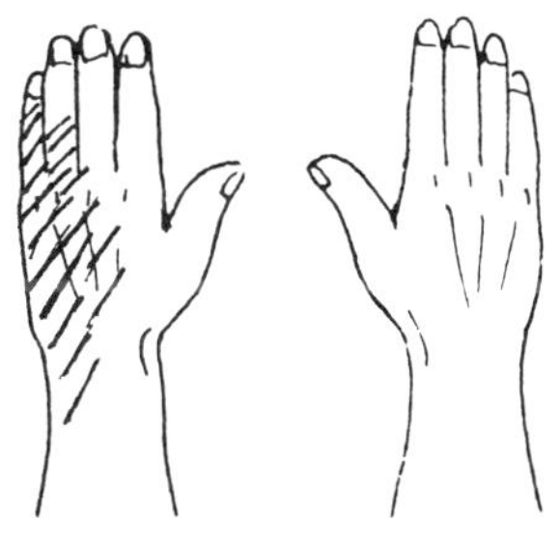

Range of Motion (degrees)

	Ring		Little	
	Active	Passive	Active	Passive
MP	+10/40	+10/40	+25/35	+25/35
PIP	5/95	0/95	20/85	10/85
DIP	0/65	0/65	+15/55	+5/55

Wrist					
Extension	70°	Radial Deviation	0°	Pronation	75°
Flexion	30°	Ulnar Deviation	15°	Supination	75°

Special Tests

Wrist flexion with fingers relaxed	= 30°
Wrist flexion with the fingers flexed	= 15°
MP joint flexion angles with wrist extended 70°	= 50° ring; 45° little
MP joint flexion angles with wrist flexed 30°	= 10° ring; 5° little
IP joint flexion angles with MP joints extended	= 110° PIPs; 80° DIPs

Exercise during the remodeling phase is multifaceted and has as its primary goal the restoration of hand function. Tissues should have healed sufficiently to begin mobilization. The "one wound–one scar" concept is quite apparent during this phase of management. During this phase, tissue interfaces heal together as one unit. This concept is evidenced by taut skin or scar, stiff joints, loss of tendon gliding, and the progression of joint deformities secondary to scar banding. Exercises during the remodeling phase are designed to regain gliding and mobility of the skin, periarticular structures, and tendons. Richard and associates[58] reported on the role of passive exercise versus static wrapping on finger range of motion of six burned hands. Their findings suggested that MP joint flexion was better achieved with passive joint exercises versus use of the multijoint stretch offered by the composite flexion wrap technique. However, IP joint flexion was best achieved using the composite flexion wrap technique.[58] A composite flexion wrap places maximum stretch on the finger extensor mechanism, so it should be used only when the tendons are able to tolerate this force.

At this time, many of the patient's ADL requirements should be addressed by the therapist to influence the remodeling of the tissues by frequent repeated stresses.

Therapeutic Modalities in Burned Hand Management

HYDROTHERAPY

The most commonly used modality to aid in wound care of the burned hand is hydrotherapy. However, an increase in edema, which may be both water temperature and position-dependent, has been reported following whirlpool therapy.[59,60] Because edema control is especially difficult during the inflammatory phase in burned hand management, careful consideration should be given to using the whirlpool during this time. To avoid dependent edema, an alternative to whirlpool therapy is the use of a low-pressure rinse.[61–64] Using 98°F (36.7°C) tap water, the hand can be rinsed off for 5 to 10 minutes in an elevated position.

SUPERFICIAL HEAT

Following closure of the burn wound, the most commonly used superficial heat modalities for the hand are paraffin, moist heat, and Fluidotherapy. Although new skin and scar are quite fragile, superficial heat is not a contraindication. Hermanson[22] reported impairment of hand temperature sensation in hand burns of all depths. Therefore, adequate precautions such as additional padding for insulation under hot packs, reducing the Fluidotherapy temperature setting to 100 to 105°F, and ladling paraffin into a separate bowl to cool before application should be considered.

Hand stiffness is a good indication for the use of superficial heat, and heat can be used to precondition tissues prior to exercise. Hot packs or paraffin can be used in combination with a composite flexion wrap prior to exercise for greater extensibility of the tissues.

A technique that can be used to reduce an IP joint flexion contracture is as follows: (1) a wooden tongue blade is insulated with self-adherent wrap before the blade is positioned under the finger; (2) the length of the blade should extend from the MP joint to the finger tip in order to obtain maximum leverage; (3) an additional length of self-adherent elastic tape is used to secure the finger to the tongue blade; (4) the finger and blade are wrapped together with enough compression to create a gentle force to extend the contracted IP joint; (5) paraffin or a hot pack then can be applied for 15 to 20 minutes in combination with the stretch technique; (6) joint mobilization using distraction and dorsal glides should follow heat and stretch prior to application of the next serial cast.

CONTINUOUS PASSIVE MOTION

Continuous passive motion (CPM) used on the hand has been suggested following flexor tendon repair and thermal injury involving the hand.[65,66] Because Salter and associates[67] research documented only the effect of CPM on cartilage, the effect of CPM on tendon and skin healing is speculation. Theoretically, CPM may support the concept of Wolff's law in healing skin, in that greater tensile strength and better alignment of the collagen may result.[68]

In a study that described the efficacy of CPM with burned hands, the authors hypothesized that the following may be indications for the use of CPM: patients with large total burn surface area requiring extensive therapist time; patients who are unable to actively participate in exercise; and patients who are in pain or apprehensive.[66] The study evaluated the use of CPM with 10 patients who had bilateral partial- and full-thickness hand burns. One hand received traditional exercises and the other a maximum of 8 hours of CPM and exercises. Most hands regained more than 220° of TAM within 3 weeks postburn.[66] Several limitations to CPM were cited, such as a need to closely monitor setup of the CPM, patients who resisted the movement of the machine, and the inability to use the machine with extensor tendon involvement.[65] Also, the therapist should consider cost and the effectiveness of traditional therapy when contemplating the use of CPM for a patient with a hand burn.

ELECTRICAL STIMULATION

The use of high-voltage pulsed current (HVPC) has been recommended to reduce posttraumatic edema formation.[69] HVPC, which does not evoke a mild muscular contraction, is used during the inflammatory phase and can be combined with active muscle contraction. To help reduce hand edema HVPC may need to be used more than once per day.[70]

Neuromuscular electrical stimulation (NMES) can be used during the postacute and reconstructive phases of burned hand management as an adjunct to exercise and ADL to promote active tendon glide. Ideally, NMES can be considered for use as early as 3 weeks postburn or 1 week following reconstructive surgery that involves skin grafts to promote active tendon gliding. Remodeling of dense adherent scar occurs during the first 3 months postburn; however, limited improvement with the use of NMES has been documented in burned hands as late as 5.5 months postburn.[71] NMES of the long finger flexor muscles during grasping exercises and activities often enhances fisting if used several times daily for 15 to 30 minutes. Following release of joint contractures, NMES can be used to improve muscle performance. For example, NMES could be used with a patient who, following surgical release of a wrist flexion contracture, is unable to maintain wrist extension during grasp activities. In this case, not only are the wrist extensor muscles weak but the patient cannot break the habit of grasping with the wrist flexed. To restore wrist joint kinematics and strength, NMES could be applied to the wrist extensors during grasp activities while the patient is encouraged to keep the wrist in an extended position. This procedure should be repeated four to six times each day, for 15 to 20 minutes, until muscle strength is functional. Until a normal grasp posture occurs, a wrist extension splint should be worn between NMES sessions to prevent muscle fatigue and abnormal grasp patterns.

CASE STUDY: APPLICATION OF BURNED HAND MANAGEMENT CONCEPTS

The case study presented in Table 19–11 is designed to illustrate key concepts in burned hand management. There are many ways to approach the restoration of function in burned hand. Creativity and the integration of the principles of wound healing, hand anatomy and kinesiology, exercise, and therapeutic modalities will produce optimal results.

FACTORS TO CONSIDER

A patient with a postacute burned hand in this case study has been referred for outpatient therapy. As part of the initial interview process, the therapist has answered the following questions.

How was the wound closed? Primary excision and split-thickness skin grafting.

Which surfaces of the hand were involved? The dorsum of the little and ring fingers, ulnar hand, and wrist. The area is sketched on the hand burn chart in Table 19–11.

When did the burn occur and when was wound closure complete? The burn was sustained 25 days ago. Primary excision and skin grafting was performed on the same day.

What do the measurements and observations reveal? See Table 19–11 for specific measurements and test results. Following are identified problems and suggested treatments.

Problem 1: Restricted Wrist Flexion and Radial Deviation

Active and passive wrist flexion is 30°. Wrist flexion decreases to 15° with the fingers flexed. Radial deviation is limited to 0° and the scar tissue over the wrist and hand blanches when stretched in a radial direction. Taut skin over the dorsal wrist and hand appears to be primarily responsible for these limitations in range of motion.

Problem 2: Restricted Composite Flexion of the Ring and Little Fingers

Composite active and passive motion of the little and ring fingers is limited. Type I MP joint extension contractures are present in both fingers, because MP joint flexion is limited but greater than 30° with the wrist in 70° of extension.

However, with the wrist positioned in maximum flexion, there is a loss of passive MP joint motion. Evaluation by this method suggests that MP joint restrictions are due primarily to the taut dorsal scar and not to MP joint capsule tightness. Further impact of the taut dorsal scar is noted when the MP joints are held in full extension and the IP joints are compositely flexed.

Problem 3: Dorsal Hood Deformities of the Third and Fourth Web Space

The expansion of the third and fourth web spaces also is limited by the taut dorsal scar. Passively, the web spaces cannot be spread more than actively. When the hand is traced with the web spaces maximally stretched, blanching of the skin graft is observed. Scar hypertrophy across the digital web space and borders of the skin graft also is noted.

Problem 4: Boutonnière Deformity of the Ring and Little Fingers

The boutonnière posture of both fingers appears to be a response to the taut dorsal scar, which restricts wrist and digital joint flexion. If the wrist is held passively in full extension and the MP joint passively flexed, full passive PIP joint extension can be obtained. Full active PIP and DIP joint motion also can be attained in this position, indicating no problem with the extensor tendon systems.

TREATMENTS TO CONSIDER

Taut Dorsal Scar

To initiate gentle stretch of the taut dorsal scar, moist heat is applied with the wrist positioned in full flexion and the fingers relaxed. Gentle stretching of the warmed rigid scar should be done by actively flexing the wrist with the fingers in a relaxed position. This stretch should be maintained for 5 to 10 seconds and repeated 10 to 15 times. Following this stretch of the scar over the wrist joint, the wrist is positioned in extension so that the scar over the MP joints and articular structures of the MP joints can be stretched. This isolated single joint stretch is repeated as outlined for the wrist joint stretch. To perform a multijoint stretch of the taut dorsal scar, the MP joints are maintained in passive flexion while the wrist is actively flexed to the point that further wrist flexion could not be accomplished without changing the position of the MP joints. This gentle multijoint stretch should be held for 5 to 10 seconds and the entire routine repeated 10 to 15 times.

To progress this exercise, the patient can grasp a cylindrically shaped object with the fingers and repeat the previously described exercise. The scar gradually will regain flexibility, as noted by an improvement in the angle of wrist flexion during this exercise. As improvement occurs, the diameter of the cylinder is decreased and the routine repeated.

To increase radial deviation by stretching the dorsal ulnar scar, the palm of the hand is placed on a tabletop with the forearm parallel to the trunk. The opposite hand is used to stabilize the position of the hand on the tabletop. The elbow is brought in toward the trunk, held on stretch for 5 to 10 seconds, and repeated 10 to 15 times.

Composite flexion of the ring and little fingers also is restricted by the taut dorsal scar. The results of the special tests suggest that IP joint flexion can be improved when the MP joints are positioned in extension. As a result, flexion of the MP joint is the first priority. The hand can be superficially heated while each MP joint is maintained in a flexed position. Thermotherapy is followed by passive flexion exercises. As passive flexion of the MP joints improves, this motion is combined with wrist flexion or radial deviation for a multijoint stretch of the scar tissue. The stretch is repeated 10 to 15 times. As passive MP joint flexion improves, the cylinder grasps as outlined previously can be used to address digital composite flexion. Ultimately, wrist, MP, and IP joint flexion exercises are combined for maximum multijoint stretch. Any activity, such as the weight-well, BTE with cylindrical tools, or neuromuscular electrical stimulation, which encourages the combination of digital flexion with wrist flexion for a prolonged period, would complement this program.

Restricted Web Spaces

Passive stretching of the web spaces with the opposite hand for 5 to 10 seconds should precede active digital abduction exercises. This exercise program can be combined with elastomer putty web spacers to give a longer-duration stretch and apply pressure into the dorsal scar. The dynamic type of elastomer putty web spacers or static web spacers held in place with an Isotoner glove as shown in Figure 19–15 would be indicated for this situation. Caution should be taken not to impede flexion of the digit or mobility of the longitudinal metacarpal arch of the hand.

Metacarpophalangeal Hyperextension and Boutonnière Deformity

If exercise alone does not adequately address the taut dorsal scar, splinting at night or intermittently during the day for a low load–long duration stretch may be needed. Several splints would achieve the objective of maximizing MP joint flexion and facilitating IP joint extension. A static splint can be fabricated to position the wrist in extension to permit maximum MP joint flexion and IP joint extension of the little and ring fingers. A self-adherent elastic wrap could be used to keep the hand in the splint. The splint should be worn at night for a long-duration stretch, and if needed, for several hours three times each day. As the range of motion of the MP and IP joints improves, the splint could be serially remolded to position the wrist in greater flexion. If an improvement is not noted with the use of a static splint, a figure-of-8 splint, which positions the MP joints in flexion, could be worn over an Isotoner glove. This splint maintains the MP joints of the little and ring finger in maximum flexion so that PIP joint extension can occur as the patient actively uses the hand. As the skin graft gains tensile strength, dynamic MP flexion slings can be used to provide a gentle stretch to the dorsal scar.

The restrictions in this case study have existed for less than 1 month, which indicates that the tissues are still remodeling and should respond to the above-outlined treatment plan. Repeating the initial baseline measurements will assist the clinician in judging the effectiveness of this treatment plan. If the scar tissue does not respond to intervention during the next 2 months, the surgeon should be informed of the patient's progress for possible surgical intervention.

SUMMARY

Hands are the most frequent site of burn injury, and proper management is essential to assure that optimum functional recovery is achieved. Problems to be anticipated with the burned hand, including edema formation, common hand deformities and loss of skin functions, are reviewed. This information is followed by factors to consider when managing the burned hand through the various stages of wound healing. In addition, guidelines for the use of splints, pressure, exercise, and modalities with the burned hand are presented. Case presentations throughout the chapter illustrate potential hand burn problems and their management.

REFERENCES

1. Kelsey, J, et al: Upper Extremity Disorders: A Survey of Their Frequency and Cost in the United States. CV Mosby, St Louis, 1980, p 7.
2. Kaplan, EB: The hand is an organ. In Spinner, M (ed): Kaplan's Functional Anatomy of the Hand. JB Lippincott, Philadelphia, 1983, pp 3–19.
3. Witte, CL, Witte, MH, and Dumont, AE: Significance of protein in edema fluid. Lymphology 4:29–31, 1971.
4. Salisbury, RE and Dingeldein, GP: The burned hand and upper extremity. In Green, DP (ed): Operative Hand Surgery. Churchill Livingstone, New York, 1982, vol 1, p 1523.
5. Salisbury, RE: Burns of the upper extremity. In Artz, CP, et al (eds): Burns: A Team Approach. WB Saunders, Philadelphia, 1979, p 320.
6. Peacock, EE: Wound Repair, ed 3. WB Saunders, Philadelphia, 1984, pp 1, 35, 54, 107, 108, 114, 196, 199.
7. Littler, JGW: The digital extensor-flexor system. In Converse, JM (ed): Reconstructive Plastic Surgery, ed 2. WB Saunders, Philadelphia, 1977, vol 6, p 3166.
8. Hunter, JW and Mackin, EJ: Edema and bandaging. In Hunter, JW, et al (eds): Rehabilitation of the Hand, ed 3. CV Mosby, St Louis, 1990, p 187.
9. Graham, TJ, Stern, PJ, and True, MS: Classification and treatment of postburn metacarpophalangeal extension contractures in children. J Hand Surg 15A:450–456, 1990.
10. Maisels, DO: The middle slip or boutonnière deformity in burned hands. Br J Plast Surg 18:117–129, 1965.
11. Hunt, JL and Sato, RM: Early excision of full thickness hand and digit burns: Factors affecting morbidity. J Trauma 22:414, 1982.
12. Valentin, P: Physiology of extension of the fingers. In Tubiana R (ed): The Hand. WB Saunders, Philadelphia, 1981, vol 1, p 389.
13. Stern, PJ, et al: Classification and treatment of postburn proximal interphalangeal joint flexion contractures in children. J Hand Surg 12A:450–457, 1987.
14. Sherif, MM and Boswick, JA: Postburn proximal interphalangeal joint hyperextension deformity of the fingers. Bull Clin Rev Burn Inj 3:32–35, 1985.
15. Salisbury, RE, McKeel, DW, and Mason, AD: Ischemic necrosis of the intrinsic muscles of the hand after thermal injury. J Bone Joint Surg 56:1701–1707, 1974.
16. Storch, MD, et al: Impending ischemic contracture in the burned hand and upper extremity. Bull Hosp Joint Dis 37:63–75, 1976.

17. Madden, JW, Carlson, EE, and Hines, J: Presence of modified fibroblast in ischemic contracture of the intrinsic muscles of the hand. Surg Gynecol Obstet 140:509–516, 1975.
18. Smith, RJ: Nonischemic contracture of the intrinsic muscles of the hand. J Bone Joint Surg 53:1313–1331, 1971.
19. Peacock, EE: Preservation of proximal interphalangeal joint function. South Med J 56:56–63, 1963.
20. Stern, PJ, et al: Classification and management of burned thumb contractures in children. Burns 11:168–174, 1985.
21. Warden, GD: The pediatric burn patient: Issues in wound management. In Boots Burn Management Report, vol 1. Boots Pharmaceuticals, Lincolnshire, 1991.
22. Hermanson, A, Jonsson, CE, and Lindblom, U: Sensibility after burn injury. Clin Physiol 6:507, 1986.
23. Ward, RS, et al: Sensory loss over grafted areas in patients with burns. J Burn Care Rehabil 10:536–538, 1989.
24. Folkerts, JF, Sneep, AJ, and Meihling, HA: Comparative investigation of the return of sensation to skin grafts. In Biemont, A, et al (eds): Recent Neurological Research. Amsterdam, 1959, p 521.
25. Warwick, W: Gray's Anatomy, 35th ed. WB Saunders, Philadelphia, 1972, p 1167.
26. Donelan, MB: Nailfold reconstruction for correction of postburn fingernail deformities. Proc Am Burn Assoc 23:142, 1991.
27. Dufourmentel, C: Nail prostheses. In Pierre, M (ed): The Nail. Churchill Livingstone, Edinburgh, 1981, p 85.
28. Barfod, B: Reconstruction of the Nail Fold. In Pierre, M (ed): The Nail. Churchill Livingstone, Edinburgh, 1981, p 114.
29. Pillet, J: Prostheses in amputated fingertips. In Pierre, M (ed): The Nail. Churchill Livingstone, Edinburgh, 1981, p 90.
30. Warwick, R and Williams, PL: Gray's Anatomy, 35th ed. WB Saunders, Philadelphia, 1972, p 1160.
31. Dobbs, ER and Curreri, PW: Burns: Analysis of results of physical therapy in 681 patients. J Trauma 12:242–248, 1972.
32. Goodwin, CW, et al: Prospective study of burn wound excision of the hands. J Trauma 23:510–517, 1983.
33. Moncreif, JA: Third-degree burns of the dorsum of the hand. Am J Surg 96:535–544, 1958.
34. Janzekovic, Z: A new concept in early excision and immediate grafting of burns. J Trauma 10:1103–1108, 1970.
35. Levine, BA, et al: Efficacy of tangential excision and immediate autografting of deep dermal burns of the hand. J Trauma 19:670–673, 1979.
36. Habal, MB: The burned hand: A planned treatment program. J Trauma 18:587–595, 1978.
37. Habal, MB: Follow-up report on burned hands, treatment plans. J Burn Care Rehabil 8:213–215, 1987.
38. Apfel, LM, et al: Functional hand assessment after enzymatic debridement and early autografting. J Burn Care Rehabil 5:438–445, 1984.
39. Edstrom, LE, et al: Prospective randomized treatments for burned hands: Non-operative vs operative. Scand J Plast Reconstr Surg 13:131–135, 1979.
40. Salisbury, RE and Wright, P: Evaluation of early excision of dorsal burns of the hand. Plast Reconstr Surg 69:670–675, 1982.
41. Rudolph, R: Construction and control of contraction. World J Surg 4:279–287, 1980.
42. American Society for Surgery of the Hand: The Hand: Examination and Diagnosis. Churchill Livingstone, New York, 1983, pp 104–107.
43. Brand, PW: Clinical Biomechanics of the Hand. CV Mosby, St Louis, 1985, pp 68–86.
44. Salisbury, RE, et al: Postburn edema of the upper extremity: Evaluation of present treatment. J Trauma 13:857–862, 1973.
45. Barnett, PH and Stafford, FS: Use of plastic air bands for edema and scar contracture. J Burn Care Rehabil 5:469–473, 1984.
46. Moberg, E: Objective methods of determining the functional value of sensibility of the hand. J Bone Joint Surg 40B:454–476, 1958.
47. Tiffin, J: Purdue Pegboard Examiner Manual. Science Research Associates, Chicago, 1968.
48. Salisbury, RE, Reeves, S, and Wright, P: Acute care and rehabilitation of the burned hand. In Hunter, JM, et al (eds): Rehabilitation of the Hand, ed 3. CV Mosby, St Louis, 1990, p 831.
49. Malick, MH and Carr, JA: Management of the Burn Patient. Harmarville Rehabilitation Center, Education Resource Center, Pittsburgh, 1982, p 246.
50. Stone, PA and Madden, JW: Effect of primary and delayed split grafting on wound contraction. Surg Forum 25:41–44, 1974.
51. Larson, DL, et al: Repair of boutonnière deformity of the burned hand. J Trauma 10:481–487, 1970.
52. Howell, JW: Post-hospitalization care of the burn patient. In DeGregorio, W (ed): Rehabilitation of the Burn Patient. Churchill Livingstone, New York, 1982, p 151.
53. Schumann, L and Gaston, S: Common sense guide to topical burn therapy. Nursing 3:345, 1979.
54. Kealey, GP and Jensen, KT: Aggressive approach to physical therapy management of the burned hand: A clinical report. Phys Ther 68:683–685, 1988.

55. Gabbiani, G, Ryan, GB, and Majno, G: Presence of modified fibroblasts in granulation tissue and their possible role in wound contraction. Experientia 27:549–550, 1971.
56. Ward, RS: Pressure therapy for the control of hypertrophic scar formation after burn injury. J Burn Care Rehabil 12:257–262, 1991.
57. Tanigawa, MC, O'Donnell, OK, and Graham, PL: The burned hand: A physical therapy protocol. Phys Ther 54:953–958, 1974.
58. Richard, RL, et al: Comparison of the effect of passive exercise versus static wrapping on finger range of motion in the burned hand. J Burn Care Rehabil 8:576–578, 1987.
59. Shultz, K: The effect of active exercise during whirlpool on the hand. Master's thesis. San Jose, San Jose State University, 1982.
60. Walsh, M: Relationship of hand edema to upper extremity position and water temperature during whirlpool. J Hand Surg 9A:609, 1984.
61. Gross, A, Cutright, DE, and Bhaskar, SN: Effectiveness of pulsating jet lavage in treatment of contaminated crushed wounds. Am J Surg 124:373–377, 1972.
62. Hamer, MI, et al: Quantitative bacterial analysis of comparative wound irrigations. Ann Surg 181:819–822, 1975.
63. Rodeheaver, GT, et al: Wound cleansing by high pressure irrigation. Surg Gynecol Obstet 141:357–362, 1975.
64. Wheeler, CB, et al: Side-effects of high pressure irrigation. Surg Gynecol Obstet 143:775–778, 1976.
65. Gelberman, RH, et al: Flexor tendon healing: A prospective clinical trial evaluating controlled passive motion rehabilitation. Proceedings American Society for Surgery of the Hand. Baltimore, 1990, p 46.
66. Covey, MH, et al: Efficacy of continuous passive motion (CPM) devices with hand burns. J Burn Care Rehabil 9:397–400, 1988.
67. Salter, RB, et al: The effects of continuous passive motion on the healing of articular cartilage defects: An experimental investigation in rabbits. J Bone Joint Surg 57A:570, 1975.
68. Forrester, JC, et al: Wolff's law in relation to the healing skin wound. J Trauma 10:770–779, 1970.
69. Reed, BV: Effect of high voltage pulsed electrical stimulation on microvascular permeability to plasma proteins: A possible mechanism in minimizing edema. Phys Ther 68:491–495, 1988.
70. Taylor, K, et al: Effect of a single 30-minute treatment of high voltage pulsed current on edema formation in frog hind limbs. Phys Ther 72:63–68, 1992.
71. Apfel, LM, et al: Function electrical stimulation in intrinsic/extrinsic imbalanced burned hands. J Burn Care Rehabil 8:97–102, 1987.

CHAPTER 20

Neuromuscular and Musculoskeletal Complications

Kristi Dutcher, PT
Carole Johnson, PhD, PT

Prevention of neuromuscular and musculoskeletal complications in patients must be a continuing goal of the burn therapist. Such complications not only lengthen a patient's rehabilitation process but also frequently impair the patient's functional outcome. The purpose of this chapter is to provide information regarding neuromuscular and musculoskeletal complications that may occur following a burn injury to aid therapists in their ability to recognize and manage these conditions. Although both neuromuscular and musculoskeletal complications may occur simultaneously in a patient, they will be discussed separately.

NEUROMUSCULAR COMPLICATIONS

A burn injury can have devastating effects on the neuromuscular system. Patient complaints regarding weakness or lack of sensation often are rationalized as generalized sequelae of the injury and healing process. However, these symptoms may be due to peripheral neuropathies resulting from either impaired peripheral nerve axons, or myelin sheaths, or both. Therefore, several causes should be considered by the burn therapist as potential explanations for any such complaints.

The incidence of peripheral neuropathy in burn patients ranges from 15 to 29 percent. Peripheral neuropathies usually are seen in patients with burns greater than 20 percent total body surface area; however, they can develop in patients with a high-voltage electrical burn of lesser area.[1,2] Certain patients are more susceptible to peripheral neuropathies: alcoholics and diabetics because of diseased nerves and the aged because they are less mobile and their nerves do not tolerate pressure well.

Peripheral neuropathy can be either generalized or local in nature. Patients with a generalized peripheral neuropathy, termed *polyneuropathy,* often complain of fatigue and lack of endurance.[2] This condition is characterized by distal weakness in the upper and lower extremities and may affect both burned and nonburned extremities without localization to a specific nerve. Sensory deficits may be present. Motor and sensory symptoms usually improve over several months, although patients may experience decreased endurance for years. The exact etiology of peripheral polyneuropathy is unknown; however, neurotoxicities from the numerous drugs used in the treatment of burn patients has been suggested.

In contrast, local neuropathies are caused by a stretch or compression injury to a single nerve. They can result from improper treatment techniques applied to a burn patient.[2] The therapist should understand that these complications can be either prevented or promoted. Unfortunately, local neuropathies and peripheral polyneuropathies can occur simultaneously, creating an even greater functional deficit for the patient.

Knowledge about the etiologies of these deficits can guide a burn therapist in prevention and intervention strategies. Neuropathies directly related to a burn injury and its management as well as common pre-existing neuropathies are described in the following section.

Review of Nerve Structure and Function

A basic understanding of nerve structure and function is necessary to effectively treat patients who have neurologic complications. The nerve cell, or *neuron,* consists of a cell body from which extends a number of short highly branched processes called *dendrites* and a single elongated process known as an *axon* (Fig. 20–1). Dendrites carry electrical signals from other neurons to cell body and the axon conducts these signals to nerves and muscles. Near its origin, the axon acquires a sheath of myelin, a protein-lipid complex made up of many layers. The myelin sheath envelops the axon except at its ending and at periodic constrictions about 1 mm apart, known as *the nodes of Ranvier.* Conduction along the axon is related to the diameter of the myelin sheath.

Within a muscle, the axon from a single motor nerve cell divides into many terminal branches.[4] Each branch is attached to an individual muscle fiber. The branching of the axon permits a single neuron to stimulate a group of muscle fibers. The functional unit, defined as a *motor unit,* consists of a neuron, its axon, and all the muscle fibers innervated by that axon.

Injuries to a nerve have been classified into three types: neuropraxia, axonotmesis, and neurotmesis. *Neuropraxia* refers to a temporary compression of a nerve. The structure of the axon remains intact but there may be segmental demyelination. Depending upon the time course and severity of compression and subsequent need for remyelinization, neuropraxia may last for minutes to weeks. *Axonotmesis* refers to nerve cell injury in which the myelin remains intact, but axonal continuity is lost. Recovery from axonal lesions depends upon the regeneration rate of axon nerve fibers, which is about 1 to 3 mm/day. Patients may require many months to improve and may not recover fully. *Neurotmesis* refers to complete functional transection of a nerve with Wallerian degeneration occurring distal to the site of the lesion. Regeneration that occurs is incomplete and poorly organized with frequent neuroma formation.

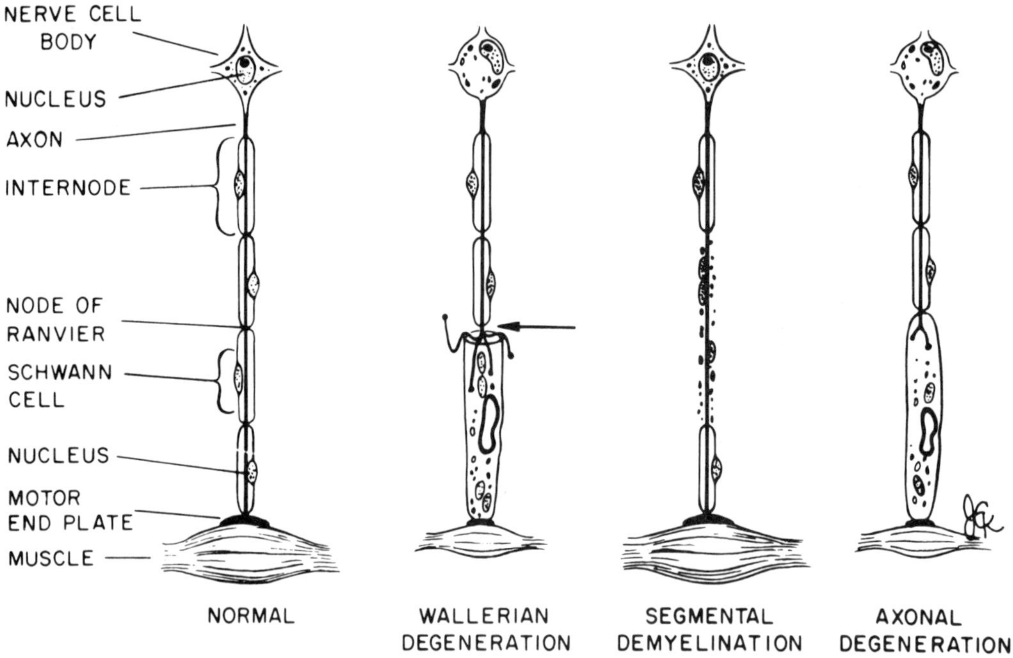

FIGURE 20–1. The basic pathologic processes affecting peripheral nerves. Degeneration of the axis cylinder and myelin distal to the site of axonal interruption occurs in Wallerian degeneration. The axon is spared in segmental demyelination. Distal degeneration of the axis cylinder and myelin occurs in axonal degeneration. (From Adams,[3] p 1031, with permission.)

Electrophysiologic Testing

The diagnosis of peripheral neuropathies is aided by nerve conduction studies (NCS) and electromyography (EMG). Nerve conduction testing evaluates the speed that a nerve conducts an electrical impulse along its axon. Electromyography evaluates the integrity of a motor unit and allows localization of lesions. Pathologic findings usually are related to: (1) axonal failure, (2) damage to myelin, (3) a combination of both, and (4) pathologies in motor units (Fig. 20–2). Sequential electrophysiologic testing can help monitor reinnervation and recovery of a motor unit.

A nerve conduction velocity (NCV) is calculated by dividing distance by time. Distance is measured in millimeters between two stimulation sites and divided by the difference in conduction time in milliseconds between the distal stimulation site and the proximal stimulation site (Fig. 20–3). The most commonly tested nerves, in order of frequency, are the median, ulnar, peroneal, tibial, sural, and radial.

An EMG-needle examination typically has three stages. In the first stage, the patient rests and a needle is inserted into a muscle. Insertion itself causes irritation of the muscle, and the response is termed *insertional activity.* After the cessation of that activity, the healthy muscle is electrically silent. Abnormal muscles will show fibrillations and sharp wave potentials, which are spontaneous activities of single muscle fibers.

In the second stage, the patient contracts a muscle with minimal effort. Electrical signals arising from one or more motor units may be observed. The signal parameters

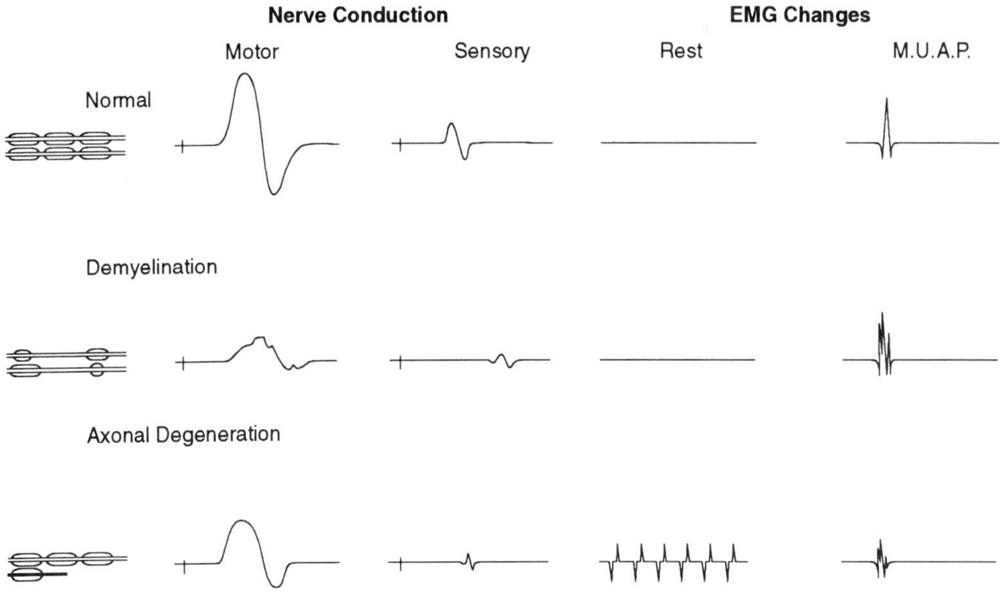

FIGURE 20–2. Different patterns are observed in both nerve conduction and EMG tests for demyelination and axonal degeneration when compared to a normal nerve. M.U.A.P. stands for motor unit action potential. (From Johnson,[6] p 156 and 159, with permission.)

evaluated include amplitude, duration, shape, and phase. Typically, a healthy motor unit exhibits fewer than four phases or intersections with the baseline.

In the third stage, the patient contracts with maximal effort and recruits or activates as many motor units as possible. The motor unit potentials begin to overlap and individual motor units can no longer be distinguished. This EMG recording is referred to as an *interference pattern.* Analysis of the interference pattern allows the electromyographer to distinguish disease states of muscle or nerve (Fig. 20–4).

Electrophysiologic testing is helpful in identifying the type and severity of nerve injuries; however, enough time must be allowed for the abnormalities to manifest themselves. Immediately after complete transection of a nerve, no motor unit activity exists with voluntary contraction; however, the distal portion of the nerve remains electrically excitable for 3 to 5 days. Subsequently, the nerve becomes unexcitable and conduction ceases. The motor end plate retains its full excitability for 5 to 10 days. Therefore, electrodiagnostic studies should be delayed a minimum of 14 days.

Electrophysiologic testing can be performed on children; however, additional care is required to ensure patient cooperation. When performing a nerve conduction velocity study, the child first should be sedated. When conducting an EMG, testing should be limited to older, more cooperative children as the exam requires active muscle contraction.

Neuropathies from Burn Injury

THERMAL INJURIES

Direct neural injury by a burn is uncommon because of the relatively protected position that peripheral nerves have in relationship to the skin and subcutaneous

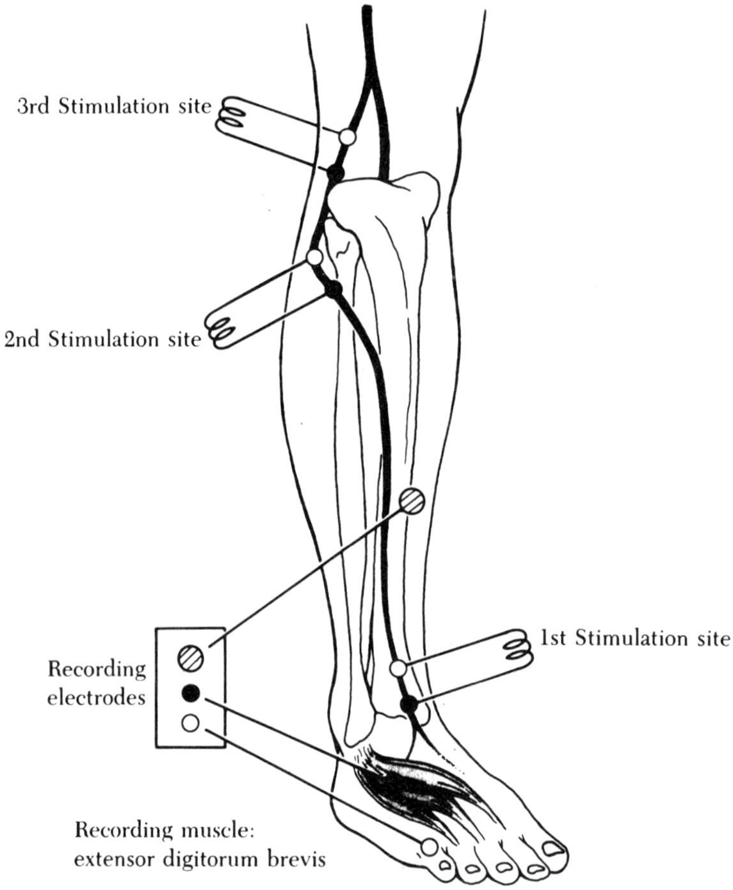

FIGURE 20–3. Example of stimulation sites for a nerve conduction test for the peroneal nerve. (From Oh,[5] p 76, with permission.)

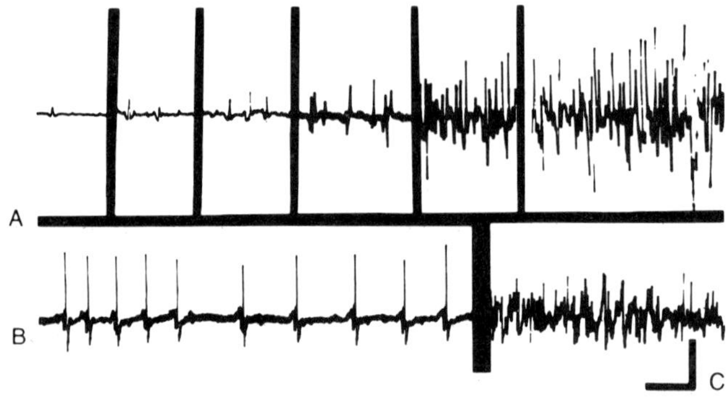

FIGURE 20–4. Examples of observations from EMG. (*A*) Normal incremental recruitment with voluntary effort. More and large units are "recruited" with increased voluntary effort until single units are no longer recognizable. (*B*) After denervation, only a single motor unit is recorded, firing repetitively, despite maximum effort. (*C*) With myopathic diseases, a normal number of units is recruited, but the amplitude is reduced. (From Adams,[3] p 1018, with permission.)

tissue.[7] Nerves that are superficial and at significant risk for damage are the *ulnar nerve* at the elbow and superficial branch of the *radial nerve* on the dorsum of the hand. However, nerve tissue can coagulate when the wound extends into the subcutaneous fat and underlying structures. These nerve injuries are rarely amenable to primary repair.[7]

ELECTRICAL BURNS

The prevalence of neuromuscular complications in association with high-voltage electrical burns has been well documented.[1,8-11] Complications include cerebellar dysfunction, paraplegia, quadriplegia, sympathetic dystrophies, and localized nerve damage. Neural tissue has a very low resistance to electric current and is particularly susceptible to injury. Spinal cord damage may result from current that passes from one arm to another, from one arm to a leg, or from entrance and exit points around the spine. An injury may manifest itself within several hours or up to 2 years following trauma. Patients typically exhibit paraparesis or quadriparesis, with or without spasticity. Subsequent weakness and spasticity may be transient or permanent.

Peripheral nerve damage is caused by direct influence of the current on the nerve and surrounding tissues and by swelling of an involved muscle compartment. Acute sensory and motor defects usually are transient and recoverable in the absence of concomitant thermal or mechanical injury.[7] Permanent damage to peripheral nerves, due to heat generated by current flow, is limited to the area of local tissue damage. The median and ulnar nerves are the most frequently injured nerves in electrical burns, reflecting the greater frequency with which the hand is involved in such injuries.

CHEMICAL BURNS

If chemical burns lead to full-thickness wounds, underlying nerves could be involved. Damage to a nerve would then be due to direct local action of the individual chemical.

RADIATION BURNS

Information regarding radiation burns primarily has been obtained from the study of the use of radiation in treating malignancies. Although the central nervous system can be damaged by the effects of radiation, peripheral nerves appear to be highly resistant.[12]

Neuropathies from Burn Management

POSITIONING AND SPLINTING

Burn therapists usually are responsible for positioning and splinting of patients' limbs to prevent deformities. Three particular areas must be managed carefully to prevent nerve injury: the shoulder for brachial plexus injuries, the elbow for ulnar nerve lesions, and the knee for peroneal nerve lesions.

Clinical observations can provide pertinent information regarding the type of brachial plexus lesion. For lesions of the entire plexus, the upper extremity is flaccid (Fig. 20–5). With an upper brachial plexus paralysis, the extremity hangs at the side, internally rotated and extended at the elbow. With a lower brachial plexus paralysis, the hand has a characteristic claw hand deformity with weakness and atrophy of the intrinsic muscles of the hand (Table 20–1).

A brachial plexus injury may result from improper positioning of the shoulder for prolonged periods of time. Shoulder abduction greater than 90° combined with external rotation decreases the distance between the clavicle and the first rib, which may result in compression of the plexus.[2] This position, when combined with posterior displacement of the shoulder, also may cause stretching of the plexus.[2] Both stretch and compression on the plexus can be alleviated by limiting shoulder abduction to 90° and by horizontally adducting the arm 30°.[2] When a patient is in a prone

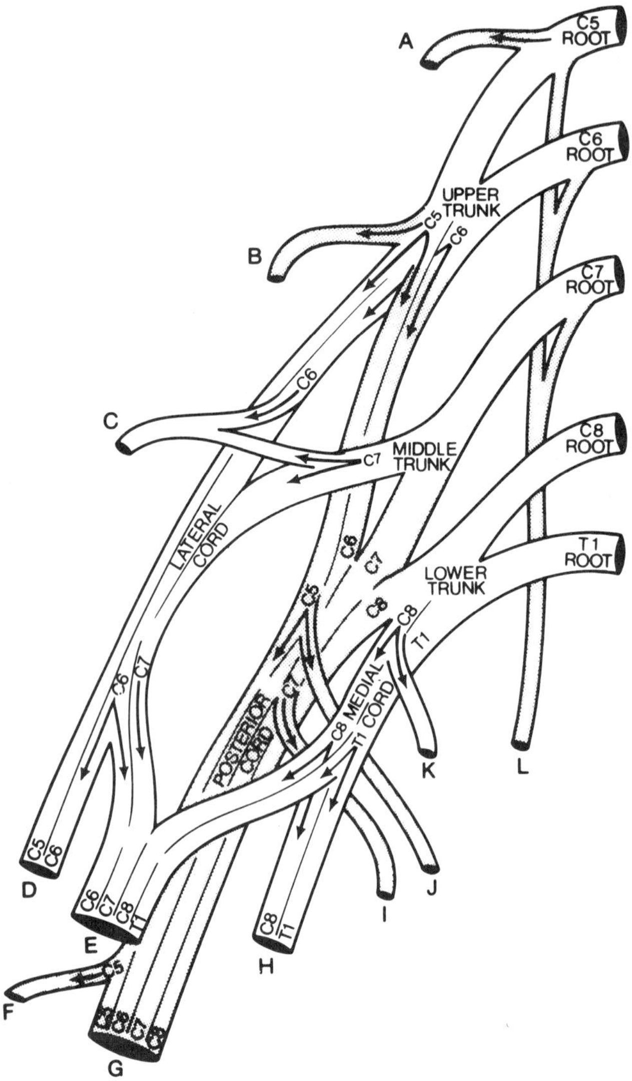

FIGURE 20–5. Anatomy of the brachial plexus with eventual destination of all root components. The posterior divisions of the trunks and their derivatives are shaded. The brachial plexus gives rise to dorsal scapular (*A*), suprascapular (*B*), lateral pectoral (*C*), musculocutaneous (*D*), median (*E*), axillary (*F*), radial (*G*), ulnar (*H*), thoracodorsal (*I*), subscapular (*J*), medial pectoral (*K*), and long thoracic (*L*) nerves. (From Kimura, J: Electrodiagnosis in Diseases of Nerve and Muscle: Principles and Practice, ed 2. FA Davis Company, Philadelphia, 1989, p 12, with permission.)

TABLE 20-1. Neurology of the Upper Extremity

Disc	Root	Reflex	Muscles	Sensation
C4-5	C5	Biceps reflex	Deltoid Biceps	*Lateral arm* Axillary nerve
C5-6	C6	Brachioradialis reflex (biceps reflex)	Wrist extension Biceps	*Lateral forearm* Musculocutaneous nerve
C6-7	C7	Triceps reflex	Wrist flexion Finger extension Triceps	*Middle finger*
C7-T1	C8	—	Finger flexion Hand intrinsics	*Medial forearm* Med. ant. brach. Cutaneous nerve
T1-2	T1	—	Hand intrinsics	*Medial arm* Med. brach. Cutaneous nerve

From: Hoppenfield,[13] p 125.

position, sufficient horizontal adduction of the shoulder can be achieved by placing pillows under the patient's chest. Frequent monitoring of a patient's position is necessary to prevent this injury from occurring.

The ulnar nerve innervates the ulnar flexor of the wrist, the ulnar half of the deep finger flexors, the adductors and abductors of the fingers, the adductor of the thumb, the third and fourth lumbricals, and the muscles of the hypothenar eminence (Fig. 20-6). The ulnar nerve supplies sensation to the ulnar aspect of the hand, the ulnar half of the ring finger, and all of the little finger. Patients with ulnar nerve lesions typically present with numbness of the fourth and fifth fingers. Complete ulnar paralysis is manifested by a characteristic claw hand deformity and wasting of the small hand muscles.

Certain arm positions put the ulnar nerve at risk for compression as the nerve runs through the cubital tunnel. When the elbow is flexed to 90°, the ulnar nerve is susceptible to "physiologic" pressure exerted by the arcuate ligament. The ligament that forms the roof of the tunnel is taut at 90° of elbow flexion but slack in elbow extension. When the forearm is pronated, the ulnar nerve is susceptible to an external compression force created by the surface on which the nerve lies. The combination of these two positions puts the nerve doubly at risk. The undesirable position of elbow flexion and forearm pronation frequently is seen when patients are positioned prone or when patients with upper extremity burns have their hands positioned on pillows. Ulnar neuropathy can be prevented by positioning the elbow in extension with the forearm supinated and positions alternated for comfort.

Branches of the peroneal nerve supply the dorsiflexors of the foot and toes and carry sensory fibers from the dorsum of the foot and lateral aspect of the lower half of the leg (Fig. 20-7). Clinically, compression of this nerve is characterized by an acute onset of foot drop and occasionally is associated with sensory impairment in the region of the superficial or deep peroneal nerve.

The peroneal nerve is frequently injured.[2] The nerve is vulnerable to compression by being exposed over the fibular head for about 4 to 5 cm, covered only by skin, fat, and superficial fascia.[2] Compression of the nerve can occur during prolonged

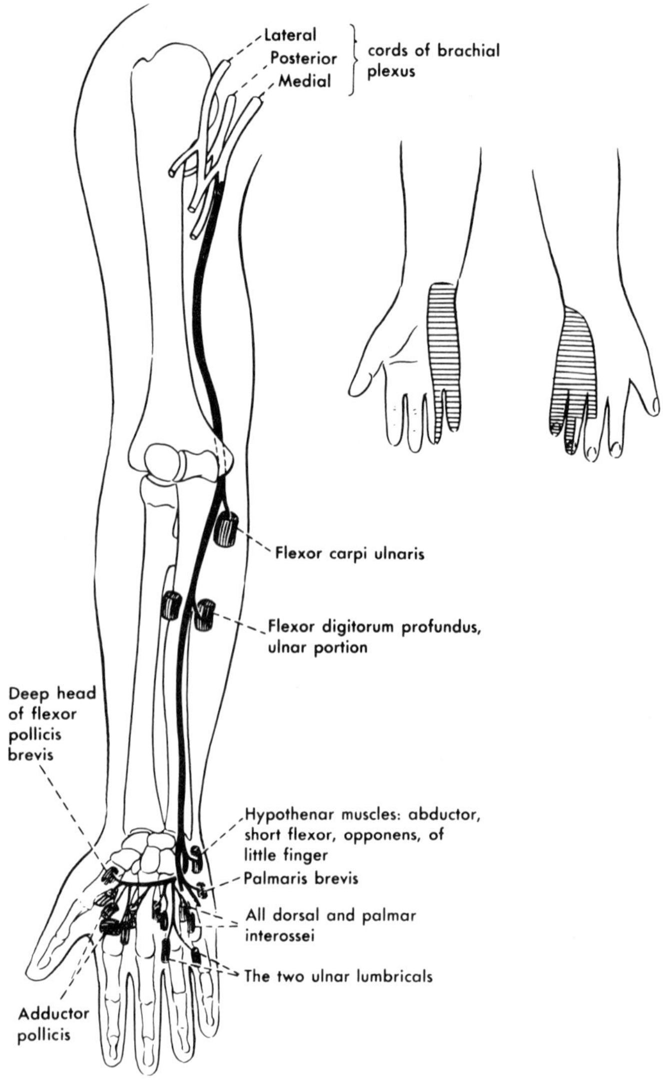

FIGURE 20–6. Motor and sensory distribution of the ulnar nerve. (From Hollinshead,[14] p 139, with permission.)

side-lying, from side rails on the bed, and from poorly fitting splints. The peroneal nerve also is susceptible to stretch injury because of limited longitudinal mobility. Prolonged "frog leg" position due to medial thigh burns or edema of the perineum can increase the stretch to the nerve. Preventive measures include alternating side-lying positions, constant vigilance to avoid the frog leg position, and positioning the knees in extension and the ankles in dorsiflexion.

OPERATING ROOM PROCEDURES

The operating room is a particularly dangerous environment for causing iatrogenic injury. Debridement of devitalized soft tissue can injure or sever nerves. With the advent of early excision and skin grafting, neurologic deficits may become more prevalent.

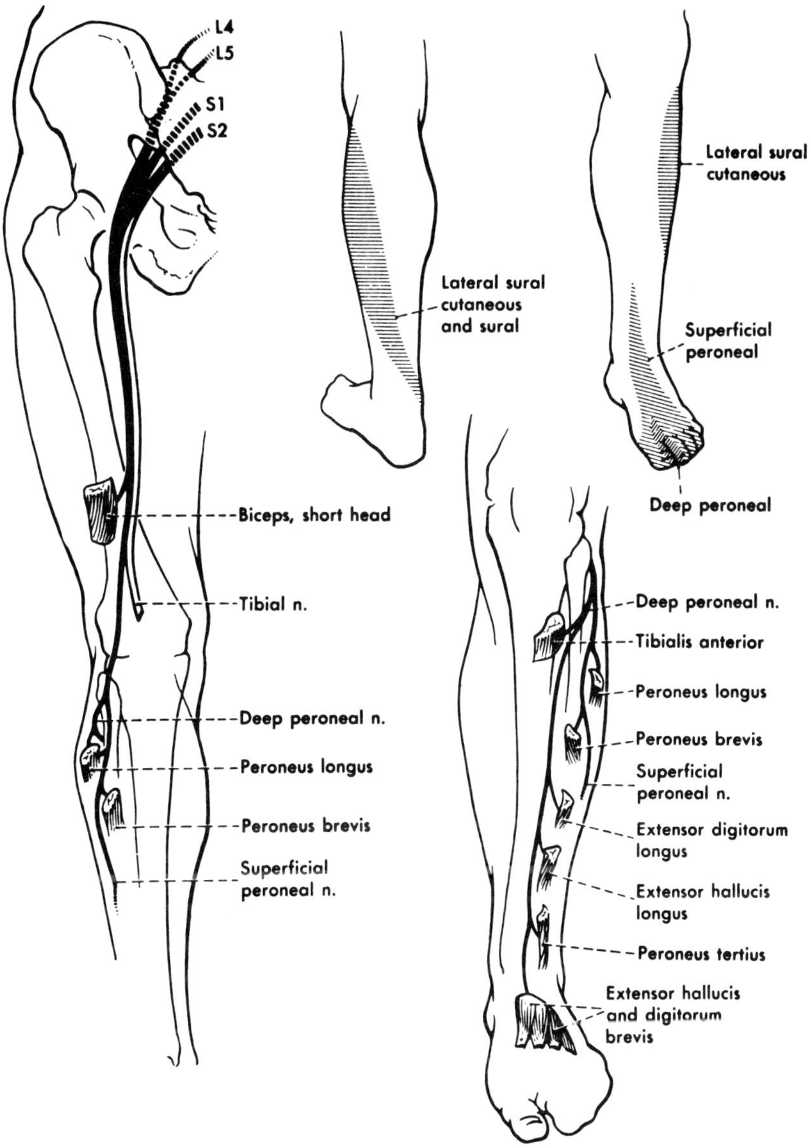

FIGURE 20–7. Motor and sensory distribution of the peroneal nerve. (From Hollinshead,[14] p 327, with permission.)

Compression neuropathies can occur during surgery from prolonged application of an elastic tourniquet to create a bloodless field.[2] Pneumatic tourniquets have decreased the incidence, but pressure of the cuff and time remain critical. Direct compression of underlying nerves and ischemic injury to tissue distal to the tourniquet are two possible mechanisms of injury.

Brachial plexus injuries also may occur during surgery.[15] Stretch or compression of the plexus appears to be the common mechanism of injury. Compression injuries, due to the clavicle being forced against the first rib, are anatomically possible in a true side-lying position, for example, when a thoracotomy is performed. Both stretch and compression injuries are preventable if careful attention is given to proper positioning techniques.

DRESSINGS

Tight, bulky dressings may cause direct pressure to various nerves, although the peroneal is affected most frequently.[2] Measures for prevention include: applying dressings with less compression; providing a window for the area; and educating personnel performing dressing changes.

INJECTIONS

Injury to muscle and small nerve fibers may occur as a result of failing to alternate sites for intramuscular injections. The deltoid muscle is a commonly affected area. Johnson and colleagues[16] postulated that damage was caused by an inflammatory reaction due to the physical trauma from the needle, pressure from the volume injected, and toxicity of the drug. If therapists observe deltoid weakness and the patient complains of pain in the shoulder where an injection was administered, an injection injury should be suspected.

SKELETAL TRACTION

Skeletal pins occasionally are used to achieve elevation and immobilization of an extremity after skin grafting. Improperly applied traction may create undue stress on the brachial plexus and peripheral nerves. In addition, changes in position may alter the traction forces. For example, raising the head of the bed may put excessive stretch on the brachial plexus if the traction device is not appropriately adjusted.

Neuropathies from Burn Complications

EDEMA

In burns greater than 25 percent of the body, capillaries of both unburned and injured tissue become abnormally permeable. Plasma escapes into the interstitial space with subsequent edema formation. Fluid resuscitation required to combat initial burn shock increases edema. Normal skin expands to accommodate swelling, but skin with denatured collagen and destroyed elastic fibers is inelastic and lacks this ability.

If a burn is circumferential on an extremity, a tourniquet effect is exerted and progressive ischemia may develop, involving peripheral nerves and soft tissue underlying and distal to the burn. Protection of neurovascular structures in such cases depends upon timely and adequate escharotomy.[17] However, during an escharotomy, nerves can be damaged if a physician does not appreciate that edema may obscure normal anatomic landmarks.[7] For example, the ulnar nerve is vulnerable particularly at the medial epicondyle and the superficial branch of the radial nerve must be avoided during the distal radial escharotomy incision. A tourniquet effect also may be caused by a normal anatomic structure such as fascia. A fasciotomy of the overlying muscle compartment is required if escharotomy alone is inadequate at decompressing the neurovascular bundles. This procedure often is performed following high-voltage electrical injuries because of the propensity for electrical current to damage subfascial tissue.

HETEROTOPIC OSSIFICATION

Heterotopic bone formation, which is discussed later in this chapter, also contributes to the development of peripheral neuropathy. This abnormal bony tissue development can compress soft nerve tissue. Bony encasement of the ulnar nerve along with signs and symptoms of ulnar nerve compression frequently are found when heterotopic bone is located about the elbow.[18]

Concurrent and Pre-existing Neuropathies

A therapist should be aware that there may be pre-existing neuropathies in a burn patient. This section focuses on those neuropathies most likely to be encountered. Further readings in clinical neurology texts will provide detailed explanations of less frequent neuropathies.

DIABETIC NEUROPATHY

Diabetes mellitus (DM) is the most common metabolic disorder with substantial neurologic complications.[19] Any involvement of the peripheral nervous system in DM is referred to as a *diabetic neuropathy.* Unlike other complications of DM, neuropathy is thought to be metabolic in origin. The most consistent finding of damage in the peripheral nerve is demyelination.[5] Axonal degeneration may be present in severe cases. Patients exhibit a symmetrical loss of sensation and to a lesser extent loss of motor control. Distal muscles, such as the intrinsic foot muscles, are affected most frequently.

ALCOHOLIC NEUROPATHY

Alcoholic neuropathy is an insidious disorder found in people who have imbibed a large quantity of alcoholic beverages for several years. Nutritional deficiency, particularly of B vitamins and direct toxic effects of alcohol, are examples of probable etiology. The earliest pathologic change noted on NCV studies is axonal degeneration and subsequent marked reduction in amplitude. Virtually all muscles in patients with alcoholic polyneuropathies show some evidence of denervation. Symptoms occur initially in the lower extremities.

UREMIC NEUROPATHY

Peripheral neuropathy is a common complication in patients with chronic renal failure. Clinical and electrophysiologic observations have shown that uremic polyneuropathy progresses with worsening chronic renal failure, stabilizes during chronic hemodialysis, and consistently improves following renal transplantation. Electrophysiologic testing reveals axonal degeneration and secondary segmental demyelination.[6]

Anastakis and colleagues[20] published a case report of a patient with a 45 percent mixed deep partial- and full-thickness flame burn who developed a severe polyneuropathy.[20] The authors suggested the most likely cause of the polyneuropathy was the development of uremia diagnosed on the 33rd postburn day.

MUSCULOSKELETAL COMPLICATIONS

The frequency of musculoskeletal complications is lower than those involving the neuromuscular system, but the effects can be equally devastating. This section describes the direct and indirect effects of burns to bone, joint, and tendon. Heterotopic bone formation has been a major topic in the literature and makes up a large portion of this section.

Heterotopic Ossification

Heterotopic ossification (HO) can be defined as "the formation of new bone in tissues that normally do not ossify."[21] HO may occur in soft tissue surrounding a joint, within a joint capsule and ligaments, or may form a bony bridge across a joint[22] (Fig. 20–8). In addition to burns, HO is a complication associated with other injuries and paralytic diseases, including spinal cord injury, head injury, cerebral vascular accidents, and musculoskeletal trauma. In some instances, this abnormal deposition of bone resolves spontaneously. In other cases, the continued presence of HO limits the functional abilities of a patient so severely that surgical excision is necessary.

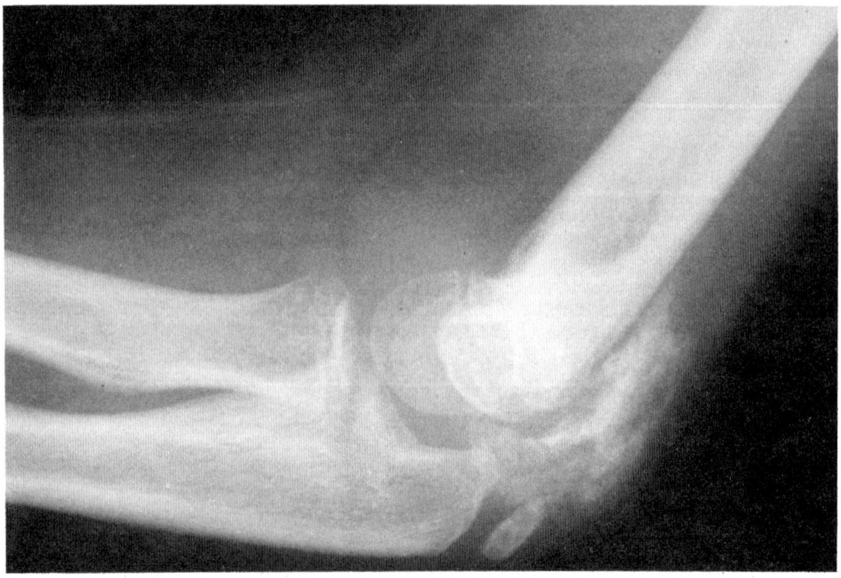

FIGURE 20–8. Heterotopic ossification present at the posterior aspect of the elbow. Ectopic bone first appears on radiograph as an amorphous cloudy mass.

INCIDENCE

The incidence of HO in burn patients ranges from 0.1 percent to 3.3 percent in retrospective studies and 13.6 percent to 23 percent in prospective studies.[23-26] The high incidence in prospective studies might be explained by the investigators' increased awareness of the problem and increased use of diagnostic techniques. HO may occur in a single joint or in multiple joints, and frequently occurs bilaterally. In burn patients, HO occurs in the temporomandibular joint, shoulder, elbow, wrist, hand, hip, knee, and ankle.[27,28] The posteromedial aspect of the elbow joint is most frequently affected followed by the shoulder and the hip.[27]

The formation of HO is not related to age, gender, race, or cause of burn injury. The location of a burn does not necessarily dictate the formation of new bone, as joints remote from the injury may become involved. However, HO is found more commonly in patients with a greater than 20 percent full-thickness burn and in patients whose wounds remain ungrafted for long periods of time.[29]

ETIOLOGY

The absolute pathogenesis of HO formation has not been identified, but many theories about its etiology exist. One theory attributed the formation of HO to a disturbance in calcium metabolism.[30] Prolonged immobility and trauma have been shown to increase calcium mobilization from bone and increase caluresis. High protein intake (greater than 150 g/day) also has been shown to double calcium mobilization and its excretion, possibly due to an alteration in calcium transport by the kidney.[30] Proponents of this theory claim that excessive calcium mobilization and hypercaluresis may lead to focal ectopic calcium deposits.

A more popular theory attributes HO formation to superimposed trauma and repeated microtrauma that results in local hemorrhage.[31] Using a rabbit model, both Izumi[32] and Michelsson and colleagues[33] were able to demonstrate that immobilization followed by a forcible mobilization resulted in the development of HO. The longer a joint remains immobilized, the less flexible it becomes and more soft tissue damage will occur if the joint is taken abruptly through a range of motion. Patients who are uncooperative or restless may inadvertently add increased stress on their joints by resisting therapy or restraints.[27,31] Supporters of this theory maintain that "quality" of joint motion along with the relative stiffness of the joint or intrinsic resistance of soft tissue may play a role in the development of HO.

Other etiologic possibilities include ischemia and antigen/antibody and hormonal disorders.[34] Additional information gained about the etiology of HO will assist in prevention and management in the future.

DIAGNOSTIC AIDS

The onset of HO usually occurs within the first few months following a burn injury. However, the recognition of ossification can be as late as several years.[22] The first clinical symptom is pain followed by a rapid loss of ROM in a joint. Redness and swelling typically associated with HO may not be recognized as easily due to the overlying or surrounding burned tissue.

Radiologic evidence of calcification frequently is not present in the early phase of development, but is present usually within a few weeks after the patient begins ex-

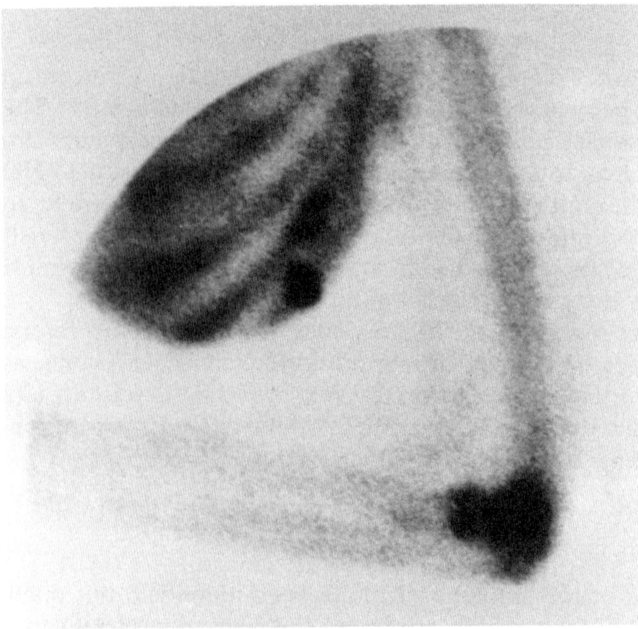

FIGURE 20–9. Bone scan of the left upper extremity. Patient had circumferential full-thickness arm burns with complete loss of elbow motion. Increased uptake at the elbow suggests the presence of heterotopic ossification.

periencing symptoms.[25] HO first appears on radiograph as an amorphous cloudy mass in close proximity to a joint. This calcification may shrink and be absorbed or ossify and be viewed as mature bone on radiograph.[31]

Radionuclear imaging (bone scan) detects the onset of HO as much as 3 weeks before clinical radiographic evidence is present, thereby aiding in a prompt diagnosis[35] (Fig. 20–9). However, while bone scans are sensitive, they are not specific.[27] Vanlaken and associates[27] demonstrated that many joints with a positive scan did not develop HO. They suggested that bone scans might be used better to identify joints at risk.

Laboratory tests are of little value for diagnosis. Serum calcium and phosphorus levels usually are normal.[25] Serum alkaline phosphatase levels, which are greatly elevated with HO in spinal cord and head injury patients, are elevated infrequently in burn patients.[22]

THERAPEUTIC MANAGEMENT

The management of HO is frustrating for the physical and occupational therapist. As joint ROM decreases, the tendency for the therapist is to become more aggressive in passive exercises and in splinting. However, this tendency should be avoided. Serial splinting or casting is ineffective. A ROM gain in one direction results in a loss of ROM in the opposite direction. Splinting first in flexion and then in extension also has been ineffective.[22] The efficacy of ultrasound and continuous passive motion (CPM) devices in the treatment of HO is not well documented.

Crawford and associates[34] demonstrated that patients with HO who were treated with active-assisted exercises and with passive exercises developed joint ankylosis requiring surgical excision.[34] Patients who performed active exercise within the pain-free range demonstrated spontaneous resolution of their HO. These findings suggest that patient participation and cooperation is necessary to maximize recovery. Patients should be encouraged to perform active exercise of the affected joint within a pain-free range. Unconscious patients or patients otherwise unable to participate in their rehabilitation program should be treated with very gentle passive range of motion (PROM).[27] PROM should never be performed beyond resistance of any kind. Care should be taken to minimize joint trauma in the agitated and uncooperative patient. VanLaeken and colleagues[27] suggested sedating patients to prevent them from fighting against restraints and procedures.

Low-dose radiation has been advocated to prevent the recurrence of ossification in surgical patients by inhibiting mesenchymal cells from turning into osteoblasts.[28,36] However, the effect of radiation on existing HO, or in preventing HO in the burn patient, is not well documented.

PHARMACOLOGIC MANAGEMENT

The use of etidronate disodium diphosphate (EDP) in the treatment of HO in burn injury has been suggested, because this usage has been effective in spinal cord injury, closed head injury, and total hip arthroplasty.[37-39] EDP inhibits the growth of hydroxyapatite crystals in vitro, and may lessen the incidence of HO in vivo.[40] The severity of calcification in the latter case depends upon when the drug is administered. Orzel and Rudd[40] concluded that medication was most effective when administered before soft tissue calcification was observed radiographically.

SURGICAL MANAGEMENT

Many patients respond positively to the conservative treatment of active exercise advocated for HO. This approach is beneficial especially for children, who reportedly have a high incidence of spontaneous resolution.[22] In other patients, the condition progresses with deleterious effects. Loss of functional joint ROM and joint ankylosis may occur. Entrapment of the ulnar nerve is common when HO affects the elbow.

Surgical excision of ectopic bone should be performed when a significant limitation in ROM or nerve entrapment is present. However, the optimal time for surgical excision is controversial. Excision usually should be delayed to minimize the chance of recurrence.[41] Surgery should be postponed until all wounds are healed, skin grafts are mature, the patient is free of infection, and a bone scan of the affected joint is negative (usually 1 to 1.5 years after detection).[42] However, Peters[43] reported on a patient who underwent excision of HO in both elbows with "strongly positive bone scans" and maintained full ROM postoperatively.[43]

When nerve entrapment occurs, early surgical excision of HO is necessary to prevent progressive neurologic loss, despite the risk of recurrent bone formation.[18] In the elbow joint, a posterior longitudinal incision is used. The ulnar nerve is carefully freed, transposed anteriorly, and buried into adjacent soft tissue to prevent recurrent entrapment.

Postoperative treatment includes immobilization of the joint for 2 to 7 days to allow the incision to heal.[31,41] Immobilization in the position opposite of the original deformity is preferred. Following healing of the incision, active exercise in a pain-free range is advocated.[41]

Complications Involving Bone

In addition to heterotopic bone formation, a number of other musculoskeletal complications can occur, either as direct or indirect sequelae to the burn injury itself.

EXPOSED BONE

A burn of bone tissue is possible in severe thermal injuries. In some cases necrosis of the periosteum and cortex has been found,[21] especially in superficially located bone such as the skull, tibia, and olecranon process. In electrical injuries, the extreme temperatures resulting from current may cause necrosis of the periosteum and matrix. Treatment of burned bone is determined by the area involved and the extent of bony and soft tissue damage. In some cases, management may include amputation. Exposed bone optimally is closed by a variety of flaps[44] (Fig. 20–10). If flap coverage is not possible, dead bone sequesters and may become infected. If this event occurs, the sequestrum is removed and the wound is allowed to close by contraction. In larger wounds, the cortex of the bone is removed or holes are drilled into the remaining bone to stimulate growth of granulation tissue, thus facilitating closure of the wound with a skin graft.[44]

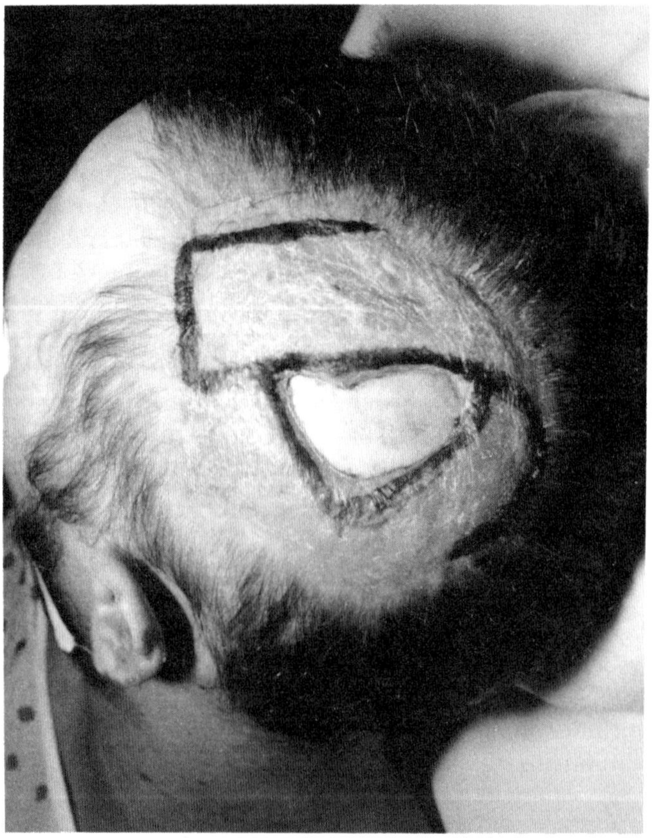

FIGURE 20–10. Exposed skull ready for closure with a local rotation flap.

FRACTURES

Fractures present a very serious problem when they accompany a burn injury. Concurrent burn injury and fractures are commonly a result of motor vehicle accidents and of electrical injuries due to a fall or tetanic muscle contracture.

A careful initial evaluation must be performed by the therapist because fractures often are difficult to identify in an anesthetic and edematous limb.[45] The simultaneous management of fractures and burn wounds is difficult and appropriate treatment of both injuries is vital. The task is complicated further when a fracture lies beneath burned tissue. Saffle and colleagues,[45] in deciding on the best fracture management plan, considered the following factors: (1) necessity for reduction and immobilization of the fracture, (2) access to the burn wound for hydrotherapy and dressings, (3) need for excision and grafting of associated burn wounds, and (4) ability to institute aggressive physical therapy as soon as possible.

The advantages and disadvantages of the treatment options also must be considered. While a cast or brace may adequately immobilize a fracture under normal circumstances, these devices make wound care, skin grafting, and therapy very difficult when they are placed over the burn wound. Skeletal traction increases access to extremity burns but decreases access to back wounds and limits the patient's overall mobility. The placement of external fixators permits wound access and patient mobility but may interfere with movement of joints adjacent to the fracture. Internal fixation interferes minimally with wound care and a patient's mobility status; however, careful attention must be given both to timing of the operation and to the appropriateness of surgical intervention to prevent infectious complications.[45]

OSTEOPOROSIS

Osteoporosis is the most common change in bone observed in a burn patient and may be present in up to 36 percent of severely burned patients. This complication is indistinguishable on radiograph from other types of disuse poroses.[26] In a burn patient, porosis may be due to prolonged immobility, hyperemia, infection, malnutrition, or adrenocortical hyperactivity.[44] Osteoporosis has been found mainly in areas underlying a burn; however, if proximal areas of the body are burned, distal sites may be involved as well.[44] Pathologic fractures due to progressive bone atrophy have been reported.[31] Early mobilization of a patient with frequent weight-bearing activities has been advocated to prevent demineralization.[21]

BONE SPURS

New bone formation at amputation sites is another skeletal complication (Fig. 20-11). Spurs protruding from the distal surface of a bone can cause residual limb pain, ulcerations, and significant problems with prosthetic fitting.[46] New bone formation typically is found in amputated areas where the bones have been transected, but seldom seen in cases of disarticulation or in amputations involving small bones of the hands and feet.[46] With flame burns, spurs are seen more commonly in children and adolescents and their presence is explained as normal bony growth secondary to maturation. In electrical burns, bone spurs can be found in both children and adults, but the exact etiology of the spurs is unknown.

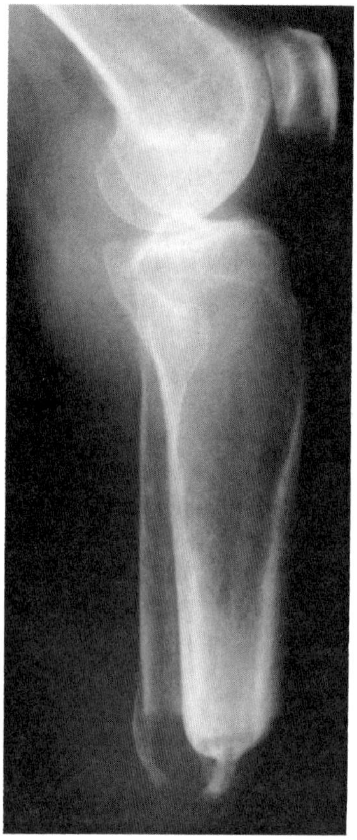

FIGURE 20–11. Bone spurs at the distal end of the tibia and fibula.

CALCINOSIS CUTIS

Several cases of abnormal calcification distant from a bone also have been documented.[42] Appearing on radiograph as masses of calcification in the skin, this condition typically is detected 30 years after a burn injury and is found exclusively in areas of neglected burn scar. The initial presentation may be as bone fragments protruding through a scar or as an ulcer or sinus tract within a scar.

BONE GROWTH RETARDATION

The epiphyseal plate is responsible for most of the longitudinal growth of bone. If damage occurs to the epiphyseal cartilage, growth can be arrested in the young or adolescent patient. If only part of the cartilage is damaged, the undamaged portion will continue to grow and an angulation deformity may result.[23]

Rigid pressure devices, when used on the head and neck, can disturb bone growth in children. The mandible particularly is susceptible to deformation by such devices and forces to the skull should be closely monitored (Fig. 20–12). Regular follow-up with an orthodontist, during and after pressure garment wear, is recommended to prevent serious dental complications.[47]

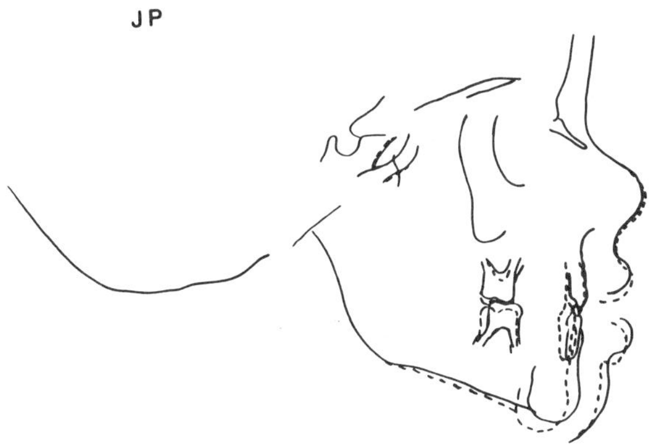

FIGURE 20–12. Superimposition of two cephalograms taken of a 9-year-old girl with full-thickness burns to her entire face. Patient wore a hard-plastic face mask during the day and an elastic face mask at night for a total of one year. The solid line represents the initial cephalogram taken after grafting and the broken line represents a tracing of the cephalogram taken six months later. Note the backward and downward rotation of the mandible.

Complications Involving Joints

Problems involving joints are found in deep burn injuries. Early treatment should be limited to splinting to protect the joint from further insult (Fig. 20–13). Definitive management of the wound is determined by the extent of tissue destruction. Flap closure of the wound, arthrodesis of the joint, and even amputation of the extremity may be necessary.

SEPTIC ARTHRITIS

Septic arthritis is a rapidly progressing infection of a joint that can result in severe destruction. This complication may occur in an unburned joint as a result of uncontrolled bacteremia associated with cases of systemic infection.[48,49] Septic arthritis also may occur in a burned or exposed joint as open wounds contain bacteria, and bacteria carry the risk of infection. The onset of septic arthritis is insidious. The usual

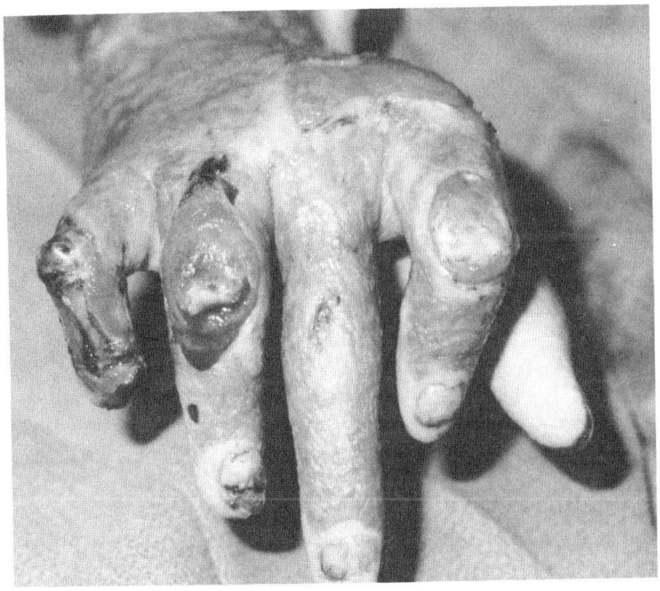

FIGURE 20–13. Open PIP joints are preventable through the use of protective splinting.

symptoms of fever; chills; and a painful, hot, swollen joint may be masked in the burn patient.[48] Attention to this complication must be immediate because articular cartilage has a poor blood supply and a limited resistance to the infectious process. Treatment includes the administration of appropriate systemic antibiotics, an arthrotomy with extensive cleansing of the joint, and closure of the wound over irrigation and suction drains.[50] If the involved joint lies beneath a burn wound, closure of the wound may present a significant problem. The joint should be splinted in an antideformity position for protection. Once a positive response to treatment has been attained, gentle passive movement, followed by active movement of the involved joint is advocated to prevent intra-articular adhesions.[50] Prognosis for this burn complication depends upon the amount of destruction of articular cartilage and surrounding bone. Joint dislocation, degenerative joint disease, and even joint ankylosis can occur.

CAPSULAR TIGHTNESS

Traumatic injuries can cause damage to isolated parts of a joint capsule followed by specific areas of capsular tightening and adherence to adjacent tissues during the healing process.[51] More often, a therapist is faced with cases in which the entire joint capsule is tight as evidenced by a capsular pattern of restriction during PROM of a joint. Conditions that can cause a capsular pattern of restriction include joint effusion, in which the joint capsule is distended by excessive intra-articular synovial fluid, and relative capsular fibrosis as seen in cases of prolonged immobilization.[51] Management of capsular conditions varies according to the cause of the restriction. In cases of capsular tightness due to joint effusion, stretching the capsule to restore movement is contraindicated and efforts should be aimed at diminishing the acute inflammatory process. When capsular tightness is caused by capsular fibrosis, movement can be restored through the use of specific joint mobilization techniques in combination with ultrasound.[51]

DISLOCATIONS

Dislocation of a joint due to a burn injury is rare. When dislocations do occur, they are usually the result of trauma (caused by a tetanic muscle contraction), a change in articular surfaces (as seen in septic arthritis), capsular injury (boutonnière deformity), faulty positioning, or scar contracture. Management of traumatic and positional dislocations includes relocation of the joint and prevention of recurring deformity with appropriate splinting or pinning.[29] Management of dislocations due to a change in articular surfaces frequently is unsatisfactory and may require reconstructive procedures.[48] Efforts should be aimed at splinting the joint in an antideformity position.

Complications Involving Tendons

EXPOSED TENDONS

Burns involving tendons may not be apparent due to overlying necrotic tissue. If tendon involvement is suspected, all attempts should be made to prevent desiccation of the tendon through the use of appropriate wound coverings and to prevent tendon rupture by following specific ROM and splinting protocols (Fig. 20–14).

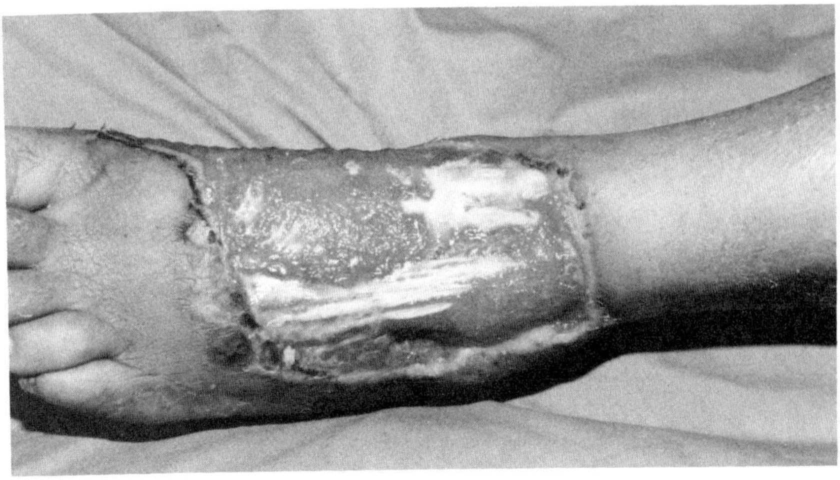

FIGURE 20–14. Exposed extensor tendons of left-dorsal foot which were kept viable through the vigilant use of wet dressings. The wound was closed eventually with a free flap.

Therapy protocols are tailored to the specifics of the tendon involved and to the amount of tissue damage present. For example, exposed but viable extensor tendons of the proximal interphalangeal joints in the hand are treated with isolated joint motion (no combined joint flexion), and the fingers are splinted in finger extension at all times except during exercise. For an exposed but viable patellar tendon, motion is limited to gentle knee ROM, the knee is splinted in extension except during exercise, and the patient is allowed to ambulate with full weight bearing with the knee splinted in extension. For an exposed but viable Achilles tendon, motion is limited to gentle ankle ROM, the ankle is splinted in a neutral position at night, and the patient is allowed to ambulate with full weight bearing with precautions not to perform vigorous lower extremity activities involving the ankles, such as running and jumping.

TENDONITIS

The presence of tendonitis should be assessed during the therapist's evaluation of joint pain. Increased stress to tendons can occur due to the burn injury itself and during management of the burn injury. Tendonitis can be found in children and adults and the supraspinatus tendon is a frequent location.[51] Typical management includes: 1) ultrasound to the area to decrease inflammation; 2) transverse friction massage to the site of the lesion to keep the scar mobile; 3) strict avoidance of activities that cause pain; and 4) progressive restrengthening of involved muscles to restore normal joint mechanics.[51] Open wounds or new skin grafts over the site of the lesion may delay the initiation of friction massage.

Structural Deformities Subsequent to Scarring and Scar Management

Hypertrophic scarring is discussed in Chapter 14. However, the potential structural deformities that can be created by scarring and by the management of scarring should be emphasized.

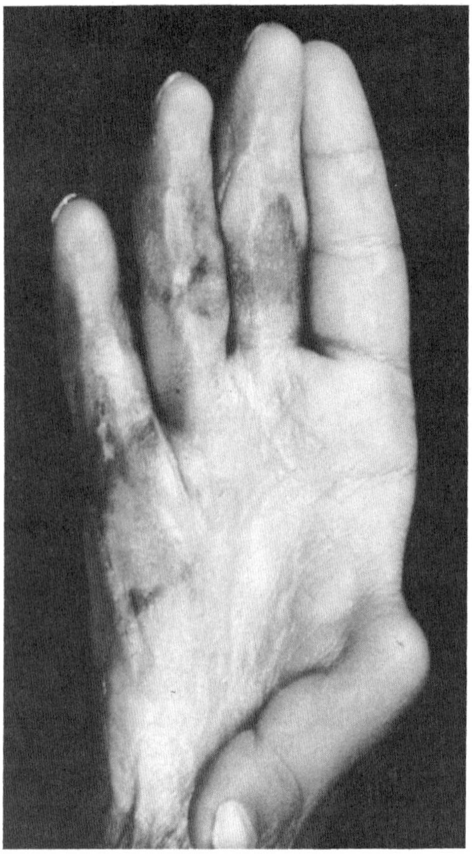

FIGURE 20–15. Severe dislocation of the thumb caused by scar contracture.

Joint subluxation and dislocation in young children can be caused by the powerful contractile forces of hypertrophic scarring (Fig. 20–15). The small joints of the hands and feet are affected most frequently; however, cases of hip joint involvement also have been documented.[31] Scoliosis, with the concavity on the side of scar contracture, may occur in children with asymmetrical trunk burns and in children with leg length discrepancies created by hip and knee flexion contractures.[21] Thoracic kyphosis can occur in patients with anterior neck and trunk burns. This problem is intensified when a patient also has anterior shoulder burns that tend to contract causing scapular protraction.[21]

Management of these deformities includes elongating the tight structures on the concave side of the curve; symmetrical stretching exercises to elongate the trunk, strengthening of musculature on the convex side of the curve, symmetrical strengthening of trunk musculature necessary for posture control, and posture training.[52] Early recognition, combined with aggressive positioning, ROM, and splinting will aid the burn therapist to prevent or minimize these potential deformities.

Splints and positioning devices often are used for extended periods of time to prevent deformities. Frequent exercise with these devices removed is necessary to maintain full joint motion. Tight pressure garments often are perceived as restrictive, limiting the patient's ROM. Although wearing these garments during exercise sessions does not create an overall difference in ROM achieved, some patients may be more compliant with exercise when allowed to do so with their garments removed.[53]

CASE STUDY

HISTORY

MJ was a 10-year-old boy who was burned in a house fire and sustained a smoke inhalation injury and a 55 percent total body surface area burn. The patient became extremely edematous and lost pulses in his hands and feet. Escharotomies were performed on all four extremities. The patient received standard wound care and was treated twice daily by a physical and occupational therapist for active and gentle passive exercise for his face, neck, and extremities during the first week.

The patient was taken to the operating room for excision and autografting of both arms during the second week. His elbows were immobilized in extension with anterior splints for 5 days after surgery to prevent disruption of his grafts.

Over the course of the third to fifth weeks, the patient developed a serious fungal infection. He became septic and the skin grafts on his arms sloughed. The patient became very confused and agitated and frequently required the use of soft arm restraints. He physically resisted most medical care procedures including gentle passive range-of-motion exercises performed by the therapists. His elbows remained splinted in extension except during exercise sessions and dressing changes. Aggressive antibiotic and surgical interventions were used that eventually controlled the infection.

The patient's arms were autografted once again during the sixth week. His elbow splints were discontinued on the fifth postoperative day following successful skin graft adherence. At this time, the patient was alert enough to participate in his exercise program. He was able to demonstrate 0° to 135° elbow motion and complete forearm supination and pronation bilaterally.

During the eighth week of hospitalization, the patient began to complain of elbow pain during end-range flexion and extension. Radiographs taken of the elbows were negative.

By the tenth week, the patient became very reluctant to move his elbows due to pain. Active range of motion had decreased to 0° to 70° of flexion and neutral supination bilaterally. Repeat radiographs of the elbows revealed small calcium deposits posteriorly. Calcification increased significantly during the next 2 weeks with a further concomitant loss of elbow range of motion.

PROBLEM LIST

Progressive loss of motion in elbows and forearms
Heterotopic calcification of bilateral elbows
Elbow pain with motion

GOALS

Minimal elbow pain
Increase elbow and forearm active range of motion to within normal limits

INTERVENTIONS

Surgical excision of heterotopic ossification
Postoperative use of elbow continuous passive motion device with range of motion adjusted to patient comfort
Pain-free active range of motion
Gross and fine motor activities within available range of motion
Functional equipment adaptations (e.g., long handle utensils) to promote active use of elbows and forearms

RATIONALE

With a suspected, or surgically corrected, condition of heterotopic ossification, only active range-of-motion exercise and interventions in a pain-free range of joint motion is indicated.

SUMMARY

This chapter provides a comprehensive review of neuromuscular and musculoskeletal complications that can follow burn injuries. The reader is provided with a brief review of neuroscience and of electrophysiologic testing to better understand neurologic complications. Neuropathies from burn injury, burn management, burn complications, and concurrent disease processes are described in detail.

Heterotopic ossification is defined and its incidence in burn injuries is presented. Popular theories about the etiology of HO are included. Key clinical symptoms and radiologic findings are presented as diagnostic aids. Various therapeutic, pharmacologic, and surgical management strategies are reviewed.

Complications involving bone, joints, and tendons are discussed. Guidelines for the management of exposed bone, fractures, osteoporosis, bone spurs, calcinosis cutis, septic arthritis, capsular tightness, dislocations, exposed tendons, and tendonitis are outlined. Prevention strategies for structural deformities that occur subsequent to scarring and scar management also are included.

REFERENCES

1. Henderson, B, Koepke, GH, and Feller, I: Peripheral polyneuropathy among patients with burns. Arch Phys Med Rehabil 52:149–151, 1971.
2. Helm, PA: Neuromuscular considerations. In Fisher, SV and Helm, PA (eds): Comprehensive Rehabilitation of Burns. Williams & Wilkins, Baltimore, 1984, pp 235–241.
3. Adams, RD and Victor, MD: Principles of Neurology. McGraw-Hill, New York, 1989, pp 1009–1077.
4. Goodgold, J and Eberstein, A: Electrodiagnosis of Neuromuscular Diseases. Williams & Wilkins, Baltimore, 1978, p 8.
5. Oh, S: Clinical Electromyography Nerve Conduction Studies. University Park Press, Baltimore, 1984, pp 481–498.
6. Johnson, E: Practical Electromyography. Williams & Wilkins, Baltimore, 1980, pp 155–205.
7. Salisbury, R and Dingeldein, P: Peripheral nerve complications following burn injury. Clin Orthopaed Rel Res 163:92–97, 1982.
8. Helm, PA, Johnson, ER, and Carlton, AM: Peripheral neurological problems in acute burn patients. Burns Therm Inj 3:122–125, 1977.

9. Esses, SI and Peters, WJ: Electrical burns: Pathophysiology and complications. Can J Surg 24:11-14, 1981.
10. Silversides, J: The neurological sequelae of electrical injury. Canad Med Assoc J 91:195-204, 1964.
11. Rosenberg, DB: Neurologic sequelae of minor burns. Arch Phys Med Rehabil 70:914-915, 1989.
12. Prasad, KN: Human Radiation Biology. Harper & Row, New York, 1974, p 264.
13. Hoppenfield, S: Physical Examination of the Spine and Extremities. Appleton-Century-Crofts, New York, 1976, pp 119, 125.
14. Hollinshead, WH: Functional Anatomy of the Limbs and Back. WB Saunders, Philadelphia, 1969, pp 139, 327.
15. Jackson, L and Keats, AS: Mechanism of brachial plexus palsy following anesthesia. Anesthesiology 26:190-194, 1965.
16. Johnson, EW, Braddom, R, and Watson, R: Electromyographic abnormalities after intramuscular injection. Arch Phys Med Rehabil 52:250-252, 1971.
17. Siegel, JH: Trauma: Emergency Surgery and Critical Care. Churchill Livingstone, New York, 1987, pp 1108-1109.
18. Vorenkamp, SE and Nelson, TL: Ulnar nerve entrapment due to heterotopic bone formation after a severe burn. J Hand Surg 12A:378-380, 1987.
19. Robins, S and Cotran, R: Pathologic Basis of Disease. WB Saunders, Philadelphia, 1979.
20. Anastakis, DJ, Peters, WJ, and Lee, KC: Severe peripheral burn polyneuropathy: A case report. Burns Therm Inj 13:232-235, 1987.
21. Varghese, GV: Musculoskeletal considerations. In Fisher, SV and Helm, PA (eds): Comprehensive Rehab of Burns. Williams & Wilkins, Baltimore, 1984, pp 242-248.
22. Hoffer, MM, Brody, G, and Ferlic, F: Excision of heterotopic ossification about elbows in patients with thermal injury. J Trauma 18:667-670, 1978.
23. Jackson, DM: Destructive burns. Some orthopaedic complications. Burns Therm Inj 7:105-122, 1980.
24. Kolar, J and Vrabec, R: Periarticular soft tissue changes as a late consequence of burns. J Bone Joint Surg 41A:103-111, 1959.
25. Munster, AM, et al: Heterotopic ossification following burns: A prospective study. J Trauma 12:1071-1074, 1972.
26. Schiele, HP, Hubbard, RB, and Bruck, HM: Radiographic changes in burns of the upper extremity. Radiology 104:13-17, 1972.
27. VanLaeken, N, et al: Heterotopic bone formation in the patient with burn injuries. A retrospective assessment of contributing factors and methods of investigation. J Burn Care Rehabil 10:331-335, 1989.
28. Rubin, MM and Cozzi, GM: Heterotopic ossification of the temporomandibular joint in a burn patient. J Oral Maxillofac Surg 44:897-899, 1986.
29. Jay, MS, et al: Bone and joint changes following burn injury. Clin Pediatr 20:734-736, 1981.
30. November-Duskansky, A, et al: Caliuretic response to protein loading in burn patients. Burns Incl Therm Inj 6:198-201, 1980.
31. Evans, EB: Orthopedic measures in the treatment of severe burns. J Bone Joint Surg 48A:643-669, 1966.
32. Izumi, L: Study of ectopic bone formation in experimental spinal cord injured rabbits. Paraplegia 21:351-363, 1983.
33. Michelson, JE, Granroth, G, and Andersson, LC: Myositis ossificans following forcible manipulation of the leg. J Bone Joint Surg 62A:811-815, 1980.
34. Crawford, CM, et al: Heterotopic ossification: Are range of motion exercises contraindicated? J Burn Care Rehabil 7:323-325, 1986.
35. Tepperman, PS, et al: Heterotopic ossification in burns. J Burn Care Rehabil 5:283-287, 1984.
36. Ayers, DC, Evarts, CM, and Parkinson, JR: The prevention of heterotopic ossification in high-risk patients by low-dose radiation therapy after total hip arthroplasty. J Bone Joint Surg 68A:1423-1430, 1986.
37. Stover, SL, Hahn, HR, and Miller, JM: Disodium etidronate in the prevention of heterotopic ossification following spinal cord injury. Paraplegia 14:146-158, 1976.
38. Spielman, G, Gennarelli, TA, and Rogers, CR: Disodium etidronate: Its role in preventing heterotopic ossification in severe head injury. Arch Phys Med Rehabil 64:539-542, 1983.
39. Finerman, GA, and Stover, SL: Heterotopic ossification following hip replacement or spinal cord injury. Metab Bone Dis Rel Res 4:337-342, 1981.
40. Orzel, JA and Rudd, TG: Heterotopic bone formation: Clinical, laboratory and imaging correlation. J Nucl Med 26:125-132, 1985.
41. Peterson, SL, et al: Postburn heterotopic ossification: Insights for management decision making. J Trauma 29:365-369, 1989.
42. Edlich, RF, et al: Heterotopic calcification and ossification in the burn patient. J Burn Care Rehabil 6:363-368, 1985.
43. Peters, WJ: Heterotopic ossification: Can early surgery be performed, with a positive bone scan? J Burn Care Rehabil 11:318-321, 1990.
44. Trapnell, DH and Jackson, D: Bone and joint changes following burns. Clin Radiol 16:180-186, 1965.

45. Saffle, JR, et al: The management of fractures in thermally injured patients. J Trauma 23:902–910, 1983.
46. Helm, PA and Walker, SC: New bone formation at amputation sites in electrically burn-injured patients (abstr). Arch Phys Med Rehabil 68:284–285, 1987.
47. Fricke, NB, et al: Effects of pressure garment wear on facial and dental development. Proc American Burn Association 24:15, 1992.
48. Evans, EB, Larson, DL, and Yates, S: Preservation and restoration of joint function in patients with severe burns. JAMA 204:91–96, 1968.
49. Miller, SF, Finley, RK, and Alkire, SA: Intervertebral disc space infection: A late sequelae of burn wound sepsis. Bull Clin Rev Burn Inj 1:41, 1984.
50. Salter, RB: Textbook of Disorders and Injuries of the Musculoskeletal System. Williams & Wilkins, Baltimore, 1983, p 178.
51. Hertling, D and Kessler, RM: Management of Common Musculoskeletal Disorders. JB Lippincott, Philadelphia, 1990, pp 36, 68, 195.
52. Kisner, C and Colby, LA: Therapeutic Exercise: Foundations and Techniques. FA Davis, Philadelphia, 1990, pp 535–542.
53. Ward, RS, et al: Influence of pressure support on joint range of motion. Proc American Burn Association 23:182, 1991.

CHAPTER 21

Electrical and Chemical Burns

Margaret I. Wittman, PT

ELECTRICAL BURNS

Electrical burns can be devastating injuries and account for 6 percent of burn unit admissions in the United States with approximately 760 deaths per year.[1,2] Unlike thermal burns, electrical burns involve a relatively small amount of body surface area. The sites where the electric current enters and exits the body are usually the only surface areas of tissue involved, except when sparks cause clothing to ignite. In fact, the damage done by electricity often is described using the iceberg metaphor. In comparison to a scald or flame burn, the cutaneous damage associated with an electrical burn injury may be deceptively benign, while the damage below the skin surface may be catastrophic, often leading to limb loss. Also, survivors may be faced with any number of additional complications, including cataracts and neurologic deficits. Despite a plethora of research, the effects of electricity on the human body are still not fully understood. Some of the current yet divergent theories will be discussed here but it is beyond the scope of this chapter to determine the validity of conflicting data. The purpose of this section is to provide the therapist with an overview of the pathophysiology of electrical burns, how specific systems in the body are affected, and issues to address in the rehabilitation of these patients.

Electrical energy occurs in different forms: lightning, low voltage (under 1000 volts), high voltage, and alternating or direct current. Most low-voltage accidents occur in the home, while high-voltage accidents usually occur in the workplace around high-tension wires. Alternating current is the electrical form used in homes and industry in the United States; direct current is found primarily in connection with battery power. Typically, individuals injured by electricity are male, in their mid-30s, and injured on the job. The total body surface area burned averages 12 percent, and the mean length of hospitalization is 32 days.[3]

In addition to the high-voltage electrical injury with one entrance and one exit wound, there are other varieties of injury. Electricity, for example, may arc from an electrical source to a person and/or between two adjacent body parts (such as the arm and forearm). When lightning that is the culprit in an electrical accident it will be in one of four forms: direct strike, flash discharge, ground current, or shock wave.[4] The energy of a single lightning bolt ranges from 10,000 and 20,000 amperes and contains anywhere between 1 to 20 million volts. The overall survival rate for these injuries is estimated at 70 percent.[4] A burn also may result from an electrical flash. This type of injury occurs most often when a person works on an electrical fuse box or panel with metal tools. The correct combination of elements results in a sudden flash that may cause thermal cutaneous burns to the face, hands, and upper body but does not cause internal damage.

Pathophysiology

To begin to understand electrical injuries, one should have a knowledge of Ohm's and Joule's laws. Ohm's law illustrates the relationship of voltage, resistance and current.

$$I = \frac{E}{R}$$

where E = voltage
I = current in amperes
R = resistance in ohms

Voltage is an electric potential, resistance is the opposition offered by an object to the passage of a steady flow of electricity, and current is the flow of the electric charge. Ohm's law states that electric current is directly proportional to voltage and inversely proportional to resistance. If a high voltage meets with a high resistance, the current will be small, but if the voltage is high and meets little resistance, the resulting current also will be high. It is commonly believed that high voltage is exclusively responsible for the extent of injury in an electrical burn. Often survivors proudly boast about the amount of voltage involved in their accident. However, voltage is only one part of the formula.

As previously stated, the most commonly accepted theory of tissue damage in electrical injuries deals with thermal or heat energy. Joule's law depicts the relationship between heat production, current, and resistance.

$$J = I^2RT$$

where J = heat in joules
I = current in amperes
R = resistance in ohms
T = time in seconds

From Joule's law it can be seen that heat is produced when an electric current meets resistance over time. Note that the amount of heat produced is directly related to current, resistance, and time; if any of these increase, the amount of heat produced also will increase. Each type of body tissue offers its own resistance to current flow. Table 21–1 lists the body tissues in order from greatest to least resistance and there-

TABLE 21–1. Tissue Resistance to Electricity, Greatest to Least

Bone
Fat
Tendon
Skin
Muscle
Blood vessels
Nerve

fore it may be presumed that bone generates more heat than other tissues. Figure 21-1 illustrates a common result of electrical injury, thermal damage near and around the long bones. The most common explanation for this has been that the heat generated in the bone is responsible for causing the thermal damage to the surrounding tissues.

Rarely is thermal damage found near the ribs and pelvis. A review of the literature indicated that these areas were subject to thermal damage only when they were the actual entrance or exit sites.[5] What accounts for these areas being spared? In actuality, the body acts as a volume conductor and individual differences in tissue resistance may be insignificant. The crucial factor instead is the cross-sectional area of the body part. As the cross-sectional area decreases, current density increases.[6–8]

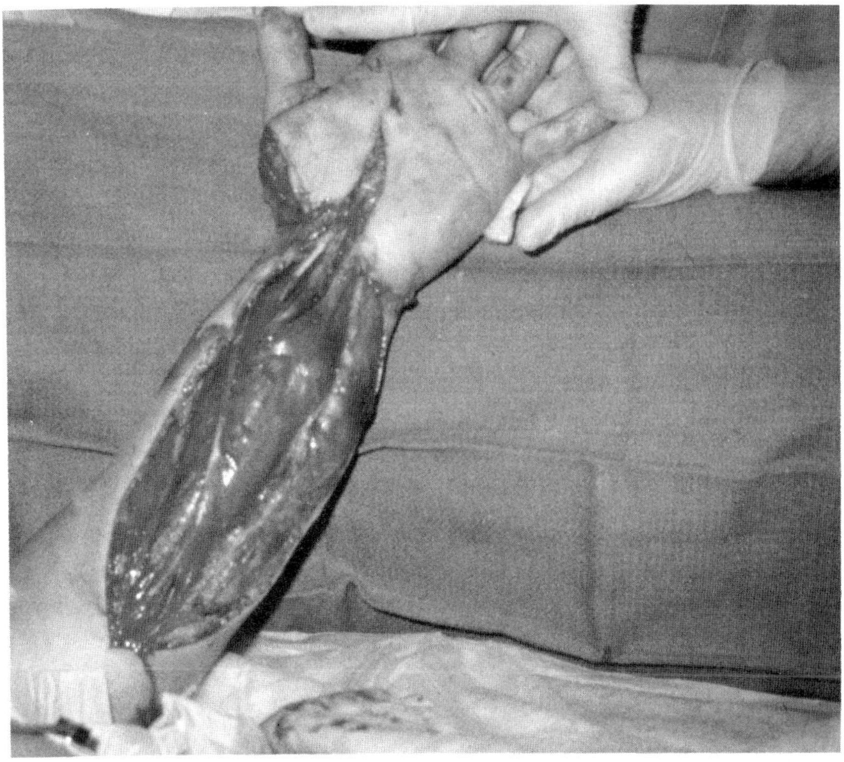

FIGURE 21–1. A fasciotomy allows the expansion of severely injured deep tissues.

Joule's law states that as the current increases, so does the amount of heat produced; therefore, the smaller the cross-sectional area, the greater the amount of thermal damage.

Electrical Pathway

Electric current entering the body meets an initial resistance at the surface of the skin. Moist skin offers less resistance than dry, calloused skin. The difference may be as much as 999,000 ohms/cm^2.[9] The significance of this difference, in relationship to Joule's law, is that more cutaneous damage may occur where the skin is dry and tough. As electricity meets the skin's resistance, the heat produced creates an *entrance site* wound. Clinicians often find this point to be relatively small, round, and charred. The point where the electricity leaves the body to find its ground is also a point of resistance which is called the *exit site.* This site may have a more explosive appearance than the entrance site but also may cover only a small area.

Areas of Injury

NERVOUS SYSTEM

Of all the areas involved in an electrical injury, the nervous system is most often the site of major complication.[10] Permanent neurologic damage due to electrical injury is well documented,[8,11-16] but there is an ongoing controversy as to the pathophysiology of damage.

Neurologic involvement can be categorized by either the time of onset, immediate or delayed; or by the anatomic site, peripheral or central. Nerve tissue offers the least resistance of all body tissues and is considered the most conductive tissue as well. In addition, some investigators contend that nerve tissue is the most susceptible to thermal injury.[17]

Immediate Neurologic Complications

The incidence of immediate neurologic findings from high-voltage injuries ranges from 29 to 67 percent.[10,14,18,19] The most frequently described immediate neurologic symptom resulting from an electric current is a depressed level of consciousness. This condition usually resolves in a matter of hours or days.[20] Peripheral and spinal cord symptoms also may be apparent immediately following injury.[20] Patients may experience paraplegia, quadriplegia, or focal paralysis, but they usually recover in a matter of days.[21]

Most clinicians agree that immediate neurologic syndromes have the best prognosis for recovery. The exception is when peripheral nerves are injured at an entrance or exit site. Peripheral nerves can necrose as a result of thermal damage or from pressure of the swelling tissues. Early surgical decompression may improve a patient's functional outcome.[22,23]

Delayed Neurologic Complications

The most serious neurologic sequelae have a delayed onset, as they are particularly devastating and usually are permanent.[8,11-16,20] Delayed neurologic symptoms may appear in the first days after injury or may take as long as 3 years to evolve.[8,21,24]

TABLE 21–2. Delayed Neurologic Symptoms Following an Electrical Burn Injury

Ascending Paralysis
Amyotrophic Lateral Sclerosis
Transverse Myelitis[15,21]
General Balance Deficits
Difficulty with Ambulation[19]
Seizures
Agitation
Confusion
Amnesia
Learning Impairment
Headaches[10]
Post-Traumatic Depression[14,46]
Paraplegia
Quadriplegia[12,15,21]
Hemiplegia
Aphasia
Striatal Symptoms[21]

The various symptoms are listed in Table 21–2. Nontraumatic spinal cord involvement occurs in 2 to 27 percent of electrical injuries, with the average being 6 percent.[8] Spinal cord injury is the most common permanent sequela and occurs regardless of the current pathway, whether from arm to arm or arm to leg.[12]

Obviously, delayed neurologic complications can have serious implications for patients with electrical injuries. Therefore, therapists should be aware that a patient who is initially symptom-free may develop serious complications and these manifestations may be permanent.

Pathophysiology of Delayed Neurologic Complications. Until recently, damage from electricity was thought to be solely from the conversion of electrical energy into heat energy. The area of delayed neurologic manifestations challenges this theory most. Delayed neurologic damage may be caused by direct thermal damage to nerves[21,24,25] resulting in demyelinization and neural death[21]; vascular compromise of nutrient blood vessels supplying the brain and spinal cord[8,13,15,21,24–26]; or accumulation of electrostatic force in ungrounded persons leading to tissue disruption.[24,25]

Lesions associated with delayed onset may develop in any number of areas, including the extrapyramidal tract–cerebral cortex (areas controlling voluntary movements), anterior horn cells in the spinal cord (similar to progressive muscle atrophies), or the brain's association areas.[21] Animal models showed spinal cord damage occurring mostly in the white matter of the posterior columns.[13] If there is complete necrosis of the spinal cord, the lesion is comparable to a transverse lesion.[24] Postmortem evaluation of criminals who were put to death by electrocution revealed damage in the brain's gray matter.[12] There is not a definitive location of injury that causes neurologic deficits, and there is usually no sensory deficit nor involvement of bowel and bladder function associated with electrical injuries.[8,21]

Peripheral Neurologic Complications

Permanent damage to peripheral nerves due to direct destruction by contact with electric current occurs in approximately 22 to 34 percent of electrically injured pa-

TABLE 21–3. Peripheral Symptoms Associated with an Electrical Burn Injury

Sensorimotor Loss
Paresthesia
Paralysis
Paresis
Dysesthesia
Causalgia
Reflex Sympathetic Dystrophy[10]

tients.[10,14] Peripheral symptoms are listed in Table 21–3. In addition, there is evidence that electricity may initiate a demyelinating process in peripheral nerves.[16] The most frequently injured peripheral nerve is the median, followed by the ulnar, radial, and peroneal nerves.[10] This sequence is not surprising, since 88 percent of entrance sites are in the upper extremity.[18] Grube[10] found that 64 percent of patients with peripheral nerve damage improved, while 36 percent of neuropathies persisted or worsened. DiVincenti[14] supports the hypothesis that peripheral nerves that are not directly damaged by the injury usually recover, however, he noted that 22 percent of patients had permanent damage to peripheral nerves due to direct destruction.

Local nerve damage is assumed to be related to both the heat generated and the immediate or delayed thrombosis of local vessels.[20] Critchley[27] found fragmentation and twisting of axons, breakdown of Schwann cell sheaths, fusion of cell nuclei, and fibrous tissue infiltration of the epineuron of peripheral nerves injured by electric current. Ugland[28] suggested that peripheral nerve injury depends upon the current pathway. If the pathway is along the nerve's longitudinal axis, there is damage to axons and myelin sheaths for almost the entire length of the nerve. If, on the other hand, the pathway is transverse, there is only localized damage.[28] Ugland further suggested that the patient be tested every 3 months to isolate the lesion. If localized, repair involves nerve grafting or neurolysis.[28] There is one reported case study utilizing a nerve grafting technique,[29] and no reported repair for longitudinal damage.

BONE

An occasional by-product of electrical injury is long bone fracture. Many injuries occur above ground level (on utility poles and roofs) and are associated with falls, and thus fractures. But bony damage can occur in the absence of a fall. Fractures have been reported at bilateral femoral necks,[30] (Figs. 21–2 and 21–3), bilateral humeral heads,[31] and in the spine at cervical and thoracic levels.[32] All of these fractures resulted from severe tetanic muscle contraction that occurred at the time of electric contact. When there is an electric injury in the absence of a fall or other trauma, a possible fracture is easily overlooked. As therapists mobilize patients, sources of unusual pain must be evaluated and fractures ruled out.

Many electrical injuries result in amputations. In addition, Helm and Walker[33] reported that 82 percent of patients with electrical injuries who required long bone amputations developed new bone formation (i.e., spurs). The average time to diagnosis was 38 weeks following injury. This bone formation can be painful and interfere with prosthetic wear and normal activity. Surgical excision may be necessary, and for

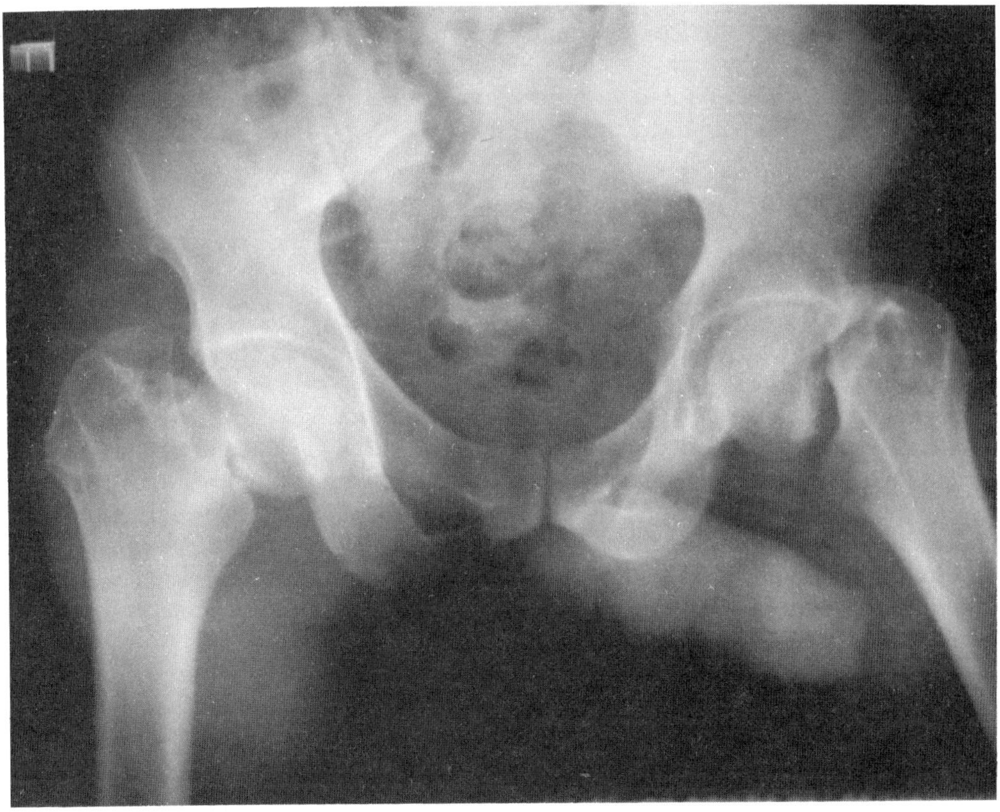

FIGURE 21–2. Radiograph showing bilateral femoral neck fractures.

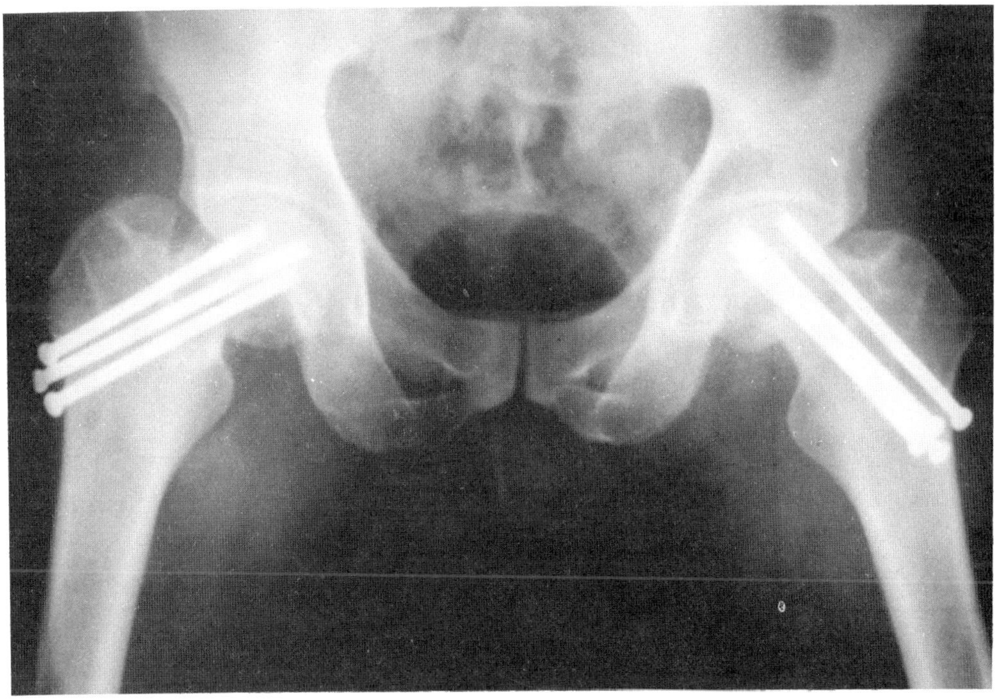

FIGURE 21–3. Radiograph showing reduced and fixated femoral neck fractures.

this reason the long bone length should be maximized at the time of initial amputation.[33] No new bone growth was reported after surgical revision. Therapists should be aware of the pain associated with new bone formation and request a radiographic evaluation prior to prosthetic fitting.

MUSCLES AND BLOOD VESSELS

The most graphic illustration of electricity's power of destruction is found in the muscles, especially the muscles of the extremities. The vast majority of entrance and exit sites are in the upper and lower extremities.[34] Because these areas have relatively small cross-sectional diameters and a large bone to tissue ratio, they are quite susceptible to thermal injury (Fig. 21–4). Possibly, the conversion of electrical energy to thermal energy can render entire muscle groups nonviable.

In response to the initial trauma, capillary permeability increases and involved areas swell. Increased compartment pressure causes damage to otherwise viable tissue, so fasciotomies are performed routinely to help preserve tissue in the extremity. Unfortunately, early fasciotomies may not prevent ensuing muscle necrosis,[18] and multiple debridement sessions frequently are needed to remove all nonviable tissue. The extent of muscle damage is a significant difference between electrical and thermal burns.

Debridement procedures usually are done in series. Initially discerning which muscles are viable and which ones are not is difficult.[18,35] Some diagnostic tests, including frozen section biopsies, xenon scans, and technetium-99 pyrophosphate scans may help make this determination.[35,36] However, there is no substitute for mul-

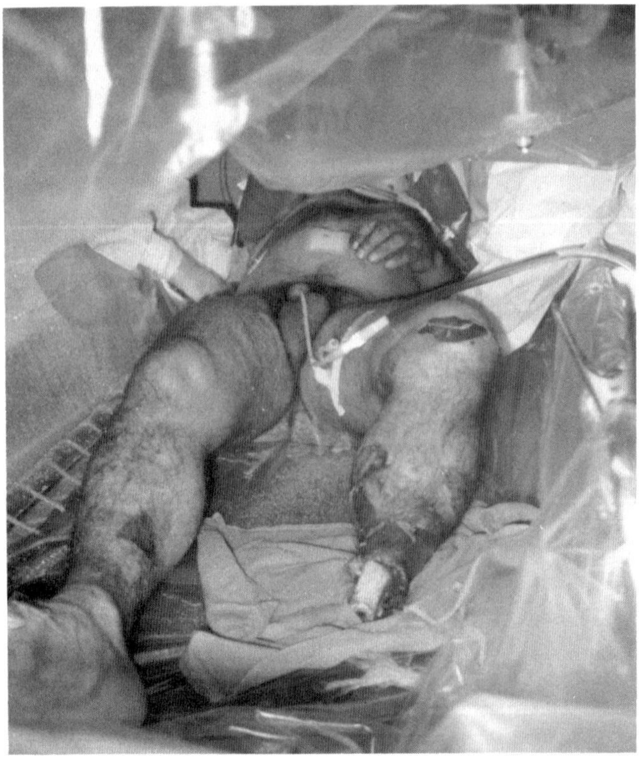

FIGURE 21–4. Traumatic amputation of the left ankle and foot which occurred at the time of injury due to the small cross-sectional area.

tiple debridements.[18] Electric stimulation to muscles during operative debridement can be utilized. A muscle with no response to stimulation is nonviable and requires debridement.

Massive muscle damage generally leads to amputation. The number of electrically injured patients who undergo at least one amputation ranges from 24[3] to 71 percent.[34] The most common site of amputation is the upper extremity.[3,17]

Muscles that are not obviously damaged at the time of injury still may be susceptible to necrosis because of vascular damage in the form of thrombosis. Such damage may begin to manifest itself as early as 15 minutes after injury or up to 10 days later.[6,8] Larger vessels tend to escape damage, as greater blood flow helps dissipate heat. Smaller nutrient vessels have a lesser blood flow, they coagulate and thrombose more readily, and therefore the muscles they supply necrose.[8,11]

In some cases muscles become damaged at sites distant from the current pathway. In these situations the mechanism of tissue injury is in question. There is a recent postulation that nonthermal electrical forces frequently contribute to rhabdomyolysis.[37] Rhabdomyolysis, which is the disintegration or dissolution of muscle, may occur from either heating or electroporation.[37] Electroporation drives otherwise homeostatic water molecules into small defects in a cell membrane, causing it to enlarge and rupture. Researchers theorize that if an electric contact is brief, nonthermal mechanisms of cell damage are more destructive.[37]

CARDIOPULMONARY SYSTEM

When a person dies immediately after electric contact, the cardiopulmonary system is involved. The most commonly accepted theory is that immediate mortality results from respiratory arrest.[13,18,38,39] Data in the literature support suggestions that current strength may determine the extent of injury within the cardiopulmonary system.[40,41] Tetanic spasm of the respiratory muscles occurs at 30 mA. At a total current of 60 mA the current density in the heart is high enough to cause fibrillation or asystole.[40,41] As the voltage exceeds 7200 V, respiratory arrest occurs from severe muscle contraction, but cardiac fibrillation does not occur.[40] Therefore, cardiopulmonary resuscitation (CPR) may be more successful for victims of higher-voltage injuries than lower-voltage injuries.[40]

Clinicians unfamiliar with electrical injuries often concern themselves with monitoring the acute cardiac status of patients surviving these injuries. Some clinicians postulate that alternating current can affect the normal conduction of electrical impulses through the myocardium.[39] Housinger and colleagues[42] found that there is indeed a low incidence of myocardial damage associated with electrical injuries. Usually there are no electrocardiogram (ECG) changes in these patients,[42,43] however, MB is not an abbreviation simply a term. Elevated MB creatine kinase (CK) isoenzyme fractions, consistent with myocardial damage, can be the result of significant skeletal muscle damage.[42]

EYE

The pathophysiology of cataract formation after electrical injury is unknown. The reported incidence in electrically burned patients is approximately 6 percent.[44] Cataracts may appear as early as 2 to 6 months following injury, or be delayed for as long as 11 years.[44] Some researchers have suggested that the incidence of cataracts is greater if there was electric contact at the head or neck.[6,45] Patients usually respond well to surgery.[44]

RENAL SYSTEM

Massive muscle damage from an electrical injury results in a significant release of myoglobin. The assault of myoglobin on the kidneys can lead to tubular necrosis and renal failure if patients are not properly resuscitated. Aggressive fluid resuscitation can avert renal failure[18,39] (see Chapter 6).

Psychologic Concerns

Posttraumatic stress disorder has been reported to occur more often in electrically burned patients than in patients with nonelectric burns[46] (see Chapter 17). Symptoms may include insomnia, headaches, difficulty in concentrating, nightmares, and anxiety.[3] Hooshmand and associates[38] studied neurologic and psychologic patterns in a group of patients for 5 years and found that generalized cerebral dysfunction led to depression, divorce, and unemployment. He also reported a high incidence of atypical seizures that were not detected on electroencephalogram (EEG) or computerized tomography (CT) studies. Evoked potentials revealed disturbances in the upper cervical spine and lower brainstem so the lesions may have been too deep for recording by EEG.[38]

The therapist is responsible for noting and reporting psychiatric or psychologic changes. Anxiety, depression, and a decrease in a patient's pain threshold are common reactions to burn trauma.[46] Patients often will need help discovering appropriate coping mechanisms. Psychiatrists and psychologists can be a vital part of the burn care team in these instances. They can offer help to a patient and provide other team members with ideas for providing support. All caregivers should be sensitive to a patient's needs and offer encouragement while directing the patient forward to an optimal recovery.

Rehabilitation

Survivors of electrical burns may face multiple complications and must confront unique rehabilitation challenges. As with all burn injuries, rehabilitation should begin early in the acute stage. Early intervention allows a therapist to evaluate immediate versus delayed neurologic symptoms and helps to decrease the patient's time in a sick role. The patient should be involved in his or her own program planning and goal setting. This involvement helps ensure a patient-specific program and creates an atmosphere in which the patient plays an active role in his or her own success. The challenging aspect of helping to rehabilitate a patient with an electrical injury comes when there is more than one system involved.

A patient whose injury has resulted in an upper extremity amputation as well as paraplegia may need a prosthesis adapted with a terminal device suitable for use during transfers, and a wheelchair with a manual drive on the unaffected side. Because the patient will rely on the upper extremities for more weight bearing than normal, skin integrity of the residual limb will have to be monitored very closely.

Strength in the residual limb, unaffected limb, and all other innervated muscle groups must be substantial enough for the new requirements of transfers and mobility. Additional areas that affect rehabilitation are soft tissue deficits and amputations.

SOFT TISSUE

When there has been muscle loss, residual muscle groups must be strengthened to compensate for the loss if possible (Fig. 21–5). Sometimes, the amount of muscle tissue lost to necrosis and debridement is so great that the normal function and rhythm of a joint may be impaired. The therapist must be aware of the extent of muscle damage when teaching early mobility because some movements may be awkward and stressful to the joint. A patient should be educated in long-term joint preservation techniques. For example, the patient should avoid prolonged or repetitive weight bearing through the joint, especially when in an extreme end range of motion. A patient who has lost wrist flexors and/or extensors and has had a traumatic below-knee amputation may require the use of a platform crutch because weight bearing through the unstable wrist would be harmful. Sometimes, the loss of muscle and subcutaneous tissue poses a long-term safety issue as seen in Figure 21–6. Helmets, like the one pictured in Figure 21–7, can be fabricated out of a heavyweight splinting material and easily concealed under a baseball cap.

Early range of motion of involved areas is advocated. Richard and colleagues[47] described aggressive range of motion to herniated quadriceps muscles and recovered full active motion in an average of 27.4 days. The use of continuous passive motion machines has proven effective in certain thermally burned patients, as well as with electrically burned patients.[48]

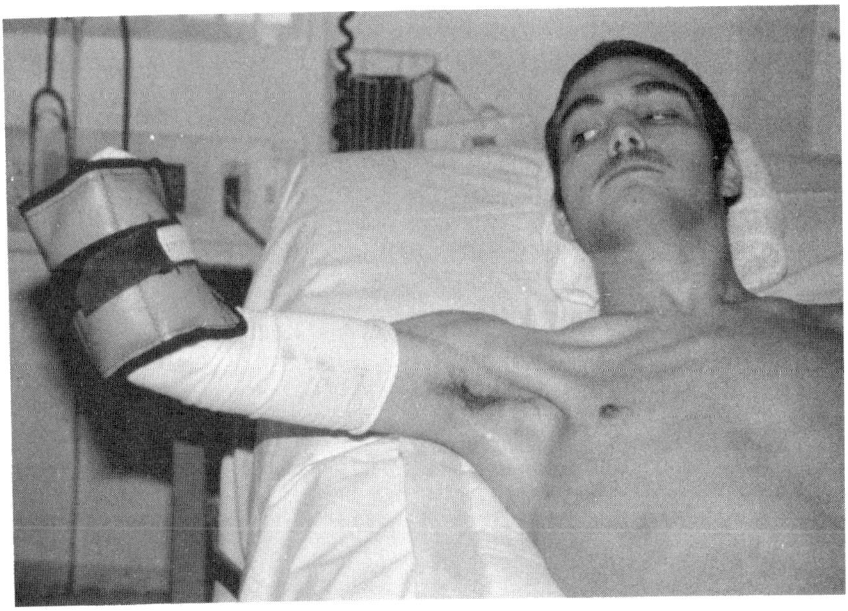

FIGURE 21–5. Strengthening the residual limb while on bed rest.

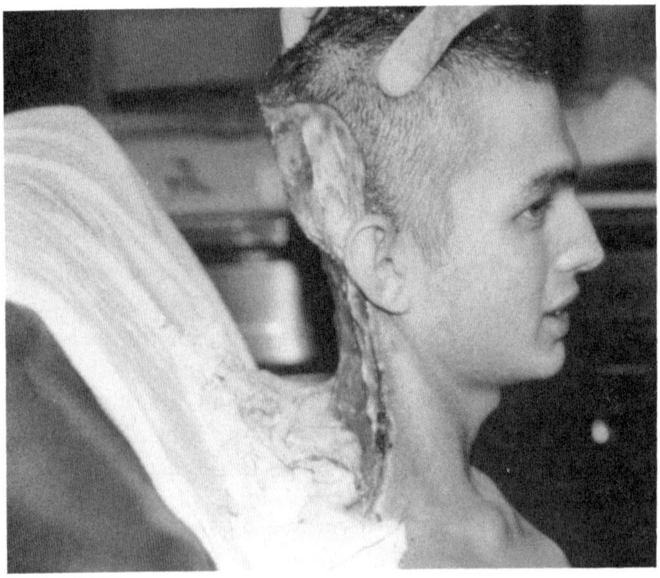

FIGURE 21–6. Extensive soft tissue and bony loss without major loss of local function.

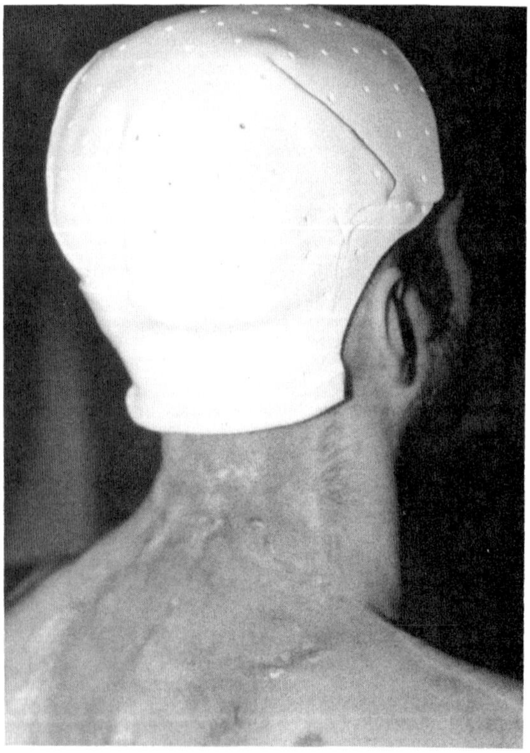

FIGURE 21–7. Orthoplast helmet can be secured with velcro and worn to protect structures which have lost their bony cover.

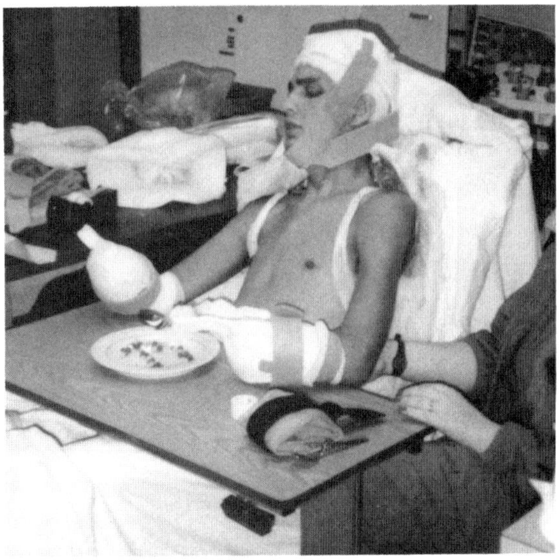

FIGURE 21–8. Patient using orthoplast prostheses for early self-feeding skills.

AMPUTATIONS

Treatment programs for patients with amputations should include traditional residual limb and preprosthetic exercises. Range of motion of the residual joints must be maximized, surrounding muscle groups must be strengthened, and the residual limb should be shaped and desensitized. There may be complications with the residual limb and adjacent joints because skin integrity may be impaired due to cutaneous burns. Range of motion can be accomplished with the same methods and modalities discussed elsewhere in this text. However, caution must be used because compromised skin covering the residual limb may break down easily.

Prosthetic training may begin early, even before a residual limb has been well shaped. For the upper extremity, temporary Orthoplast prostheses can be fabricated to initiate gross motor training (Fig. 21–8). Johansen and associates[45] discussed special rehabilitation techniques for a patient with bilateral short above-elbow amputations. These methods included balance training and using the lower extremities for some activities of daily living. Patients with lower extremity amputations should begin ambulation before there is closure of the residual limb. If possible, an appliance that offers the patient a weight-bearing platform is ideal. A pneumatic sleeve and pylon system works well when there is drainage from suture sites (Figs. 21–9 and 21–10). Rigid pylons with temporary plaster or orthoplast sockets also can be constructed.

CHEMICAL BURNS

Although chemical burns comprise a small proportion of all burn injuries,[49-52] they can be more damaging than thermal burns. This section will briefly review the incidence, action, and management of chemical burns.

Chemical burns are caused by contact with any substance that causes a chemical reaction with the cutaneous and subcutaneous tissues. Agents continue to destroy

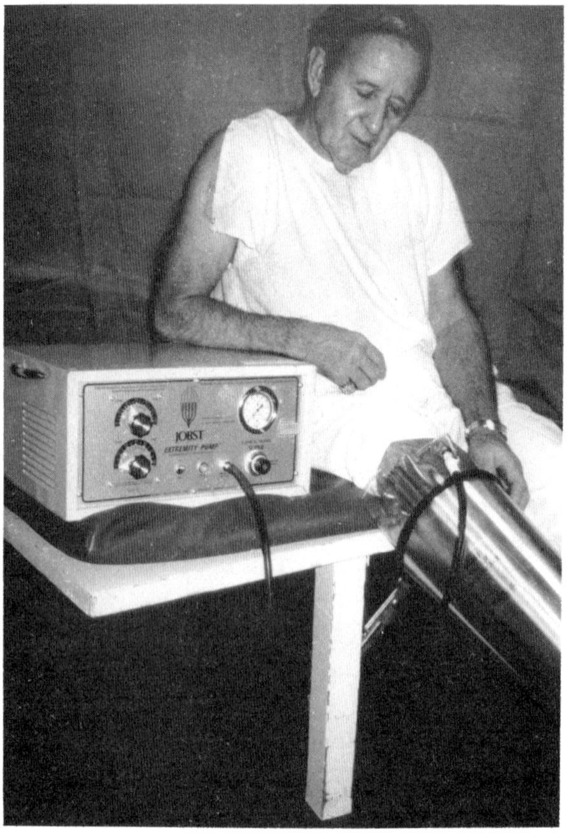

FIGURE 21–9. Donning a pneumatic sleeve and pylon.

tissue until the noxious substance depletes its capacity to damage the cellular protoplasm or until the chemical is removed from the skin.[53]

Approximately 79 percent of people injured with chemicals are between the ages of 21 and 50.[54] Sixty-nine percent of all males injured by chemicals are hurt in work-related accidents.[54] Mortality of patients with chemical burns is roughly 13 percent compared to 15 percent for all burn center admissions.[54] Approximately 95 percent of all chemical injuries involve the head, upper trunk, and shoulders.[50] Eighty-five percent of the cases involve the forearms and hands, and only 15 percent of all reported injuries have involvement below the waist. Serious ocular damage is an unfortunate and common occurrence in chemical injuries.[49,50]

There are over 25,000 different products that can cause chemical damage.[49,53] These products can be divided into two major groups: alkalis and acids. Although acid burns may cause a more severe injury, alkali chemicals are the more destructive. Acids are water-soluble and penetrate easily into subcutaneous tissue. Acids cause a coagulation necrosis with precipitation of proteins.[49] The leathery eschar that forms may actually help to limit the spread of the chemical agent.[53] Some acids, such as sulfuric acid, cause damage by desiccating the cells. Alkalis, such as lye, cause a liquefication necrosis and loosening of the tissue that may allow the agent to penetrate deeper.[49] Upon contact with subcutaneous fat, a saponification reaction occurs; in other words, soap is formed.[53] The result resembles a soapy coagulum and no leathery eschar is formed.

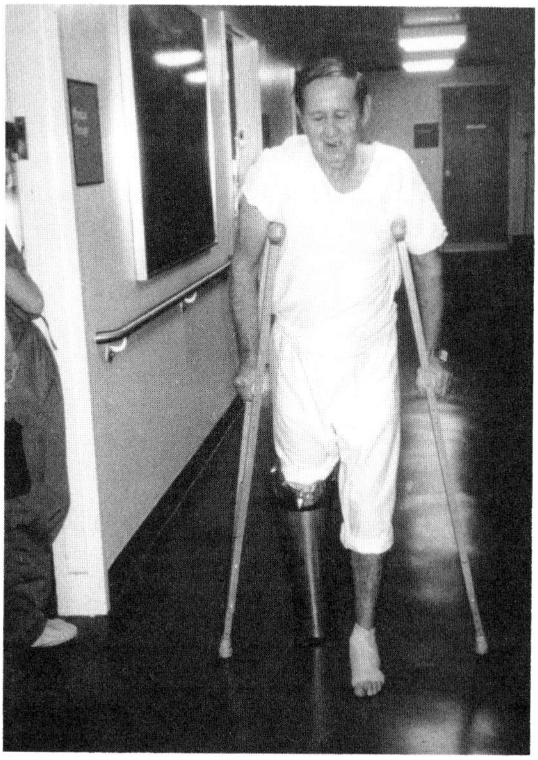

FIGURE 21–10. Partial weight bearing with a pneumatic sleeve and rigid pylon allows early ambulation before complete wound closure.

All chemical agents will continue to destroy tissue until they have been diluted, neutralized, or have finished destroying available tissue.[49,53] Some chemical injuries may appear benign at admission but necrosis may continue for 24 to 72 hours.[49,53] Although chemists teach that bases are neutralized with acids and vice versa, this treatment is not chosen for the vast majority of chemical burns. Trying to find a neutralizing agent wastes valuable time. Immediate irrigation with copious amounts of water is the recommended initial treatment.[49,53,54] Sykes and colleagues[54] found that in a group of patients who initially received adequate irrigation with water, 19 percent required skin grafting and there was a 9.5 percent mortality rate. In a group treated with delayed or inadequate irrigation, 36 percent required skin grafting and 21 percent of the patients died.

Usually, chemical burns can be treated like thermal burns after emergency care has been performed. Some chemicals, however, have a systemic impact as well. Hydrofluoric acid can cause hypocalcemia.[49] Exposure to phosphorus, tannic, chromic, or formic acids may lead to hepatic necrosis.[49] Immersion in gasoline may result in multisystem injuries because of the absorption of the aromatic hydrocarbon components.[50] Despite these sequelae, the wounds themselves are treated as they would be for thermal wounds. This treatment includes the use of baths or showers, topical agents, and excision and skin grafting.

The rehabilitation needs of the chemically burned patient are similar to the thermally burned patient; however, the extent of cutaneous damage may be greater. Because of the depth of injury, excision to fascia can result in poor tendon glide, binding of the skin to fascia, and marked cosmetic changes. Healing scar will have a propensity toward contractures and perhaps hypertrophic scarring. Aggressive range of motion and strengthening programs are vital to a patient's long-term function. Multiple grafting procedures may result in periods of bed rest and immobility, the effects of which must be reversed through steady, rigorous exercise. If an accident occurred in the workplace, the patient may be fearful of returning to his or her former job and may blame his or her boss or co-workers for the accident. Psychologic and/or psychiatric support could prove to be an important part of the successful rehabilitation of these patients.

CASE STUDY

HISTORY

SJ was a previously healthy 19-year-old male who was helping to move a house. He was standing on the roof when the transport truck drove under some low electrical wires carrying 7600 V of electricity which contacted the back of the patient's head. Thus, SJ's head became the entrance site for the electricity, which exited both of his hands.

Prior to the therapist's initial evaluation, bilateral fasciotomies of the volar forearm and hand intrinsic muscles and carpal tunnel releases had been performed. The patient was intubated and unable to follow commands but was responsive to pain and demonstrated movement in all four extremities. His cutaneous burns only accounted for 10 percent total body surface area but were full-thickness and included both hands, left anterior thigh, and an area of his upper back. The most significant area of damage was an area of subdermal burn at the entrance site on the occiput which exposed the calvarium.

Within 48 hours, the patient began to demonstrate motor neurologic problems. By the eighth day following the accident, the patient had developed a complete transverse myelitis at the tenth thoracic level. No voluntary motor control was present below the lesion but the patient retained sensation along with bowel and bladder control. Approximately one month after the injury, the patient developed spasticity in his lower extremities and trunk.

The patient underwent five surgical debridements and skin graftings to remove necrotic tissue and cover his wounds. In the process, a significant portion of the calvarium was debrided revealing unprotected dura mater. Eventually the patient necessitated below-elbow amputations bilaterally and the need for a more extensive rehabilitation training program.

PROBLEM LIST

Cranial defect
Partial loss of upper extremities
Loss of voluntary motor control below T 10

GOALS

Prevent further damage to the patient's head
Preserve extremity range of motion
Independent mobility
Independent in functional activities

INTERVENTIONS

To protect the patient's exposed skull, a helmet was fashioned from splinting material and was worn for all out-of-bed activities. Prior to the patient's amputations, he was fitted with bilateral antideformity hand splints. He also was fitted with bilateral footdrop splints. Passive range of motion was initiated to his bilateral lower extremities. By the end of the first week post burn, the patient was transferred out of bed into a reclining wheelchair. Eventually, the increased tone in the patient's lower extremities allowed him to participate in stand-pivot transfers. An emphasis was placed on performing much of his rehabilitation in a wheelchair, which included upper extremity strengthening, neck range of motion, trunk stability exercises, and wheelchair mobility. The combination of strengthening and mobility led to the patient being able to propel a manual wheelchair 30 feet by the time he was discharged. Following amputation of the bilateral forearms, temporary sockets with prosthetic terminal devices were fabricated from splinting material for the patient's upper extremities so the patient could begin practicing hygiene and feeding skills, which the patient ultimately was able to accomplish independently with a feeding setup.

RATIONALE

A helmet was fabricated to protect the cranium from possible further damage. Range of motion and strengthening exercises were performed to preserve the integrity of the patient's residual limbs. Realizing the patient eventually would be transferred to a comprehensive rehabilitation setting, all interventions were performed to physically prepare the patient for this experience based on his needs and abilities. Transfers were practiced to decrease the patient's dependence in bed and to increase mobility. Temporary prosthetic devices were constructed to allow the patient to begin training for independence in functional activities. The use of the temporary prosthesis and beginning mobility in the wheelchair gave the patient a sense of accomplishment and provided him with some control over his care and activities.

SUMMARY

Electrical and chemical burns occur less frequently than thermal burns and often involve males who are injured on the job. Electrical burns, however, frequently result in damage to more than one body system and pose a unique challenge to patients and therapists. A patient who has an amputation coupled with poor skin integrity and loss of muscle mass because of necrosis will require more than a standard range-of-motion and strengthening program. Preprosthetic training must begin early and incorporate functional activities. Contractures at residual joints could prove disastrous to prosthetic training and a surgical release may result in a scar that interferes with wearing of a prosthesis. Meanwhile the patient and therapist need to be conscious of delayed and potentially devastating complications, such as neurologic deficits and cataracts.

Survivors of electrical and chemical injury may require expanded rehabilitation programs, but the principles that apply to patients with thermal burns also apply to these patients. The therapist must be aggressive and sympathetic, creative and practical, and the patient must play an active role in his or her own recovery.

REFERENCES

1. Hummel, RP (ed): Clinical Burn Therapy. John Wright-PSG, Littleton, Massachusetts, 1982, pp 194–214.
2. Accident Facts. National Safety Council, 1990.
3. Hammond, JS and Ward, CG: High-voltage electrical injuries: Management and outcome of 60 cases. South Med J 81:1351–1352, 1988.
4. Demling, RH and LaLonde, C: Burn Trauma. Thieme, New York, 1989, pp 221–244.
5. Branday, JM, et al: Visceral complications of electrical burn injury. A report of two cases and review of the literature. West Indian Med J 38:110–113, 1989.
6. Zelt, RG, et al: High-voltage electrical injury: Chronic wound evolution. Plast Reconstr Surg 82:1027–1039, 1988.
7. Pruitt, BA and Mason, AD: Letter to the editor. Lancet 1:371, 1979.
8. Koller, J and Orsagh, J: Delayed neurological sequelae of high-tension electrical burns. Burns Therm Inj 15:175–178, 1989.
9. Martyn, JAJ: Acute Management of the Burned Patient. WB Saunders, Philadelphia, 1990, pp 66–86.
10. Grube, BJ, et al: Neurologic consequences of electrical burns. J Trauma 30:254–258, 1990.
11. Hunt, JL, et al: The pathophysiology of acute electric injury. J Trauma 16:335–340, 1976.
12. Silversides, J: The neurological sequelae of electrical injury. Can Med Assoc J 17:195–204, 1964.
13. Petty, PG and Parkin, G: Electrical injury to the central nervous system. Neurosurgery 19:282–284, 1986.
14. Divincenti, FC, Moncrief, JA, and Pruitt, BA: Electrical injuries: A review of 65 cases. J Trauma 9:497–507, 1969.
15. Farrell, DF and Starr, A: Delayed neurological sequelae of electrical injuries. Neurology 18:601–606, 1968.
16. Rosenberg, DB: Neurologic sequelae of minor electric burns. Arch Phys Med Rehabil 70:914–915, 1989.
17. Salisbury, RE and Pruitt, BA: Burns of the upper extremity. Major Probl Clin Surg XIX:72–83, 1976.
18. Solem, L, Fisher, RP, and Strate, RG: The natural history of electrical injury. J Trauma 17:487–492, 1977.
19. Wilkinson, C and Wood, M: High voltage electric injury. Am J Surg 136:693–696, 1978.
20. White, JW, et al: Cerebellar ataxia after an electrical injury: report of a case review of the literature. J Burn Care Rehabil 4:191–193, 1983.
21. Levine, NS, Atkins, H, and McKeel, DW, Jr: Spinal cord injury following electrical accidents. J Trauma 15:459–463, 1975.
22. Holliman, CJ, Saffle, JR, and Kravitz, M: Early surgical decompression in the management of electrical injuries. Am J Surg 144:733–739, 1982.
23. Mann, H, Kozic, Z, and Boulos, M: CT of lightning injury. AJNR 4:976–977, 1983.
24. Christenson, JA: Delayed neurologic injury secondary to high voltage current, with recovery. J Trauma 29:166–168, 1980.
25. Kanitkar, S and Roberts, AHW: Paraplegia in electrical burn: A case report. Burns Therm Inj 14:49–50, 1988.
26. Langworthy, OR: Abnormalities produced in the central nervous system by electrical injuries. J Exp Med 51:943–962, 1930.
27. Critchley, M: Electrical Injuries. Trans Med Soc, London 59:19, 1936.
28. Ugland, OM: Electrical injuries to peripheral nerves in animals: A preliminary report. Acta Chir Scand 131:432–437, 1966.
29. Stevenson, JH and Zuket, RM: Considerations in nerve reconstruction in electric burn injury: Case report. J Burn Care Rehabil 4:408–410, 1983.

30. Slater, RR, Jr and Peterson, HD: Bilateral femoral neck fractures after electrical injury: A case report and literature review. J Burn Care Rehabil 11:240–243, 1990.
31. Stueland, DT, et al: Bilateral humeral fractures from electrically induced muscular spasm. J Emerg Med 7:457–459, 1989.
32. Layton, TR, et al: Multiple spine fractures from electric injury. J Burn Care Rehabil 5:373–375, 1984.
33. Helm, PA and Walker, SC: New bone formation at amputation sites in electrically burn-injured patients. Arch Phys Med Rehabil 68:284–286, 1987.
34. Haberal, M: Electrical burns: A five year experience—1985 Evans Lecture. J Trauma 26:103–109, 1986.
35. Hunt, JL: Electrical injuries. In Fisher, SV and Helm, PA (eds): Comprehensive Rehabilitation of Burns. Williams & Wilkins, Baltimore, 1984, pp 249–266.
36. Hammond, J and Ward, CG: The use of technetium-99 pyrophosphate scanning in management of high-voltage electrical injuries. Proc American Burn Association 23:60, 1991.
37. Bhatt, DL, Gaylor, DC, and Lee, RC: Rhabdomyolysis due to pulsed electric fields. Plast Reconstr Surg 86:1–11, 1990.
38. Hooshmand, H, Radfar, F, and Beckner, E: The neurophysiological aspects of electrical injuries. Clin Electroencephalogr 20:111–120, 1989.
39. Essess, SI and Peters, WJ: Electrical burns: Pathophysiology and complications. Can J Surg 24:11–14, 1981.
40. Hodgkin, BC: Some consequences of electric shock. J Maine Med Assoc 69:1–3, 1974.
41. Cooper, MA: Lightning injuries: Prognostic signs for death. Ann Emerg Med 9:134–138, 1980.
42. Housinger, TA, et al: A prospective study of myocardial damage in electrical injuries. J Trauma 25:122–124, 1985.
43. Chandra, NC, Siu, CO, and Munster, AM: Clinical predictors of myocardial damage after high voltage electrical injury. Crit Care Med 18:293–297, 1990.
44. Van-Johnson, E, Kline, LB, and Skalka, HW: Electrical cataracts: A case report and review of the literature. Ophthalmic Surg 18:283–285, 1987.
45. Johansen, PB, et al: Prosthetic rehabilitation in bilateral high above elbow amputation. Scand J Rehabil Med 19:85–87, 1987.
46. Mancusi-Ungaro, HR, et al: Posttraumatic stress disorder in electric burn patients. J Burn Care Rehabil 7:521–525, 1986.
47. Richard, RL, Miller, SF, and Finely, RK, Jr: Restoration of normal function involving herniated quadriceps muscles following electric burn. J Burn Care Rehabil 6:347–349, 1985.
48. McAllister, LP and Salazar, CA: Case report on the use of CPM on an electrical burn. J Burn Care Rehabil 9:401, 1988.
49. Luterman, A and Curreri, PW: Chemical burn injury. In Boswick, J (ed): The Art and Science of Burn Care. Aspen, Rockville, 1987, pp 241–253.
50. Sawhney, CP and Kaushish, R: Acid and alkali burns: Considerations in management. Burns 15:132–137, 1989.
51. Sinha, S, Sinha, JK, and Bhattacharya, V: Chemical burns—our experience over eleven years. Ann MBC 3:203–205, 1990.
52. Mozingo, DW, et al: Chemical burns. J Trauma 28:642–647, 1988.
53. Stewart, CE: Chemical skin burns. Am Fam Physician 31:149–157, 1985.
54. Sykes, RA, Mani, MM, and Hieber, JM: Chemical burns: Retrospective review. J Burn Care Rehabil 7:343–347, 1986.

CHAPTER 22

Additional Skin Disruptions: Stevens-Johnson Syndrome, Toxic Epidermal Necrolysis, and Frostbite

Kevin McDonald, RPT

STEVENS-JOHNSON SYNDROME (SJS) AND TOXIC EPIDERMAL NECROLYSIS (TEN)

Stevens-Johnson syndrome (SJS) and toxic epidermal necrolysis (TEN) are relatively rare dermatologic disorders that have pathophysiologic similarities to a partial-thickness thermal injury. Patients diagnosed with these conditions may require treatment in a burn center because the resources for treatment on general medical floors and other intensive care units may be inadequate. In particular, members of the general health care team may be unfamiliar with the management of extensive wounds and the consequent complications that are known to members of the burn team.[1] Care of these patients should be multidisciplinary and include rehabilitative therapy.[2-5] Although several publications advocate participation by the therapist in caring for these patients, specific therapy treatment guidelines are not identified. Therapists who are unfamiliar with the characteristics and clinical course of SJS/TEN may not be aware of the potential rehabilitative complications associated with these conditions. In some burn care facilities, therapists are routinely involved and familiar with the care of patients who have been admitted with these disorders.

The purpose of this section is to: (1) review the etiology, clinical manifestations, and medical management of SJS/TEN; (2) identify complications that affect therapy management; and (3) describe guidelines for therapy intervention for patients with SJS/TEN.

Etiology, Clinical Manifestations, and Medical Management

ETIOLOGY

Although the exact etiology of SJS/TEN is unknown, the two primary causative agents that have been identified are drugs, including antibiotics, anticonvulsives, acetominophen, and aspirin; and nonstaphylococcal infectious organisms.[1-10] Frequently, no definitive cause can be isolated or determined.

CLINICAL MANIFESTATIONS

The early signs and symptoms of SJS/TEN include upper respiratory infection, headache, malaise, fatigue, and fever.[1-10] There is no definitive predilection for males or females, and both adults and children have been affected by these conditions. Skin rash and bullae formation become evident and progress to epidermal necrolysis and sloughing, at which point the wound resembles a partial-thickness thermal injury[1,5-7] (Fig. 22–1). Although the scalp is usually spared, lesions often are present on the head, trunk, face, hands, and feet.[10] The epidermal destruction associated with SJS/TEN interferes with the intended functions of the skin. Therefore, the pathophysiologic complications observed in these patients are identical to those exhibited by patients with extensive partial-thickness burns.[5] Complications directly attributable to skin loss include:

1. *Infection:* Because the skin is the primary defense mechanism against microbial invasion into the body, disturbances in epidermal integrity associated with SJS/TEN create a port of entry for bacterial contaminants.[11] Infection from bacterial

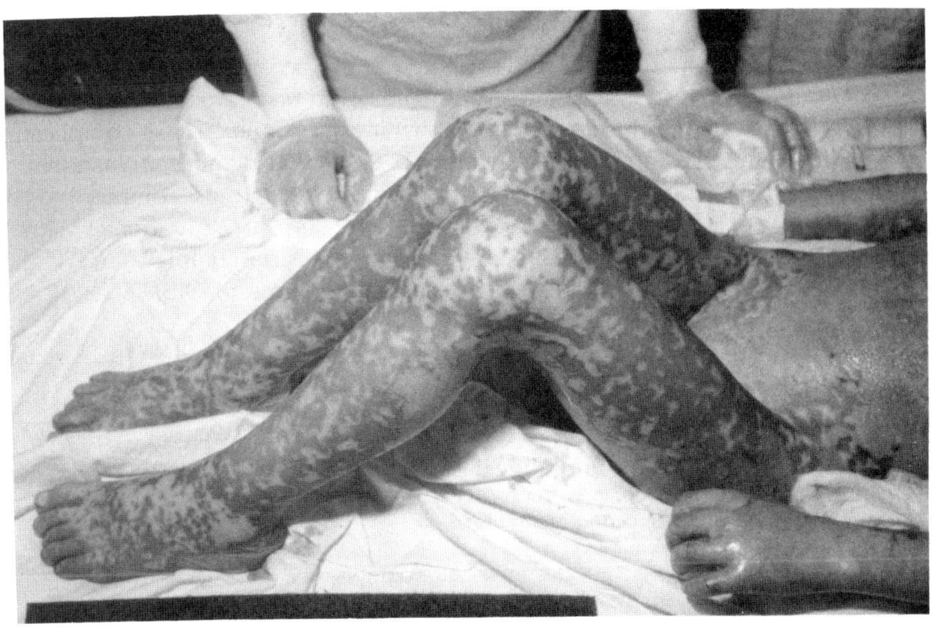

FIGURE 22–1. Skin rash and bullae formation (lower extremities) progressing to epidermal necrolysis (trunk and upper extremities) as seen in patients with SJS/TEN.

contamination accounts for 60 to 75 percent of the complications associated with SJS/TEN and is the most common cause of death in these patients.[2,3,5]

2. *Fluid, electrolyte, and metabolic derangement:* Disruption of epidermal integrity results in increased capillary permeability and a redistribution of body fluid from the intravascular to the interstitial space. Unlike the massive fluid shift observed in patients with extensive thermal injury, a small fluid shift does occur.[2,3,5] Evaporative fluid loss through the open wound surface compounds this pathologic alteration in fluid regulation and it must be monitored.[4,12]
3. *Immunologic alterations:* An unsolved, complex derangement of the immune system is associated with extensive injuries involving the skin.[13] Additional alteration and impairment in mechanisms of local and systemic immunity may expose these patients to potentially debilitating or life-threatening infectious complications.[14]
4. *Pain:* Partial-thickness wounds involving the dermal-epidermal junction result in exposure of free nerve endings. As expected, these wounds prove extremely painful when manipulated, exposed to air currents, or subjected to changes in temperature.[1]
5. *Scarring and contracture:* The incidence and severity of scarrring associated with SJS/TEN vary widely, ranging from complete absence in some reports, to presence in all but very mild cases.[2,3,7,8] Previous research on scarring in burn patients has suggested that the depth of the wound and length of time before wound closure is obtained are the most influential variables on the incidence and severity of hypertrophic scarring.[15,16] Hypertrophic scarring and contractures are most commonly associated with deep partial-thickness wounds (injuries damaging the reticular dermis) and wounds that are not healed or grafted within 21 days of injury. In SJS/TEN, these variables influence the presence and severity of hypertrophic scar formation.

Other clinical manifestations that accompany SJS/TEN, but which are not directly associated with disruption of the skin, involve the respiratory system, eyes, and oropharynx. Respiratory complications frequently accompany SJS/TEN and include pneumonitis, bronchopneumonia, bronchitis, and respiratory failure.[2-5] Intubation and ventilatory support often are necessary interventions.[5] These complications are due to the numerous causes listed in Table 22–1. Ocular manifestations identified in patients with SJS/TEN vary in severity from conjunctivitis (most common) to complete blindness.[8,12,18,19] The degree of ocular damage appears to correlate with the systemic severity of the disease. Usually visual recovery is complete and without long-term complications in patients with less severe forms of SJS/TEN.[18,19] Acute

TABLE 22–1. Causes of Respiratory Complication in Patients with SJS/TEN

1. Sloughing of the tracheobronchial mucosa
2. Secondary infection
3. Impaired mentation
4. Aspiration
5. Narcotic and anesthetic sedation
6. Immobilization
7. Shallow breathing associated with pain
8. Inability to volitionally clear secretions

inflammation or erosion of the oropharyngeal mucosal surfaces is one of the most characteristic findings in patients with SJS/TEN. Consequently, dysphagia, dehydration, and inadequate caloric intake may occur.[20] In some instances this condition progresses to involve the mucosa of the entire gastrointestinal tract. The most severe gastrointestinal complication is bleeding, and although it is rarely associated with increased mortality it may require treatment throughout and beyond hospitalization.[2,8,20]

MEDICAL MANAGEMENT

Basic management considerations for patients with SJS/TEN include the administration of intravenous fluid, antibiotics for specific infections, nutritional support, pulmonary hygiene, rigorous monitoring of opthalmalogic and gastrointestinal systems, pharmacologic and behavioral pain management, and emotional support from the burn team.[1-9]

The single most critical factor influencing the course of the SJS/TEN patient appears to be protection of the dermis from infection, dehydration, and dessication, thereby avoiding infectious complications and conversion to deep partial- or full-thickness wounds. Ideally, dermal preservation is accomplished by denuding loose skin and cleansing the wound following admission to the burn center. Immediately after wound cleansing, a biologic dressing such as amnion or homograft should be applied (Figs. 22–2 and 22–3). Recently, the effectiveness of biologic dressings in treating patients with SJS/TEN has been well documented.[1,3-7] Placing a biologic dressing over a partial-thickness wound creates a barrier to bacterial invasion and may control bacterial proliferation.[21-23] The evaporative water loss that occurs through open wounds can be reduced by 15 to 91 percent with the application of biologic dressings.[23] Biologic dressings provide pain relief by restoring a physiologic barrier over nerve endings.[21-23] The adherent properties of biologic dressings also increase the rapidity and quality of wound re-epithelialization and healing.[21-23] With uncomplicated adherence of a biologic dressing, re-epithelialization and wound healing generally occur within 7 to 14 days. If amnion is used it then can be gently peeled away (Fig. 22–4).

Following the application of a biologic dressing, a patient must be immobilized from 1 to 3 days to promote and allow its adherence. The use of air-fluidized or air-suspension beds have proven beneficial in the management of the SJS/TEN patient by reducing support pressures at select anatomic sites.[24] Thus, the mechanical disruption of freshly placed biologic dressings due to shear forces associated with patient movement can be minimized. Air-suspension or air-fluidized beds are useful in managing debilitated patients confined to bed, patients susceptible to pressure sores, and those with large and painful posterior wounds.[24]

Unfortunately, the application of biologic dressings is not always successful and their use requires meticulous daily observation and monitoring.[21-23] Typically, patients with severe forms of SJS/TEN, where the initial application of the biologic dressing fails to adhere, develop systemic sepsis and multisystemic complications. If subsequent attempts to apply biologic dressings are unsuccessful, dermal dessication to variable depths occurs. Depending on their size, these wounds may require autografting to achieve closure, preserve cosmesis, and maximize function (Fig. 22–5). Associated long-term morbidity and mortality in patients with delayed wound closure are high.[1-7] A patient's period of hospitalization is invariably prolonged greatly.

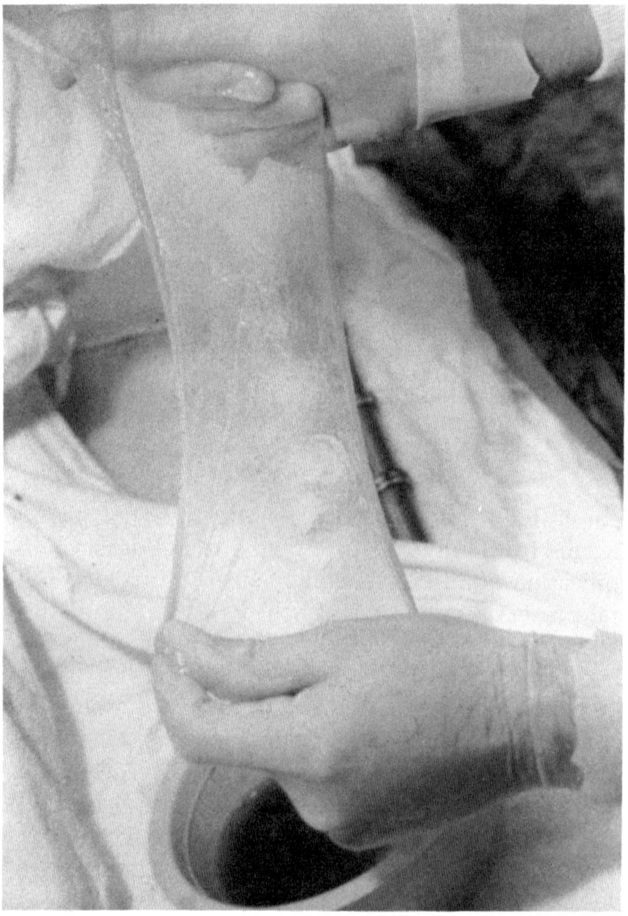

FIGURE 22–2. Amniotic membrane prior to application.

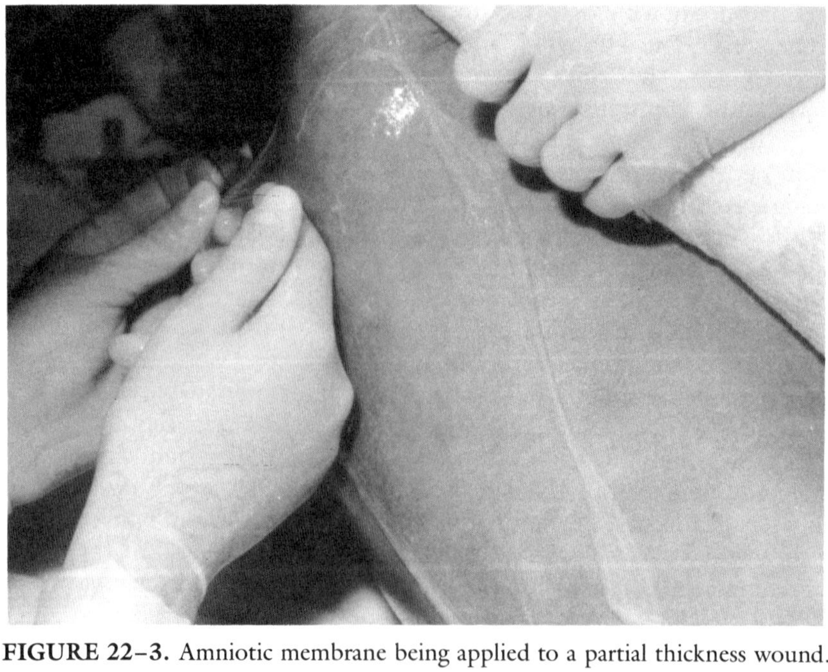

FIGURE 22–3. Amniotic membrane being applied to a partial thickness wound.

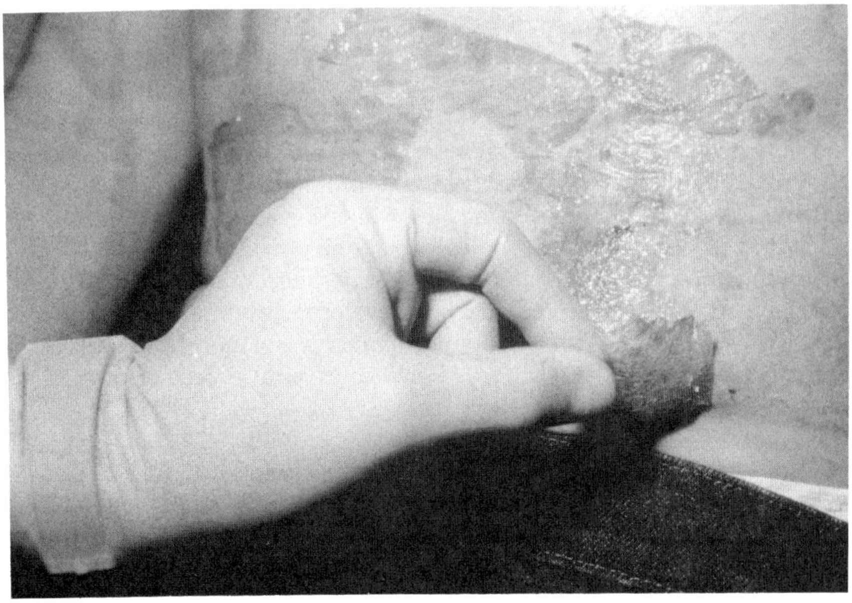

FIGURE 22–4. Removal of amniotic membrane following re-epithelialization of the underlying partial thickness wound.

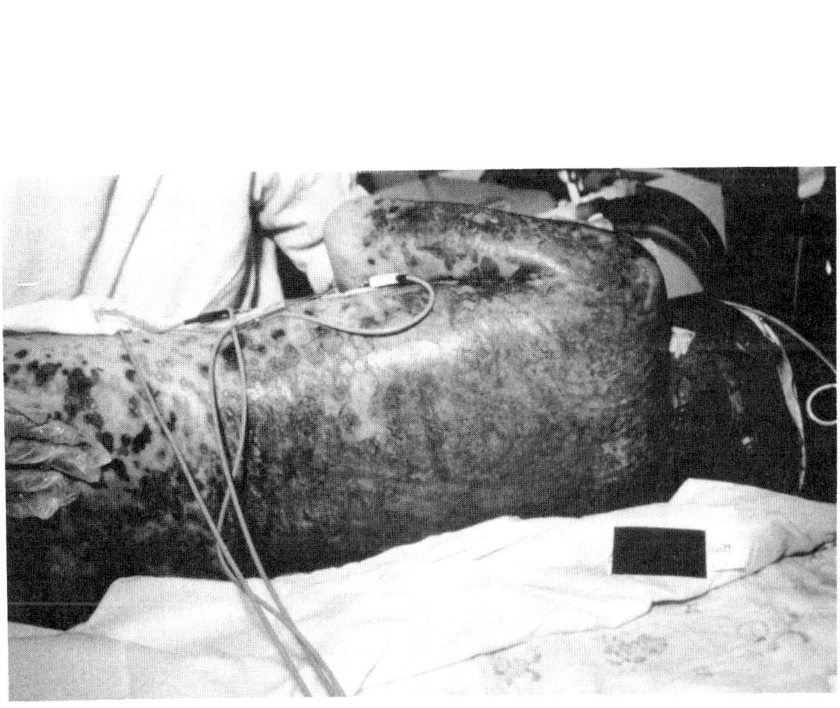

FIGURE 22–5. Dermal dessication associated with severe sepsis following an unsuccessful application of biologic dressing.

Therapy Evaluation and Treatment

EVALUATION

Upon admission, a comprehensive therapy evaluation should be completed to identify immediate and potential rehabilitative problems. A patient's baseline functional capabilities can be obtained. Daily re-evaluations should be performed. Early anticipation and recognition of musculoskeletal and functional abnormalities associated with pain, immobilization, and active tissue shortening secondary to wound healing are key components to recognize for developing and implementing a successful therapy treatment plan. With all patient treatment, isolation and sterile techniques should be used in compliance with established burn unit policies and procedures.

TREATMENT

The goals and principles of therapy management for patients with SJS/TEN essentially are identical to those established in caring for patients with burns. The necessity and intensity of therapy will vary with the severity, extent, and stage of the disease process. The rapidity and severity of the toxic onset in conjunction with the pain and emotional distress associated with SJS/TEN will determine the level of activity appropriate for the patient. Education and clear explanations to the patient regarding the type and extent of therapeutic interventions are essential. "Patients can tolerate a considerable amount of pain if they understand its cause, and the time course of recovery. Once cooperation is lost because of excessive pain and fear, recovery is greatly prolonged."[1]

The extent and intensity of therapy intervention for patients with SJS/TEN can be directly influenced and related to the success or failure of the application of a biologic dressing (Fig. 22–6). If a biologic dressing adheres, then rapid wound closure and immediate pain relief is obtained. The period of immobilization, protective posturing, and movement dysfunction is minimized, and concerns about cutaneous, soft tissue, and muscle contractures are reduced. When rapid wound closure is achieved, therapy management includes education and daily monitoring of range of motion, mobility, strength, and endurance. Clinical experience suggests that treatment, in mild cases, is confined to one or two daily visits throughout the patient's hospitalization, which typically ranges between 9 and 30 days. Outpatient therapy, other than follow-up visits to the burn clinic, usually is not indicated (Fig. 22–7).

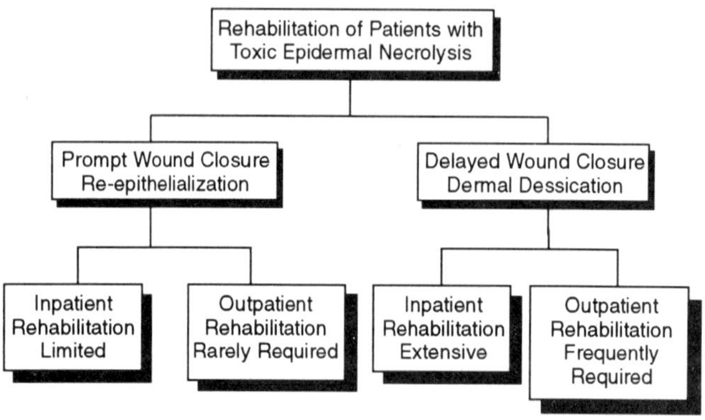

FIGURE 22–6. Flow chart differentiating effect of wound closure on rehabilitative intervention required for patients with SJS/TEN.

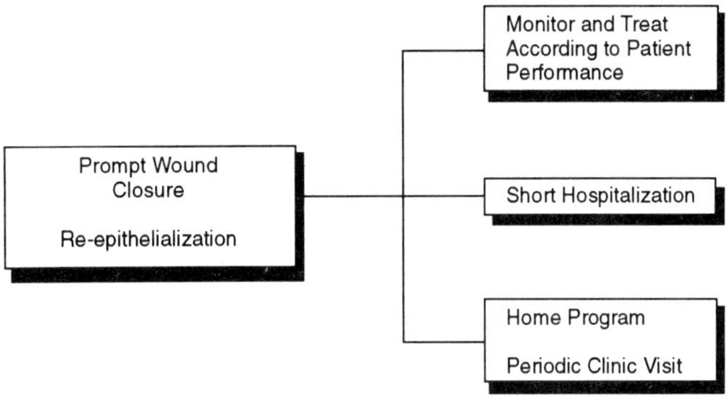

FIGURE 22–7. Diagram identifying rehabilitative interventions when prompt wound closure and rapid re-epithelialization occur.

In contrast, the inability to prevent infection and subsequent dessication of the dermis in patients with severe SJS/TEN complicates therapy management significantly. Definitive short- and long-term treatment challenges arise from complications commonly associated with open wounds (Fig. 22–8). Hospitalization is lengthy and therapy intervention may be extensive. In these cases, problem identification and treatment is directed at the following areas: pain, respiratory dysfunction, immobility, peripheral neuropathy, and hypertrophic scarring.

Pain

Pain is a major obstacle to treatment and increases physical dysfunction in the SJS/TEN patient. The patient's response to pain is influenced by nocioceptive stimuli associated with open wounds, and environmental and personality factors. Pain behaviors are variable and individualized but frequently include anxiety, apprehension, depression, regression, hostility, and noncompliance.[25] Typically these behaviors are exacerbated by wound care, dressing changes, exercise, and requests to engage in activity. Minimizing pain associated with therapy procedures requires pharmacologic and behavioral interventions.[26] These interventions include: (1) explaining the rationale for procedures and gaining the patient's cooperation; (2) scheduling and coordi-

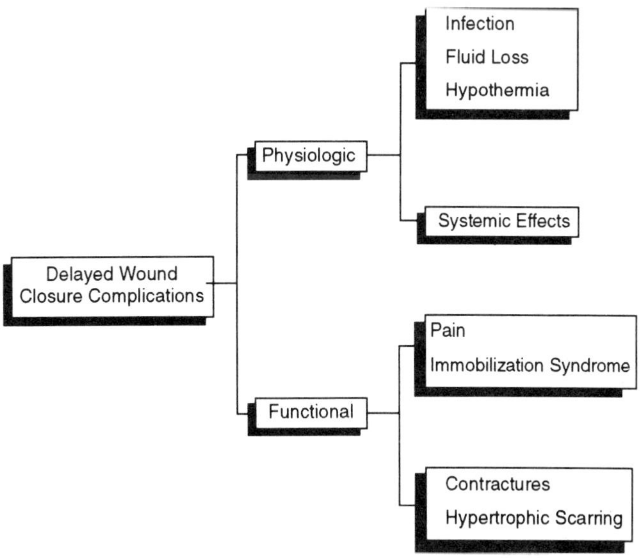

FIGURE 22–8. Flow chart indicating complications which commonly accompany large open wounds.

nating exercise and activity with the administration of pain medications and other daily patient care; (3) exercising during hydrotherapy to take advantage of the decreased friction and buoyancy of aquatic exercise; (4) if possible, encouraging patient participation in treatment procedures; and (5) maintaining consistency in approach and expectations of patient performance.

Respiratory Dysfunction

Chest physical therapy is effective in prevention and treatment of respiratory complications similar to those seen in patients with SJS/TEN.[27] Mental status permitting, patients routinely are instructed in deep breathing and coughing. The use of an incentive spirometer is reinforced by the therapist and nursing staff. Selective positioning (erect, lean-forward, supine, lateral, prone) of the patient markedly can effect physiologic lung function by manipulating and matching alveolar ventilation to capillary blood flow and should be routinely incorporated into the care plan of patients with SJS/TEN.[28] In spite of the pain associated with these conditions, a patient who is medically stable should be encouraged or required to sit in a chair frequently throughout the day and evening.

Immobility

Immobilization of patients with SJS/TEN may be related to systemic illness, impaired sensorium, pain, fear, or skin grafting. The general deleterious effects of immobilization, including contracture, weakness, orthostatic hypotension, impaired ambulation and decreased aerobic capacity, have been well documented.[29-31] The pain, discomfort, and weakness associated with SJS/TEN can make the patient reluctant or unable to move from the position of comfort (fetal position). Unfortunately, long-term failure to oppose the forces of wound contracture by active movement compounds the problem. Prolonged immobility should be recognized and avoided when possible. Patients with delayed or complicated wound closure demonstrate a definitive tendency to develop contractures as chronic wounds cause an increase in collagen deposition.[32] Specifically, weakness of the cervical, posterior shoulder, lumbar, hip, and knee extensor musculature has been noted. Weakness contributes to a patient's dependence in bed mobility, transfers, and ambulation. The combined effects of contracture formation and the onset of muscular weakness can result in significant postural and gait deviations. Postural deviations include forward head, protracted and adducted shoulders (Fig. 22–9), flexed hips, and flexed knees. Patients generally demonstrate a shuffle gait with decreased arm swing and trunk rotation. Many therapists have reported that deterioration in cardiovascular endurance and aerobic capacity occurs in this particular patient population. These observations have not been confirmed in the literature.

Treatment of the "immobilization syndrome"[31] associated with severe SJS/TEN is directed at avoiding or minimizing the length and extent of physical and "psychologic" immobility and inactivity. Therapists should immediately introduce exercise, mobility retraining, and conditioning as well as provide intellectual stimuli and challenges to the patient. Specific active, active-assistive, and passive range-of-motion exercises should be selected based on a patient's limitations and capabilities in an attempt to prevent contracture. These exercises are routinely performed with the patient in bed, in the patient's room, in hydrotherapy, and eventually in the therapy treatment areas. For noncompliant patients, patients with particularly problematic contractures, or patients with poor pain tolerance, consideration should be given to

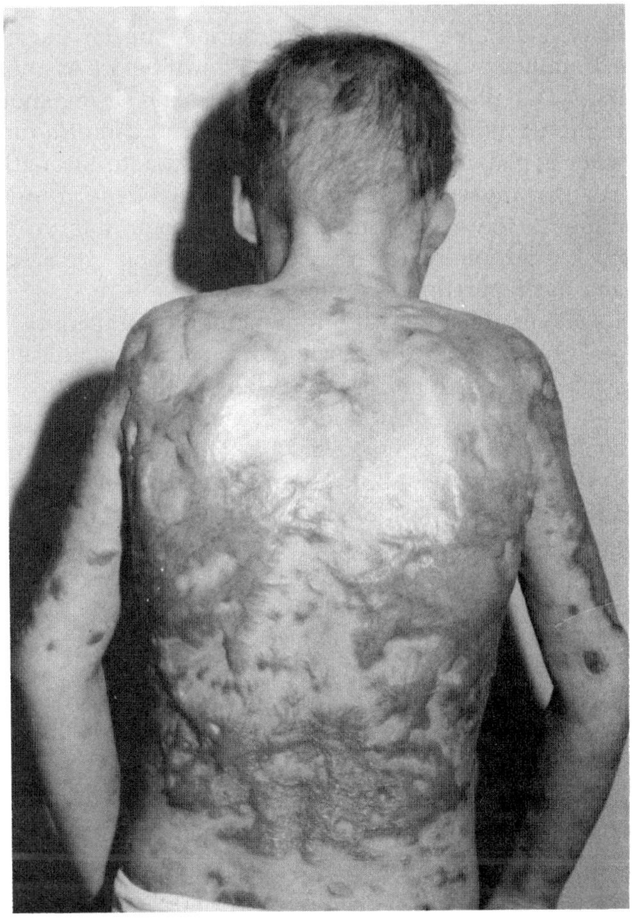

FIGURE 22–9. Postural deviation associated with weakness from prolonged recumbency, contracture, and disuse atrophy. Also note significant hypertrophic scarring from deep dermal wounds.

performing range-of-motion exercises or passive stretching under anesthesia. Range-of-motion exercise can be coordinated with a scheduled surgical procedure. This adjunctive intervention should be planned in consultation with the physician and anesthesiologist. Guidelines and precautions to be observed when implementing these procedures with burn patients have been identified by Nicosia and associates[33] and can be applied to patients with SJS/TEN. Prevention of contracture also requires discretionary use of a positioning and splinting program. Splints and techniques of anticontracture positioning should be applied selectively to patients who are disoriented or too ill to participate actively in an exercise program and who demonstrate losses in range of motion. Alert patients who can actively participate in an exercise program should be considered candidates for splints and therapeutic positioning only if deficits in range of motion remain apparent after the initial daily exercise session.

Exercise or activities to maintain and restore patient strength and mobility should occur simultaneously. Assistance from the patient with bed mobility should be encouraged throughout hospitalization. Use of an overhead trapeze may assist in promoting independence and should be considered in select cases, especially in those patients with large or extremely painful posterior wounds. Orthostatic hypotension and lower extremity extensor muscle weakness frequently impair patient mobility. Elastic bandages or appropriate support hose should be applied to the lower extremities to assist with venous return before assumption of upright sitting or standing.[34] Dangling in short-duration bedside sitting should be performed until tolerance to the upright position is obtained. The use of a tilt table or prone stander to acclimate a patient to upright standing and to strengthen the lumbar, hip, and knee extensor musculature may be indicated. Self-propulsion of a wheelchair with either upper or lower extremities can serve as an interim means of strengthening, improving cardiopulmonary function and aerobic capacity, and restoring mobility before, and in preparation for ambulation.

Re-establishing safe, independent ambulation is a major therapeutic goal. Progression through the normal ambulatory sequence is followed with the goal of re-establishing safe and independent ambulation. Avoidance and prompt discontinuation of assistive devices encourage patient self-confidence and independence. Gait analysis and feedback from the therapist, in conjunction with visual cues through use of a mirror, can be used to assist patients to establish a normal heel-toe gait pattern with equal stride length, arm swing, and trunk rotation. Progressing the distance and intensity of ambulation with the addition of ergometry, stationary biking and a treadmill will improve a patient's strength and aerobic capacity. When these activities are performed the patient's vital signs and clinical response should be monitored to evaluate the tolerance to, and the effectiveness of the exercise program.

Peripheral Neuropathy

The only reported incident of peripheral nerve involvement in patients with SJS/TEN found in the literature was one case of bilateral facial paralysis.[35] This chapter author has treated two patients who developed bilateral peroneal nerve palsy and associated foot drop requiring treatment. Due to the diverse causes of this condition, determining if a peripheral neuropathy was a direct result of SJS/TEN or if an iatrogenic cause, such as pressure or compression, was responsible is difficult.

Intervention for these two patients consisted of baseline electrodiagnostic testing, dynamic splinting, the use of an ankle foot orthosis, exercise, and electrical stimulation. Follow-up with serial electromyographic examinations and nerve conduction velocity tests in conjunction with clinical examinations documented patient progress. Within 9 months full return of function occurred for both of these patients.

Hypertrophic Scarring

Skin sloughing with the SJS/TEN patient occurs at the epidermal-dermal junction. When prompt wound closure is achieved, hypertrophic scarring is rarely present. If dermal dessication occurs, the presence of hypertrophic scarring will have a higher probability (see Fig. 22–9). Treatment of hypertrophic scar in patients with SJS/TEN is exactly the same as in patients with thermal injury because the pathophysiology of the hypertrophic scar is identical. The type of intervention varies and ranges from no intervention to the use of elaborate custom-fabricated pressure garments, silicone gel sheets, flexible elastomer inserts, and masks that apply total contact pressure to the scar.[36-40] Not all SJS/TEN patients require or are candidates for pressure therapy for scar management. Prescription of commercially available pressure garments and pressure techniques should take into account the expected compliance of the patient as well as the anticipated cosmetic and functional severity of the scar. The patient's concern with and psychosocial ability to adjust to the scars should be discussed and considered when deciding whether to intervene with pressure therapy. Complications such as blistering, abrasions, ulceration, swelling, and deformity from sustained pressure have been associated with the use of pressure garments and clinicians should be observant for these potential problems.[41,42]

Discharge Planning and Outpatient Follow-up

Patients with severe SJS/TEN may require extensive home programs and outpatient therapy for up to 1 year after discharge. Patients with significant hypertrophic scars or contractures should visit the burn clinic frequently as outpatients for multidisciplinary evaluation and treatment planning. Children, in particular, may require serial reconstructive operative procedures to correct growth-related deficiencies due to scar tissue.

FROSTBITE

Frostbite is a common thermal injury that causes destruction of the affected skin to varying depths.[43] Throughout the centuries cold exposure has been predominantly associated with military operations and wartime. During the past decade, however, an increased interest in outdoor activities (e.g., snowmobiling, mountain climbing, skiing) has led to cold exposure in the general population.[44] Other factors commonly associated with frostbite include an altered mental status due to alcohol or drug use, depression, and psychosis. The application of current treatment methods requires that therapists have skills in wound care and functional restoration of frostbitten extremities.[45] This section will: (1) review the etiology, clinical manifestations, and medical management of frostbite; (2) identify complications that affect therapy management; and (3) describe guidelines for rehabilitative therapy intervention following frostbite injury.

Etiology, Clinical Manifestations, and Medical Management

ETIOLOGY

Frostbite most commonly is caused by exposure of the skin to below freezing temperatures but also may occur at temperatures above freezing depending on humidity, wind velocity, vascular integrity, cardiac output, altitude, and duration of exposure.[46] These precipitating factors may be categorized as host factors (vascular status, smoking history, alcohol consumption, clothing, fatigue, psychologic disorders) or environmental factors (wind velocity, altitude, humidity).[45]

CLINICAL MANIFESTATIONS

The exact pathophysiology of frostbite remains unknown; however, several theories have been proposed. Whether the injury results from the actual freezing of involved tissues or from decreased local blood flow and associated tissue ischemia probably depends on variables associated with the condition of the host and presence and severity of the environmental variables. Regardless of the pathogenesis of frostbite, the clinical presentation of a patient will depend on the depth of injury. A *superficial injury* produces hyperemic skin, mild edema without blister formation, and hypersensitivity that diminishes over time. A *partial-thickness injury* is distinguished by hyperemia, edema, and blisters or peeling. A *full-thickness* frostbite injury is characterized by a waxy white or cyanotic blue-gray discoloration of the skin, which indicates skin and subcutaneous tissue involvement. *Subdermal frostbite* infers gangrene formation of subcutaneous tissue or damage to bone and nerve. Early classification of the severity of a frostbite injury can be done, but is less than 50 percent accurate. Therefore, a conservative approach to the management of frostbite patients has evolved.[47] Recent technological advances in the evaluation of an injured area with angiography and thermography appear to be helpful to distinguish the level of tissue loss.[44]

MEDICAL MANAGEMENT

Treatment of frostbite is controversial and only two principles appear to be accepted universally. These principles indicate that the patient should be removed from the cold environment and a rapid rewarming of the involved body part in a water bath or whirlpool should follow. These procedures are performed to decrease the duration of the frozen state and facilitate the restoration of blood flow. Under no circumstances should these procedures be initiated if there is a chance of re-exposing a patient to the cold. Experimental studies have documented that increased tissue damage occurs with refreezing.[48] The affected extremity should be elevated to minimize edema. Pain and discomfort may be extreme during the rewarming process and may continue throughout the acute phase of care. Narcotics often are used for pain management. Dressing changes and hydrotherapy should be performed daily unless specified otherwise. Loosely applied, unrestrictive sterile bandages commonly are applied to ulcerated areas. Loose, nonadherent superficial epithelium should be removed gently or debrided away. Bullae aspiration or removal should be considered if the fluidlike content becomes cloudy and thick. As a general rule, amputation and surgical debridement should be delayed as long as possible unless infection or the presence of subcutaneous air, diagnostic of gangrene, indicate the need for immediate amputation.[49] Medical interventions for the treatment of frostbite that have not been accepted universally but are under investigation include anticoagulation, "medical" or surgical sympathectomy, and the use of hyperbaric oxygen.[44] Education and other preventive measures provide the best mechanisms to avoid the devastating effects of frostbite.

Therapy Evaluation and Treatment

EVALUATION

Upon admission, a prompt comprehensive therapy evaluation should be initiated and completed. Identification of immediate and potential future rehabilitative problems are essential to guide appropriate therapeutic intervention. The evaluation should include a review of the host and environmental factors that contributed to the injury. These facts, along with the findings of an objective evaluation, will aid the therapist in developing short- and long-term treatment goals and a treatment plan that meets the individual needs of the patient. The therapist's evaluation should include objective information regarding sensation, pain tolerance, range of motion, mobility, strength, and potential for future musculoskeletal complications. The experienced therapist may be inclined to perform gentle passive range of motion of the joints to assist with the assessment of soft tissue restriction. However, some authors emphasize that range of motion should not be attempted by anyone but the patient and should be done very carefully to avoid friction or further injury to the damaged extremity.[48] When the lower extremity or feet are involved, early ambulation can damage adjacent viable tissues and increase swelling and thus should be avoided.[48]

TREATMENT

With the exception of the precautions noted above, therapy intervention for the frostbite patient incorporates the general strategies identified earlier in this text that were used for treating patients with thermal injuries or other skin disruptions. The primary objectives of therapy are to limit soft tissue contracture and to restore function and mobility.

Daily hydrotherapy sessions of 15 to 20 minutes duration at 38°C to 42°C (100°F to 107°F) provide an ideal time for a patient to perform prescribed active range of motion exercises. Wound dressings, if used, should be removed to allow the therapist to assess accurately the patient's active range of motion. Additional exercises also may be performed immediately after a hydrotherapy session (Fig. 22–10). Dependency of

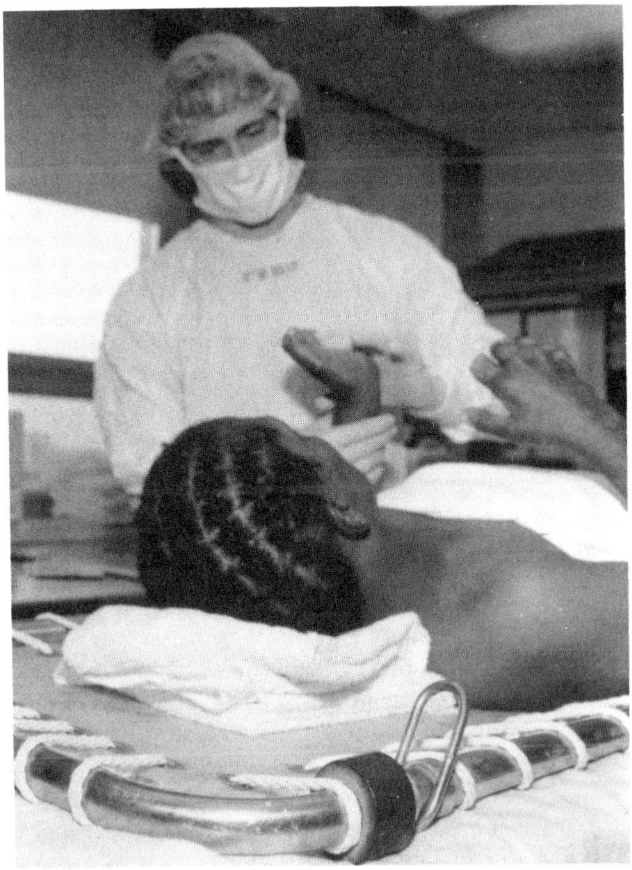

FIGURE 22–10. Gentle active assistive range of motion exercises are performed following hydrotherapy on a frostbite patient with amputated digits.

the involved body part should be minimized if edema is present. The prescribed exercises should promote edema reduction while opposing the forces directing soft tissue contracture. Washburn[48] has stated, "Great care must be exercised to distinguish between movements that may endanger the injured part and real immobility. The latter if total and prolonged can do much harm. Voluntary, careful movement of the joints at regular intervals is an important part of modern treatment. This is done in a whirlpool bath in hospitals for maximum effectiveness and safety."

Cold-injured joints are extremely vulnerable to deformity and rigidity.[45] If the extent of the injury is severe or the patient demonstrates limitation of motion, an aggressive splinting program should be initiated immediately. During the fabrication and application of splints caution must be taken to minimize pressure and friction on the involved tissues.

If amputation of the involved body part is unavoidable, appropriate prosthetic intervention should occur. Adaptive equipment to maximize function also may be indicated. For example, when a foot is involved, custom-fabricated orthotic shoes or shoe inserts may be essential to restore patient mobility. As noted previously, ambulation may be contraindicated initially, but when it is permitted, ambulatory aids may be required to reduce weight bearing on painful or hypersensitive feet. Regardless of location of a frostbite injury, basic desensitization techniques should be implemented to assist in overcoming this common problem.

Finally, the patient must be warned of the susceptibility to future reinjury. The individual host and environmental factors that place the patient at risk for recurrent injury should be reviewed and emphasized by all members of the burn care team.

CASE STUDY 1

HISTORY

A 37-year-old man developed a sore throat, cervical lymphadenopathy, and low-grade fever that was treated with aspirin, acetaminophen, and bed rest. Over the ensuing 4 days, fever persisted and he developed an erythematous maculopapular rash on the forehead and cheeks, subsequently spreading to the trunk and extremities. Conjunctival and oral lesions appeared and his temperature rose to 103°F. The maculopapular rash progressed to epidermal skin sloughing affecting 80 percent of the body surface area and the patient was diagnosed with Stevens-Johnson syndrome (SJS).

On admission, the patient had full active-assistive range of motion (ROM) of all joints. He was unable to roll side to side or achieve sitting from a supine position without moderate to maximal assistance. On his fifth hospital day, the patient developed gram-negative sepsis. He was intubated and 2 days later therapy was reinitiated. The patient now required mechanical ventilatory support. Dermal desiccation and conversion of the neck, shoulder, chest, and back wounds had occurred. Passive shoulder flexion and abduction had decreased 25° bilaterally.

The patient underwent several surgeries for debridement and skin grafting. Intraoperative passive ROM was within normal limits except at the shoulders where the onset of scar banding of the anterior and posterior axillary folds restricted flexion and abduction to 160°. The ankles could be dorsiflexed to −8° of neutral. Following each operative procedure, the patient remained confined to bed for approximately 3 days.

By hospital day 26, available bilateral shoulder flexion and left ankle dorsiflexion were now 100° and −5°, respectively, when tested by passive ROM. The patient's strength had deteriorated significantly. He had developed a peroneal nerve palsy that left him with poor dorsiflexion on the left. On hospital day 33, the patient required maximal assistance from two people to come to stand and tolerated standing for only 1 minute.

PROBLEM LIST

Decreased bilateral shoulder flexion with anterior and posterior axillary banding
Decreased ROM and strength in left ankle dorsiflexors
General deconditioning
Inability to perform activities of daily living (ADLs)
Active scarring

GOALS

Bilateral shoulder flexion to 165° actively
Left ankle dorsiflexion to 10° actively
Left ankle dorsiflexion strength rated good
Overall strength rated good
Independent ambulation on flat surfaces and stairs
Avascular, pliable, flat scars

INTERVENTIONS

Early during the patient's hospitalization, he was transferred from bed to chair with maximal assistance of one so he could sit supported. He was instructed in deep breathing, coughing, and the use of an incentive spirometer. A turning and positioning schedule was established with the nursing staff. The patient was instructed in an active ROM (AROM) exercise program. Amnion was applied to all open wounds. The patient subsequently became septic and passive ROM (PROM) was instituted.

During surgical procedures PROM was performed on the patient. Three days following each operation, AROM and active-assistive ROM exercises were performed twice daily. Positioning and splints also were used. Transfers from bed to wheelchair and back, as well as coming to stand from a wheelchair, were practiced. Within 1 week, the patient's strength and endurance improved such that he could come to stand independently and stand for three 3-minute periods during one therapy session. Active and active-assistive exercises and gait training continued until the patient's strength and endurance was rated as good. His left ankle remained weak and treatment included electrical stimulation, exercise, and the use of a custom-fabricated ankle-foot orthosis. The patient was fitted with a custom-made compression vest and panty girdle and he and his family were instructed in a home exercise program.

RATIONALE

Since sloughing of the epidermis is extremely painful and generally does not lead to long-term ROM deficits, AROM is the exercise of choice for SJS patients. However, in this case, the patient's wounds and medical status deteriorated and skin grafting along with long-term bed rest resulted in significant ROM deficits and strength loss. PROM was necessary when the patient was unable to assist with the exercise program and performing PROM under anesthesia allowed the therapist to evaluate the patient's true ROM without causing excessive pain to the patient. The turning and positioning schedule promoted pulmonary hygiene and prevented pressure sores. The initiation of an active and active-assistive exercise program soon after surgery, along with a positioning program and the use of splints, prevented contracture formation. Instructing the patient and family in an exercise program enhanced his progress in regaining ROM, strength, and endurance. Although patients with SJS generally do not require pressure garments because scarring is more a dermal phenomenon, garments were required for this patient due to the dermal destruction that occurred with his septic episode.

CASE STUDY 2

HISTORY

A 44-year-old man with a past medical history of psychiatric disorder, hypertension, peripheral vascular disease, and alcoholism was found outside, unconscious from acute alcohol intoxication at 1:15 A.M. The patient was heavily dressed except for his feet, which were protected only by thin cotton socks and canvas tennis shoes. The temperature was below freezing with a wind chill factor of −5°F.

Examination of the patient revealed mildly edematous and hyperemic hands and fingers except for the left thumb, which had a large blister on the ventral surface. Toes 3, 4, and 5 of both feet were waxy white or cyanotic blue-gray in color. The great toe of the left foot also was blistered, hyperemic, and edematous. The patient reported intense pain in his hands and feet. No other body part demonstrated signs of cold injury.

Bilateral wrist range of motion demonstrated 10° limitations in flexion and extension. Full metacarpophalangeal (MP) joint extension of digits 2 through 5 on both hands was achieved, but only 40° flexion could be obtained. The proximal and distal interphalangeal (PIP and DIP) joints of digits 2 through 5 demonstrated 0° to 50° of motion. Cautious gentle PROM by the therapist of these joints revealed mild resistance. The right thumb could be actively moved through a full arc of motion with minimal pain but bullae formation on the left thumb significantly restricted active motion. The patient was able to actively move only the right great toe. Gentle, cautious PROM of the toes revealed significant stiffening and resistance indicative of deep tissue destruction. The patient's hands healed in 2 weeks without surgical intervention; however, he continued to report hypersensitivity of his finger tips.

After approximately 1 month, subcutaneous air, diagnostic of wet gangrene, was noted in the left foot and an immediate surgical transmetatarsal amputation was performed. Definitive wound closure was obtained using split-thickness skin grafts.

On hospital day 45, the patient returned to the operating room for amputation of the right toes 2 through 5 and permanent skin closure with split-thickness skin grafts.

PROBLEM LIST

Significant past medical history for peripheral vascular disease and hypertension

Limitation in ROM of bilateral wrists and hands

Transmetatarsal amputation of left foot and amputation of digits 2 through 5 on right foot

Hypersensitivity of fingertips

GOALS

Prevent further tissue destruction

Full active ROM (AROM) of bilateral wrists and hands

Independent ambulation on flat surfaces and stairs with adapted shoes

Minimal hypersensitivity of finger tips

INTERVENTIONS

After admission to the hospital, rapid rewarming of the hands and feet in a water bath at 40°C (104°F) was initiated and continued for 20 minutes followed by elevation of the extremities. Pressure and friction to the hands were minimized by placing them on pillows. Wound care consisted of cleansing the hands and feet, selectively debriding blisters, application of silver sulfadiazine cream, and wrapping delicately with gauze. The next day, an AROM exercise program was initiated after the patient received his pain medication. Active-assistive exercise was performed gently to help improve ROM. Custom-fabricated thermoplastic palmar hand splints were fabricated and applied at night when the patient was sleeping and unable to actively monitor the position of his hands. Extreme caution was used with splint application to avoid pressure-induced ischemic necrosis of viable tissue. Due to the condition of the patient's feet, he was not allowed to ambulate but demonstrated independent mobility using a standard wheelchair.

Five days after the patient underwent a left transmetatarsal amputation, ambulation was initiated with a standard adult walker. Full AROM had been re-established in both hands, but the fingertips remained hypersensitive. Splints were discontinued and desensitization techniques, progressing from soft textures to abrasive tactile stimulation were used to decrease his symptoms. Five days following the amputation of the right toes, ambulation was reinitiated. The patient was progressed from a walker to a cane and he was fit with adapted shoes due to the absence of his left forefoot and right toes. Outpatient therapy was required to assist him in re-establishing a normal gait pattern.

RATIONALE

Rapid rewarming of frostbitten parts is necessary to prevent further tissue trauma. In addition, the tissues are susceptible to additional damage if not handled with extreme care. AROM is the preferred exercise method to minimize contact with the fragile, painful tissue. With less severe frostbite injuries, such as seen in this patient's hands, wound care can be conservative and therapeutic intervention can be directed toward maintaining ROM and desensitizing the area. With more severe frostbite injuries, the patient's feet being an example, amputation is common. Rehabilitation is more involved and adaptive or assistive devices often are necessary.

SUMMARY

Stevens-Johnson syndrome and toxic epidermal necrolysis are dermatologic disorders that have pathophysiologic similarities to partial-thickness thermal injury. The early signs and symptoms of SJS/TEN include upper respiratory infection, headache, malaise, fatigue, and fever. Skin rash and bullae formation become evident and may progress to epidermal necrolysis and sloughing, at which point the wound resembles a partial-thickness thermal injury. Other clinical manifestations that accompany SJS/TEN, which are not directly associated with disruption of the skin, involve the respiratory system, eyes, and oropharynx. Therapy treatment, in mild cases, is limited to one or two daily visits throughout the patient's hospitalization, which is typically 9 to 30 days. Rapid wound closure and prevention of dermal dessication are basic goals of wound management of these patients. If dermal dessication occurs, the therapist should direct and focus short- and long-term treatment goals to prevent or minimize pain, respiratory dysfunction, immobility, peripheral neuropathy, weakness, contracture, and hypertrophic scarring (Fig. 22–11). Hospitalization may be

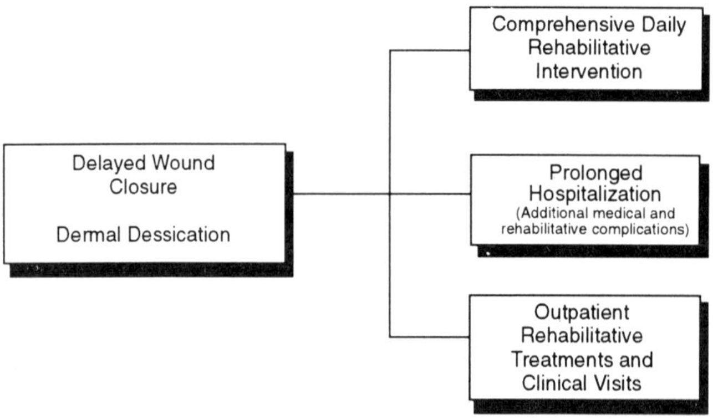

FIGURE 22–11. Diagram identifying rehabilitative requirements when wound closure is delayed and dermal dessication occurs.

prolonged and the therapist's knowledge of the treatment of these disorders may help decrease patient morbidity.

Unlike SJS/TEN, frostbite is a thermally induced injury but, like SJS/TEN, its exact pathophysiology remains unknown. Whether the injury results from actual freezing of involved tissues or from decreased local blood flow and associated tissue ischemia seems to depend on variables associated with the condition of the host and various environmental factors. The depth of frostbite injury is difficult to predict. Initial management includes removal of the patient from the cold environment and rapid rewarming of the involved body part in a water bath or whirlpool. The therapist's evaluation should include objective information regarding sensation, pain tolerance, range of motion, mobility, strength, and potential for future musculoskeletal complications. When evaluating and introducing treatment interventions, the therapist must be cautious to avoid further damage to fragile tissue. Range of motion and ambulation must be instituted cautiously and judiciously progressed based on the medical condition of the patient. Desensitization programs and prosthetic or orthotic intervention are common aspects of care for frostbite patients.

REFERENCES

1. Demling, R, Ellerbe, S, and Lowe, N: Burn unit management of toxic epidermal necrolysis. J Burn Care Rehabil 4:176–183, 1983.
2. Crosby, S, et al: Management of Stevens-Johnson syndrome. Clin Pharm 5:682–689, 1986.
3. Marvin, J, et al: Improved treatment of the Stevens-Johnson Syndrome. Arch Surg 119:601–605, 1984.
4. Heimbach, D, et al: Toxic epidermal necrolysis, a step forward in treatment. JAMA 257:2171–2208, 1987.
5. Kim, P, et al: Stevens-Johnson syndrome and toxic epidermal necrolysis: A pathophysiologic review with recommendations for a treatment protocol. J Burn Care Rehabil 4:91–100, 1983.
6. Prasad, J, Feller, I, and Thompson, P: Use of amnion for the treatment of Stevens-Johnson syndrome. J Trauma 26:945–946, 1986.
7. Davidson, B and Hunt, J: Human cadaver homograft in toxic epidermal necrolysis. J Burn Care Rehabil 2:94–96, 1981.
8. Edlich, R, et al: Toxic epidermal necrolysis. Cur Concepts Trauma Care. Spring:10–15, 1985.
9. Araujo, V and Flowers, F: Stevens-Johnson syndrome. J Emerg Med 2:129–135, 1984.
10. Ting, H and Aram, B: Stevens-Johnson syndrome: A review of 34 cases. Int J Dermatol 24:587–591, 1985.
11. Feller, I and Archambeault, C: Nursing the Burned Patient, ed 1. National Institute for Burn Medicine, Ann Arbor, 1974.
12. Halebian, P, et al: A burn center experience with toxic epidermal necrolysis. J Burn Care Rehabil 4:176–183, 1983.
13. Warden, G: Immunologic response to burn injury. In Boswick, J (ed): The Art and Science of Burn Care. Aspen, Rockville, 1987, pp 113–119.
14. Harnar, T, et al: Toxic epidermal necrolysis complicated by severe wound sepsis. A case study. J Burn Care Rehabil 8:554–557, 1987.
15. Lawrence, J (ed): Workshop on scar management. Burns Incl Therm Inj 13:553–556, 1987.
16. Dietch, E, et al: Hypertrophic burn scars: Analysis of variables. J Trauma 23:895–898, 1983.
17. Virant, F, Redding, G, and Novak, A: Multiple pulmonary complications in a patient with Stevens-Johnson syndrome. Clin Pediatr 23:412–414, 1984.
18. Howard, G: The Stevens-Johnson syndrome: Ocular prognosis and treatment. Am J Opthamol 55:893–900, 1963.
19. Arstikaitis, M: Ocular aftermath of Stevens-Johnson syndrome. Arch Opthalmol 90:376–379, 1973.
20. Nathan, M: Stevens-Johnson syndrome: 23 cases and their otolaryngolic significance. Laryngoscope 85:1713–1724, 1975.
21. Thompson, P and Parks, D: Amnion as a Burn Wound Dressing. In Wise, D (ed): Burn Wound Coverings. CRC Press, Boca Raton, 1984, pp 47–53.
22. Walker, A: Use of amniotic membranes for burn wound coverage. In Wise, D (ed): Burn Wound Coverings. CRC Press, Boca Raton, 1984, pp 55–75.
23. Remensnyder, J: Burn Wound Coverings and Biologic Dressings. In Carvajal, H and Parks, D (eds): Burns in Children: Pediatric Management. Yearbook, Chicago, 1988, pp 182–191.

24. Peltier, G, Poppe, S, and Twomey, J: Controlled air suspension: An advantage in burn care. J Burn Care Rehabil 8:558–560, 1987.
25. Marvin, J and Heimbach, D: Pain management. In Fisher, S and Helm, P (eds): Comprehensive Rehabilitation of Burns. Williams & Wilkins, Baltimore, 1984, pp 311–329.
26. Friedmann, J, Shapiro, J, and Plon, L: Psychosocial Treatment and Pain Control. In Achaeur, B (ed): Management of the Burned Patient. Appleton & Lange, Norwalk, 1987, pp 247–255.
27. Irwin, S and Tecklin, J (eds): Cardiopulmonary Physical Therapy. CV Mosby, St. Louis, 1985.
28. Dean, E: Effects of body position on pulmonary function. Phys Ther 65:613–618, 1985.
29. Spencer, W, Valbona, C, Carter, R: Physiologic concepts of immobilization. Arch Phys Med Rehabil 46:89–100, 1965.
30. Steinberg, F: The Immobilized Patient: Functional Pathology and Management. Plenum, New York, 1980.
31. Valbona, C: The immobilization syndrome. In Halstead, L, et al (eds): Medical Rehabilitation. Raven Press, New York, 1985, p 289.
32. Johnson, C: Wound healing and scar formation. Topics Acute Care Trauma Rehabil 1:1–114, 1987.
33. Nicosia, J, Stein, ED, Stein, JM: The advantages of physiotherapy for burn patients under anesthesia. Burns Incl Therm Inj 6:202–204, 1979.
34. Kozerefski, P: Exercise and Ambulation in the Burned Patient. In DiGrigorio, V (ed): Rehabilitation of the Burn Patient. Churchill Livingstone, New York, 1984, pp 55–73.
35. Friedman, J, Challeon, Y, and Brust, J: Bilateral facial palsy associated with Stevens-Johnson Syndrome. Neurology 29:1304–1306, 1979.
36. Johnson, C: Physical therapists as scar modifiers. Phys Ther 64:1381–1387, 1984.
37. Jenson, L and Parshly, P: Postburn scar contractures: Histology and effects of pressure treatment. J Burn Care Rehabil 5:119–123, 1984.
38. Rose, M and Dietch, E: The clinical use of a tubular compression bandage, Tubigrip for burn scar therapy: A critical analysis. Burns Incl Therm Inj 12:58–64, 1985.
39. Malick, M and Carr, J: Flexible elastomere molds in burn scar control. Am J Occup Ther 34:603–608, 1980.
40. Perkins, K, Davey, R, and Wallis, K: Silicone gel: A treatment for burn scars and contractures. Burn Incl Therm Inj 9:201–204, 1982.
41. Cheng, J, et al: Pressure therapy in the treatment of postburn hypertrophic scars: A critical look into its usefulness and fallacies by pressure monitoring. Burns Incl Therm Inj 9:201–204, 1982.
42. Leung, K, Cheng, J, and Ma, G: Complications of pressure therapy for postburn hypertrophic scars: Biomechanical analysis based on 5 cases. Burns Incl Therm Inj 10:434–438, 1983.
43. Rasmusen, D and Zook, E: Frostbite: A review of pathophysiology and newest treatments. J Indiana State Med Assoc 65:1237–1241, 1972.
44. Purdue, G and Hunt, J: Cold injury: A collective review. J Burn Care Rehabil 7:331–342, 1986.
45. Thorman, M: The pathology and management of frostbite. Clin Mgmt 5:12–15, 1985.
46. Welch, G: Frostbite. Practitioner 213:801–804, 1974.
47. Erickson, U and Ponten, B: The possible value of arteriography supplemented by a vasodilator agent in the early assessment of tissue viability in frostbite. Injury 6:150–153, 1974.
48. Washburn, B: Frostbite. N Engl J Med 266:974, 1962.
49. Tischler, J: The soft tissue and bone changes in frostbite injuries. Radiology 102:511–513, 1972.

APPENDIX A

Burn Wound Care Products

TOPICAL AGENTS

Topical Antibiotics

MAFENIDE ACETATE

Sulfamylon Cream
Winthrop-Breon Pharmaceuticals
90 Park Avenue
New York, NY 10016

SILVER SULFADIAZINE

SSD-AE
Boots-Flints, Inc.
300 Tri-State International Center
Suite 200
Lincolnshire, IL 60069-4415
(800) 537-8087

Silvadene
Marion Merrell Dow, Inc.
Kansas City, MO 64114
(800) 362-7466

Thermazene
Sherwood Medical
St. Louis, MO 63103
(800) 325-7472

Antifungal Agents

Mycostatin (Nystatin)
Westwood-Squibb Pharmaceuticals, Inc.
100 Forest Avenue
Buffalo, NY
(716) 887-3773

Nilstat
Professional Services Department
Lederle Laboratories
Pearl River, NY 10965
(914) 735-2815

Nystex
Savage Laboratories
Division of Altana, Inc.
60 Baylis Road
Melvil, NY 11747
(800) 231-0206

Additional Ointments

Bacitracin Ointment
E. Fougera & Company
Division of Altana, Inc.
Melvil, NY 11747

Bactroban (Mupirocin)
Beecham Laboratories
Bristol, TN 37620
(615) 764-5141

Furacin Cream
Norwich Eaton Pharmaceuticals, Inc.
P.O. Box 191
Norwich, NY 13815-0191
(607) 335-2565

Garamycin Ointment
Schering Corporation
Galloping Hill Road
Kennilworth, NJ 07033
(800) 526-4099

Neosporin
Burroughs Wellcome Company
3030 Cornwallis Road
Research Triangle Park, NC 27709

Vitamin A & D Ointment
Available from local pharmacys

Enzymatic Debriding Agents

Elase
Parke-Davis
Division of Warner-Lambert Company
201 Tabor Road
Morris Plains, NJ 07950
(800) 223-0432

Travase
Boots-Flint, Inc.
300 Tri-State International Center
Suite 200
Lincolnshire, IL 60069-4415
(800) 537-8087

Whirlpool Additives

Betadine Whirlpool Concentrate
Purdue Frederick Company
100 Connecticut Avenue
Norwalk, CT 06856
(203) 853-0123

Chlorazene
Wisconsin Pharmaceutical Company
Jackson, WI 53037
(414) 677-4121

Hibiclens
Stuart Pharmaceuticals
Division of ICI Americas, Inc.
Wilmington, DE 19897
(302) 575-2231

Disinfectants

A-500 Dry
Airkem
Division of Ecolab
Ecolab Center
St. Paul, MN 55102
(800) 247-5362

Sanizene
Ferno-Washington, Inc.
Wilmington, OH 44177-9371
(513) 382-1451

Cleansers and Solvents

CLEANSERS

Cara-Klenz
Carrington Laboratories, Inc.
Irving, TX 75062
(214) 541-2278

Shur-Clens
Calgon Vestal Laboratories
Merck and Company
Health Care Market Group
P.O. Box 147
St. Louis, MO 63166
(314) 535-1810

Tar Removing Solvent

Orange-Sol
Orange-Sol, Inc.
Chandler, AZ 85244

APPENDIX **B**

Wound Dressings and Bandaging Material

WOUND DRESSINGS

Biosynthetic Occlusive and Semiocclusive Dressings

COLLAGEN-IMPREGNATED GAUZE

Biobrane II
Dow-Hickam Pharmaceuticals
Wound Care Division
Division of Sterling Drug
New York, NY 10016

SEMIPERMEABLE POLYURETHANE FILM

Mitraflex
Calgon Vestal
Merck & Company, Inc.
St. Louis, MO 63133
(314) 535-1910

OpSite
Smith & Nephew
Largo, FL 34643
(800) 876-1261

HYDROCOLLOID DRESSINGS

Comfeel
Kendall Health Care Products Company
15 Hampshire Street
Mansfield, MA 02048
(800) 422-8811

Duoderm
ConvaTec, Squibb Company
P.O. Box 4000
Princeton, NJ 08543-5254
(800) 346-7197

Intrasite
Smith & Nephew
Massillon, OH 44646-7199
(800) 321-9752

HYDROGEL DRESSINGS

Elasto-Gel
Southwest Technologies, Inc.
Kansas City, MO 64108
(800) 247-9951

Vigilon
Bard Home Health Division
C.R. Bard, Inc.
111 Spring Street
Murray Hill, NJ 07974
(800) 526-4493

SEMIPERMEABLE FOAM

LyoFoam
Acme United Corporation
Fairfield, CT 06430
(800) 835-2263

BANDAGING MATERIAL

Elastic Netting

Flexinet
Bioplasty, Inc.
1385 Centennial Drive
St. Paul, MN 55113
(800) 328-9105

Stretch Net
Division of DeRoyal Industries, Inc.
200 DeBusk Lane
Powell, TN 37849
(800) 251-9864

Surgifix
Fispin Corporation
P.O. Box 499
Elmsford, NY 10523
(914) 347-5727

Surg-O-Flex
P.O. Box 262
Lyman, NE 69352
(800) 334-2592

X span Tubular Dressing Retainer
Baxter Healthcare Corporation
Hospital Supply Division
Deerfield, IL 60015

Impregnated Gauze Bandage

Adaptic
Johnson & Johnson
Arlington, TX 76004-0130
(800) 433-5009

Aquaphor
Beiersdorf Corporation
Norwalk, CT

UNNA boot kit
Blenwood, Inc.
P.O. Box 518
Tenafly, NJ 07670
(201) 569-0050

Nonadherent Wound Dressing

N-Terface
Winfield Laboratories, Inc.
Richardson, TX 75080

APPENDIX C

Moisturizers

Compat
Jobst Institute, Inc.
P.O. Box 653
Toledo, OH 43694-4511
(800) 537-1063

Corrective Concepts
Pattee Products, Inc.
3045 Park Lane, Suite 1084
Dallas, TX 75220
(214) 352-9880

Curel
S.C. Johnson & Son, Inc.
Racine, WI 53403
(800) 558-5252

Dermaide
Dermaide Research Corporation
P.O. Box 562
Palos Heights, IL 60463
(800) 344-2563

Eucerin
Beiersdorf, Inc.
Norwalk, CT 06856-5529

Eutra
Swiss-American Products, Inc.
4315 Alpha Road
Dallas, TX 75244
(800) 633-8872

Lymphazome
Fountain Pharmaceuticals, Inc.
11201 Concept Boulevard
Suite A
Largo, FL 34643
(800) 253-5115

Nivea Cream
Beiersdorf Corporation
Norwalk, CT 06856-5529

Third Step
Bio-Concepts, Inc.
2424 East University Drive
Phoenix, AZ 85034
(800) 421-5647

Vaseline Intensive Care Lotion
Chesebrough Pond's Inc.
33 Benedict Place
Greenwich, CT 06830
(800) 243-5804

Water Babies Sunblock
Plough, Inc.
Memphis, TN 38151

APPENDIX D

Pressure-Reducing Beds

Clinitron
Flexicare
Support Systems International, Inc.
4349 Corporate Road
Charleston, SC 29405
(800) 845-2478

Fluid-Aire
Kinair
Kinetic Concepts, Inc.
3440 East Huston Street
San Antonio, TX 78208-0588
(800) 531-5346

Mediscus
Mediscus Products, Inc.
13135 Champions Drive
Suite 120
Houston, TX 77069
(800) 922-9065

Pegasus Airwave System
Pegasus Airwave
640 S Military Trail
Deerfield Beach, FL 33442
(800) 443-4325

APPENDIX E

Positioning Devices

Arm Troughs

Regular bed
Genetic Laboratories, Inc.
1385 Centennial Drive
St. Paul, MN 55113
(800) 328-9105

Air bed
Kinetic Concept Therapeutic Services, Inc.
3440 East Huston Street
San Antonio, TX 78208-0588

Donuts

Ali-Med, Inc.
297 High Street
Dedham, MA 02026
(800) 225-2610

Foam (precut wedge or customized pieces)

Ali-Med, Inc.
297 High Street
Dedham, MA 02026
(800) 225-2610

Mobile IV Stand

Abbey Medical
17390 Brookhurst Street
Suite 200
Fountain Valley, CA 92708

Sandbags

AliMed, Inc.
297 High Street
Dedham, MA 02026
(800) 225-2610

Velfoam

Northcoast Medical, Inc.
187 Stauffer Boulevard
San Jose, CA 95125-1042
(800) 821-9319

APPENDIX **F**

Commercially Available Splints

Splint type	1	2	3	4	5	6	7	8	9	10	11	12	13	14
	Source													
Air splint	•	•		•		•					•			
Ankle immobilization		•				•								
Back brace, spinal	•													
Clavical brace	•	•									•		•	
Collar, cervical	•	•								•	•			
Collar, Philadelphia	•									•	•			
Dynamic: low-load, prolonged stretch			•					•	•					•
Elbow extension		•	•	•	•	•	•				•			•
Flexion mitt/glove		•	•			•								
Knee extension					•	•								•
MPA													•	
Shoulder abduction	•					•					•			

SOURCES

1. ACOR Orthopaedic
   4129 Mayfield Road
   Cleveland, OH 44121
   (216) 381-1717
   (800) 237-ACOR

2. Fred Sammons, Inc.
   Box 32
   Brookfield, IL 60513-0032
   (800) 323-5547

3. LMB Hand Rehab Products, Inc.
   P.O. Box 1181
   San Luis Obispo, CA 93406
   (800) 541-3992

4. North Coast Medical, Inc.
   187 Stauffer Boulevard
   San Jose, CA 95125-1042
   (408) 283-1900
   (800) 821-9319

5. Contour Fabricators, Inc.
   P.O. Box 56
   Grand Blanc, MI 48439
   (313) 695-2910
6. Smith & Nephew Rolyan, Inc.
   N93 W14475 Whittaker Way
   P.O. Box 555
   Menomonee Falls, WI 53052-0555
   (800) 558-8633
7. Unlimited Functional Orthoses
   10679 California Street
   Redlands, CA 92373
   (714) 792-5466
8. Ultraflex Systems, Inc.
   95 Great Valley Parkway
   Malvern, PA 19355
   (800) 220-6670
9. Dynasplint
   Landmark Medical
   6655 Amberton Drive
   Suite A
   Baltimore, MD 21227
   (800) 624-9169
10. Zimmer
    Warsaw, IN 46580-0708
    (800) 348-2759
11. Ali-Med
    297 High Street
    Dedham, MA 02026-9135
    (800) 225-2610
12. MPA Company
    13720 Hillcrest Rd.
    Dallas, TX 75240
    (214) 458-0757
13. Abby Medical
    17390 Brookhurst St.
    Suite 200
    Fountain Valley, CA 92708
14. Empi, Inc.
    1275 Grey Fox Road
    St. Paul, MN 55112-6989
    (800) 328-2536

APPENDIX G

Patient Communication Aids

POSITIONING STICKERS

Therapy Skill Builders
3830 East Bellevue
P.O. Box 42050
Tucson, AZ 85733

COMMUNICATION AIDS FOR CHILDREN AND ADULTS

Crestwood Company
6625 North Sidney Place
Milwaukee, WI 53209
(414) 352-5678

OTHER DEVICES

Fred Sammons, Inc.
P.O. Box 32
Brookfield, IL 60513
(800) 323-5547

North Coast Medical
187 Stauffer Boulevard
San Jose, CA 95125
(800) 821-9319

J A Preston Corporation
P.O. Box 89
Jackson, MI 49204
(800) 631-7277

APPENDIX H

Splinting Materials

CHARACTERISTICS

Aquaplast—Original or T

Vendors: 1, 2, 5, 6
Color available: Ivory
Softening temperature: 160°-180°F
Heating time: 1 min (until transparent)
Work time: 3-4 min
Edge finishing: Trims or smooths easily (save until final step due to elastic memory)
Coating/bonding: Original: no coating—self bonding when hot
T: acrylic coating—scrape off with scissors or dissolve with solvent
Rigidity (quality when cold): + +
Moldability: + + +
Drape: + +
Memory: + + + (elastic)
Shrinkage: 2%
Fingerprinting: Resistant
Recommended uses: Hand splint, finger splint, large orthosis
Other: Transparent when heated; easier to work with if fingers are wet

Blue Stripe—T

Vendors: 1, 2, 5, 6
Color available: Ivory
Softening temperature: 160°-180°F
Heating time: 1 min (until transparent)
Work time: 3-4 min
Edge finishing: Trims or smooths easily (save until final step due to elastic memory)

*Key: + = minimal display; + + = moderate display; + + + = maximal display.

Coating/bonding: Acrylic coating—scrape off with scissors or dissolve with solvent
Rigidity (quality when cold): + +
Moldability: + + +
Drape: + + +
Memory: + + (elastic)
Shrinkage: 2%
Fingerprinting: Resistant
Recommended uses: Face/neck conformer, highly detailed splints, splint for scar control
Other: Duplicates soft tissue details

Clinic/Clinic D

Vendor: 5
Color available: Off-white
Softening temperature: 160°F
Heating time: 45 sec/30 sec
Work time: Up to 4 min
Edge finishing: Self-finishing if cut while warm
Coating/bonding: Coated—scrape off with scissors or dissolve with solvent
Rigidity (quality when cold): + + +
Moldability: + + +
Drape: + + / + + +
Memory: None
Shrinkage: None
Fingerprinting: Less susceptible
Recommended uses: Hand splint, finger splint

Ezeform/Ezeform Light

Vendors: 1, 6
Colors available: White, beige, blue/white
Softening temperature: 160°–170°F/150°–160°F
Heating time: 1 min/30 sec
Work time: 4–5 min/1 min
Edge finishing: Smooths or rolls easily; self-finishing if cut while warm
Coating/bonding: No coating—self-bonding when hot
Rigidity (quality when cold): + + + / +
Moldability: + + / + + +
Drape: + / + +
Memory: None
Shrinkage: None
Fingerprinting: Resistant
Recommended uses: Immobilization/pediatric splint; full-contact axillary splint/finger splint
Other: Translucent to x-rays; resistive stretch makes it ideal for uncooperative patients

*Key: + = minimal display; + + = moderate display; + + + = maximal display.

Kay-Splint Series I/Kay-Splint Isoprene

Vendor: 2
Colors available: White
Softening temperature: 150°F
Heating time: 1 min
Work time: 3–4 min
Edge finishing: Smooths or rolls easily; self-finishing if cut while warm
Coating/bonding: Coated—scrape off with scissors or dissolve with solvent
Rigidity (quality when cold): + + +
Moldability: + + +
Drape: + + +/+ +
Memory: Information unavailable
Shrinkage: <10%
Fingerprinting: Susceptible
Recommended uses: Hand splint/elbow splint; outrigger; finger splint
Other: Very stretchable and self-adhering when overheated

Kay-Splint Series III

Vendor: 2
Color available: White
Softening temperature: 170°F
Heating time: 1 min
Work time: 3–5 min
Edge finishing: Trims or rolls easily
Coating/bonding: No coating—self-bonding when hot
Rigidity (quality when cold): + + +
Moldability: +
Drape: +
Memory: Information unavailable
Shrinkage: <10%
Fingerprinting: Resistant
Recommended uses: Hand splint/immobilization
Other: Rubberlike feel, matte finish

Multiform I and II

Vendor: 1
Color available: White
Softening temperature: 160°F
Heating time: 45–60 sec
Work time: 1 min
Edge finishing: Smooths or rolls easily

*Key: + = minimal display; + + = moderate display; + + + = maximal display.

Coating/bonding: I: No coating—self-bonding when hot
II: Coated—scrape with scissors or dissolve with solvent
Rigidity (quality when cold): + + +
Moldability: + + +
Drape: + + +
Memory: + (if not bonded)
Shrinkage: +
Fingerprinting: Resistant
Recommended uses: Thumb spica; hand outriggers; foot orthotics
Other: Also available as isoprene or thin materials

Orfit (soft)/Orfit (stiff)

Vendor: 5
Colors available: Red, blue, orange, pink
Softening temperature: 135°F
Heating time: 1–2 min
Work time: $2\frac{1}{2}$–3 min
Edge finishing: Rolls easily
Coating/bonding: No coating—self-bonding when hot
Rigidity (quality when cold): + +
Moldability: + + +
Drape: + +/+
Memory: + + +
Shrinkage: None
Fingerprinting: Resistant
Recommended uses: Protective splint; pediatric splint; finger or toe splint/ airplane splint; back support
Other: Becomes transparent when heated; good teaching tool as it can be reused several times

Orthoplast

Vendors: 1, 2, 3, 5
Color available: White
Softening temperature: 140°–170°F
Heating time: 1 min
Work time: 5–8 min
Edge finishing: Smooths or rolls easily; self-finishing if cut while warm
Coating/bonding: No coating—self-bonding when both surfaces are hot and dry
Rigidity (quality when cold): + +
Moldability: +
Drape: +
Memory: +

*Key: + = minimal display; + + = moderate display; + + + = maximal display.

Shrinkage: +
Fingerprinting: Resistant
Recommended uses: Hand splint; immobilization; large orthoses
Other: Porous; soils easily; susceptible to yellowing if left out in air and light

Orthoplast II

Vendors: 2, 3, 5
Color available: White
Softening temperature: 150°–170°F
Heating time: 1 min
Work time: 3–4 min
Edge finishing: Self-finishing if cut while warm
Coating/bonding: Wax coating—scrape off with scissors or dissolve with solvent
Rigidity (quality when cold): + + +
Moldability: + + +
Drape: + + +
Memory: +
Shrinkage: None
Fingerprinting: Resistant
Recommended uses: Upper extremity splint
Other: Reported to be rigid, but slightly less so than Orthoplast

Polyflex II/Polyflex Light

Vendors: 1, 6
Colors available: White, beige/white
Softening temperature: 150°–160°F
Heating time: 1 min/30 sec
Work time: 3–5 min/1 min
Edge finishing: Smooths or rolls easily; self-finishing if cut while warm
Coating/bonding: Coated—scrape off with scissors or dissolve with solvent
Rigidity (quality when cold): + + / +
Moldability: + + +
Drape: + + / + + +
Memory: None
Shrinkage: None
Fingerprinting: Susceptible
Recommended uses: Hand splint; larger orthoses, i.e., elbow splint/infant splint; finger splint; insert over scar
Other: Translucent to x-rays

---

*Key: + = minimal display; + + = moderate display; + + + = maximal display.

Polyform/Polyform Light

Vendors: 1, 6
Colors available: White, beige/white
Softening temperature: 150°–160°F
Heating time: 1 min/30 sec
Work time: 3–5 min/1 min
Edge finishing: Smooths or rolls easily; self-finishing if cut while warm
Coating/bonding: Coated—scrape off with scissors or dissolve with solvent
Rigidity (quality when cold): + + +/+
Moldability: + + +
Drape: + + +
Memory: None
Shrinkage: None
Fingerprinting: Susceptible
Recommended uses: Hand splint, outriggers, finger splint, neck collar/finger splint; insert over scar; infant splint
Other: Translucent to x-rays/fast cooling

NCM Preferred

Vendor: 5
Color available: Beige
Softening temperature: 160°F
Heating time: 45 sec
Work time: Up to 4 min
Edge finishing: Self-finishing if cut while warm
Coating/bonding: Coated—scrape off with scissors or dissolve with solvent
Rigidity (quality when cold): + +
Moldability: + +
Drape: + +
Memory: +
Shrinkage: None
Fingerprinting: Resistant
Recommended uses: Dynamic splint; hand- or arm-based splint; lower extremity splint

NCM Spectrum

Vendor: 5
Colors available: White, pink, blue, beige
Softening temperature: 160°F
Heating time: 1 min

*Key: + = minimal display; + + = moderate display; + + + = maximal display.

Work time: 1–2 min
Edge finishing: Self-finishing if cut while warm
Coating/bonding: Coated—scrape off with scissors or dissolve with solvent
Rigidity (quality when cold): + + +
Moldability: + +
Drape: +
Memory: + +
Shrinkage: None
Fingerprinting: Resistant
Recommended uses: Positioning splint; serial splinting

Synergy

Vendor: 6
Colors available: White, beige, pastel pink, light blue
Softening temperature: 160°F
Heating time: 1 min
Work time: 3–5 min
Edge finishing: Trims or smooths easily
Coating/bonding: No coating—self-bonding when both surfaces are hot and dry
Rigidity (quality when cold): + + +
Moldability: +
Drape: +
Memory: None
Shrinkage: None
Fingerprinting: Resistant
Recommended uses: Hand splint; immobilization

Ultra-Form

Vendor: 2
Colors available: White, beige
Softening temperature: 140°–160°F
Heating time: 1 min
Work time: 3–4 min
Edge finishing: Trims or rolls easily
Coating/bonding: Coated—scrape off with scissors or dissolve with solvent
Rigidity (quality when cold): + +
Moldability: + + +
Drape: + + +
Memory: None
Shrinkage: <3%
Fingerprinting: Resistant
Recommended uses: Hand splint, outriggers, finger splint, burn pressure splint, face mask, neck collar

*Key: + = minimal display; + + = moderate display; + + + = maximal display.

Ultra-Form 294

Vendor: 2
Colors available: White, beige
Softening temperature: 160°–170°F
Heating time: 1 min
Work time: 4–6 min
Edge finishing: Trims or rolls easily
Coating/bonding: Coated—scrape off with scissors or dissolve with solvent
Rigidity (quality when cold): + + +
Moldability: + + +
Drape: +
Memory: Information unavailable
Shrinkage: <3%
Fingerprinting: Resistant
Recommended uses: Hand splint, positioning splint, lower extremity splint

Watercolors

Vendors: 1, 2, 5, 6
Colors available: Electric blue, medium blue, pastel blue, hot pink, medium pink, pastel pink, light brown, medium brown, dark brown, blush, burnt orange, brick
Softening temperature: 160°–180°F
Heating time: 1 min (until semi-transparent)
Work time: 3–4 min
Edge finishing: Trims or smooths easily (save until final step due to elastic memory)
Coating/bonding: Acrylic coating—self bonding when hot; for more permanent bond, scrape with scissors or dissolve with solvent
Rigidity (quality when cold): + +
Moldability: + +
Drape: +
Memory: + + + (elastic)
Shrinkage: 2%
Fingerprinting: Resistant
Recommended uses: Hand splint; basic positioning splint
Other: Bright colors for: (1) pediatrics; (2) adult neurologic patients with visual field deficits; (3) reduces possibility of splint being lost in linens, (4) color code (R) and (L)

X-Lite Plus

Vendors: 1, 2, 4, 5
Color available: White
Softening temperature: 160°F

---

*Key: + = minimal display; + + = moderate display; + + + = maximal display.

Heating time: 1 min
Work time: 5 min
Edge finishing: Fold edges or line with padding
Coating/bonding: No coating—self-bonding when hot
Rigidity (quality when cold): + (increased by addition of layers)
Moldability: + +
Drape: + +
Memory: + + +
Shrinkage: +
Fingerprinting: Minimal surface area to fingerprint
Recommended uses: Post-op splint; immobilization
Other: Marketed as casting material; used to be named Hexcelite Plus

VENDORS

1. *Alimed*
   297 High Street
   Dedham, MA 02026-9135
   (800) 225-2610

2. *Fred Sammons, Inc.*
   Box 32
   Brookfield, IL 60513-0032
   (800) 323-5547

3. *Johnson & Johnson Orthopaedics*
   501 George Street
   New Brunswick, NJ 08903-2400
   (800) 526-2459

4. *Kirschner Medical Corp.*
   10 W. Aylesbury
   Timonium, MD 21093
   (301) 252-2000

5. *North Coast Medical, Inc.*
   187 Stauffer Blvd.
   San Jose, CA 95125-1042
   (800) 821-9319

6. *Smith & Nephew Rolyan, Inc.*
   P.O. Box 555
   N93 W14475 Whittaker Way
   Menomonee Falls, WI 53051
   (800) 558-8633

*Key: + = minimal display; + + = moderate display; + + + = maximal display.

APPENDIX I

Casting Materials

	Source					
	1	2	3	4	5	6
Plaster	•	•	•	•	•	•
Synthetic	•	•	•	•	•	•
Synthetic, colors			•	•	•	•

1. *ACOR Orthopaedic*
   4129 Mayfield Road
   Cleveland, OH 44121
   (216) 381-1717
   (800) 237-ACOR
2. *Ali-Med*
   297 High Street
   Dedham, MA 02026-9135
   (800) 225-2610
3. *Crocker Fels*
   990 Dalton Avenue
   Cincinnati, Ohio 45203
   (513) 381-7700
   (800) 582-7065
4. *DePuy*
   P.O. Box 988
   Warsaw, IN 46581-0988
   (800) 366-8143
5. *Fred Sammons, Inc.*
   Box 32
   Brookfield, IL 60513-0032
   (800) 323-5547
6. *Smith & Nephew Rolyan, Inc.*
   N93 W14475 Whittaker Way
   P.O. Box 555
   Menomonee Falls, WI 53052-0555
   (800) 558-8633

APPENDIX J

Compression Bandages

Characteristics	Vendors									
	1	2	3	4	5	6	7	8	9	10
Self-adherent elastic wraps										
Coban		•					•	•	•	•
Co-wrap		•				•	•	•	•	
Medi-rip		•							•	
Rol-Flex								•		
Tubular support bandage										
Compressogrip			•				•			
Dermafit				•						
No-Wrap					•					
Tensogrip								•		
Tubigrip	•	•					•	•	•	
Tubiton		•					•	•	•	
Other bandages										
Elastic bandages*							•	•		
Isotoner gloves*		•					•	•	•	
Tubigrip gloves							•	•		

*Available at local pharmacies or at local drug stores.

VENDORS

1. *Acme United Corporation*
   Medical Products Division
   Fairfield, CT 06430
   (800) 243-9852

2. *AliMed, Inc.*
   297 High Street
   Dedham, MA 02026
   (800) 225-2610

3. *All Orthopedic Appliances*
   74 Northeast 75th Street
   P.O. Box 380939
   Miami, FL 33138
   (800) 327-3288

4. *Bioplasty Inc.*
   1385 Centennial Drive
   St. Paul, MN 02026
   (800) 328-9105

5. *Brecon Knitting Mill, Inc.*
   P.O. Box 478
   Talladega, AL 35160
   (800) 841-2821
6. *Conco Medical Company*
   Bridgeport, CT 06610
   (800) 243-2294
7. *North Coast Medical, Inc.*
   187 Stauffer Boulevard
   San Jose, CA 95125-1042
   (800) 821-9319
8. *Smith & Nephew Rolyan, Inc.*
   N93 W14475 Whittaker Way
   P.O. Box 555
   Menomonee Falls, WI 53052
   (800) 558-8633
9. *Fred Sammons, Inc.*
   P.O. Box 32
   Brookfield, IL 60513-0032
   (800) 323-5547
10. *3M Health Care Group*
    Medical-Surgical Division
    St. Paul, MN 55144-1000

APPENDIX K

Pressure Garment Manufacturers

Barton Carey Compression Garments
P.O. Box 421
Perrysburg, OH 43551
(800) 421-0444

Bio-Concepts, Inc.
2424 East University Drive
Phoenix, AZ 85034
(800) 421-5647

Gottfried Medical, Inc.
P.O. Box 8966
Toledo, OH 43623
(800) 537-1968

Jobst Institute, Inc.
P.O. Box 653
Toledo, OH 43694-4511
(800) 537-1063

Medical—Z
709 South Lane Street
Seattle, WA 98104
(800) 368-7478

APPENDIX L

Pressure Garment Insert and Padding Material

Characteristics	Vendors 1	2	3	4	5	6	7	8
Contour self-adhesive foam padding	•		•			•		
Elastogel pads			•		•	•		
Elastomer putty	•		•			•		
Luxafoam			•					
Orthopaedic felt			•					
Otoform-K silicone elastomer putty	•		•		•	•		
Polycushion	•					•		
Prosthetic foam	•	•			•	•		
Silicone elastomer	•	•	•		•	•		
Silicone gel sheets	•		•			•		
Skin care pads	•		•		•	•	•	
T foam	•							
Velfoam-2 padding	•		•	•	•	•		•

VENDORS

1. *AliMed*
   297 High Street
   Dedham, MA 02026
   (800) 225-2610

2. *Dow Corning*
   P.O. Box 100
   Arlington, TN 38002
   (901) 867-9971

3. *North Coast Medical, Inc.*
   187 Stauffer Boulevard
   San Jose, CA 95125-1042
   (800) 821-9319

4. *J.A. Preston Corporation*
   P.O. Box 89
   Jackson, MI 49204
   (800) 631-7277

5. *Fred Sammons, Inc.*
   P.O. Box 32
   Brookfield, IL 60513
   (800) 323-5547
6. *Smith & Nephew Rolyan*
   N 93 W 14475 Whittaker Way
   P.O. Box 555
   Menomonee Falls, WI 53052
   (800) 558-8633
7. *Spenco*
   P.O. Box 2501
   Waco, TX 76702-2501
8. *Velcro USA, Inc.*
   Manchester, NH 03103

APPENDIX M

Camouflage Cosmetics

Center for Image Enhancement
Rancho Los Amigos Medical Center
7601 E. Imperial Highway
Downey, CA 90242

Cinema Secrets, Inc.
4400 Riverside Drive
Burbank, CA 91505
(818) 846-0579

Lydia O'Leary
1 Anderson Avenue
Moonachie, NJ 07074
(800) 524-1120

Oncolotech Prosthesis
169 South Main Street
Centerville, OH 45459
(800) 753-4247

Paramedical Camouflage
3121 B Farr Hill Avenue
Kettering, OH 45429
(513) 296-0047

APPENDIX **N**

Physical Agents Manufacturers

BIOFEEDBACK

Davicon
79 2nd Avenue
Burlington, MA 01803
(800) 328-4266

J & J Enterprises
22797 Holgar Court, N.E.
Poulsbo, WA 98370
(206) 779-3853

Verimed
1001 NW 62nd Street
Suite 212
Fort Lauderdale, FL 33309
(800) 999-9797

COMPRESSION THERAPY

CAMP
P.O. Box 89
Jackson, MI 49204-0089

Jobst Institute, Inc.
P.O. Box 71407
Toledo, OH 43694-4511
(800) 537-1063

Wright Linear Pump
185A Robinson Road
Imperial, PA 15126
(412) 695-0800

CONTINUOUS PASSIVE MOTION

Chattanooga Corporation
P.O. Box 4287
Chattanooga, TN 37405
(800) 592-7329

Daninger
4140 Fisher Road
Columbus, OH 43228
(800) 225-1814

J.A.C.E.
1300 Route 73
Mount Laurel, NJ 08054
(800) 234-0900

Stryker
420 East Alcott Street
Kalamazoo, MI 49001-6197
(800) 854-2216

Sutter
9425 Chesapeake Drive
San Diego, CA 92123
(800) 854-2216

Toronto Medical
901 Dillingham Road
Pickering, Ontario, Canada
(800) 289-5139

ELECTROTHERAPY EQUIPMENT

Chattanooga Corporation
P.O. Box 4287
Chattanooga, TN 37405
(800) 592-7329

EMPI
1275 Grey Fox Road
St. Paul, MN 55112
(800) 328-2536

Henley International, Inc.
10518 Kinghurst
Houston, TX 77099
(800) 237-8749

Medical Designs
929 Eastwind Drive S-201
Westerville, OH 43081
(800) 551-1959

Medtronics
10237 Flanders Court
San Diego, CA 92121
(800) 854-1915

Mettler Electronics Corporation
1333 South Claudina Street
Anaheim, CA 92805
(714) 533-2221

Rich-Mar
P.O. Box 879
Inola, OK
(800) 762-4665

Stayodyne
1225 Florida Avenue
Longmont, CO 80501
(800) 525-2114

Tru Trac
P.O. Box 880
Temecula, CA 92390
(800) 321-0918

HYPERBARIC OXYGEN EQUIPMENT

B & F Medical Products, Inc.
1421 North Expressway Drive
Toledo, OH 43608
(419) 729-0606

Concord Laboratories, Inc.
Keene, NH 03431
(800) 258-5361

Topox Therapeutic Rentals, Inc.
634 Summit Avenue
Jersey City, NJ 07306
(201) 798-0636

THERMAL AGENT MANUFACTURERS

Amrex-Zectron, Inc.
12583 Crenshaw Boulevard
Hawthorne, CA 90250
(800) 221-9069

Arjo
6380 West Oakton Street
Morton Grove, IL 60053
(800) 323-1245

Bosch Medical Products
861 Turnpike Street
North Andover, MA 01845
(800) 633-5463

Chattanooga Corporation
P.O. Box 4287
Chattanooga, TN 37405
(800) 592-7329

Dynaware
2520 Kaneville Court
Geneva, IL 60134
(312) 232-4945

Ferno-Ille
70 Weil Way
Wilmington, OH 45177
(800) 733-3766

Henley International, Inc.
10518 Kinghurst
Houston, TX 77099
(800) 237-8749

International Medical Electronics
2805 Main Street
Kansas City, MO 64108
(816) 221-0115

Logan
3041 South Shannon Street
Santa Ana, CA 92704
(714) 556-6441

Mettler Electronics Corporation
1333 South Claudina Street
Anaheim, CA 92805
(714) 533-2221

Rich-Mar
P.O. Box 879
Inola, OK
(800) 762-4665

Talcott Laboratories
301 East Barr Street
McDonald, PA 15057
(412) 926-3011

Thermo Electric
1948 Columbus Road
Cleveland, OH 44113
(216) 241-6762

Tru Trac
P.O. Box 880
Temecula, CA 92390
(800) 321-0918

Whitehall
P.O. Box 3527
15125 Proctor Avenue
City of Industry, CA
(800) 782-7706

APPENDIX **O**

Home Exercise Equipment Use by Body Area

Mouth, Neck, Trunk	Axilla	Elbow
Tongue blades Bed Couch pillows Door frame Corner of wall	Pulleys Chin-up bar Towel, rope, belt Door knob Pediatric growth chart Paint roller Scrub brush Grasping top of door	Milk jugs Barbells

Forearm	Wrist	Hand, Fingers
Hammer Milk jug	Milk jug Purse Barbell Scrub brush Wash cloth Wrist roller	Cans, bottles Bowl of beans Balls Silly putty Mobile Clothes pins on coffee can rim Busy box

Knee	Ankle	Cardiorespiratory
Chair Belt and milk jug Old purse Weighted sock	Towel Chair Telephone book 2 × 4 Stairs Step stool	Step stool Rope Stairs

APPENDIX P

Additional Exercise Equipment Ideas

1. Step ladder on floor for gait
2. Vegetable shortening for massage cream
3. Pillows on floor to stretch ankle inversion/eversion
4. Mirror for biofeedback
5. Ice cups
6. Home paraffin
7. Screw lightbulb in and out of socket
8. Hammer nails in a board
9. Crack nuts with nut cracker
10. Kneading dough
11. Pop bubbles of packing material for pinch
12. Blow-up balloons for respiratory effect
13. Sit on towel and "walk" across floor
14. Attach belt or rope to overhead bar or hook and pull self up
15. Dust the ceiling
16. Rubber bands
17. Sweeping the floor
18. Using scissors

APPENDIX Q

Easy Home Exercise Equipment Fabrication

SHOULDER PULLEYS*

Materials

7-foot piece of rope
Foam pipe insulation
Ceiling hook (1)
Single pulley (1)
Cable clamps (2)

Directions

1. Securely fasten the ceiling hook to a *solid* overhead strut (e.g., exposed support beam or doorframe).
2. Cut two pieces of pipe insulation the width of the hand plus 1 inch.
3. Thread one end of the rope through the center hole of one cylindrical pipe insulation handle.
4. Fasten the free end of the rope to the main piece of the rope with a cable clamp.
5. Run the free end of the rope through and around the wheel of the pulley.
6. Thread the free rope end through the second handle and clamp as described in steps 3 and 4.
7. Place the eye of the pulley over the open end of the ceiling hook.

*Richard, RL, et al: Home exercise kit for the shoulder. J Burn Care Rehabil 8:144, 1987.

CHIN-UP BAR

Materials

Dowel rod at least 1 inch thick
End sockets (2)
Screws
Screw driver
Saw

Directions

1. Fasten the end sockets to each side of a door frame 15 inches from the top of a door frame.
2. Cut a length of dowel rod to fit between and rest within the end sockets.
3. Place dowel rod securely on shelves of end sockets.
4. Grasp rod with one or both hands to stretch axillas.

WRIST ROLLER

Materials

Broom or mop handle 12 inches long
4-foot piece of rope
Milk jug with cap
Drill and $\frac{3}{8}$-inch drill bit
(If drill not available, hammer and nail)

Directions

1. In the center length of the handle, drill a hole through the thickness of the handle (or drive nail into center).
2. Thread one end of the rope through the hole and tie a knot on top of the handle (or tie knot around nail).
3. Fill the milk jug with water to the desired weight.*
4. Tie the remaining free end of the rope around the handle of the jug.
5. Grasp bar with both hands and hold in front at shoulder height.
6. Alternately flex and extend the opposite wrist to wind the rope around the handle.
7. Repeat exercise to unwrap the rope.

*Each inch of water weighs approximately 1 pound; each filled gallon jug weighs approximately 9 pounds.

BARBELLS AND DUMBBELLS

Materials

Old broom or mop handle approximately 5 feet long
Two to four old milk jugs with caps
Four to eight 2-inch wood screws
Screwdriver
Water
Saw

Directions

1. One inch from each end of the broom or mop handle, screw-in a 2-inch wood screw approximately $\frac{3}{4}$ inch deep.
2. Screw in another 2-inch wood screw approximately $1\frac{1}{4}$ inch in closer from the first screw.
3. Fill two jugs with water to a height equal to one half the desired weight needed for exercise.*
4. Replace cap on jug.
5. Slide jug handle over screws on each side until jug handle is in between each of the two screws.
6. Grasp wood handle in middle with hands evenly spaced apart.
7. Perform desired exercise.
8. If more weight is required, repeat above steps by placing additional set of screws 6 inches in from innermost screw on handle.
9. If construction of a dumbbell is desired, cut the handle to the needed length, leaving enough space in the middle for the width of one hand and sufficient length at the ends to place two screws. The length of the dumbbell handle will be approximately 10 to 12 inches.

---

*Each inch of water weighs approximately 1 pound; each filled gallon jug weighs approximately 9 pounds.

APPENDIX **R**

Work Conditioning Equipment Manufacturers

BTE Work Simulator
Baltimore Therapeutics Equipment Company
Hanover, MD 21076
(800) 331-8845

Valpar Work Samples
Valpar International Corporation
P.O. Box 5767
Tucson, AZ 85703-5767
(800) 528-7070

Work Evaluation Systems Technology
16400 Pacific Coast Highway
Huntington Beach, CA 92649
(213) 592-4348

APPENDIX S

Burn Camps

UNITED STATES

Foundation for Burns and Trauma
PO Box 80055
Phoenix, AZ 85060

Alisa Ann Ruch Burn Foundation
20944 Sherman Way, Suite 115
Canoga Park, CA 91303

The Cheley Children's Hospital Burn Camp
1056 East 19th Avenue
Denver, CO 80218

The Illinois Fire Safety Alliance Burn Camp
PO Box 7
Skokie, IL 60076

St. Paul-Ramsey Burn Center
640 Jackson Street
St. Paul, MN 55101

St. Barnabas Burn Foundation
Old Short Hills Road
Livingston, NJ 07039

Northwest Burn Foundation
PO Box 3183
Seattle, WA 98114

Kern County Burn Council
2109 Earlene Court
Bakersfield, CA 93304

Chico Community Hospital Burn Center
560 Cohasset Avenue
Chico, CA 95926

Connecticut Burns Care Foundation
21 Wentworth Street
Milford, CT 06460

Baltimore Regional Burn Center
4940 Eastern Avenue
Baltimore, MD 21224

North Carolina Jaycee, Department of Recreation Therapy
101 Manning Drive
Chapel Hill, NC 27514

Houston Phoenix Society
8787 Brae Acres Road
Houston, TX 77074

CANADA

University of Alberta Hospital
8440 112th Street
Edmonton, Alberta T6G 2B7
Canada

Burn Unit—Children Hospital
840 Sherbrook
Winnipeg, Manitoba R3A 1S1
Canada

AUSTRALIA

Royal Children's Hospital Brisbane
9 Roseby Avenue
Clayfield, Queensland
4011 Australia

EUROPE

University Hospital, Leuven
U.Z. St. Pieter
Brusselsestraat 69
B3000 Leuven
Belgium

NEW ZEALAND

Burn Support Group
Charitable Trust, Inc.
92 Wallace Road
Papatoetoe, Auckland
New Zealand

Glossary of Burn Terminology

Abscess: Nodule or tumor containing pus.
Acidosis: Excessive acidity of body fluids due to an accumulation of acids or an excessive loss of bicarbonate.
Allograft: A graft of tissue between individuals of the same species but of disparate genotype; also called a *homograft*.
Alopecia: Baldness; absence of hair from skin areas where it normally is present.
Amnion: The thin but tough extraembryonic membrane of mammals that lines the chorion and contains the fetus and fluid around it.
Angiogenesis: Migration, proliferation, and differentiation of endothelial cells to create new vasculature.
Anoxia: Oxygen deficiency.
Aspirate: Aspiration; to draw in or out by suction.
Atelectasis: Imperfect expansion or collapse of the lung.
Autograft: A graft of tissue derived from another site in or on the body of the organism receiving it.
Autorelease: The sudden separation of tissue usually from an applied force.
Basal: Pertaining to or situated near a base; the most interior cell layer of the epidermis from which all other layers evolve.
Basement membrane: The extracellular matrix layer that separates an epithelium from the underlying tissue.
Biologic dressing: Biologic tissue used to cover an open wound.
Blanching: To make or become white or pale.
Blebs: Any bulla or skin vesicle filled with fluid.
Bronchoscopy: Examination of the bronchi through a bronchoscope.
Burn: The coagulative necrosis of skin and underlying tissue caused by contact with heat.
Burn severity index: The cumulative effect of several burn factors relating the rate of patient morbidity or mortality.
Cannula: A tube for insertion into the body.
Cellulitis: Diffuse inflammation of cells.
Central venous pressure: The pressure within the superior vena cava that reflects the pressure of the blood volume returned to the right atrium.

Chemotaxis: Directed migration of cells toward a chemical stimulus.
Chondritis: Inflammation of cartilage, especially that of the ear in burns.
Circatrix: A scar.
Collagen: An albuminoid; a main supportive protein of skin, tendon, bone, cartilage, and connective tissue.
Collagenase: An enzyme that breaks down collagen.
Commissure: The coming together of two structures such as the lips.
Concomitant: Accessory; taking place at the same time.
Contraction: The process whereby wound edges migrate toward the center of a wound to shrink it in size.
Contracture: The shrinkage of a scar through maturation of collagen; a condition of fixed high resistance to passive elongation of a connective tissue.
Conjunctiva: The delicate membrane that lines the eyelids and covers the eye in front.
Corium: The dermis.
Corneum: The horny outermost layer of the epidermis.
Curling's ulcer: An ulcer of the duodenum following a severe burn.
Cyanosis: Blueness of the skin indicating insufficient oxygenation of the blood.
Cytokine: A protein produced by a cell to induce an action on itself or another cell.
Debridement: The removal of foreign material and devitalized or contaminated tissue from a traumatic or infected lesion until surrounding healthy tissue is exposed.
Denaturation: The destruction of the usual nature of a substance.
Dermatome: Instrument for incising the skin or cutting thin slices for transplantation of skin.
Dermis: Layer of skin underlying the epidermis composed of connective tissue.
Devitalized: Deprived of vitality or of life.
Diapedesis: A process of cellular migration.
Donor site: Area from which skin is taken for use as a skin graft elsewhere on the body.
Ectropion: The turning outward (eversion) of an edge or margin, as of the eyelid or lip.
Edema: The presence of abnormally large amounts of fluid in the intercellular or interstitial tissue spaces of the body.
Elastin: A fibrous and stretchy protein that gives elasticity to tissue.
Electrolytes: Ionized salts in blood, tissue fluids, and cells.
Endothelial cells: Cells lining the inner surface of blood vessels.
Endothelium: The layer of epithelial cells that lines the cavities of the heart, blood, and lymph vessels.
Endotracheal tube: Tube used to provide an airway through the trachea and prevent the aspiration of foreign material into the bronchus.
Epidermis: The outermost and nonvascular layer of the skin, derived from the embryonic ectoderm, and made up of five layers.
Epithelialization: Healing by the growth of epithelium over a denuded surface.
Epithelium: An aggregate of cells that form a protective barrier over a large surface of tissue.
Erythema: Name applied to redness of the skin produced by inflammation and congestion of capillaries.
Eschar: A slough or coagulum of necrotic tissue produced by a burn.
Escharotomy: An incision made through devitalized eschar.

Excision: Removal by cutting, generally under anesthesia.
Excoriation: An abrasion of the epidermis or surface of other tissue.
Exogenous: Developed or originating outside the organism or organ.
Extracellular: Pertaining to the space that exists outside of cells.
Extracellular matrix: Noncellular structural molecules that make up the support and framework of tissues.
Exudate: Material, such as fluid, cells, or cellular debris, which has escaped from blood vessels and has been deposited in tissue or on tissue surfaces, usually as a result of inflammation.
Fasciotomy: Incision through the fascia.
Fibrillation: Spontaneous contraction of individual muscle fibers usually associated with the heart.
Fibroblast: A connective tissue cell that forms the fibrous tissues in the body.
Fibronectin: A complex molecule that binds both cells and many components of the extracellular matrix.
Fibroplasia: The formation of fibrous tissue as occurs in the healing of wounds.
Fibrosis: Excessive scar formation in a tissue or organ.
Full-thickness burn: Necrosis of tissue through the entire thickness of the skin.
Full-thickness skin graft: Transplantation of all skin elements from one body site to another.
Glycosaminoglycans: Complex extracellular matrix of molecules that are composed of a protein core with multiple polysaccharide side chains.
Graft: Portion of tissue used to replace a defect in the body.
Granulation tissue: The formation in wounds of small rounded masses of tissue composed largely of capillaries and fibroblasts, often with inflammatory cells present.
Granulosum: An intermediate, waterproofing layer of the epidermis.
Growth factor: A subclass of cytokines that stimulate cell proliferation.
Helix: Rounded, convex margin of the pinna of the ear.
Hematocrit: The percent of centrifuged blood composed of red cells.
Hemoglobin: The iron-containing pigment of the red blood cells.
Hemolysis: The destruction of red blood cells.
Heterograft: Graft taken from another individual or an animal of a different species from the one for whom it is intended; xenograft, e.g., pigskin.
Heterotopic ossification: Bone formation occurring at an abnormal place or upon the wrong part of the body.
Homograft: Tissue taken from a person other than the recipient; allograft, e.g., cadaver skin.
Hydrostatic pressure: The pressure exerted by a column of water.
Hyperemia: An excess of blood in a part; engorgement.
Hyperpigmentation: Darkening of skin color due to excessive production of normal pigment.
Hypertonic: Having a higher osmotic pressure than a compared solution.
Hypertrophic scar: Excessive scar formation that rises above the level of the skin plane but staying within the boundary of the wound.
Hypokalemia: Low in potassium.
Hypotension: Low blood pressure.
Hypovolemia: Low or decreased blood volume.

Hypoxia: Condition similar to anoxia but with less reduction of oxygen tension in the blood.
Hypopigmentation: Lightening of skin color due to loss of normal pigment.
Hypotonic: A solution of lower osmotic pressure than another.
Ileus: Intestinal obstruction.
Immunosuppressive: Acting to suppress the body's natural immune response to an antigen.
Inflammation: A localized response elicited by injury or destruction of tissues, which serves to protect the injured tissue.
Inosculation: Union of two vessels.
Interstitial: Space between cells of tissue or organ.
Intracellular: Pertaining to that space within a cell.
Intravascular: Pertaining to that space within a vessel.
Ischemia: Local diminution in blood supply due to obstruction of inflow of arterial blood.
Isotonic: Having the same tension; same osmotic pressure.
Keloid: Excessive scar formation elevated above the plane of the skin and extending beyond the boundary of the original wound.
Keratin: A scleroprotein that is the principal constituent of the epidermis.
Keratinocyte: Epidermal cell that synthesizes keratin and constituting the majority of epidermal cells.
Kwashiorkor: Malnutrition caused by poor protein intake despite adequate calorie consumption.
Lucidum: Epidermal cell layer found in thick skin areas such as the palms and soles.
Maceration: Softening of a tissue.
Marasmus: Malnutrition caused by inadequate protein and calorie intake.
Mesh graft: A skin graft expanded to cover a larger surface area than is otherwise possible, usually has a cross-hatched appearance.
Melanin: The dark amorphous pigment of the skin.
Melanocyte: The cell responsible for the synthesis of melanin.
Microstomia: A defect in which the mouth is unusually small.
Mitogen: A protein or other type of molecule that stimulates cellular proliferation.
Mitosis: Type of somatic cell division.
Murphy slings: Slings that are cut from a tubular support bandage, placed over the bandages of a burned extremity and tied to an overhead device to keep an extremity elevated.
Myofibroblast: A fibroblast having smooth muscle characteristics; involved in wound contraction.
Myoglobin: A respiratory pigment in muscle tissue that serves as an oxygen carrier.
Nasogastric tube: Tube passed through the nasal passage to the stomach for the purpose of alleviating gastric distention, dilatation, or vomiting.
Nasolabial: Pertaining to the nose and lip.
Necrosis: Death of areas of tissue or bone surrounded by healthy tissue.
Neutrophil: A polymorphonuclear white blood cell.
Osmotic pressure: The difference in pressure that develops when two solutions of different concentrations are separated by a semipermeable membrane.
Odoriferous: Having an odor, smell, or fragrance.
Oliguria: Reduced daily output of urine.

Papillary: Pertaining to or resembling a papilla, or nipple; superficial layer of the dermis.

Partial-thickness burn: A burn injury extending through the epidermis, down into the dermis.

Patent: Wide open.

Pneumothorax: A collection of air or gas in the pleural cavity.

Primary closure: Closure of a wound with suture or other means to approximate the wound margins.

Pruritus: Itching.

Purulent: Consisting of or containing pus; associated with the formation of or caused by pus.

Resuscitation: The restoration to life or consciousness.

Rete pegs: A network of ridges forming the epidermal-dermal junction.

Reticular: Pertaining to or resembling a net; the deeper layer of the dermis.

Reverse Trendelenburg: A position where the patient's head is higher than the feet while supine.

Sanguineous: Bloody.

Serosanguineous: Watery blood.

Scar: Mark left in skin or other tissue by wound healing because of replacement by connective tissue.

Scar maturation: Progressive remodeling of a scar characterized by softening and flattening of the scar texture, decreased wound tension, and progressive devascularization with complete resolution of erythema.

Sepsis: Poisoning caused by the products of a putrefactive process.

Septicemia: A morbid condition due to the presence of pathogenic bacteria and their associated poisons in the blood.

Serous: Watery, clear.

Serum osmolality: Osmotic concentration of ions in the serum of blood.

Sharp debridement: Use of scissors and forceps to remove devitalized tissue.

Shock: A condition of acute peripheral circulatory failure due to derangement of circulatory control or loss of circulatory fluid brought about by injury.

Slough: Dead matter or necrosed tissue separated from living tissue or an ulceration.

Skin: The outer covering of the body (corium—true skin; contains nerve endings and capillaries).

Spinosum: Cellular layer of epidermis having spinous projections.

Split-thickness skin graft: A skin graft containing all of the epidermis and a portion of the dermis.

Stasis: Stagnation of normal flow of fluids.

Superficial burn: An injury involving only the epidermal layer of skin.

Suppuration: The formation of pus.

Swan-Ganz catheter: Catheter that measures the pressure of the left side of the heart.

Syndactyly: Anomaly of the fingers or toes marked by webbing between adjacent digits.

Tarsorrhaphy: The suturing together of the eyelids.

Thermoregulatory: Pertaining to the regulation of temperature, especially body temperature.

Tracheostomy: Operation of cutting into the trachea through the neck usually for insertion of a tube to overcome tracheal obstruction.

Tracheotomy: The formation of an artificial opening into the trachea.

Transudate: A fluid substance that has passed through a membrane or has been extruded from a tissue.
Vasoconstriction: Narrowing of blood vessels.
Viscous: Gel-like.
Vesicle: A small bladder or sac containing liquid.
Xenograft: Skin donation from another species of animal; heterograft.
Z-plasty: An operation for the relaxation of contractures.

Index

An "f" following a page number indicates a figure; a "t" indicates a table.